AF900230

Lymphoproliferative and Granulomatous Disorders of the Oral Cavity

Felipe Paiva Fonseca
Hélder Antônio Rebelo Pontes
Pablo Agustin Vargas
Guilherme Rossi Assis de Mendonça
Javier Rendon Henao
Editors

Lymphoproliferative and Granulomatous Disorders of the Oral Cavity

A Clinical and Microscopic Approach

Springer

Editors
Felipe Paiva Fonseca
Department of Oral Surgery and Pathology,
School of Dentistry
Universidade Federal de Minas Gerais
Belo Horizonte, Brazil

Hélder Antônio Rebelo Pontes
Service of Oral Pathology
João de Barros Barreto University Hospital,
Federal University of Pará
Belém, Brazil

Pablo Agustin Vargas
Oral and Maxillofacial Division,
Piracicaba Dental School
State University of Campinas (UNICAMP)
Piracicaba, Brazil

Guilherme Rossi Assis de Mendonça
Department of Pathology,
School of Medical Sciences
University of Campinas
Campinas, Brazil

Javier Rendon Henao
Department of Hematopathology
and Flow Cytometry
Ayudas Diagnósticas Sura Center
Cartagena, Colombia

ISBN 978-3-031-98843-1 ISBN 978-3-031-98844-8 (eBook)
https://doi.org/10.1007/978-3-031-98844-8

© The Editor(s) (if applicable) and The Author(s), under exclusive license to Springer Nature Switzerland AG 2025

This work is subject to copyright. All rights are solely and exclusively licensed by the Publisher, whether the whole or part of the material is concerned, specifically the rights of reprinting, reuse of illustrations, recitation, broadcasting, reproduction on microfilms or in any other physical way, and transmission or information storage and retrieval, electronic adaptation, computer software, or by similar or dissimilar methodology now known or hereafter developed.
The use of general descriptive names, registered names, trademarks, service marks, etc. in this publication does not imply, even in the absence of a specific statement, that such names are exempt from the relevant protective laws and regulations and therefore free for general use.
The publisher, the authors and the editors are safe to assume that the advice and information in this book are believed to be true and accurate at the date of publication. Neither the publisher nor the authors or the editors give a warranty, expressed or implied, with respect to the material contained herein or for any errors or omissions that may have been made. The publisher remains neutral with regard to jurisdictional claims in published maps and institutional affiliations.

This Springer imprint is published by the registered company Springer Nature Switzerland AG
The registered company address is: Gewerbestrasse 11, 6330 Cham, Switzerland

If disposing of this product, please recycle the paper.

I dedicate this book to my dear parents (Juares Fonseca and Clotilde Paiva), my brother (Rafael Fonseca), and my sister (Valeria Fonseca). And to my lovely wife (Aline Sampaio) and kids (Clara and Pedro), the meaning of my life. Their continuous support and kindness make any project less challenging.
Felipe Paiva Fonseca, DDS.

To God, always.
To my parents, Ariosto and Marizete, for introducing me to unconditional love.
To my daughters, Analu and Duda, the best blessings I have received.
To Flávia, my wife, my safe haven.
Hélder Antônio Rebelo Pontes, DDS.

To the patients whose lives have been affected by lymphoproliferative and granulomatous disorders of the oral cavity, this book is dedicated to you. Your strength and resilience inspire us to explore these complex conditions, with commitment, working tirelessly to improve diagnostics, treatments, and, your quality of life. To my family, your love and generosity have allowed me to pursue this goal with purpose and determination. And finally, to the oral pathologists and the broader scientific community, may this book serve as a valuable resource in your pursuit of excellence for diagnosing these diseases. With gratitude and dedication.
Pablo Agustin Vargas, DDS.

To my mother Lúcia, my wife Juliana and my daughter Alice for the daily love, support, and trust.
To my mentor, friend, and eternal reference José Vassallo (in memoriam), who guided my initial steps in Hematopathology and taught me much beyond.
Guilherme Rossi Assis de Mendonça, MD.

Foreword

The American Academy of Oral Medicine (AAOM) defines Oral Medicine as a dental specialty that focuses on diagnosing, managing, and treating medically related conditions and diseases affecting the mouth, jaws, and surrounding structures. This field involves managing various oral health issues often connected to systemic conditions, such as autoimmune diseases, infections, and oral manifestations of systemic diseases.

In addition to managing the oral care of patients receiving medical treatments like chemotherapy or organ transplantation, oral medicine specialists are trained to diagnose and treat conditions like temporomandibular joint disorders (TMJ), burning mouth syndrome, salivary gland disorders, and oral mucosal diseases like lichen planus, aphthous stomatitis, chronic oral candidiasis, and early diagnosis of oral cancer.

To provide a more thorough approach to patient care, they collaborate closely with other medical specialists like dermatologists, rheumatologists, head and neck surgeons, and oncologists. Additionally, they help patients manage oral complications from systemic treatments, such as chemotherapy-induced mucositis or bisphosphonate-related osteonecrosis of the jaws.

From a preventative standpoint, oral medicine practitioners create and implement patient education programs for patients with systemic conditions, like Sjögren's syndrome, or during and following radiation therapy for head and neck cancers.

Certain systemic diseases, like lymphoproliferative disorders, including lymphoma or leukemia, and different types of granulomatous diseases frequently begin in the mouth before spreading to other areas of the body. As a result, oral medicine specialists are occasionally able to diagnose these conditions or serious illnesses early.

In conclusion, oral medicine contributes to the multidisciplinary care of patients suffering from both oral and systemic conditions. In addition to assisting other medical professionals with early diagnosis, comprehensive treatment, and long-term maintenance, oral medicine specialists make sure patients receive the best oral care possible. Apart from aiding in accurate diagnosis, their expertise fosters better outcomes through early intervention, enhanced patient education, and better symptom management of oral disorders.

Emeritus Professor of Oral Medicine – University of Valencia
Valencia, Spain

Jose Bagan

Foreword

This new book is the first I have seen that is entirely devoted to a comprehensive account of hematological and lymphoproliferative disorders that may arise in, or affect, the oral and maxillofacial regions. These disorders present a significant diagnostic challenge to the dentist or oral physician since they often present as minor swellings or ulcers that, even on histological examination, may show nonspecific features resembling a simple inflammatory response. For many, an early diagnosis is essential for effective management, and may even be lifesaving. Accurate diagnosis starts with an awareness of the wide range of disorders that may affect the oral regions, but also with an open mind, careful correlation of clinical, radiological and pathological findings, and a willingness to adopt a multidisciplinary approach and to consult colleagues from different disciplines. Many of these lesions will first be encountered by an oral physician or oral pathologist who must be therefore be familiar with this heterogeneous group of lesions.

The editors of this admirable book exemplify this approach by bringing together clinicians from a range of diverse and relevant medical and dental specialties, including Oral Pathologists, Oral Physicians, Oral and Maxillofacial Surgeons, Hematologists, Hematopathologists, Dermatologists, and Oncologists. The editors and all the contributors are senior clinicians and scientists, many with world-leading reputations in their field of expertise.

The book includes a full and comprehensive consideration of lymphoproliferative disorders that may be encountered in the oral and maxillofacial regions. As well as common conditions that affect the oral cavity, such as gingival and periodontal inflammation, the book considers infections and systemic conditions including, for example, tuberculosis, infectious mononucleosis, leishmaniasis, sarcoidosis, Rosai-Dorfman disease, and Langerhans cell histiocytosis. The final three sections of the book give an account of leukemias and lymphomas that frequently present in the mouth, or regional lymph nodes.

Each chapter is short and concise, logically laid out, and well-illustrated with high-quality clinical and microscopic photographs. This makes the book easily accessible, and it should be essential reading for trainees in head and neck specialties as well as a work of reference for experienced clinicians of any specialty.

Professor of Oral Pathology – University of Sheffield
Sheffield, UK

Paul M. Speight

Foreword

This comprehensive series highlights the diverse spectrum of lymphoproliferative and granulomatous diseases affecting the mouth, emphasizing the pivotal role of oral pathology and oral medicine in the diagnosis of these conditions.

The United States and England are pioneering models for these specialties and dentistry in general, exemplified by the Baltimore College of Dental Surgery, the world's first dental school, established in 1840. Brazil and other countries adopted this model for training dental surgeons, fostering oral pathology and oral medicine as essential specialties within dentistry. It is important to consider that more than other dental disciplines, oral pathology, and oral medicine require close collaboration with medical specialties, ensuring accurate diagnoses and treatment for patients. Usually, the diagnosis of lymphoproliferative diseases needs the expertise of medical pathologists with rigorous training in hematopathology, and in fact, two of the editors of this series, Dr. Javier Rendon Henao and Dr. Guilherme Rossi Assis de Mendonça, are expert hematopathologists, which further demonstrates the commitment to ensure a high quality and scientific reliability for the book.

This collection also honors contributions from renowned international contributors, who significantly impacted the formation of a new generation of Brazilian specialists in oral diagnosis, now renowned worldwide by their high-quality international scientific publications.

The other three editors, Dr. Felipe Paiva Fonseca, Dr. Pablo Agustin Vargas, and Dr. Hélder Antônio Rebelo Pontes, represent Brazil's enthusiastic group of oral pathologists. They brought together in this book Brazilian and international experts to create a comprehensive and authoritative resource on granulomatous and lymphoproliferative oral diseases. This valuable work benefits oral and medical specialists who work in this area, but also dental surgeons in general, who play a crucial role in diagnosing oral diseases, as they frequently are the first to see patients with mouth diseases.

I am confident that this group will address additional relevant themes in oral pathology and oral medicine in the near future.

Professor of Oral Pathology – University of Campinas
Campinas, Brazil

Oslei Paes de Almeida

Preface

Lymphoproliferative and granulomatous disorders comprise a very complex and heterogeneous group of lesions that may be diagnosed in any part of the body, and that may also very often occur in the oral and maxillofacial region, demanding from pathologists and clinicians a high level of training and knowledge to be able to appropriately recognize each disorder and to make the correct diagnoses.

A diverse number of infectious processes may develop in the oral cavity and gnathic bones, often leading to severe reactive lymphoproliferative and/or granulomatous proliferations that may hamper the identification of the etiologic microorganisms in routine microscopic evaluations. Moreover, a large number of noninfectious and nonneoplastic lymphoproliferative conditions and granulomatous diseases can also be diagnosed in the oral cavity, representing localized processes or oral manifestations of systemic disorders. Their diversity and heterogeneous microscopic presentation also demand a detailed clinicopathological correlation. Histiocytic disorders represent another group of lesions that can be diagnosed in the oral and maxillofacial region, and pathologists should now be familiarized not only with their microscopic findings, but also with the newly recognized pathogenetic events that have been shown to carry important diagnostic roles. Finally, lymphoproliferative neoplasms, typically exemplified by lymphomas and leukemic infiltrations, are always recognized as some of the most challenging diagnoses to be made in the oral cavity and the jaws.

Despite the large number of leukemia and lymphoma subtypes currently recognized in the classification of hematolymphoid tumors (HAEME-5) of the World Health Organization and in the International Consensus Classification position paper, the number of variants that are more often diagnosed in the oral cavity and gnathic bones is much reduced, although virtually any subtype can spread to this anatomical region. Therefore, the joint work of oral pathologists, oral medicine specialists, hematopathologists, dermatopathologists, among others, as exemplified in the collaborative contribution of this textbook, is recommended to obtain the most accurate diagnoses.

The objective of this work is to provide pathologists and clinicians with a high-quality and reliable scientific source for the study of lymphoproliferative and granulomatous disorders that more often affect the oral cavity and the jaws.

Belo Horizonte, Brazil	Felipe Paiva Fonseca
Belém, Brazil	Hélder Antônio Rebelo Pontes
Piracicaba, Brazil	Pablo Agustin Vargas
Campinas, Brazil	Guilherme Rossi Assis de Mendonça
Cartagena, Colombia	Javier Rendon Henao

Acknowledgments

The editors acknowledge the support of the following Brazilian agencies: Coordination for the Improvement of Higher Education Personnel (CAPES), National Council for Scientific and Technological Development (CNPq), São Paulo Research Foundation (FAPESP), and Minas Gerais State Research Foundation (FAPEMIG).

We are very grateful for the editorial assistance of Érica de Cássia Ferraz (Springer Nature) who very kindly and efficiently supported us in every step of the writing process of this book, making it much easier and delightful.

The editors acknowledge the important contribution of Dr. Roman Carlos (Guatemala City/Guatemala) to the improvement of oral pathology by the publication of hundreds of scientific articles, the training of many international oral pathology students and the organization of important scientific meetings. Since 2022, the Slide seminar session of the Annual Congresses of the Brazilian Society of Oral Medicine and Oral Pathology (SOBEP) has been named Dr. Roman Carlos Slide Seminar in honor of his outstanding contributions, which are also recognized by the Roman Carlos Challenging Cases online seminar that has occured since 2020 and gathers prestigious oral pathologists from different countries. Dr. Celeste Sánchez Romero (Mexico City/Mexico) is recognized as a talented young oral pathologist who, in her brief career, significantly contributed to the better understanding of the oral manifestations of different lymphoproliferative disorders and is remembered for having helped her colleagues to achieve their best academic performances. Finally, the editors acknowledge the great contribution of Dr. José Vassallo (Campinas/Brazil) to the development of hematopathology, acting as a leader in this specialty and representing a respected reference for hematopathologists from all over the world, especially from Latin America and Brazil. Dr. José Vassallo published many high-quality scientific articles and was responsible for the training of many talented Brazilian hematopathologists. All of them also contributed to the development of this textbook, and their academic contributions and lovely friendship will never be forgotten. (*in memorian*).

Contents

Editors and Contributors

About the Editors

Felipe Paiva Fonseca, DDS Oral pathologist at the Department of Oral Surgery and Pathology at the School of Dentistry of the Universidade Federal de Minas Gerais (Brazil). Oral pathology and Oral medicine MSc and PhD degrees from the University of Campinas (Brazil), with training periods in the University of Sheffield (UK), the University of Pretoria (South Africa) and the University of São Paulo (Brazil). Fellow of the National Council for Scientific and Technological Development (CNPq/Brazil) and General Secretary of the Brazilian Society of Oral Medicine and Oral Pathology (SOBEP). Editor-in-chief of the J Oral Diagn and Associate editor of the J Oral Pathol Med and Med Oral Patol Oral Cir Bucal.
e-Mail: felipepfonseca@hotmail.com

Hélder Antônio Rebelo Pontes, DDS Oral pathologist and Head of the Service of Oral Pathology and Oral Surgery of the João de Barros Barreto University Hospital of the Federal University of Pará (Brazil). Oral pathology MSc degree from the Universidade Federal de Minas Gerais (Brazil) and Oral pathology PhD degree from the University of São Paulo (Brazil). Fellow of the National Council for Scientific and Technological Development (CNPq/Brazil).
e-Mail: harp@ufpa.br

Pablo Agustin Vargas, DDS Oral pathologist of the Department of Oral Diagnosis (Pathology) at the Piracicaba Dental School of the University of Campinas (Brazil). Bucodental biology and pathology MSc and PhD degrees from the University of Campinas (Brazil) with training periods in the School of Medicine of the University of São Paulo (Brazil). Post-doctoral fellowship from the University of Sheffield (UK), Fellow of the Royal College of Pathologists (FRCPath/UK), President of the International Association of Oral Pathologists (IAOP) and of the Brazilian Society of Oral Medicine and Oral Pathology (SOBEP) and Fellow of the National Council for Scientific and Technological Development (CNPq/Brazil). Associate editor of the journal Oral Surg Oral Med Oral Pathol Oral Radiol.
e-Mail: pavargas@fop.unicamp.br

Guilherme Rossi Assis de Mendonça, MD Guilherme Rossi Assis de Mendonça, MD Pathologist at the School of Medical Sciences of the University of Campinas (Brazil). Pathology PhD degree from the University of Campinas (Brazil) and Specialist in Pathology from the University of Campinas (Brazil). Awarded the prize of best Brazilian Doctorate Thesis in Medicine from the Coordination for the Improvement of Higher Education Personnel (CAPES/Brazil). Training period at the Institut Universitaire du Cancer de Toulouse (ONCOPOLE) (France).
e-Mail: gui.rossiam@gmail.com

Javier Rendon Henao, MD Pathologist at the Department of Hematopathology and Flow Cytometry of the Ayudas Diagnósticas Sura Center (Colombia). Former professor of Hematopathology at the Medical School of the University of Antioquia (Colombia). Specialist in Hematopathology by the Instituto Lorenzo Ariosto Seragnoli (Italy).
e-Mail: jrendonh1@yahoo.es

Contributors

Maria Cassia Ferreira Aguiar Department of Oral Surgery and Pathology, School of Dentistry, Universidade Federal de Minas Gerais, Belo Horizonte, Brazil

Pablo Aguirre-Echevarría Pathological Anatomy Service, Donostia University Hospital Osakidetza, University of the Basque Country (UPV/EHU), Donostia, Spain

José Manuel Aguirre Urizar Department of Stomatology, University of the Basque Country (UPV/EHU), Leioa, Spain

Fábio Abreu Alves Department of Stomatology, A.C. Camargo Cancer Center, São Paulo, Brazil

Department of Stomatology, São Paulo University, São Paulo, Brazil

Ana Lia Anbinder Department of Biosciences and Oral Diagnosis, Institute of Science and Technology, São Paulo State University (UNESP), São José dos Campos, Brazil

José Narciso Rosa Assunção Júnior Serviço de Estomatologia do Hospital Infantil Gonzaga, Santos, Brazil

Serviço de Estomatologia da Santa Casa da Misericórdia de Santos, Santos, Brazil

Faculdade de Odontologia da Universidade São Judas Tadeu – Campus Unimonte, Santos, Brazil

Jose Bagan Oral Medicine, University of Valencia, Valencia, Spain

Daniel Galera Bernabé Oral Oncology Center and Department of Diagnosis and Surgery, São Paulo State University (Unesp), School of Dentistry, Araçatuba, São Paulo, Brazil

Hélen Kaline Farias Bezerra Department of Oral Diagnosis (Pathology), Piracicaba Dental School, University of Campinas (UNICAMP), Piracicaba, Brazil

Department of Oral Diagnosis (Semiology), Piracicaba Dental School, University of Campinas (UNICAMP), Piracicaba, Brazil

Lynne Bingle Academic Unit of Oral and Maxillofacial Medicine and Pathology, Department of Clinical Dentistry, School of Clinical Dentistry, University of Sheffield, Sheffield, UK

Leticia Ferreira Cabido Department of Diagnostic Sciences, College of Dentistry, Texas A&M University (TAMU), Dallas, TX, USA

Patrícia Carlos Caldeira Department of Oral Surgery and Pathology, School of Dentistry, Universidade Federal de Minas Gerais, Belo Horizonte, Brazil

Fábio Luiz Coracin Department of Dentistry and Department of Pathology, Barretos Cancer Hospital, Barretos, São Paulo, Brazil

João Adolfo Costa Hanemann School of Dentistry, Federal University of Alfenas, Alfenas, Brazil

Danyel Elias da Cruz Perez Department of Clinical and Preventive Dentistry, Oral Pathology Unit, Universidade Federal de Pernambuco, Recife, Pernambuco, Brazil

Tarcilia Aparecida da Silva Department of Oral Surgery and Pathology, School of Dentistry, Universidade Federal de Minas Gerais, Belo Horizonte, Brazil

Oslei Paes de Almeida Oral Pathology, University of Campinas, Campinas, Brazil

Juliana Diogo de Almeida Sampaio Prefeitura Municipal de Belo Horizonte – SMSA – Centro de Treinamento e Referência em Doenças Infecto-Parasitárias Orestes Diniz, Belo Horizonte, Brazil

Bruno Augusto Benevenuto de Andrade Department of Oral Diagnosis and Pathology, School of Dentistry, Universidade Federal do Rio de Janeiro, Rio de Janeiro, Brazil

José Alcides Almeida de Arruda Department of Oral Diagnosis and Pathology, School of Dentistry, Universidade Federal do Rio de Janeiro, Rio de Janeiro, Brazil

Cinthia Veronica Bardalez Lopez de Caceres Department of Oral Surgery and Pathology, School of Dentistry, Universidade Federal de Minas Gerais, Belo Horizonte, Brazil

Mauricio Augusto Aquino de Castro Department of Oral Surgery and Pathology, School of Dentistry, Universidade Federal de Minas Gerais, Belo Horizonte, Brazil

Wagner Henriques de Castro Department of Oral Surgery and Pathology, School of Dentistry, Universidade Federal de Minas Gerais, Belo Horizonte, Brazil

Júlio Cesar Tanos de Lacerda Department of Oral Medicine, Hospital Metropolitano Odilon Behrens (Odilon Behrens Metropolitan Hospital), Belo Horizonte, Brazil

Elismauro Francisco de Mendonça School of Dentistry, Federal University of Goiás, Goiânia, Brazil

Guilherme Rossi Assis de Mendonça Department of Pathology, School of Medical Sciences, University of Campinas, Campinas, Brazil

Irene Lafuente Ibáñez de Mendoza Department of Stomatology, University of the Basque Country (UPV/EHU), Leioa, Spain

Renata Gonçalves de Resende Department of Oral Medicine, Hospital Metropolitano Odilon Behrens (Odilon Behrens Metropolitan Hospital), Belo Horizonte, Brazil

Silvia Ferreira de Sousa Department of Oral Surgery and Pathology, School of Dentistry, Universidade Federal de Minas Gerais, Belo Horizonte, Brazil

Lucas Lacerda de Souza Department of Oral Diagnosis, Piracicaba Dental School, University of Campinas, Piracicaba, Brazil

Marianne de Vasconcelos Carvalho Department of Oral Pathology, School of Dentistry, Universidade de Pernambuco, Recife, Brazil

Integrated Center for Pathological Anatomy, Oswaldo Cruz University Hospital, Universidade de Pernambuco, Recife, Brazil

Wilson Delgado-Azañero Department of Oral Pathology, Oral Medicine and Oral Surgery, School of Dentistry, Universidad Peruana Cayetano Heredia, Lima, Peru

Gleyson Kleber do Amaral-Silva Department of Oral Pathology, School of Dentistry, Federal University of Mato Grosso do Sul, Campo Grande, Brazil

Leonardo Amaral dos Reis School of Dentistry, Federal University of Alfenas, Alfenas, Brazil

Jean Nunes dos Santos Department of Oral Pathology, School of Dentistry, Federal University of Bahia, Salvador, Brazil

Sara Ferreira dos Santos Costa Department of Pathology and Parasitology, Institute of Biomedical Sciences, Federal University of Alfenas, Alfenas, Brazil

Victor Zanetti Drumond Department of Oral Surgery and Pathology, School of Dentistry, Universidade Federal de Minas Gerais, Belo Horizonte, Brazil

Raquel Conceição Ferreira Department of Social and Community Dentistry, School of Dentistry, Universidade Federal de Minas Gerais, Belo Horizonte, Brazil

Felipe Paiva Fonseca Department of Oral Surgery and Pathology, School of Dentistry, Universidade Federal de Minas Gerais, Belo Horizonte, Brazil

Nathalia Rodrigues Gomes Department of Oral Surgery and Pathology, School of Dentistry, Universidade Federal de Minas Gerais, Belo Horizonte, Brazil

Ricardo Santiago Gomez Department of Oral Surgery and Pathology, School of Dentistry, Universidade Federal de Minas Gerais, Belo Horizonte, Brazil

Medical School, Minas Gerais Medical Science, Belo Horizonte, Brazil

Wilfredo Alejandro González-Arriagada Facultad de Odontología, Universidad de Los Andes, Santiago, Chile

Luiz Alcino Monteiro Gueiros Department of Clinic and Preventive Dentistry, Federal University of Pernambuco, Recife, Pernambuco, Brazil

Javier Rendon Henao Department of Hematopathology and Flow Cytometry, Ayudas Diagnósticas Sura Center, Cartagena, Colombia

Mohammed N. Islam Department of Oral and Maxillofacial Pathology, University of Florida College of Dentistry, Gainesville, FL, USA

Syed Ali Khurram School of Clinical Dentistry, Faculty of Health, University of Sheffield, Sheffield, UK

Tatiana Nayara Libório Kimura Department of Pathology and Legal Medicine, School of Medicine, Federal University of Amazonas, Manaus, AM, Brazil

Omar Kujan UWA Dental School, The University of Western Australia, Nedlands, WA, Australia

Igor Mesquita Lameira Service of Oral Pathology, João de Barros Barreto University Hospital, Federal University of Pará, Belém, Brazil

Juan Manuel Arteaga Legarrea Department of Oral Surgery and Pathology, School of Dentistry, Universidade Federal de Minas Gerais, Belo Horizonte, Brazil

Rafael Paschoal Esteves Lima Department of Oral Surgery and Pathology (Periodontics), School of Dentistry, Universidade Federal de Minas Gerais, Belo Horizonte, Brazil

Márcio Ajudarte Lopes Department of Oral Diagnosis (Semiology), Piracicaba Dental School, University of Campinas (UNICAMP), Piracicaba, Brazil

Hercílio Martelli-Júnior Health Science/Primary Care Postgraduate Program, State University of Montes Claros (Unimontes), Montes Claros, Brazil

Manoela Domingues Martins Department of Oral Pathology, School of Dentistry, Federal University of Rio Grande do Sul, Porto Alegre, Brazil

Roberta Rayra Martins-Chaves Medical School, Faculdade Ciências Médicas de Minas Gerais, Belo Horizonte, Brazil

Ricardo Alves Mesquita Department of Oral Surgery and Pathology, School of Dentistry, Universidade Federal de Minas Gerais, Belo Horizonte, Brazil

Cesar Augusto Migliorati Department of Oral and Maxillofacial Diagnostic Sciences, University of Florida College of Dentistry, Gainesville, FL, USA

Ronell Bologna Molina Department of Diagnostic in Pathology and Oral Medicine, Facultad de Odontología, Universidad de la República, Montevideo, Uruguay

Adalberto A. Mosqueda-Taylor Department of Health Care, Universidad Autónoma Metropolitana Xochimilco, Mexico City, Mexico

Felipe Nör Department of Periodontics and Oral Medicine, University of Michigan School of Dentistry, Ann Arbor, MI, USA

Ricardo Martinez Pedraza School of Dentistry, Universidad Autónoma de Nuevo León, Nuevo León, Mexico

Eduardo David Piemonte Department of Oral Medicine, Facultad de Odontología, Universidad Nacional de Córdoba, Córdoba, Argentina

Fabio Ramôa Pires Oral Pathology, School of Dentistry, Universidade do Estado do Rio de Janeiro, Rio de Janeiro, Brazil

Lucas Fabian Polti Department of Oral Surgery and Pathology, School of Dentistry, Universidade Federal de Minas Gerais, Belo Horizonte, Brazil

Department of Pathology, School of Dentistry, University of Buenos Aires, Buenos Aires, Argentina

Flávia Sirotheau Correa Pontes Service of Oral Pathology, João de Barros Barreto University Hospital, Federal University of Pará, Belém, Brazil

Hélder Antônio Rebelo Pontes Service of Oral Pathology, João de Barros Barreto University Hospital, Federal University of Pará, Belém, Brazil

Raghu Radhakrishnan Department of Oral and Maxillofacial Pathology, Manipal College of Dental Sciences, Manipal Academy of Higher Education, Manipal, India

Unit of Oral Biology and Oral Pathology, Oman Dental College, Mina Al Fahal, Muscat, Oman

Oral and Maxillofacial Pathology, School of Clinical Dentistry, University of Sheffield, Sheffield, UK

Ana Carolina Prado Ribeiro Dental Oncology Service, São Paulo State Cancer Institute (ICESP-FMUSP), São Paulo, Brazil

Liam Robinson Department of Oral and Maxillofacial Pathology, School of Dentistry, University of Pretoria, Pretoria, South Africa

André Caroli Rocha Oral and Maxillofacial Surgery and Traumatology Service, Hospital das Clínicas of the University of São Paulo Medical School, São Paulo, Brazil

Carla Isabelly Rodrigues-Fernandes Department of Clinical and Preventive Dentistry, Oral Pathology Unit, Universidade Federal de Pernambuco, Recife, Pernambuco, Brazil

Aline Araujo Sampaio Department of Oral Surgery and Pathology, School of Dentistry, Universidade Federal de Minas Gerais, Belo Horizonte, Brazil

Vanessa Santiago-Pacheco Department of Pathology, Hematopathology, University of Antioquia, Medellin, Colombia

Alan Roger Santos-Silva Department of Oral Diagnosis (Semiology), Piracicaba Dental School, University of Campinas (UNICAMP), Piracicaba, Brazil

Lauren Frenzel Schuch Department of Diagnosis in Pathology and Oral Medicine, School of Dentistry, Universidad de la República, Montevideo, Uruguay

Madhu Shrestha Department of Diagnostic Sciences, Texas A&M University, College Station (TAMU), School of Dentistry, Dallas, TX, USA

Felipe Martins Silveira Department of Diagnosis in Pathology and Oral Medicine, School of Dentistry, Universidad de la República, Montevideo, Uruguay

Chané Smit Department of Oral and Maxillofacial Pathology, School of Dentistry, University of Pretoria, Pretoria, South Africa

Ciro Dantas Soares Laboratório de Patologia Getúlio Sales, Natal, Brazil

Paul M. Speight Oral Pathology, University of Sheffield, Sheffield, UK

Jefferson R. Tenório Department of Oral Diagnosis and Pathology, School of Dentistry, Universidade Federal do Rio de Janeiro, Rio de Janeiro, Brazil

Vitor Bonetti Valente Oral Oncology Center and Department of Diagnosis and Surgery, São Paulo State University (Unesp), School of Dentistry, Araçatuba, São Paulo, Brazil

Pablo Agustin Vargas Oral and Maxillofacial Division, Piracicaba Dental School, State University of Campinas (UNICAMP), Piracicaba, Brazil

Willie F. P. van Heerden Department of Oral and Maxillofacial Pathology, School of Dentistry, University of Pretoria, Pretoria, South Africa

PathCare Vermaak Histopathology Laboratory, Pretoria, South Africa

María Elisa Vega-Memije Department of Dermatology, Hospital General "Dr. Manuel Gea González", Mexico City, Mexico

Mariana Villarroel-Dorrego Instituto de Investigaciones Odontológicas, Universidad Central de Venezuela, Caracas, Venezuela

Vivian Petersen Wagner Department of Oral Medicine, School of Dentistry, University of São Paulo, São Paulo, Brazil

John M. Wright Department of Diagnostic Sciences, Texas A&M University, College Station (TAMU), School of Dentistry, Dallas, TX, USA

José Candido Xavier-Junior School of Medicine, Centro Universitário Católico Unisalesiano Auxilium, Araçatuba, Brazil

Pathology Institute of Araçatuba, Araçatuba, Brazil

Part I

General Overview

General Overview on Lymphoproliferative and Granulomatous Disorders

1

Cinthia Veronica Bardalez Lopez de Caceres, Chané Smit, Javier Rendon Henao, and Felipe Paiva Fonseca

1.1 General Comments on Hematopathology

Hematopathology is a subspecialty of pathology especially committed to the study of blood cells and the organs and tissues responsible for hematopoiesis. It is an important and complex discipline that very often is responsible for the diagnosis of lymphomas and leukemias, as well as many other infectious and non-neoplastic diseases that may also originate from these cellular populations. The primary (bone marrow and thymus) and secondary (lymph nodes, spleen, and mucosa-associated lymphoid tissue) lymphoid organs are the most affected anatomical locations by lymphoproliferative disorders and a large number of granulomatous diseases may also involve these structures; therefore, hematopathologists should be familiarized with the microscopic architectural aspects of these organs and the morphology of the main cellular components of this system.

Given the high biological heterogeneity and complex morphological features observed among the various subtypes of lymphomas and leukemias or non-neoplastic conditions, hematopathology often demands the use of laboratory techniques as important auxiliary tools for the routine diagnostic practice. These include immunohistochemistry, flow cytometry, (fluorescent) in situ hybridization, polymerase chain reaction (PCR), and next-generation sequencing (NGS), among others. Meanwhile, understanding the epidemiological distribution of the main types of lymphomas, leukemias, non-neoplastic lymphoid diseases, and granulomatous disorders is crucial for helping clinicians and pathologists accurately recognize the most common conditions and better understand their clinical and biological behavior, ultimately improving patient care.

1.2 Hematopathology Applied to the Oral Cavity

Many diseases that affect the oral cavity are microscopically characterized by an important content of lymphoid or myeloid-derived cellular populations, like lymphocytes, plasma cells, macrophages/histiocytes, eosinophils, and neutrophils. This group of lesions comprises a wide spectrum of disorders ranging from infectious diseases like syphilis, leprosy, and leishmaniasis, to dental/periodontal inflammatory disorders associated with biofilm, to foreign body reactions. It also includes non-neoplastic disorders like eosinophilic ulcer, orofacial granulomatosis, IgG4-related disease, and malignant neoplasms like lymphomas and leukemic infiltrates. Moreover, systemic conditions like Sjögren disease, sarcoidosis, and lupus erythematosus also have an important lymphoid or granulomatous component in their microscopic features, and various histiocytic diseases can also be diagnosed in the oral cavity, like juvenile xanthogranuloma, Langerhans cell histiocytosis, and histiocytic sarcomas.

Despite the large number of oral diseases presenting lymphoproliferative and granulomatous features, lymphomas are the most important entities in the context of hematopathology applied to the oral cavity. They represent the third most common group of malignant neoplasms in the oral and maxillofacial region, following squamous cell carcinoma and malignant salivary gland tumors. In addition to lymphomas, leukemic infiltrates and/or myeloid sarcoma may also be diagnosed in these regions. This highlights the necessity of

C. V. B. L. de Caceres (✉) · F. P. Fonseca
Department of Oral Surgery and Pathology, School of Dentistry, Universidade Federal de Minas Gerais, Belo Horizonte, Brazil

C. Smit
Department of Oral and Maxillofacial Pathology, School of Dentistry, University of Pretoria, Pretoria, South Africa
e-mail: chane.smit@up.ac.za

J. R. Henao
Department of Hematopathology and flow cytometry, Ayudas Diagnósticas Sura Center, Cartagena, Colombia

F. P. Fonseca
Department of Oral Surgery and Pathology, School of Dentistry, Universidade Federal de Minas Gerais, Belo Horizonte, Brazil

© The Author(s), under exclusive license to Springer Nature Switzerland AG 2025
F. P. Fonseca et al. (eds.), *Lymphoproliferative and Granulomatous Disorders of the Oral Cavity*,
https://doi.org/10.1007/978-3-031-98844-8_1

oral pathologists and oral medicine specialists to be familiarized with the clinical and microscopic features of this highly heterogeneous group of diseases.

In the oral and maxillofacial region, Waldeyer's ring is the most frequently affected region by neoplastic and non-neoplastic lymphoid disorders, and special care should be given to the palatine tonsils. Although most oral lymphomas represent high-grade diseases, low-grade lymphoid malignancies like follicular lymphoma and marginal zone lymphoma of the mucosa-associated lymphoid tissue (MALT lymphoma) may also be diagnosed in the oral cavity. The clinical manifestations of these neoplasms, together with their microscopic diagnosis, very often elucidate the biological behavior of the tumor. High-grade oral lymphomas are more often associated with ulcerative, necrotic, and destructive ulcers/swellings with a short time of duration, whereas low-grade lymphomas are more associated with asymptomatic expansive lesions with a longer time of duration (Fig. 1.1). Leukemic infiltrates in the oral cavity more commonly manifest in the gingiva as reddish, easily bleeding, and ill-defined gingival swellings. The diagnosis of lymphomas in the oral cavity should prompt pathologists and clinicians to consider the possibility of a secondary manifestation of a disseminated disease. The presence of multiple oral lesions should also be concerning, since some lymphoma subtypes like lymphoblastic lymphoma, mantle cell lymphoma, and small lymphocytic lymphoma are very frequently associated with leukemic manifestations and/or systemic widespread disease.

The gnathic bones may also be affected by lymphomas and leukemias, either as a primary manifestation of the disease or as a secondary extension of a disseminated condition. The mandible and the maxilla may also be affected by lymphomas extending from the adjacent anatomical structures, like the maxillary sinus and the nasal cavity. When the jaws are affected, the neoplasms often represent high-grade subtypes like diffuse large B cell lymphoma, plasmablastic lymphoma, Burkitt lymphoma, and lymphoblastic lymphoma. Radiographically, they usually manifest as ill-defined radiolucent lesions, possibly causing periosteal reactions like "sun-ray" appearance and "Codman triangle." Extensive bone destruction, especially of the alveolar bone, may cause tooth mobility and/or displacement, resulting in the so-called "floating tooth" appearance, especially in Burkitt lymphoma. Dental root resorption is uncommon, but may occasionally be observed. Multiple myeloma affecting the jaws presents with "punched out" images; however, this feature is not pathognomonic of plasma cell neoplasms. Although rare, non-neoplastic lymphoid diseases like intraosseous xanthoma and intraosseous Rosai–Dorfman disease can also be diagnosed in the jaws, as well as some granulomatous processes like sarcoidosis and foreign body reactions (Fig. 1.2).

Lymphomas affecting the major salivary glands are another important clinical scenario, and these structures are more commonly associated with specific subtypes, especially MALT lymphoma, follicular lymphoma, and diffuse large B cell lymphoma not otherwise specified. Patients diagnosed with Sjögren disease have a higher risk and incidence of major salivary gland lymphomas, of which clini-

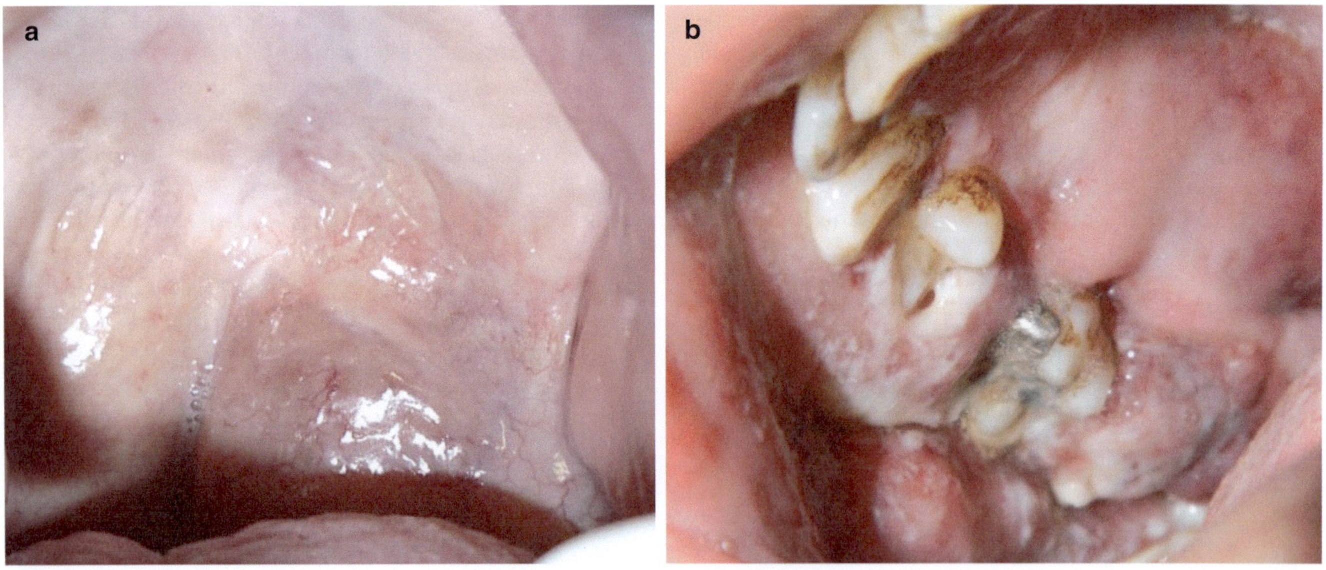

Fig. 1.1 Comparative clinical presentation of low- and high-grade lymphomas affecting the oral cavity. (**a**) Low-grade lymphoma exemplified in this image by a marginal zone lymphoma, more often manifesting as an expansive, non-ulcerated, slowly-growing swelling. (**b**) High-grade lymphoma in this case exemplified by a plasmablastic lymphoma, more typically manifesting as ulcerated, destructive, and infiltrative ulcer and swelling, often showing areas of tissue necrosis

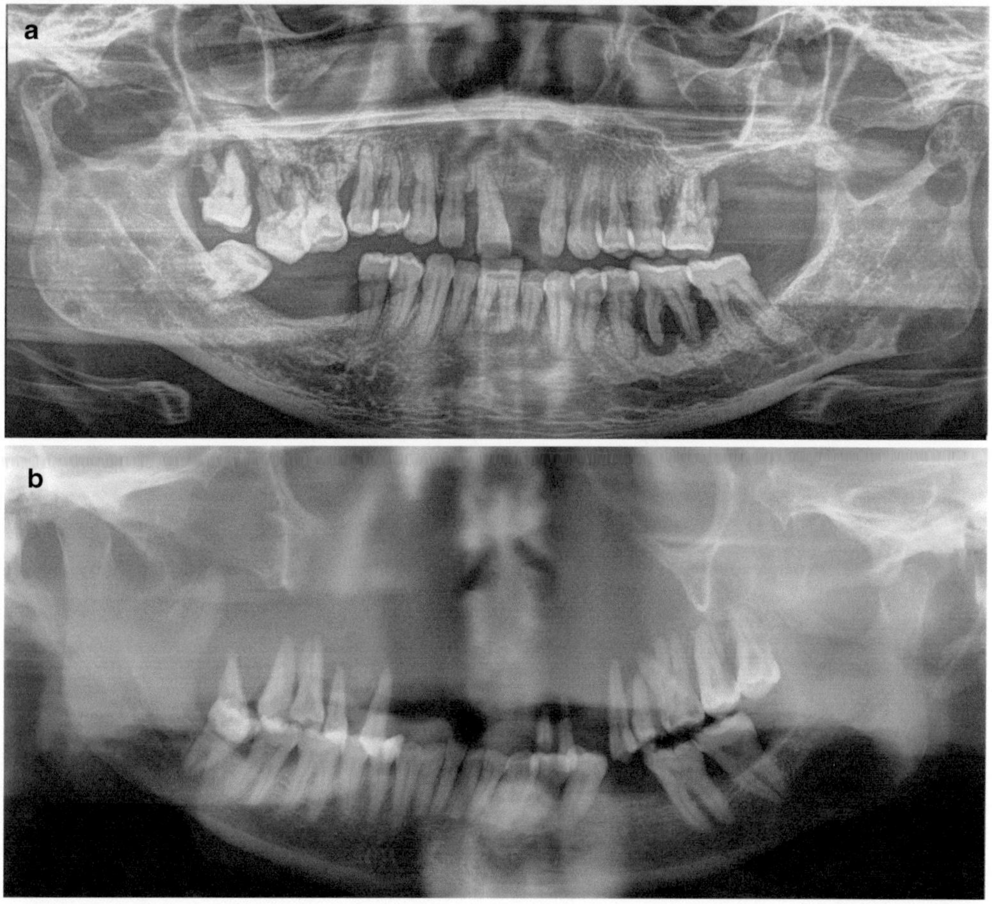

Fig. 1.2 Radiographic features of multiple myeloma and lymphomas affecting the gnathic bones. (**a**) A patient diagnosed with multiple myeloma presented multiple small, round, punched-out radiolucent lesions affecting the right and left mandible in the ramus regions. (**b**) A patient diagnosed with plasmablastic lymphoma with extensive destruction of the midface region with associated "floating teeth"

cians must be cognizant. The parotid glands are more commonly affected by lymphomas compared to the submandibular and sublingual glands, most likely because of the presence of lymph nodes in the parotid. In the sublingual glands, lymphomas usually manifest as intraoral asymptomatic swellings in the floor of the mouth, and a presumptive diagnosis of salivary gland tumor is usually the initial clinical hypothesis (Fig. 1.3).

Immunosuppressed patients are known to have an increased risk for developing lymphomas and lymphoproliferative disorders. For instance, this group of patients presents a higher incidence of plasmablastic lymphoma and diffuse large B cell lymphoma not otherwise specified; two very aggressive neoplasms associated with poor survival rates. Antiretroviral therapy is considered mandatory for HIV-positive patients, and care must be taken for the presence of other lesions frequently associated with immunosuppression like Kaposi's sarcoma, which may be simultaneously associated with lymphoma development. Moreover, the occurrence of EBV-positive mucocutaneous ulcers in the oral and oropharyngeal mucosa is more commonly found in immunosuppressed patients. It commonly affects patients under treatment with immunomodulatory agents such as methotrexate, which is very often used for the treatment of chronic diseases. Post-transplant lymphoproliferative disorders affecting the oral mucosa can also be observed and represent a very complex diagnosis needing strict clinical correlation. The differentiation of these conditions from truly neoplastic disorders may not be reliably achieved in

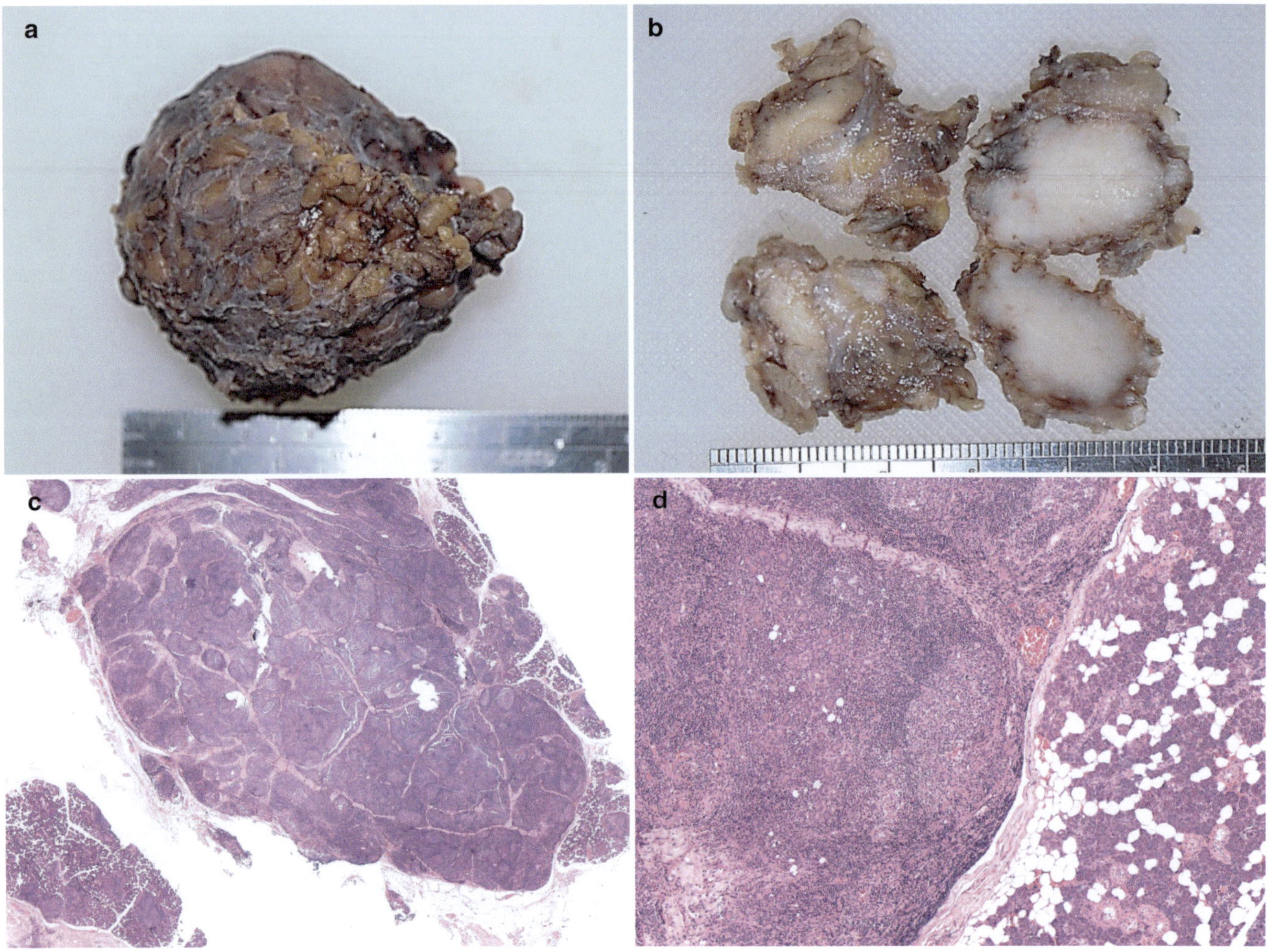

Fig. 1.3 Lymphoma affecting the parotid gland. (**a**) Gross specimen illustrating a follicular lymphoma in the parotid gland. (**b**) Cut surface of the follicular lymphoma in the parotid gland showing a pale whitish region consistent with the tumor. (**c**) Follicular lymphoma involving the parotid gland (H&E; 10×). (**d**) Observe the follicular lymphoma in the left side and the glandular parenchyma in the right side (H&E; 25×)

some instances, and follow-up is necessary to confirm the biological nature of the disease.

1.3 Historical Perspectives, Classification Schemes, and General Epidemiology of Lymphomas

Some lymphoma subtypes have been known for over a century like mycosis fungoides, Hodgkin lymphoma, and anaplastic large cell lymphoma, among many others, whereas several important subtypes like Burkitt lymphoma have been better recognized during the twentieth century. This long timeline of tumor descriptions demonstrates the complexity and ever-evolving dynamics of hematolymphoid disorders and neoplasms. This is further illustrated by the various attempts to create a reproducible and effective classification method that could be applied in different regions of the world and would facilitate the diagnosis of lymphomas (Fig. 1.4).

The majority of the first classification approaches for lymphomas focused on the morphological features of the diseases and their resemblance to normal cellular counterparts. The Rappaport classification in 1966, the Lukes–Collins classification in 1974, and the Kiel classifications in 1967 and 1978 are the most important examples of this trend. The Working formulation released in 1982 by the National Institutes of Health (USA) subsequently proposed a classification system where the clinical behavior of the tumors was used as the cornerstone for their definition, recognizing lymphomas as low, intermediate, or high-grade neoplasms. However, the integration of microscopic and clinical parameters was only achieved with the REAL (Revised European American Lymphoma) classification in 1994. This classification also considered genetics and

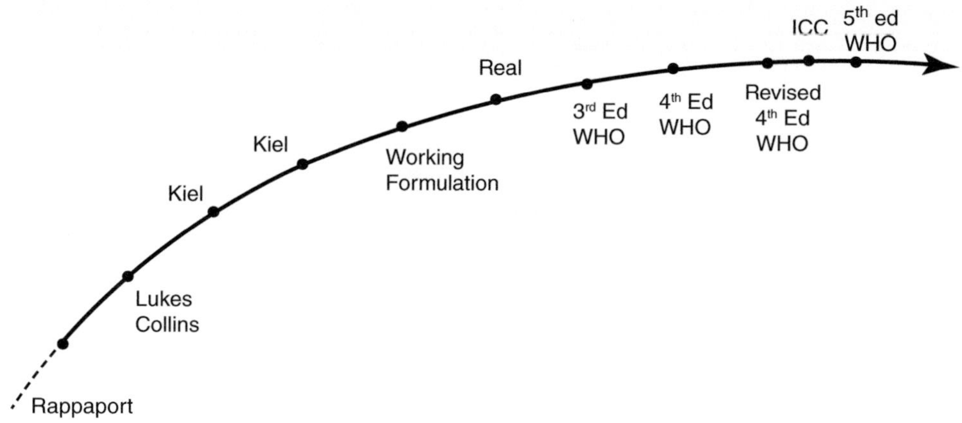

Fig. 1.4 Timeflow of the different schemes proposed for classifying lymphomas

immunohistochemical features to define entities and represented a consensus based on the knowledge available in scientific publications. This classification was used as an important reference by the World Health Organization to publish its first classification of tumors of the hematopoietic and lymphoid tissues in 2001 (third edition). This represented a joint effort of the Society for Hematopathology (SH) and the European Association for Hematopathology (EAHP), together with many hematologists, oncologists, and scientists through joint Clinical Advisory Committees. After this, new published editions by the World Health Organization followed in 2008 (fourth edition) and 2017 (revised fourth edition).

Recently, the release of the fifth edition of the World Health Organization classification of lymphoid tumors in 2023 followed the publication of the International Consensus Classification (ICC) protocol for classification of tumors of the hematopoietic and lymphoid tissues by a large group of prestigious experts in 2022. Although the ICC group and the World Health Organization classification group agreed on the majority of definitions, important differences existed, and, consequently, two classification schemes are currently available. The significance of the different classification systems on the outcome of patients' care and management remains unknown. Therefore, for consistency, throughout this textbook, the World Health Organization classification guidelines will be used as the main reference, but important comments regarding the ICC definitions will always be highlighted as necessary.

Lymphomas are broadly classified according to the cell lineage of differentiation as either B cell or NK/T cell lymphomas. Neoplasms derived from plasma cells are mostly classified as plasmacytoma or multiple myeloma, with clinical, imaging, and laboratorial data being very important to determine the exact diagnosis. To obtain a reliable and effective classification scheme, the simultaneous use of clinical data, morphological features, immunophenotype, genetics, and biological behavior is mandatory. These features should always be considered together in order to achieve the most appropriate diagnosis, although in some situations one or more of these parameters will have a stronger significance than the others.

The International Agency for Research on Cancer (IARC) reported that 82,409 new cases of Hodgkin lymphomas were estimated for 2022 worldwide, accounting for 0.4% of all cancer cases. Non-Hodgkin lymphomas were estimated to affect 553.010 new patients in the world in the same period, accounting for 2.8% of all cancers. Additionally, 486,777 new cases of leukemia were estimated, representing 2.4% of all cases of cancer. These neoplasms were estimated to be associated with 22,701, 250,475, and 305,033 new deaths, respectively, demonstrating that these diseases represent important public health issues around the world. Moreover, it is important to recognize that some lymphoma subtypes predominate in specific geographic regions, possibly because of different populations or environmental factors, and understanding this epidemiological variability may significantly contribute to improving the diagnosis of these conditions. For instance, in the oral cavity, extranodal NK/T cell lymphoma represents the most common NK/T cell lymphoma in Central and South America and is also very prevalent in many parts of Asia. In contrast, Burkitt lymphoma is very common in the so-called "lymphoma belt" region of the African continent.

Following the current World Health Organization classification of lymphomas, diffuse large B cell lymphoma not otherwise specified still represents the most common subtype, followed by follicular lymphoma. Patients are most frequently older adults, although some specific subtypes like Burkitt lymphoma may predominate among infants and adolescents. Males are usually the most affected, and lymph nodes are often the most involved anatomical sites. However, extranodal structures may also be frequently affected by non-Hodgkin lymphomas, especially the gastrointestinal tract and the skin, while leukemias usually manifest in the bone marrow and/or in the peripheral blood, but also as solid masses in extranodal tissues (myeloid sarcoma). Hodgkin lymphomas are mostly a nodal disease, and it is only very rarely diagnosed in extranodal sites.

1.4 Recognizing Important Structures and Cell Types in Lymphoproliferative and Granulomatous Disorders

The recognition of microscopic structures and cell types that are frequently present in lymphoproliferative and granulomatous disorders, either reactive or neoplastic, is very important to achieve the correct diagnoses. It also guides the decision on which immunohistochemical or genetic analyses will be necessary for each case.

The architectural growth pattern of the disease appreciated under a low-power view is the first microscopic analysis that should be done. Although most lymphoproliferative lesions will demonstrate a diffuse proliferation of lymphoid cells, some entities will be characterized by follicular or nodular growth patterns, such as in follicular and mantle cell lymphomas (Fig. 1.5). These patterns may be subtle and difficult to observe using H&E staining and therefore will be better appreciated with the support of immunohistochemical reactions against follicular dendritic cells using CD21, CD23, or CD35 antibodies. The presence of fibrous bands may also be indicative of specific conditions like IgG4-related disease. Extranodal NK/T cell lymphoma and other aggressive lymphomas are characterized by angioproliferation, angioinvasion, and angiodestruction, histological findings that, when observed in the oral cavity, are very indicative of the diagnosis. Although the "starry sky" pattern is typically associated with the diagnosis of Burkitt lymphoma, it is also present in other lymphomas with high proliferative potential like lymphoblastic lymphoma, diffuse large B cell lymphoma/high-grade B cell lymphoma, blastoid mantle cell lymphoma, and plasmablastic lymphoma. This microscopic feature is a consequence of the presence of tingible body macrophages that phagocytize apoptotic bodies and debris. Other features frequently described in cases of Burkitt lymphoma are the intimate association between neoplastic cells, giving rise to the so-called "puzzle-like" aspect, while the epithelioid appearance is observed in many cases of plasmablastic lymphomas. In lymphoblastic lymphoma, the presence of the "single line" aspect and the epitheliotropism of neoplastic cells are frequent findings, and the latter is also a typical finding in mycosis fungoides. The occurrence of lymphoepithelial lesions in MALT lymphomas is common, but it can also be observed in lymphoepithelial sialadenitis. The presence of granulomas more commonly leads to the diagnosis of granulomatous conditions, either infectious or not, but aggregates of histiocytes can also be found in some lymphomas (Fig. 1.6).

Regarding the cellular component of the lymphoid diseases, it is important to recognize the most common cell populations, which are assessed using higher-power objectives. Lymphocytes predominate in the majority of the disorders and are morphologically characterized as small round to oval cells with scant cytoplasm and hyperchromatic nuclei, and the use of immunohistochemical markers is necessary to determine the B, T, or NK lineage of these cells (Fig. 1.7). During lymphocyte maturation and differentiation, important subpopulations are morphologically recognizable, and their identification is very important for diagnostic approaches. *Immunoblasts* are described as large and round cells with dispersed chromatin and one central prominent nucleolus, while *centroblasts* are described as large and round cells with three or more nucleoli located in the periphery of the nucleus. *Centrocytes* are small and cleaved lymphocytes with hyperchromatic nuclei, inconspicuous nucleoli, and scant cytoplasm. Immature lymphocytes may give rise to lymphoblastic lymphoma/leukemia, and they are more often recognized as small to medium-sized, round, undifferentiated cells with poorly recognizable nucleoli and scant cytoplasm (Fig. 1.8).

Plasma cells are terminally differentiated cells capable of producing secreted immunoglobulins. These cells are small to medium in size with a peripherally displaced nucleus that shows four to five nucleoli located in the periphery of the nuclear membrane ("cartwheel" chromatin arrangement). Its cytoplasm is abundant and eosinophilic. In close proximity to the nuclear membrane, the prominent Golgi apparatus gives rise to the hof, a paler eosinophilic region in the perinuclear cytoplasm. Plasmablasts are larger cells than plasma cells and have one or more prominent nucleoli in a vesicular nucleus and will predominate in several types of lymphomas like plasmablastic lymphoma, primary effusion lymphoma, and ALK-positive large B cell lymphoma (Figs. 1.9 and 1.10).

Histiocytes will have a varied morphology, ranging from epithelioid macrophages to tingible body macrophages. The epithelioid macrophages will have an eosinophilic cytoplasm and a round to oval central nucleus and are commonly observed in some granulomatous infections like leprosy and tuberculosis. Tingible body macrophages present a round to oval nucleus with clear cytoplasm containing apoptotic bodies and debris inside, and it is frequently observed in some high-grade lymphomas. The occurrence of ill-defined or well-formed granulomas is always very important to be recognized and indicates a granulomatous process. Moreover, the presence of multinucleated giant cells is also very important for microscopic diagnosis of many diseases, and pathologists should be familiarized with the most frequent types of these cells: Foreign body-type (it is often found in foreign body reactions and orofacial granulomatosis), Langhans

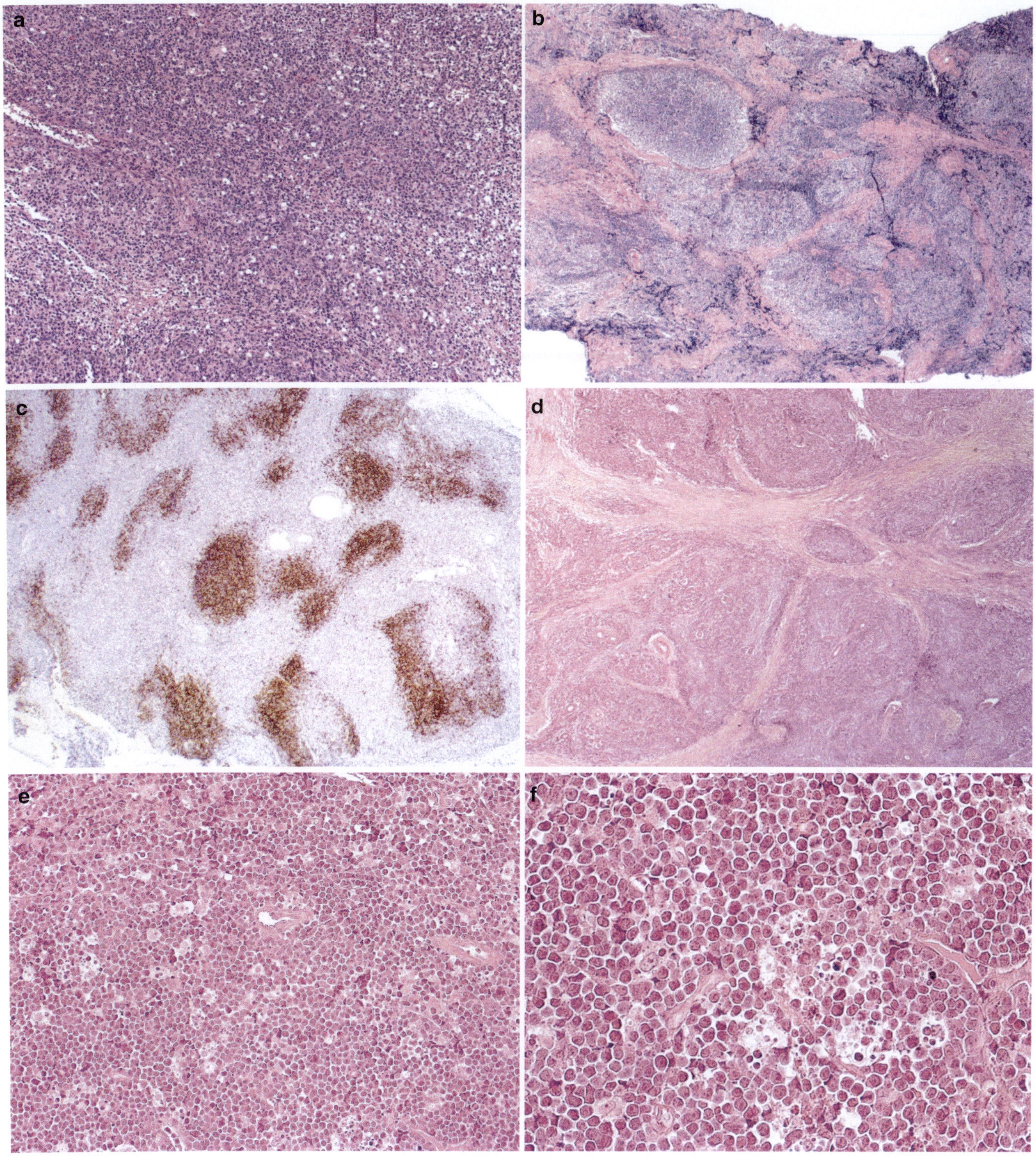

Fig. 1.5 Architectural microscopic findings important for the diagnosis of different lymphoproliferative disorders. (**a**) Diffuse growth pattern of a diffuse large B cell lymphoma not otherwise specified (H&E; 50×). (**b**) Follicular growth pattern in a follicular lymphoma (H&E; 50×). (**c**) Follicular dendritic cells network highlighted using CD23 expression (H&E; 50×). (**d**) IgG4-related disease is characterized by the presence of fibrous bands in its content (H&E; 50×). (**e**) The starry sky pattern typically observed in Burkitt lymphoma (H&E; 100×). (**f**) Under higher magnification, the tingible body macrophages phagocytizing apoptotic debris can be better appreciated (H&E; 200×)

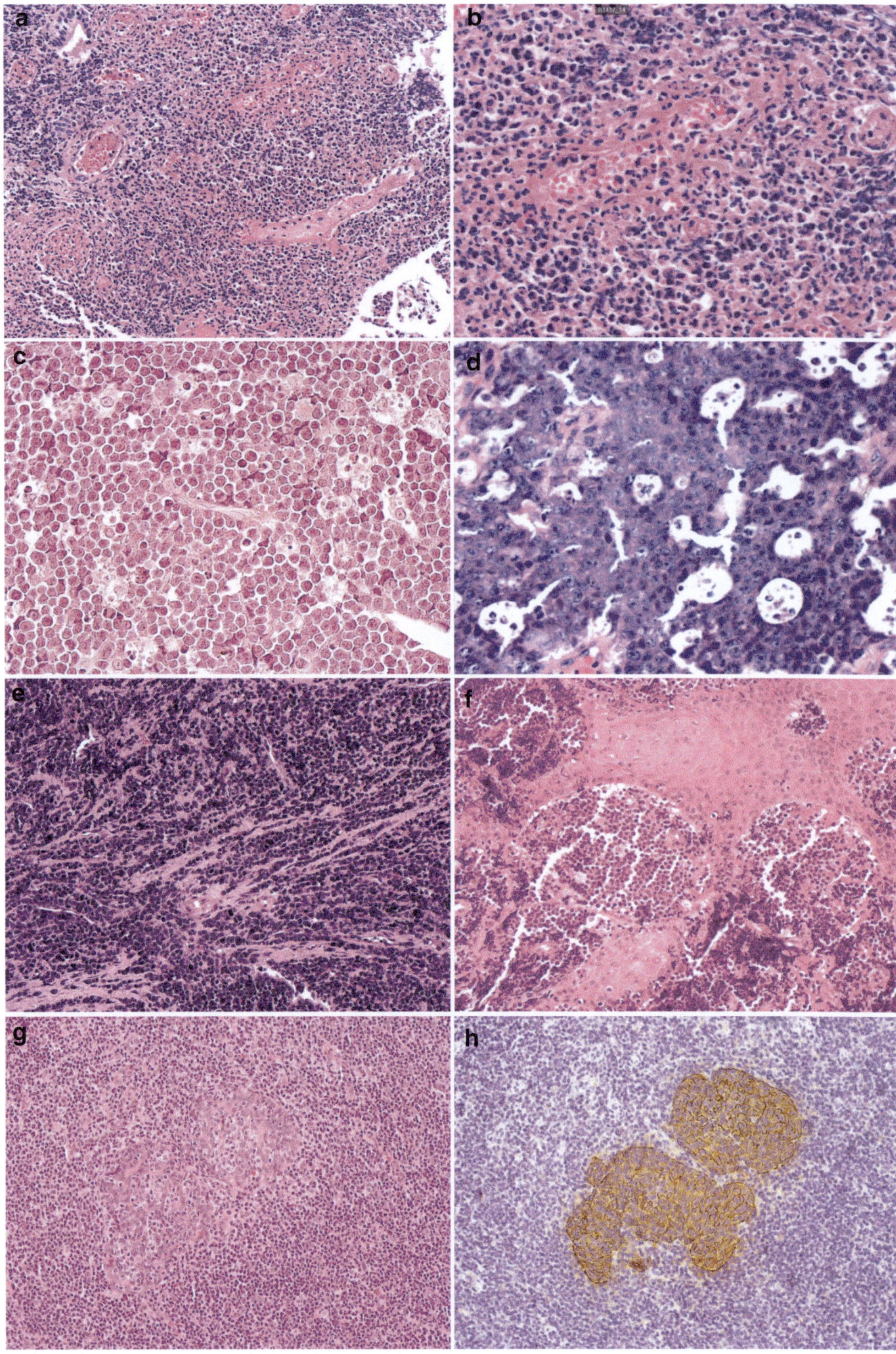

Fig. 1.6 Architectural microscopic findings important for the diagnosis of different lymphoproliferative disorders. (**a**) The occurrence of angioinvasion and angiodestruction in a case of extranodal NK/T cell lymphoma (H&E; 100×). (**b**) Observe an invaded blood vessel in the center of the image. The vessel wall is disrupted, and there is an eosinophilic fibrinoid necrosis around the vessel (H&E; 200×). (**c**) The puzzle-like aspect is often observed in Burkitt lymphoma. Observe that the cytoplasmic borders of the neoplastic cells seem to fit each other (H&E; 200×). (**d**) Plasmablastic lymphoma may reveal an epithelioid appearance of its neoplastic cells. It is not possible to observe the cytoplasmic limits of each cell (H&E; 200×). (**e**) A single line growth pattern is a frequent finding in lymphoblastic lymphoma/leukemia (H&E; 100×). (**f**) The presence of epitheliotropism is another common finding in lymphoblastic lymphoma/leukemia (H&E; 100×). (**g**) Lymphoepithelial lesion in a case of MALT lymphoma. There is a residual salivary gland duct in the center of the image that is infiltrated by the lymphoid cells (H&E; 100×). (**h**) This glandular duct can be better appreciated using AE1/AE3 reaction (DAB; 100×)

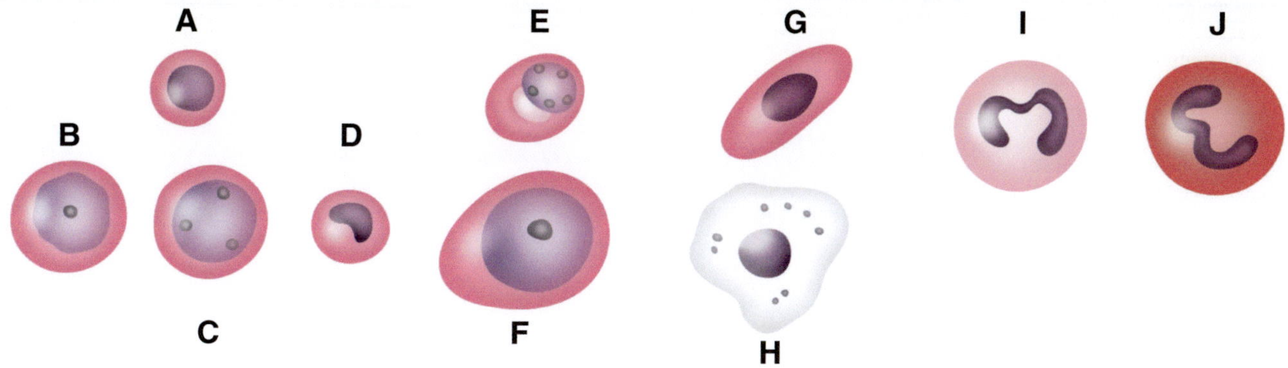

Fig. 1.7 Schematic representation of important cell populations most frequently found in different lymphoproliferative disorders. (**a**) Lymphocytes, (**b**) immunoblast, (**c**) centroblast, (**d**) centrocyte, (**e**) plasma cell, (**f**) plasmablast, (**g**) epithelioid macrophage, (**h**) tingible body macrophage, (**i**) neutrophil, and (**j**) eosinophil

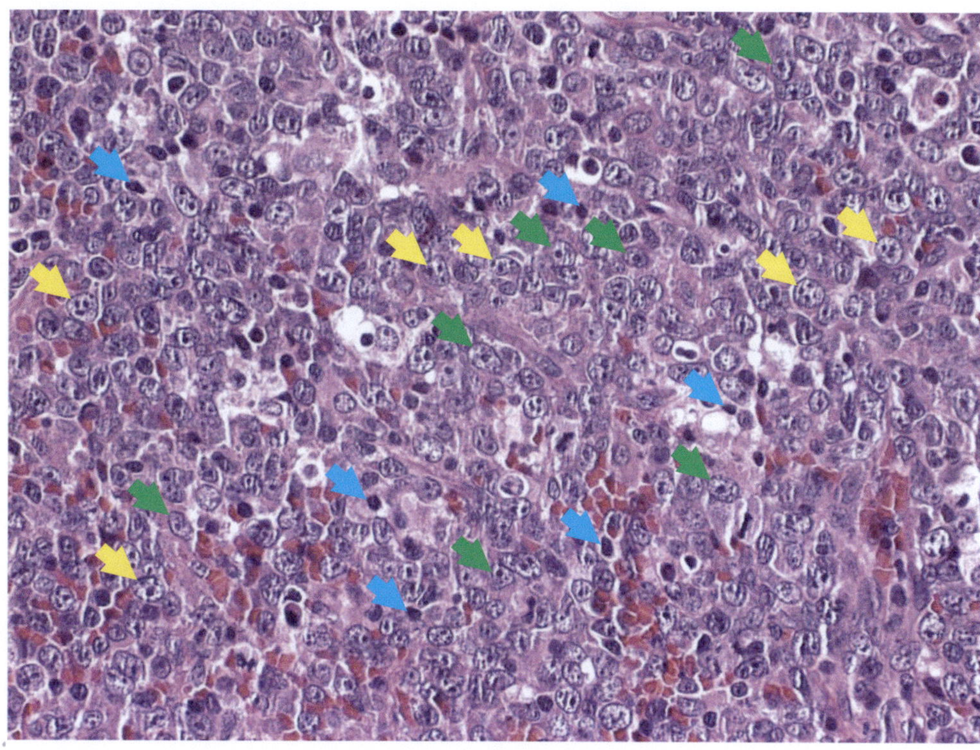

Fig. 1.8 Important cell populations frequently found in different lymphoproliferative disorders. Immunoblasts representing large and round cells with dispersed chromatin and one central prominent nucleolus (green arrows). Centroblasts are large and round cells with three or more nucleoli located in the periphery of nuclei (yellow arrows). Centrocytes are small and usually cleaved lymphocytes with hyperchromatic nuclei, inconspicuous nucleoli, and scant cytoplasm (blue arrows) (H&E; 400×)

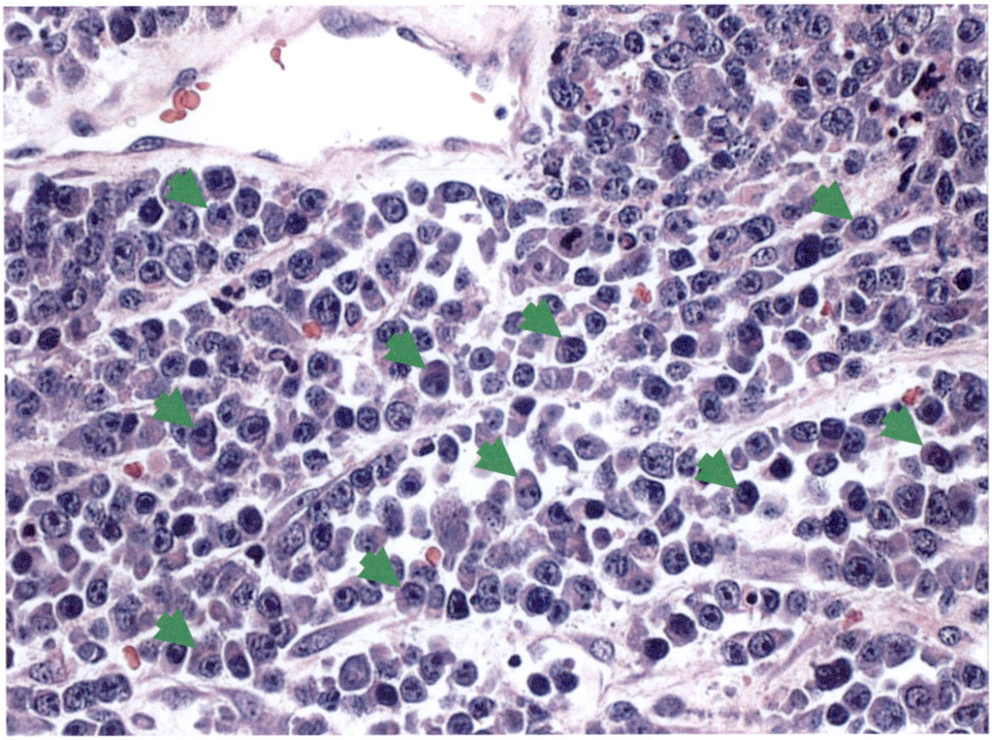

Fig. 1.9 Important cell populations frequently found in different lymphoproliferative disorders. Plasmablasts are cells larger than plasma cells, with one or more prominent nucleoli in a peripherally displaced nucleus (green arrows) (H&E; 400×)

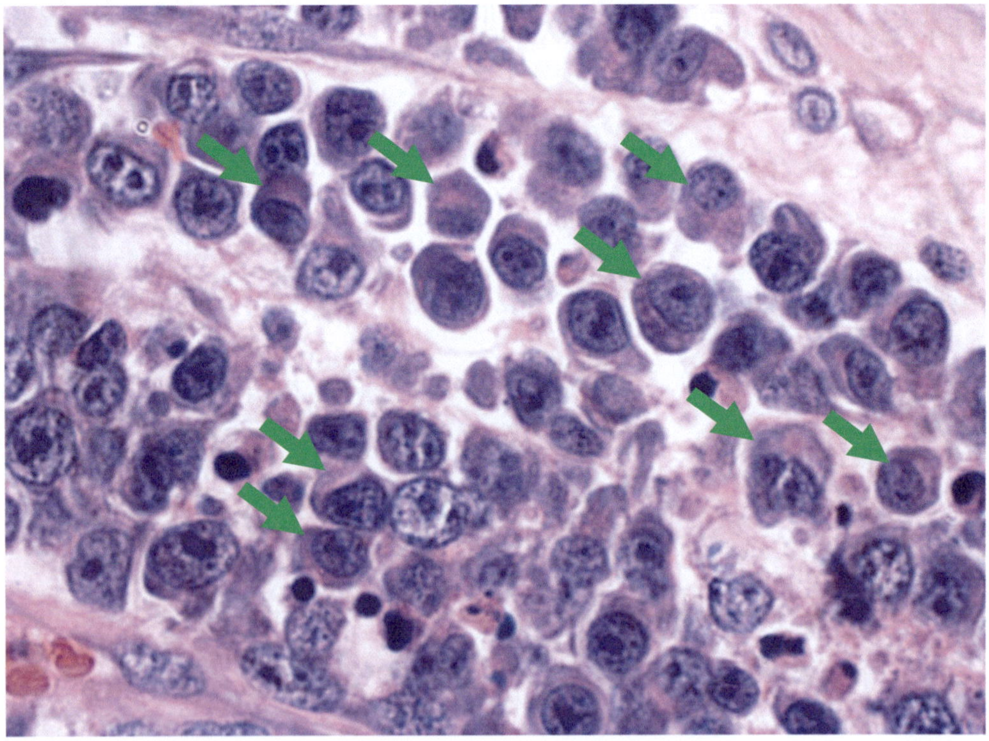

Fig. 1.10 Important cell populations frequently found in different lymphoproliferative disorders. Plasmablasts are cells larger than plasma cells, with one or more prominent nucleoli in a peripherally displaced nucleus (green arrows) (H&E; 1000×)

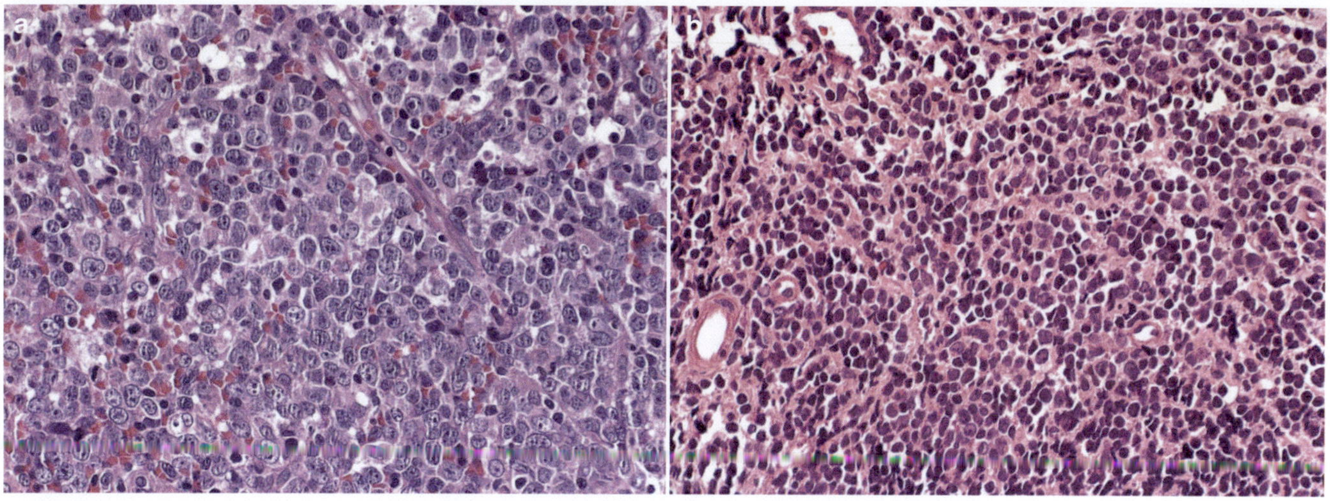

Fig. 1.11 Comparative image between a large cell lymphoma and a small cell lymphoma. (**a**) Diffuse large B cell lymphoma not otherwise specified containing centroblasts and immunoblasts (H&E; 200×). (**b**) Lymphoblastic lymphoma/leukemia with smaller cells (H&E; 200×)

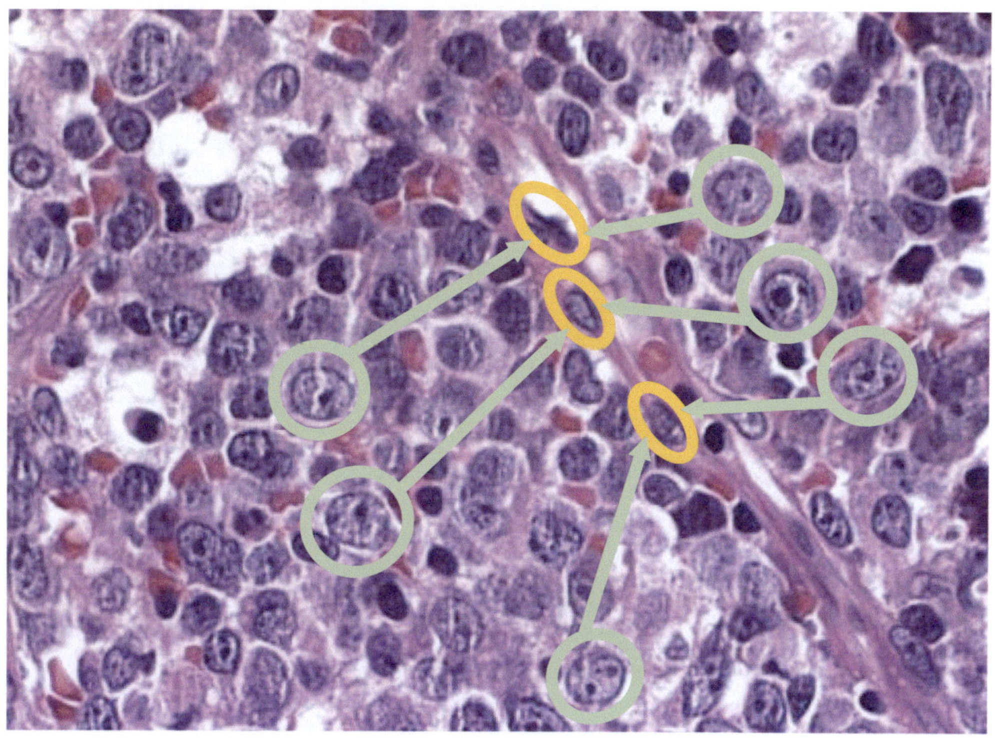

Fig. 1.12 Comparative image between a normal reference—in this case, endothelial cells (yellow circles) were used because macrophages were not reliably identified—and neoplastic cells of a diffuse large B cell lymphoma not otherwise specified (green circles). Observe that tumor cells are at least two times larger than endothelial cells. This initial comparative approach is very important to understand what type of lymphoma we are working with (H&E; 400×)

type (it is often found in different infectious processes), and Touton type (it is often found in juvenile xanthogranuloma).

Determining the predominant size of the neoplastic cells in lymphomas is important in the diagnostic process for categorizing specific subtypes, either large cell lymphomas or small cell lymphomas, or even a medium-sized cell lymphoma (Fig. 1.11). Consequently, this histological approach will also determine the initial panel of antibodies that should be used to determine the immunophenotype of the lymphoma. The predominant size of the cells is estimated by a direct comparison of the size of neoplastic cells with a physiological reference, often a macrophage. When the size of neoplastic cells is similar to, or larger than, the size of the macrophage nucleus, it is categorized as a large cell lymphoma. In contrast, the opposite is true if the neoplastic cells are smaller. When medium-sized cells predominate, both the

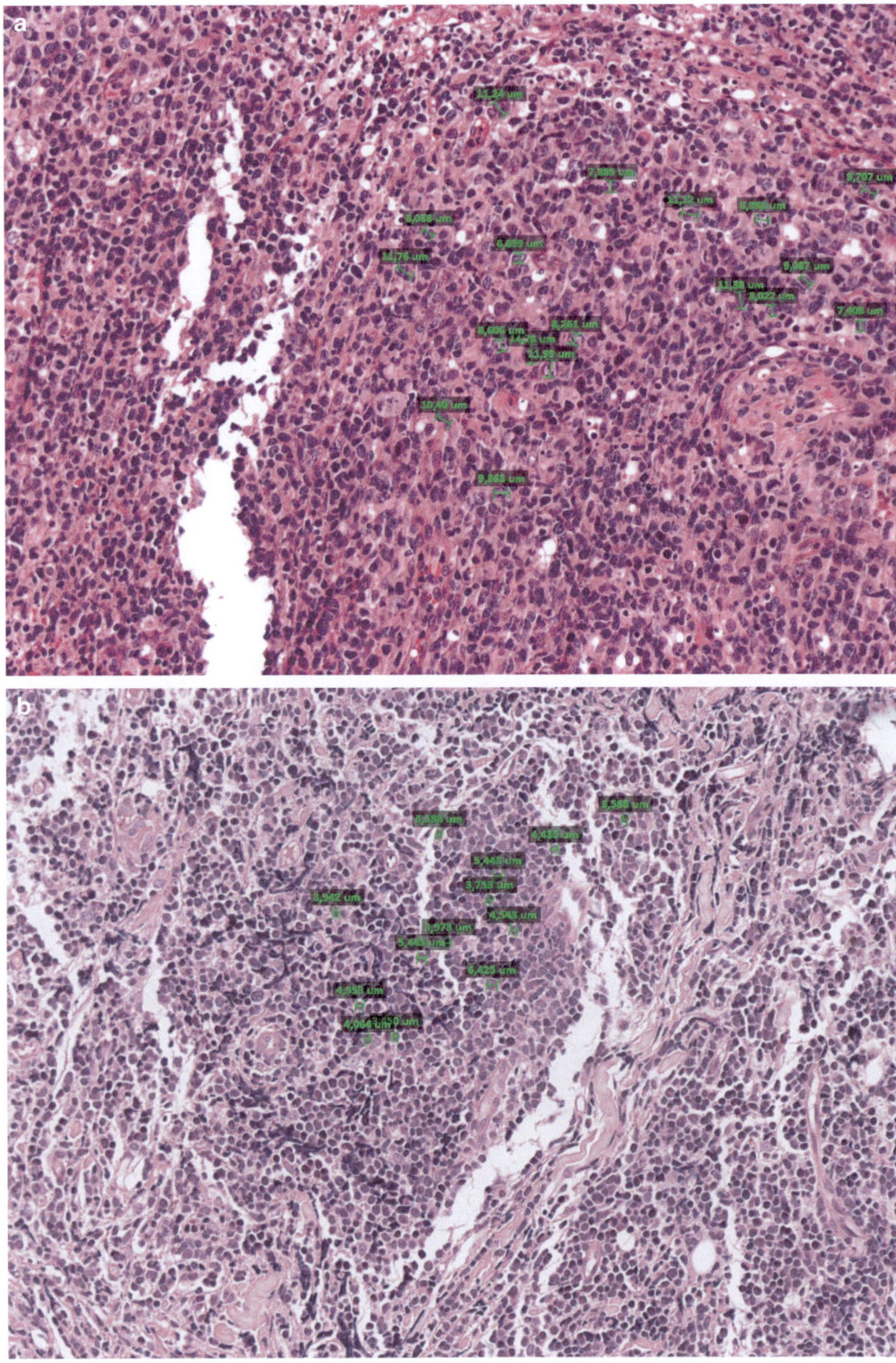

Fig. 1.13 Comparative image between a large cell lymphoma and a small cell lymphoma using scanned slides and a tool for measuring the cells. Observe the different values attributed to each cell. (**a**) Diffuse large B cell lymphoma not otherwise specified contained cells ranging from 7.8 to 11.99 μm (H&E; 100×). (**b**) Lymphoblastic lymphoma/leukemia contained cells ranging from 3.5 to 6.4 μm (H&E; 100×)

neoplastic and the macrophage nuclei have similar sizes, which is typically observed in Burkitt lymphoma. Other physiological references can be used if macrophages are not easily recognizable, like normal lymphocytes or normal endothelial cells. In these instances, the neoplastic cells will need to be two or three times larger than these references to be considered as a large cell (Figs. 1.12 and 1.13).

1.5 How to Differentiate a Reactive Lymphoid/Inflammatory Infiltrate from a Lymphoma in the Oral Cavity? A General Comment

The oral cavity is frequently affected by reactive lymphoid/inflammatory processes. Determining the biological significance of these infiltrates and differentiating them from neoplasms may be problematic, and many oral pathologists are often not confident in making this distinction. Therefore, being able to recognize key microscopic aspects and associated clinical, radiographic, and immunohistochemical data will make the diagnostic process less challenging. The specific microscopic findings of each entity will be elucidated in the subsequent chapters of this book, but as a general overview of the lymphoid disorders, some features can be useful to distinguish between non-neoplastic and neoplastic conditions.

An appropriate clinical and radiographic correlation is extremely important to reach a correct diagnosis. Oral pathologists should obtain as much clinical and radiographic data as possible from the referring clinician. As described above, in the presence of an aggressive, destructive, and infiltrative lymphoid lesion, a diagnosis of high-grade lymphoma should be suspected. In contrast, the presence of asymptomatic non-ulcerated tumoral lesions should be preferentially investigated for low-grade lymphomas. Possible local traumatic events should be evaluated and excluded. Additionally, the clinical status of the dental pulp and the periodontium around a lymphoid/inflammatory infiltrate should be considered during the microscopic analysis, since it may explain the occurrence of the disorder. Strict follow-up of patients is recommended to understand the behavior of a lymphoid/inflammatory lesion in cases of unclear diagnosis. General medical data and systemic evaluation of the patient can be very useful in some cases, and radiographic evaluation should be performed for cases with gnathic bone involvement.

From a microscopic perspective, the presence of a polymorphous infiltrate containing lymphocytes, neutrophils, plasma cells, and macrophages, with a similar distribution of B and T lymphocytes determined by immunohistochemistry, in the absence of necrosis, atypical mitotic figures, and cellular pleomorphism, usually favors a reactive process. However, many B and T cell lymphomas may also have a very rich reactive background. A dense and monotonous appearing infiltrate of lymphoid cells that invades normal surrounding structures like bone, muscles, and nerves, especially with an angiocentric growth pattern, favors a diagnosis of a neoplastic lymphoproliferative process. The presence of tingible body macrophages and the consequent "starry sky" pattern is strongly associated with a diagnosis of high-grade lymphoid neoplasm.

Immunohistochemically, the presence and distribution of each cellular component are important to differentiate a reactive from a neoplastic disorder. A clear predominance of a B cell infiltrate or a T cell infiltrate will favor a diagnosis of lymphoma. Moreover, an important approach is to carefully investigate what cellular population is expressing a given marker; for instance, T cell lymphomas frequently have a dense reactive background and misinterpretation of B cell markers may lead to an erroneous conclusion. Although there is no cut-off value for Ki67 expression, high proliferation rates will also favor a high-grade neoplasm. In cases with a high amount of plasma cells, monoclonality for immunoglobulin light chains will lead to a diagnosis of plasmacytoma/multiple myeloma. In the presence of secondary lymphoid follicles, the loss of the mantle zone, the lack of histiocytes, and the absence of the zonation pattern in the germinal centers, together with the expression of BCL2 protein in the germinal centers, will lead to a diagnosis of follicular lymphoma instead of follicular hyperplasia.

Lymphoproliferative lesions are a complex group of disorders that may affect the maxillofacial and oral region. Strict clinicopathological correlation is needed to achieve a definitive diagnosis. The subsequent chapters will discuss in detail the different entities and highlight important characteristics.

Sources

1. Triantafillidou K, Dimitrakopoulos J, Iordanidis F, Gkagkalis A. Extranodal non-hodgkin lymphomas of the oral cavity and maxillofacial region: a clinical study of 58 cases and review of the literature. J Oral Maxillofac Surg. 2012;70:2776–85. https://doi.org/10.1016/j.joms.2012.01.018.
2. Miron RJ, Bosshardt DD. Multinucleated giant cells: good guys or bad guys? Tissue Eng Part B Rev. 2018;24:53–65. https://doi.org/10.1089/ten.TEB.2017.0242.
3. de Arruda JAA, Schuch LF, Conte Neto N, de Souza LL, Rodrigues-Fernandes CI, Abreu LG, et al. Oral and oropharyngeal lymphomas: a multi-institutional collaborative study. J Oral Pathol Med. 2021;50:603–12. https://doi.org/10.1111/jop.13211.
4. Sung H, Ferlay J, Siegel RL, Laversanne M, Soerjomataram I, Jemal A, et al. Global cancer statistics 2020: GLOBOCAN estimates of incidence and mortality worldwide for 36 cancers in 185 countries. CA Cancer J Clin. 2021;71:209–49. https://doi.org/10.3322/caac.21660.

5. Ashoub M, Wali M, Noureldin N, Keraa K, El Desouky E, ElShafei MM. Oral and para-oral lymphomas: a 10-year multi-center retrospective study in Egypt with time series analysis and forecasting to 2030. BMC Oral Health. 2022;22:556. https://doi.org/10.1186/s12903-022-02582-8.
6. Uchôa DC, Pontes FS, Souza LL, Santos GS, Prado-Ribeiro AC, Brandão TB, et al. HIV-related non-Hodgkin lymphomas affecting the oral cavity: a clinicopathologic study of 11 cases. Med Oral Patol Oral Cir Bucal. 2022;27:e99–e105. https://doi.org/10.4317/medoral.24993.
7. Alaggio R, Amador C, Anagnostopoulos I, Attygalle AD, Araujo IBO, Berti E, et al. The 5th edition of the World Health Organization classification of haematolymphoid tumours: lymphoid neoplasms. Leukemia. 2022;36:1720–48. https://doi.org/10.1038/s41375-022-01620-2.
8. Ahmadzadeh K, Vanoppen M, Rose CD, Matthys P, Wouters CH. Multinucleated giant cells: current insights in phenotype, biological activities, and mechanism of formation. Front Cell Dev Biol. 2022;10:873226. https://doi.org/10.3389/fcell.2022.873226.
9. Campo E, Jaffe ES, Cook JR, Quintanilla-Martinez L, Swerdlow SH, Anderson KC, et al. The international consensus classification of mature lymphoid neoplasms: a report from the clinical advisory committee. Blood. 2022;140:1229–53. https://doi.org/10.1182/blood.2022015851.
10. Gomes NR, Lima LA, Morais-Perdigão AL, de Caceres CVBL, Sant'Ana MSP, Pontes HAR, et al. Radiological aspects of lymphomas and leukaemias affecting the jaws: a systematic review. J Oral Pathol Med. 2023;52:315–23. https://doi.org/10.1111/jop.13422.
11. de Oliveira EM, de Cáceres CVBL, Santos-Silva AR, Vargas PA, Lopes MA, Pontes HAR, et al. Clinical diagnostic approach for oral lymphomas: a multi-institutional, observational study based on 107 cases. Oral Surg Oral Med Oral Pathol Oral Radiol. 2023;136:427–35. https://doi.org/10.1016/j.oooo.2023.03.011.
12. Araújo GR, Morais-Perdigão AL, de Cáceres CVBL, Lopes MA, Aguirre-Urizar JM, Carlos R, et al. Lymphomas affecting the sublingual glands: a clinicopathological study. Head Neck Pathol. 2023;17:154–64. https://doi.org/10.1007/s12105-022-01489-8.
13. Araújo GR, Morais-Perdigão AL, Lopez-de-Cáceres CV, Almeida OP, Vargas PA, Roman-Tager EM, et al. Lymphomas affecting the submandibular glands. Med Oral Patol Oral Cir Bucal. 2024;29:e78–86. https://doi.org/10.4317/medoral.26065.
14. Al-Shahrestani F, Al-Khafaf AE, Asheer Z, Jelicic J, Chanchiri I, Blocher CE, et al. Lymphomas of the submandibular gland: a nationwide cohort study. Eur Arch Otorrinolaringol. 2025;282:2021–31. https://doi.org/10.1007/s00405-024-09008-x.
15. Lafuente-Ibáñez de Mendoza I, Vigarios E, Herbault-Barres B, Alberdi-Navarro J, Sibaud V, Maret D, Aguirre-Urizar JM. Non-infectious granulomatous disorders of the upper lip: clinicopathological analysis of 11 patients. BMC Oral Health. 2022;22:173. https://doi.org/10.1186/s12903-022-02189-z.
16. Bray F, Laversanne M, Sung H, Ferlay J, Siegel RL, Soerjomataram I, et al. Global cancer statistics 2022: GLOBOCAN estimates of incidence and mortality worldwide for 36 cancers in 185 countries. CA Cancer J Clin. 2024;74:229–63. https://doi.org/10.3322/caac.21834.
17. Fooksman DR, Jing Z, Park R. New insights into the ontogeny, diversity, maturation and survival of long-lived plasma cells. Nat Rev Immunol. 2024;24:461–70. https://doi.org/10.1038/s41577-024-00991-0.
18. Alamoudi WA, Abdelsayed RA, Sollecito TP, Alhassan GA, Kulkarni R, Bindakhil MA. Causes of oral granulomatous disorders: an update and narrative review of the literature. Head Neck Pathol. 2024;18:72. https://doi.org/10.1007/s12105-024-01678-7.
19. Anastasia A, Mazzucco W, Pipitò L, Fruscione S, Gaudiano R, Trizzino M, et al. Malignancies in people living with HIV: a 25-years observational study from a tertiary hospital in Italy. J Infect Public Health. 2025;18:102661. https://doi.org/10.1016/j.jiph.2025.102661.
20. Frauenfeld L, Campo E. Advances in the classification of aggressive B-cell lymphomas. Adv Anat Pathol. 2025;32:208–19. https://doi.org/10.1097/PAP.0000000000000484.

2 Laboratorial Tools for the Diagnosis of Lymphoproliferative and Granulomatous Disorders

Lynne Bingle, Pablo Agustin Vargas, Guilherme Rossi Assis de Mendonça, Javier Rendon Henao, and Felipe Paiva Fonseca

2.1 Immunohistochemistry and EBV Detection

Although flow cytometry is a frequently used approach to determine the immunophenotype of hematolymphoid diseases, immunohistochemistry (IHC) can provide further information concerning the immune architecture of these lesions. This feature has consolidated IHC as an invaluable tool for the diagnosis of many pathological disorders using formalin-fixed, paraffin-embedded tissue, and therefore, it is considered very useful for the diagnosis of lymphoproliferative disorders affecting the oral cavity and the jaws. The more widespread use of IHC was enabled by improved development and production of antibodies, which are not only more specific for the target of interest but more accessible for many healthcare providers in terms of cost. Immunohistochemistry is such an established method that it is now possible for automated IHC instruments to be found in many routine diagnostic laboratories. However, even where this is not possible, the method is simple to execute following basic rules of antigen retrieval, blocking unspecific staining, and antibody titration. Not surprisingly, therefore, immunohistochemistry has proved to be an important routine technique for the diagnosis of lymphoid lesions, regardless of whether they are reactive or neoplastic. This is due in part to the fact that the technique has been shown to help identify the type of lymphocytes involved in the lesion, the cell proliferation and differentiation status of the lymphocytes, and their architecture in the context of different tissue types. Moreover, it can also represent a useful auxiliary for the diagnosis of granulomatous processes in some instances.

In order to determine the biological nature of a lesion, it is necessary to demonstrate the differentiation lineage of the tumor cells, to enable identification of structures and cells not recognizable in H&E-stained sections, to determine the relationship between different cell populations, and ultimately to predict patient outcome and response to therapy. There is a considerable level of complexity in many lesions, some of which pathologists may not encounter regularly, despite the absolute requirement for an accurate diagnosis. A careful morphological study, followed by an adequate selection of IHC markers, is therefore of utmost importance. It is necessary to stress, however, that not one specific immunohistochemical panel or marker is used for all lymphoid diseases, and the selection of the most appropriate diagnostic marker(s) will depend on the specific morphological aspects of each lesion, applied to a particular clinical context. In lesions that are poorly differentiated, non-lymphoid markers may also be needed in some instances to rule out the diagnosis of a possible carcinoma, sarcoma, neuroendocrine tumor, or other disorders (Fig. 2.1).

The most frequently used immunohistochemical markers are described in Table 2.1. In general, less specific antibodies with a higher sensitivity are commonly used during the first diagnostic steps and include the pan-leucocitary antigen (LCA/CD45), followed by markers of B lymphocytes, T lymphocytes and plasma cells, and the analysis of the proliferative potential of the disease measured by Ki67 expression. Mature B lymphocytes are usually demonstrated

L. Bingle (✉)
Academic Unit of Oral and Maxillofacial Medicine and Pathology, Department of Clinical Dentistry, School of Clinical Dentistry, University of Sheffield, Sheffield, UK
e-mail: l.bingle@sheffield.ac.uk

P. A. Vargas
Oral and Maxillofacial Division, Piracicaba Dental School, State University of Campinas (UNICAMP), Piracicaba, Brazil
e-mail: pavargas@fop.unicamp.br

G. R. A. de Mendonça
Department of Pathology, School of Medical Sciences, University of Campinas, Campinas, Brazil

J. R. Henao
Department of Hematopathology and Flow Cytometry, Ayudas Diagnósticas Sura Center, Cartagena, Colombia

F. P. Fonseca
Department of Oral Surgery and Pathology, School of Dentistry, Universidade Federal de Minas Gerais, Belo Horizonte, Brazil

© The Author(s), under exclusive license to Springer Nature Switzerland AG 2025

F. P. Fonseca et al. (eds.), *Lymphoproliferative and Granulomatous Disorders of the Oral Cavity*,
https://doi.org/10.1007/978-3-031-98844-8_2

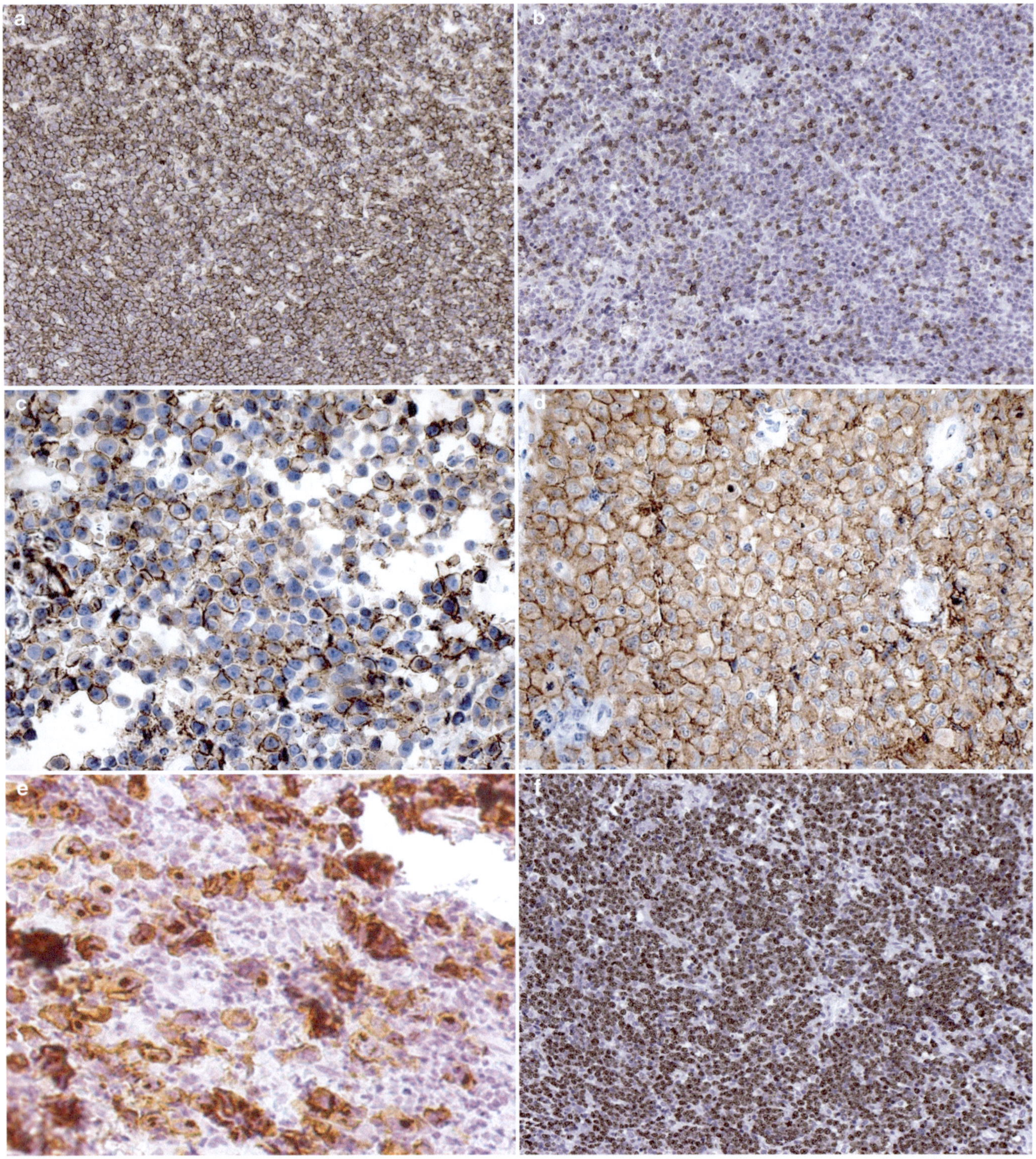

Fig. 2.1 Illustrative images of immunohistochemical markers commonly used in the diagnosis of lymphoma affecting the oral cavity. (**a**) CD20 shows mature B cell differentiation (DAB; 100×). (**b**) CD3 is used to demonstrate T cell phenotype; reactive T cells demonstrated here (DAB; 100×). (**c**) CD138 is frequently used to demonstrate plasma cell differentiation (DAB; 200×). (**d**) Langerhans cell histiocytosis is diagnosed using CD1a staining (DAB; 200×). (**e**) The characteristic dot-like staining pattern of CD30 is commonly seen in anaplastic large cell lymphoma (DAB; 200×). (**f**) Proliferative index is commonly evaluated by Ki67 nuclear expression (DAB; 100×)

by CD20, CD79a, and PAX5 expression, whereas CD3, CD2, CD5, CD7, and CD43 identify mature T lymphocyte expression. In contrast, TdT combined with CD10, CD99, and/or CD34 aids in the identification of immature lympho-

Table 2.1 Summary of the main immunohistochemical markers used for the diagnosis of the most common reactive and neoplastic lymphoproliferative disorders affecting the oral and maxillofacial region

Antibody	Most common expression pattern	Most frequent cell targets	Most frequent lymphoproliferative disorders
ALK	Cytoplasm/membrane/nucleus	ALK+ ALCL cells	ALK+ ALCL
BCL2	Cytoplasm	Different cells may express BCL2, such as B and T lymphocytes	Expressed in different lymphoma subtypes, and frequently used for follicular lymphoma diagnosis (BCL2 positive in the germinal center), in contrast with follicular lymphoid hyperplasia (BCL2 negative in the germinal center)
BCL6	Nucleus	Germinal center-derived cells	Lymphomas derived from germinal center cells
BOB	Nucleus	Mature B lymphocytes	Mature B cell lymphomas
CD1a	Membrane	Langerhans cells	Langerhans cell histiocytosis
CD3	Membrane	Mature T lymphocytes	T cell lymphomas
CD4	Membrane	Mature T lymphocytes	T cell lymphomas
CD5	Membrane	Mature T lymphocytes	T cell lymphomas and some B cell lymphomas like CLL/SLL and MCL
CD7	Membrane	Mature T lymphocytes	T cell lymphomas
CD8	Membrane	Mature T lymphocytes	T cell lymphomas
CD10	Membrane	Germinal center-derived cells Immature lymphocytes	Lymphomas derived from germinal center cells Lymphoblastic leukemia/lymphoma
CD20	Membrane	Mature B lymphocytes	Mature B cell lymphomas
CD21	Membrane	Follicular dendritic cells	Follicular dendritic cell sarcoma. Also used to demonstrate the follicular dendritic cells' meshworks of normal germinal centers and associated lymphomas, such as follicular lymphoma
CD23	Membrane	Follicular dendritic cells	Follicular dendritic cell sarcoma. Also used to demonstrate the follicular dendritic cells' meshworks of normal germinal centers and associated lymphomas, such as follicular lymphoma
CD30	Membrane/perinuclear	Different cells may express CD30	ALCL, ENKTCL, mucocutaneous ulcers, post-transplant lymphoproliferative disorders, DLBCL
CD34	Membrane	Immature B and T lymphocytes	Lymphoblastic leukemia/lymphoma
CD35	Membrane	Follicular dendritic cells	Follicular dendritic cell sarcoma. Also used to demonstrate the follicular dendritic cells' meshworks of normal germinal centers and associated lymphomas, such as follicular lymphoma
CD43	Membrane	T lymphocytes and some B lymphocytes	Expressed by T cell lymphomas, but it may also be expressed in some B cell lymphomas
CD45RO	Membrane	Mature T lymphocytes	T cell lymphomas
CD68	Cytoplasm	Macrophages	Disseminated juvenile xanthogranuloma, xanthoma, histiocytic sarcoma, RDD
CD79a	Membrane	Mature B lymphocytes	Mature B cell lymphomas
CD99	Membrane	Immature B and T lymphocytes	Lymphoblastic leukemia/lymphoma
CD138	Membrane	Plasma cells	Plasmacytoma/multiple myeloma and lymphomas with plasmablastic differentiation
CD163	Membrane	Macrophages	Disseminated juvenile xanthogranuloma, xanthoma, histiocytic sarcoma, RDD
MYC	Nucleus	Different lymphoma cells	Burkitt lymphoma, DLBCL NOS
Cyclin D1	Nucleus	Macrophages and endothelial cells	MCL, hairy cell leukemia, some multiple myelomas, and RDD
EMA	Membrane/cytoplasm	Plasma cells	Plasmacytoma/multiple myeloma and lymphomas with plasmablastic differentiation, and ALCL
Factor XIIIa	Cytoplasm	Macrophages	Disseminated juvenile xanthogranuloma
GATA3	Nucleus	T lymphocytes	PTCL
Granzyme B	Cytoplasm granular	Cytotoxic T lymphocytes and NK cells	ENKTCL
HGAL	Nucleus	Germinal center-derived cells	Lymphomas derived from germinal center cells
IgD	Membrane	Plasma cells and B lymphocytes	MCL

(continued)

Table 2.1 (continued)

Antibody	Most common expression pattern	Most frequent cell targets	Most frequent lymphoproliferative disorders
IgG	Cytoplasm	Plasma cells and B lymphocytes	Used for IgG4-related disease diagnosis
IgG4	Cytoplasm	Plasma cells and B lymphocytes	Used for IgG4-related disease diagnosis
Kappa/lambda	Cytoplasm	Plasma cells	Used to determine immunoglobulin light chain restriction (monotypic/polytypic) in lymphoid disorders
Ki67	Nucleus	Cells in general	It is used to demonstrate the proliferative feature of one lesion
LCA (CD45)	Membrane	Virtually all leukocytes	Sensitive marker, used to determine the lymphoid nature of a neoplasm, together with more lineage-specific markers
LEF1	Nucleus	B and T lymphocytes	CLL/SLL
LMO2	Nucleus	Germinal center-derived cells	Lymphomas derived from germinal center cells
LMP1	Membrane	Cells infected by EBV	Hodgkin lymphoma, a subset of EBV+ DLBCL NOS, mucocutaneous ulcers
Lysozyme	Cytoplasm	Macrophages	Disseminated juvenile xanthogranuloma, xanthoma, histiocytic sarcoma
MPO	Cytoplasm	Myeloid cells	Myeloid sarcoma
MUM1/IRF4	Nucleus	Plasma cells and B lymphocytes	Plasmacytoma/multiple myeloma and lymphomas with plasmablastic differentiation, and a subset of DLBCL
OCT2	Nucleus	Mature B lymphocytes	Mature B cell lymphomas
PAX5	Nucleus	Mature B lymphocytes	Mature B cell lymphomas
Perforin	Cytoplasm granular	Cytotoxic T lymphocytes and NK cells	ENKTCL
Plasma cell (VS38c)	Cytoplasm	Plasma cells	Plasmacytoma/multiple myeloma and lymphomas with plasmablastic differentiation
S100	Cytoplasm/nucleus	Langerhans cells and macrophages	Langerhans cell histiocytosis, RDD, and histiocytic sarcoma
SOX11	Nucleus	MCL cells	MCL
TBX21	Nucleus	T lymphocytes	PTCL
TdT	Nucleus	Immature B and T lymphocytes	Lymphoblastic leukemia/lymphoma, a subset of DLBCL
TIA-1	Cytoplasm granular	Cytotoxic T lymphocytes and NK cells	ENKTCL

LCA leukocyte common antigen, *CD* cluster of differentiation, *CLL/SLL* chronic lymphocytic leukemia/small cell lymphocytic lymphoma, *MCL* mantle cell lymphoma, *NK* natural killer, *DLBCL* diffuse large B cell lymphoma, *ALCL* anaplastic large cell lymphoma, *EMA* epithelial membrane antigen, *RDD* Rosai–Dorfman disease, *ENKTCL* extranodal NK/T cell lymphoma, *PTCL* peripheral T cell lymphoma, *EBV* Epstein–Barr virus, *NOS* not otherwise specified, *LMP1* latent membrane protein 1

[a]A summary of the most common immunohistochemical markers used in the diagnosis of the lymphoproliferative disorders that may affect the oral and maxillofacial region. The above-described markers may have other applications, both in lymphoid and non-lymphoid diseases, and specific literature must be accessed for full descriptions and applications of each marker

cytes. Histiocytes express CD68, CD163, and lysozyme, while CD1a, langerin (CD207), and S100 are used to identify Langerhans cells. Plasma cell markers include CD138, MUM1, EMA, and VS38c, while the monoclonality status of these cells can be inferred using immunoglobulin light chain restriction for kappa or lambda. Normal B and T cell markers of potential therapeutic importance include CD20, CD30, CD79, CD22, BCL2, and CD52, among others. (Fig. 2.2).

Cells derived from germinal centers express CD10, BCL6, LMO, and HGAL, but the presence of germinal centers can also be demonstrated by the presence of follicular dendritic cell meshworks using CD21, CD23, or CD35. Other markers that have a lower cellular population specificity, but are useful to diagnose specific lymphoproliferative disorders and that are frequently used in hematopathology include BCL2, GATA3, TBX21, IgG, and IgG4 (Table 2.1). The immunoexpression of some diagnostic markers like Cyclin D1 and ALK denotes the occurrence of molecular abnormalities (Fig. 2.3).

It is important to be aware that aberrant protein expression might be found in some lymphomas, such as the expression of the T-cell marker CD5 in tumor cells of mantle cell lymphoma, a mature B-cell neoplasm (Fig. 2.4). High-grade lymphomas may also frequently express aberrant proteins, including non-lymphoid markers such as cytokeratin in plasmablastic lymphomas, which may lead to a misdiagnosis of carcinoma. Moreover, lymphomas may also lose the expression of proteins, such as peripheral T-cell lymphomas that can lose expression of one or more T-cell markers. Therefore, the interpretation of immunohistochemical studies must ideally be done in an integrated approach, taking

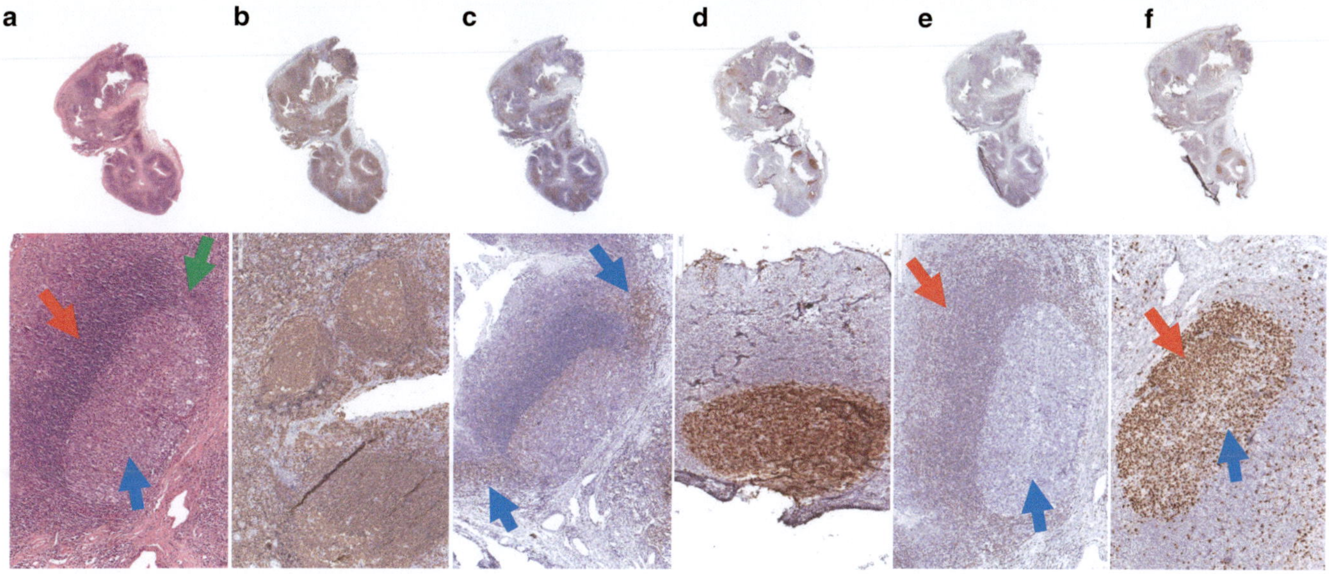

Fig. 2.2 Immunohistochemistry used to investigate the biological nature of a hyperplastic lymphoid tissue from the palatine tonsil. Note that the interpretation of immunohistochemistry reactions should always be associated with an H&E-stained morphological study. (**a**) Palatine tonsil showing lymphoid hyperplasia with the presence of secondary follicles (green arrow) containing germinal centers (blue arrow) surrounded by a darker mantle zone (red arrow) (H&E; 50×). (**b**) The expression of CD20 is used to demonstrate the B lymphocyte population predominantly located in the lymphoid follicles (DAB; 50×). (**c**) T lymphocytes express CD3 and are predominantly located in the interfollicular zones (blue arrows) (DAB; 50×). (**d**) Germinal center is highlighted using, for instance, the CD10 protein. Observe the strong expression in the germinal center cells (DAB; 50×). (**e**) The expression of BCL2 located in the interfollicular zone (red arrow) with a negative result in the germinal center cells (blue arrow) is useful to demonstrate the reactive nature of the lymphoid tissue (DAB; 50×). (**f**) Germinal centers exhibit a high proliferative index measured by Ki67 expression. Zonation is demonstrated by a higher Ki67 expression in the dark zone (red arrow) and a slightly lower expression in the light zone (blue arrow). This is also indicative of a reactive nature of the lesion (DAB; 50×). Images in the upper line represent the same markers described above, but illustrated under lower magnification to demonstrate a more general overview of each marker

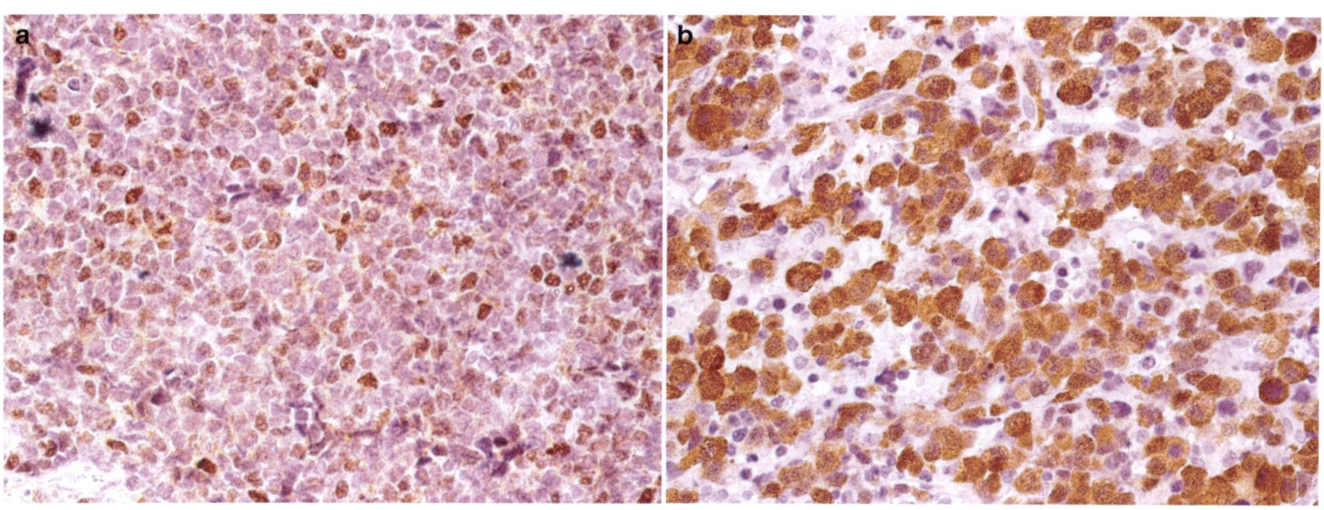

Fig. 2.3 Immunohistochemistry can also be used to indirectly demonstrate the occurrence of molecular events. (**a**) The strong and diffuse nuclear expression of Cyclin D1 in a case of mantle cell lymphoma is indicative of CCND1 abnormality (DAB; 100×). (**b**) The strong expression of ALK protein is also indicative of molecular abnormalities involving this gene, and the expression pattern in the cytoplasm and nucleus is also indicative of a t(2;5)(p23;q35) involving *NPM::ALK* genes (DAB; 100×)

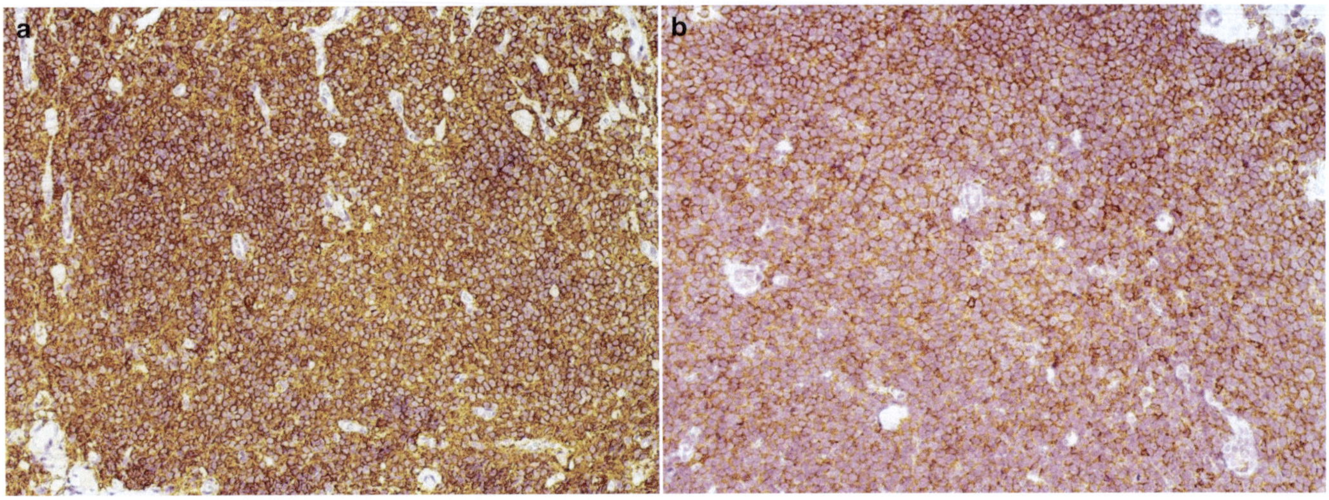

Fig. 2.4 Aberrant immunohistochemical expression of different markers that carry important diagnostic potential is well known. (**a**) Mantle cell lymphoma is a mature B cell lymphoma and therefore, strongly expresses CD20 protein (DAB; 100×). (**b**) However, this neoplasm also aberrantly expresses the T cell marker CD5, which is an important immunohistochemical signature of the neoplasm (DAB; 100×)

into account the expression pattern of a series of markers, rather than one isolated marker (Table 2.2).

The detection of virus-associated antigens may also help in the classification of lymphoid lesions. The most common virus involved in lymphomagenesis is Epstein–Barr virus (EBV), a member of the γ-herpesvirus subfamily, which, when discovered in an endemic Burkitt's lymphoma cell culture in 1964, reignited research into the role of viruses in the development of cancer. EBV represents the fourth herpesvirus to be identified, often referred to as human herpesvirus 4, and is a linear, double-stranded, enveloped DNA virus with virions 100–200 nm in diameter. EBV infection is present in over 95% of the world population, and while the majority of individuals are asymptomatic or develop only mild symptoms, EBV contributes to approximately 1.5% of all human cancers. The importance of EBV infection for the pathogenesis of lymphoid lesions is well known, and detection of this virus can be achieved by using a number of laboratory techniques. A successful detection of the virus is, however, dependent on the viral latency stage in each lesion, as described in Table 2.3. The oncogenic potential of the lytic phase of EBV has recently gained more attention and importance. However, the latent phase of EBV infection is more often associated with lymphomagenesis and, depending on the viral latent gene expression pattern, is classified as 0, I, IIa, IIb, and III.

In the routine diagnosis of oral and maxillofacial lymphoid lesions, immunohistochemistry is used to identify the EBV membrane protein, LMP1, which is known to be present in EBV+ mucocutaneous ulcers and in some cases of diffuse large B cell lymphoma not otherwise specified (DLBCL NOS). However, most EBV-positive lesions are encompassed in latency type I, and may have therefore lost structural components of the virus, including LMP1. For example, EBV-positive Burkitt lymphoma is usually negative for LMP1, but positive for EBV RNA type 1 (EBNA-1), as demonstrated by chromogenic in situ hybridization [(CISH) (Epstein-Barr encoded RNA—EBER]. Thus, the use of CISH for EBV detection is recommended, as it shows greater sensitivity than immunohistochemistry when the viral load is low. Moreover, histological interpretation of EBER is usually straightforward; the presence of nonspecific staining is less common and, importantly, a number of detection kits for EBER are available (Fig. 2.5).

Table 2.2 Summary of the most frequently observed immunohistochemical results and the most frequent EBV status in the main histiocytic neoplasms, lymphomas, and leukemic infiltrations that more commonly affect the oral and maxillofacial region

Subtype	CD20	PAX5	CD3	CD5	CD7	CD1a	S100	CD68	MPO	TdT	CD21	CD23	BCL2	BCL6	CD10	Cyclin D1	SOX11	MYC	MUM1	CD138	CD56	CD30	ALK	Gran.	Ki67	EBER
LCH	–	–	–	–	–	+	+	–/+	–	–	–	–	+	–	–	–	–	–	–	–	–	–	–	–	+	–
FDCS	–	–	–	–	–	–	–	–	–	–	+	+	–/+	–	–	–	–	–	–	–	–	–	–	–	+	–
HS	–	–	–	–	–	–	+	+	–	–	–	–	–/+	–	–	–	–	–	–	–	–	–	–	–	++	–
MS	–	–	–	–	+/–	–/+	–	+	+	–	–	–	+	–	–	–	–	–	–	–	–	–	–	–	++	–
ALL	–	+/–	+/–	+/–	+/–	–/+	–	–	–	+	–	–	+/–	–	+	–	–	–	–	–	–	–	–	–/+	+++	–
CLL/SLL	+	+	–	+	–	–	–	–	–	–	–	+	+/–	–	–	–	–	–	–	–	–	–	–	–	+	–
MZL (MALT)	+	+	–	–	–	–	–	–	–	–	–	–	+	–	–	–	–	–	–	–	–	–	–	–	+	–
FL	+	+	–	–	–	–	–	–	–	–	–	–/+	+	+	+	–	–	–	–	–	–	–	–	–	+	–
MCL	+	+	–	+	–	–	–	–	–	–	–	–	+	–	–	+	+	–	–	–	–	–	–	–	++	–
BL	+	+	–	–	–	–	–	–	–	–	–	–	–	+	+	–	–	+	–	–	–	–	–	–	++++	+/–
DLBCL NOS	+	+	–	–/+	–	–	–	–	–	–/+	–	–	+	+/–	+/–	–	–	+/–	+/–	–	–	+/–	–	–	++	–/+
PBL	–	–	–	–	–	–	–	–	–	–	–	–	+	–	+	–	–	+	+	+	+/–	+/–	–	–	+++	+/–
P/MM	–/+	–	–	–	–	–	–	–	–	–	–	–	+/–	–	+/–	–/+	–	+	+	+	–/+	–	–	–	+	/++
ENKTL	–	–	+	+	+	–	–	–	–	–	–	–	+	–/+	+	–	–	–	–	–	+	+/–	–	+	++	+
PTCL NOS	–	–	+/–	+/–	+/–	–	–	–	–	–	–	–	+	–	+/–	–	–	–	–	–	+/–	+/–	–	+/–	++	+/–
ALCL[a]	–	–	–	+/–	+/–	–	–	–	–	–	–	–	–/+	–	–	–	–	–	–	–	–/+	+	+/–	+	++	–
MF	–	–	+	–/+	–/+	–	–	–	–	–	–	–	+/–	–	–	–	–	–	–	–	–/+	–/+	–	–	+	–

A brief summary of the most commonly used antibodies for the diagnosis of hematolymphoid neoplasms that affect the oral cavity. Variability in results for each marker may occur and other markers may be required to achieve a final diagnosis. For a more detailed and complete discussion on the immunohistochemical features of each entity, please refer to the specific chapters

LCH langerhans cell histiocytosis, *FDCS* follicular dendritic cell sarcoma, *HS* histiocytic sarcoma, *MS* myeloid sarcoma, *ALL* acute lymphoblastic lymphoma/leukemia, *CLL/SLL* chronic lymphocytic leukemia/small lymphocytic lymphoma, *MALT* marginal zone lymphoma. Mucosa-associated lymphoid tissue, *FL* follicular lymphoma, *MCL* mantle cell lymphoma, *BL* Burkitt's lymphoma, *DLBCL NOS* diffuse large B cell lymphoma not otherwise specified, *PBL* plasmablastic lymphoma, *P/MM* plasmocytoma/multiple myeloma, *ENKTCL* extranodal NK/T cell lymphoma, *PTCL NOS* peripheral T cell lymphoma not otherwise specified, *ALCL* anaplastic large cell lymphoma, *MF* mycosis fungoides, *Gran.* granzyme B. – negative, + positive, –/+ or +/– variable

[a]Results may vary depending on the subtype of ALCL

Table 2.3 EBV latency and distribution in some lymphoproliferative disorders

Latency	Molecules expressed	Main lymphoid diseases
Type I	EBNA1, EBV BARTs, EBV miRNAs, EBER1, and EBER2	Burkitt lymphoma
Type II	EBNA1, LMP1, LMP2A, LMP2B, EBV BARTs, EBV miRNAs, EBER1, and EBER2	DLBCL, extranodal NK/T cell lymphoma, and HL
Type III	EBNA1, 2, 3A, 3B, 3C and EBNA LP, LMP1, 2A and 2B, EBV BART, EBV miRNAs, EBER1, and EBER2	DLBCL, PTLD, IM

DLBCL diffuse large B cell lymphoma, *HL* Hodgkin lymphoma, *PTLD* post-transplant lymphoproliferative disorder, *IM* infectious mononucleosis

2.2 Genetics

The understanding of the molecular basis of many human neoplasms over the last few decades has led to the identification of many new biomarkers with diagnostic, prognostic, and/or therapeutic potential. The search for genetic mutations is frequently used as an auxiliary diagnostic tool for different groups of neoplasms, especially in the field of lymphoproliferative disorders. Despite the importance of these genetic events for the pathogenesis of the neoplasms, it is not always necessary to demonstrate their existence if the clinicopathological and immunohistochemical correlation is considered sufficient. However, demonstration of the presence

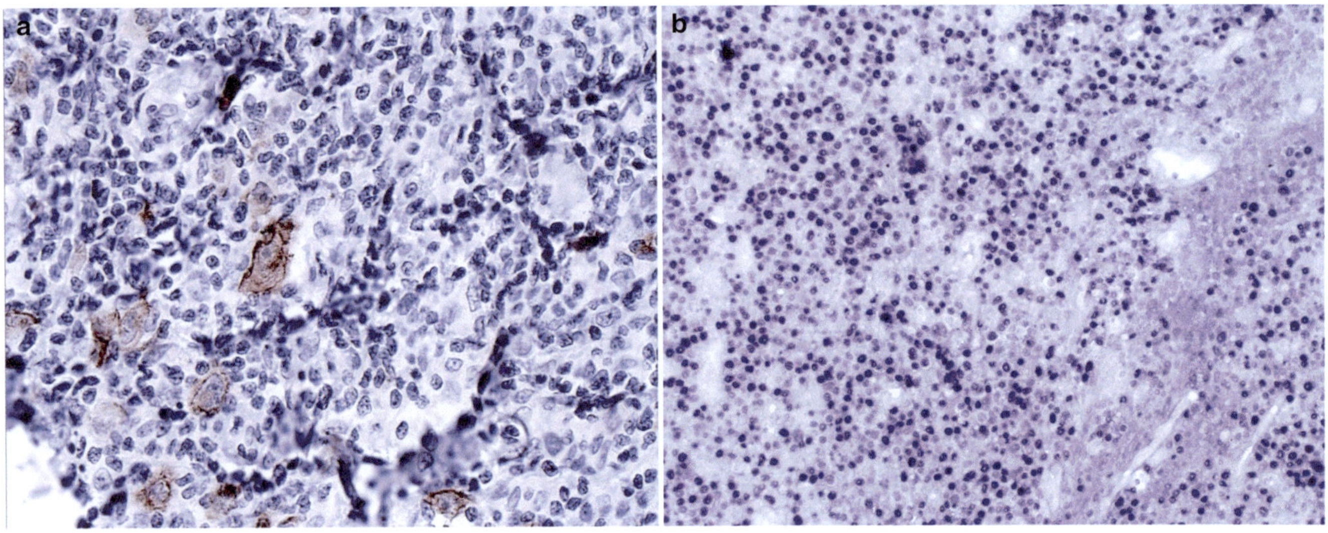

Fig. 2.5 Immunohistochemistry and in situ hybridization can be used to investigate the presence of EBV in lymphoproliferative disorders. (**a**) Immunohistochemistry demonstrates the expression of the latent membrane protein, LMP1 (DAB; 200×). (**b**) In situ hybridization for EBER covers a wider spectrum of EBV latency and is a more sensitive technique, being able to detect RNA expression. The microscopic presentation of the reaction depends on the specific kit used, ranging from dark blue on a light blue background to dark blue on a reddish background (EBER; 100×)

of genetic mutations in some lymphomas is necessary to confirm a final diagnosis, for example, the *IRF4* mutation in a specific subset of large B cell lymphomas. Concerning T-cell lymphoproliferations, the assessment of T-cell receptor (TCR) clonality with molecular methods (PCR) is also useful to favor a neoplastic process in cases with suspected morphology, but inconclusive immunohistochemical results. In addition, genetic events may also be important in determining the prognosis and/or the most appropriate therapeutic option for a patient; for instance, B cell lymphoblastic lymphoma/leukemia is categorized according to molecular events, and this determines patients' prognosis and treatment.

The most important genetic events found in oral and maxillofacial lymphomas are detailed in Table 2.4. Fluorescent in situ hybridization (FISH) is often used to identify these molecular events as this allows cytogeneticists not only to determine the presence or absence of a genetic change, but also to observe, to some extent, molecular alterations in the tumor cells (Fig. 2.6). PCR has also been used in the identification of some mutations, but this does not allow for any spatial expression information, as is the case with next-generation sequencing (NGS), which has recently been used more frequently. PCR and NGS can therefore identify molecular changes, which may be sufficient information for diagnosis, prognosis, and/or suggestions for therapeutic regimens, but they do not give the in-depth histological or spatial expression data that immunohistochemistry or FISH provide. These techniques are therefore complementary and should be used in specific contexts following a precise morphological and immunohistochemical examination.

Table 2.4 Genes often showing molecular abnormalities that can be used as auxiliaries for the diagnosis of the most common lymphoproliferative disorders in the oral and maxillofacial region

Gene	Lymphoproliferative lesions
BCL2	DLBCL, follicular lymphoma, high-grade B-cell lymphoma with *MYC/BCL2* rearrangements
BCL6	DLBCL
MYC	DLBCL, Burkitt lymphoma, high-grade B-cell lymphoma with *MYC/BCL2* rearrangements
IRF4	*IRF4*-mutated LBCL
CCND1, CCND2, CCND3	MCL, multiple myeloma
MALT1	MALT lymphoma
IGH/IGK/IGL	Main gene partners of the chromosomal translocations
STAT3, JAK3, BCOR, DDX3X, TP53	Extranodal NK/T cell lymphoma
ALK, DUSP22, TP63, STAT3	Anaplastic large cell lymphoma
BRAF-V600E	Rare DJX, histiocytic sarcoma and Langerhans cell histiocytosis
NRAS/KRAS	RDD

Practical summary of the most frequent genetic abnormalities found in lymphoproliferative disorders that more often affect the oral cavity. Variability in the presence of genetic abnormalities and other genetic events may also occur in these lesions. For a more detailed and complete discussion of the genetic features of each disorder, refer to the specific chapters

DLBCL diffuse large B cell lymphoma, *LBCL* large B cell lymphoma, *MCL* mantle cell lymphoma, *MALT* marginal zone lymphoma, mucosa-associated lymphoid tissue, *DJX* disseminated juvenile xanthogranuloma, *RDD* Rosai–Dorfman disease

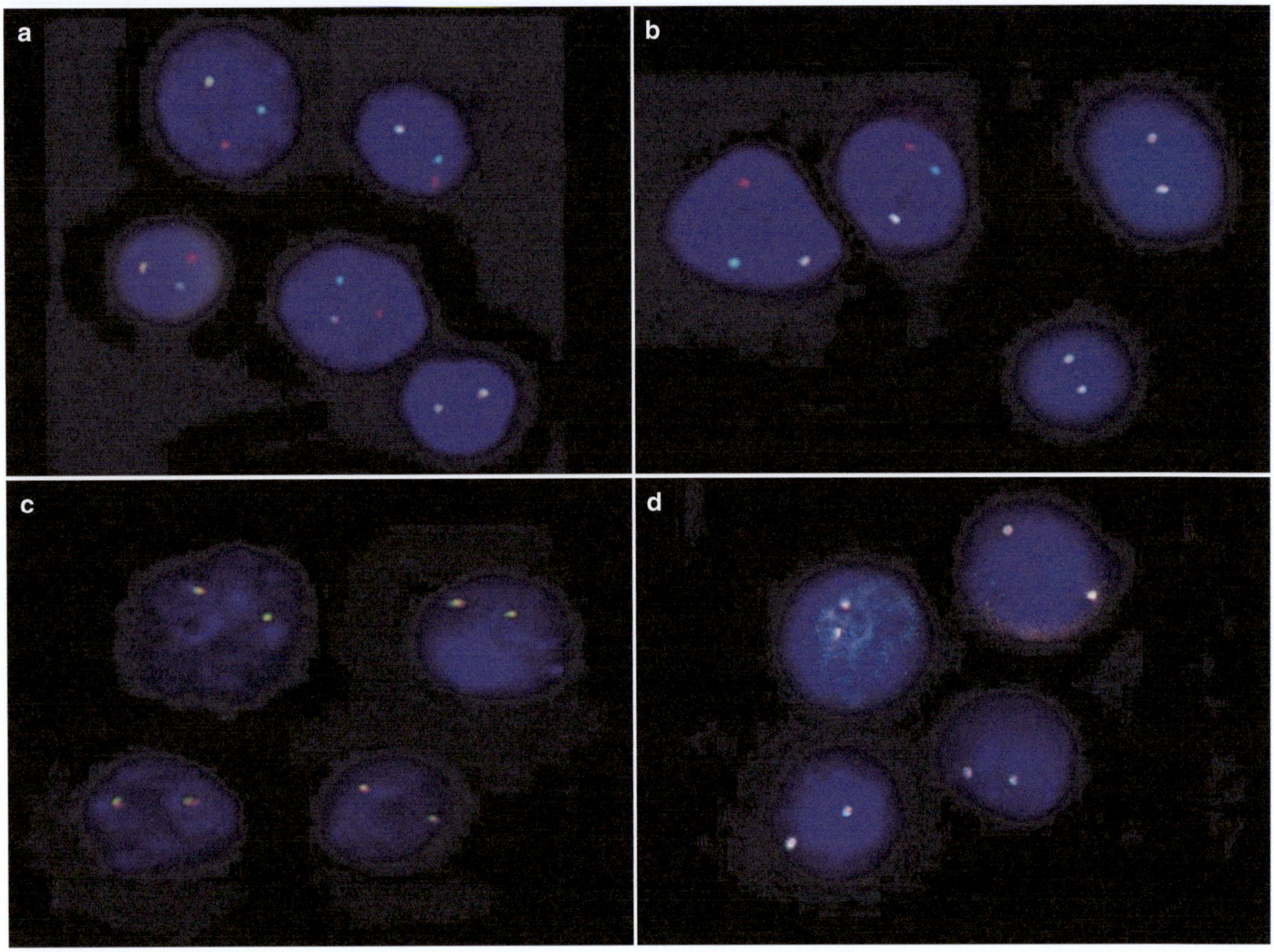

Fig. 2.6 The investigation of chromosomal translocations can be very important for the diagnosis of some lymphomas affecting the oral cavity. (**a**) Fluorescence in situ hybridization is the most frequently used technique to demonstrate the occurrence of a translocation. In this example, using a break-apart probe, the separated red and green dots illustrate a translocation involving the *BCL2* gene in a case of DLBCL NOS (DAPI; 1000×). (**b**) FISH demonstrating *MYC* gene translocation in a plasmablastic lymphoma; separated red and green dots identify the occurrence of the chromosomal translocation (DAPI; 1000×). (**c**) Using a break-apart probe joined red and green dots, resulting in a yellowish signal, demonstrates the lack of translocation in the *MYC* gene in this DLBCL NOS case (DAPI; 1000×). (**d**) Yellow dots resulting from joined red and green signals in a DLBCL NOS without *BCL2* translocation (DAPI; 1000×)

Sources

1. Kang MS, Kieff E. Epstein–Barr virus latent genes. Exp Mol Med. 2015;47:e131. https://doi.org/10.1038/emm.2014.84.
2. Rosemarie Q, Sugden B. Epstein-Barr virus: how its lytic phase contributes to oncogenesis. Microorganisms. 2020;8:1824. https://doi.org/10.3390/microorganisms8111824.
3. Rodríguez-Sevilla JJ, Salar A. Recent advances in the genetic of MALT lymphomas. Cancers (Basel). 2021;14:176. https://doi.org/10.3390/cancers14010176.
4. Kos IA, Thurner L, Bittenbring JT, Christofyllakis K, Kaddu-Mulindwa D. Advances in lymphoma molecular diagnostics. Diagnostics (Basel). 2021;11:2174. https://doi.org/10.3390/diagnostics11122174.
5. Araújo ALD, Fonsêca JM, do Amaral-Silva GK, de Lima Morais TM, Mariz BALA, Fonseca FP, et al. The role of immunohistochemistry for primary oral diagnosis in a brazilian oral pathology service. Appl Immunohistochem Mol Morphol. 2021;29:781–90. https://doi.org/10.1097/PAI.0000000000000960.
6. Sethi S, Epstein-Peterson Z, Kumar A, Ho C. Current knowledge in genetics, molecular diagnostic tools, and treatments for mantle cell lymphomas. Front Oncol. 2021;11:739441. https://doi.org/10.3389/fonc.2021.739441.
7. Xia S, Yue J, Chen X, Hu Y, Guo F, Zhang J. Clinicopathological and genetic characteristics of diffuse large B-cell lymphoma of the oropharyngeal and maxillofacial region. Oral Dis. 2021;27:448–56. https://doi.org/10.1111/odi.13578.
8. Murata T, Sugimoto A, Inagaki T, Yanagi Y, Watanabe T, Sato Y, et al. Molecular basis of Epstein-Barr virus latency establishment and lytic reactivation. Viruses. 2021;13:2344. https://doi.org/10.3390/v13122344.
9. Alaggio R, Amador C, Anagnostopoulos I, Attygalle AD, de Oliveira Araujo IB, Berti E, et al. The 5th edition of the World Health Organization classification of haematolymphoid tumours: lymphoid neoplasms. Leukemia. 2022;36(7):1720–48.

10. Campo E, Jaffe ES, Cook JR, Quintanilla-Martinez L, Swerdlow SH, Anderson KC, et al. The international consensus classification of mature lymphoid neoplasms: a report from the clinical advisory committee. Blood. 2022;140:1229–53.
11. Lefebvre C, Veronese L, Nadal N, Gaillard JB, Penther D, Daudignon A, et al. Cytogenetics in the management of mature B-cell non-Hodgkin lymphomas: guidelines from the Groupe Francophone de Cytogénétique Hematologique (GFCH). Curr Res Transl Med. 2023;71:103425. https://doi.org/10.1016/j.retram.2023.103425.
12. Bronson AS, Zhu Y, Lilley CM, Crane GM, Mirza KM. Clinicopathologic insights and molecular oncogenesis: understanding Epstein-Barr virus-induced B-cell lymphoproliferations. Int J Surg Pathol. 2024;21:10668969241266933. https://doi.org/10.1177/10668969241266933.
13. Barreto MEZ, Soares CD, de Andrade MMP, de Oliveira SA, Fonseca FP, Abreu LG, et al. Immunohistochemistry and RT-PCR as ancillary tools in the diagnosis of acquired oral syphilis. Oral Dis. 2025;31:890–8. https://doi.org/10.1111/odi.15107.
14. Zhang F, Cui Q, Du H, Lv X, Hou T, Chen Y, et al. Comparative investigation among fluorescence in situ hybridization, DNA- and RNA-sequencing on detecting MYC, BCL2, and BCL6 rearrangements in high-grade B-cell lymphomas. Neoplasma. 2024;71:490–7. https://doi.org/10.4149/neo_2024_240527N236.
15. Yoo G, Cho J, Kwon HJ, Lee T, Kim J, Kim J. Mutational profiling of Korean lymphomas and diffuse large B-cell lymphoma subtype classification using targeted panel sequencing. Arch Med Res. 2025;56:103158. https://doi.org/10.1016/j.arcmed.2024.103158.

Part II

Infectious Diseases

Syphilis

3

Maria Cassia Ferreira Aguiar, Bruno Augusto Benevenuto de Andrade, José Alcides Almeida de Arruda, Jefferson R. Tenório, Lauren Frenzel Schuch, and Felipe Paiva Fonseca

3.1 General Overview and Clinical Presentation

Syphilis is a bacterial infection caused by the spirochete *Treponema pallidum*, whose exact origin remains a topic of considerable debate with no clear consensus among specialists. The first modern record of syphilis in Europe is typically attributed to the soldiers of the French King Charles VIII, who invaded Italy in September 1494 and reached Naples in February 1495 with an army of over 30,000 mercenaries from all over Europe. These soldiers are believed to have spread the infection throughout neighboring countries at the end of the war. However, the precise introduction of syphilis to Europe remains uncertain. One of the oldest hypotheses suggests that mercenaries or conquistadors brought the infection to Spain from the West Indies in 1493. The infection was subsequently spread to other parts of the world by sailors during the European colonial expansion; however, recent findings from the remains of people who lived on the eastern coast of South America nearly 2000 years ago have uncovered the oldest known evidence of the microorganisms responsible for syphilis. This discovery challenges the already contested theory that syphilis was introduced by Christopher Columbus's crew. Initially known as *lues*, a Latin word meaning "plague" or "to suffer," its sexually transmitted nature was observed and associated with the "act of Venus," leading to the term "venereal disease." Different terms have been used for this infection, including "French disease," "disease of Naples," "venereal lues," "great pox," and "morbus gallicus." The term "syphilis" was eventually coined by the Veronese physician and poet Girolamo Fracastoro (1478–1553) in his poem *Syphilis sive morbus gallicus*.

Over the centuries, humankind has seen periods of increased incidence of syphilis, such as during the outbreak of the AIDS epidemic, as well as moments of epidemiological decline. The introduction of penicillin in the twentieth century marked a significant turning point, greatly improving treatment and prognosis for patients. Unfortunately, it is widely recognized that since the early twenty-first century, we have witnessed a resurgence of syphilis in many parts of the world, with particularly high incidences in developing countries and low-income regions of developed nations, where the number of documented cases may still be underestimated. As a result, the development of effective public health policies and efficient diagnostic strategies remains crucial.

Syphilis is transmitted through blood transfusion, oral, vaginal, and anal sex, or vertically during pregnancy, making it one of the most important sexually transmitted infections worldwide. Infected patients should also be screened for HIV. The use of serological tests is strongly recommended, combining nontreponemal assays such as venereal disease research laboratory (VDRL) or rapid plasma reagin (RPR) tests, with more specific treponemal assays like treponemal-specific enzyme immunoassay (EIA), fluorescent treponemal antibody absorption (FTA-ABS), *T. pallidum* particle agglutination (TP-PA), or microhemagglutination assay for *T. pallidum* (MHA-TP). The combined results should be accurately interpreted and correlated with the clinical presentation.

Clinically, syphilis is classified into primary, secondary, early non-primary non-secondary, and unknown duration/late-stage (tertiary) forms, as well as congenital syphilis. Although cervical lymphadenopathy and the cutaneous and genital manifestations are hallmarks of the infection, involvement of the oral cavity is also common and often leads to the

M. C. F. Aguiar (✉) · F. P. Fonseca
Department of Oral Surgery and Pathology, School of Dentistry, Universidade Federal de Minas Gerais, Belo Horizonte, Brazil

B. A. B. de Andrade · J. A. A. de Arruda · J. R. Tenório
Department of Oral Diagnosis and Pathology, School of Dentistry, Universidade Federal do Rio de Janeiro, Rio de Janeiro, Brazil

L. F. Schuch
Department of Diagnosis in Pathology and Oral Medicine, School of Dentistry, Universidad de la República, Montevideo, Uruguay

© The Author(s), under exclusive license to Springer Nature Switzerland AG 2025

F. P. Fonseca et al. (eds.), *Lymphoproliferative and Granulomatous Disorders of the Oral Cavity*,
https://doi.org/10.1007/978-3-031-98844-8_3

initial diagnosis. Acquired oral syphilis has a widely variable clinical presentation and can be differentially diagnosed with many other conditions. Therefore, syphilis is often referred to as "the great imitator." *Primary syphilis* occurs 3 weeks to 3 months after exposure and is characterized by a self-healing, painless, solitary ulcer with a red base and irregular borders (chancre) located at the site of bacterial inoculation, most commonly in the genitalia. The presence of a chancre in the oral cavity is rarely observed. *Secondary syphilis* usually occurs 6 weeks to 6 months after initial exposure and may present with constitutional signs and symptoms such as fever, malaise, and lymphadenopathy. Mucocutaneous lesions, including erythematous-brownish plaques and papules on the palms and soles, are common. The oral mucosa may be affected by grayish to whitish mucous patches, especially on the soft palate, buccal mucosa, lips, labial commissures, and tongue. The periphery of these patches is typically radiated and well-defined, which aids in diagnosis. The oral mucosa may also present with nonspecific ulcerations or erythematous lesions of varying sizes and shapes, usually multiple and painless. An asymptomatic *early non-primary non-secondary* (latent) phase can vary in duration and is classified as early latent (<2 years after infection) or late latent (>2 years after infection). This latent phase may be interrupted by the reappearance of secondary or tertiary syphilis manifestations. Following the widespread use of antibiotics, *unknown duration/late-stage (tertiary)* syphilis has become uncommon, and the presence of lesions in the oral mucosa is even more rarely observed. When oral lesions of tertiary syphilis occur, they typically appear years after the initial infection as part of a multi-organ disease, which may include neurological/psychiatric, cardiovascular, and cutaneous granulomatous manifestations. The oral mucosa may present with aggressive ulcerations that can lead to palatine perforation and nasal involvement, or as gumma affecting the dorsum of the tongue. If left untreated, these lesions can be life-threatening.

The occurrence of syphilis during pregnancy has significant clinical implications for newborns, potentially resulting in *congenital syphilis*. Untreated maternal syphilis can lead to several neonatal complications, including fetal loss, stillbirth, and premature or low birthweight infants. Congenital syphilis may also cause ocular abnormalities, hearing impairments, and dental anomalies, particularly affecting the molars and incisors, known as Hutchinson's teeth. The presence of these findings, collectively referred to as Hutchinson's triad, is often essential for the diagnosis of congenital syphilis.

The treatment of syphilis has significantly evolved over the centuries. Initially, various extracts from specific tree species were used, but these were never proven effective. For nearly 500 years, extremely toxic mercury-based treatments were used, often in the form of an ointment made from metallic mercury and grease. Unfortunately, many patients suffered from severe side effects of mercury treatment, sometimes resulting in death, rather than from the disease itself. In 1910, arsphenamine, also known as compound 606 or Salvarsan, became the primary drug for treating syphilis. Although this injectable drug contained arsenic and was considered less toxic than mercury, it was still associated with severe side effects. The treatment of syphilis became truly effective with the advent of penicillin in the 1940s, which revolutionized therapy and became the standard approach for the infection. Currently, benzathine benzylpenicillin is the first-line treatment for syphilis, with dosing varying according to the clinical stage of the infection. Primary, secondary, and early latent syphilis are treated with 2.4 million units of benzathine benzylpenicillin administered intramuscularly as one dose (two injections). For late latent and unknown duration (tertiary) syphilis, the treatment consists of 7.2 million units of benzathine benzylpenicillin given as three weekly doses (six injections). Alternative treatments include doxycycline, ceftriaxone, or azithromycin. The prognosis for syphilis has greatly improved with the advent of antibiotics, but if left untreated, the infection can be fatal (Figs. 3.1, 3.2, 3.3, 3.4, and 3.5).

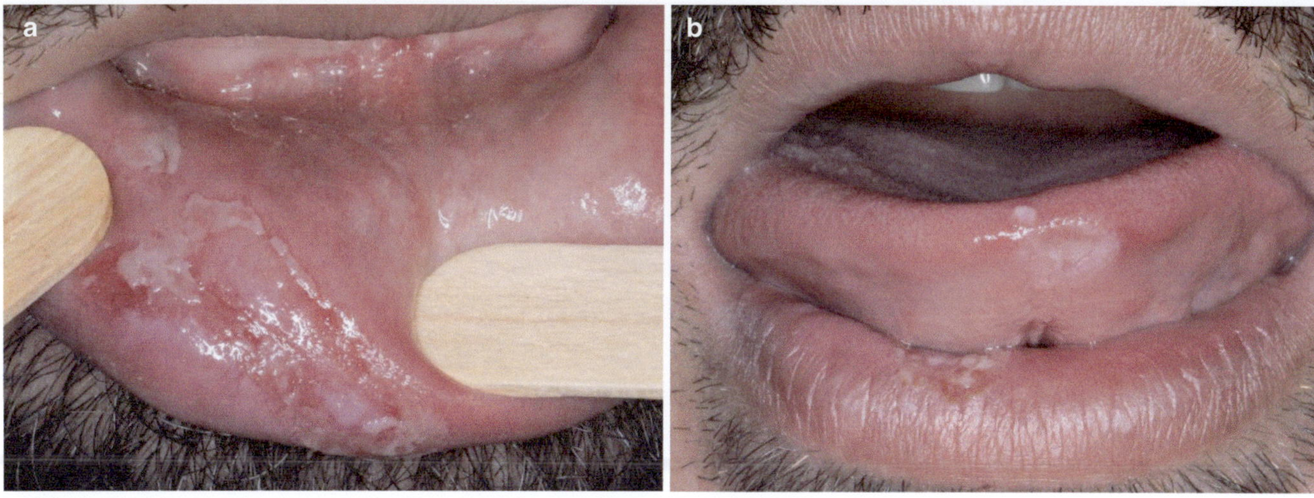

Fig. 3.1 Clinical presentation of syphilis in the oral cavity. (**a**) A male patient with multiple lesions in the oral mucosa. The lower lip shows an asymptomatic, superficial ulcer covered by a yellowish pseudomembrane, present for approximately 2 months. (**b**) The tongue exhibits a well-demarcated ulcer

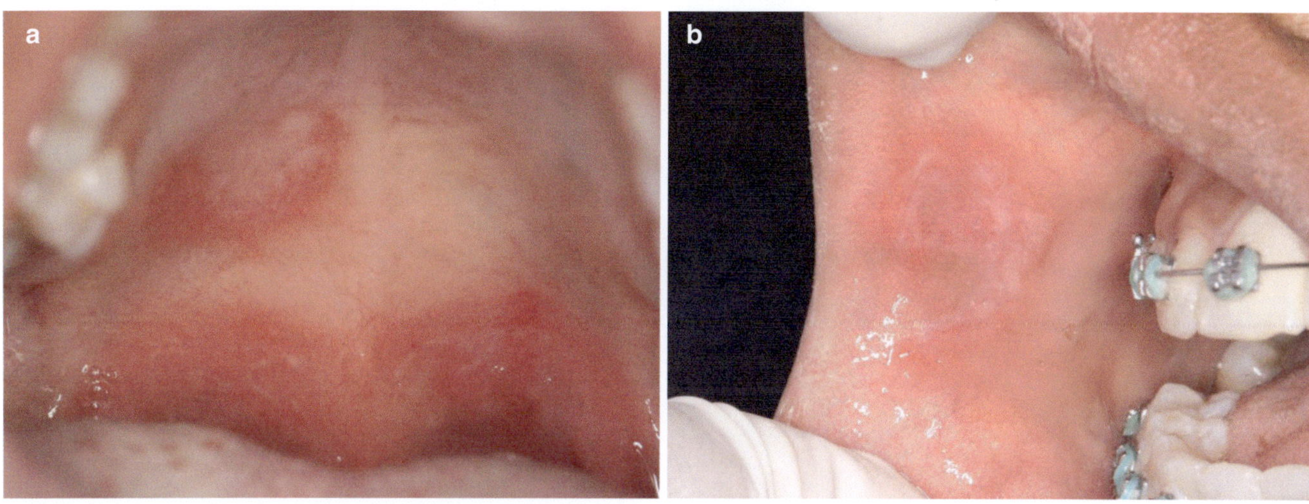

Fig. 3.2 Clinical presentation of syphilis in the oral cavity. (**a**) A female patient with multiple erythematous lesions affecting the hard and soft palate, extending toward the oropharynx. The lesions were asymptomatic and had been present for approximately 2 months. (**b**) The patient also had additional erythematous lesions in the oral mucosa. Note the presence of a reddish lesion with a superficial grayish membrane affecting the right buccal mucosa

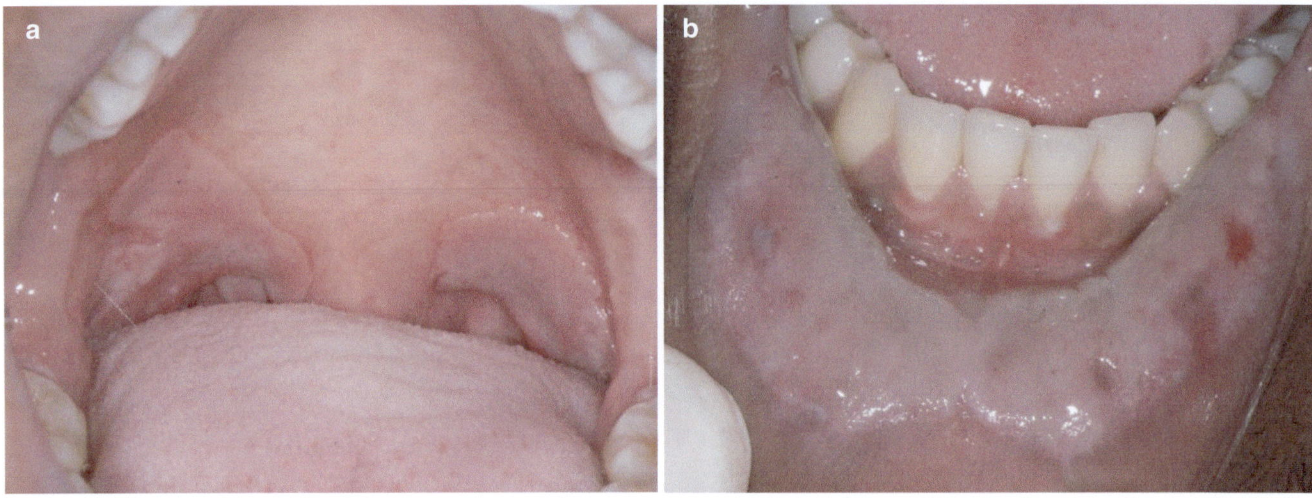

Fig. 3.3 Clinical presentation of syphilis in the oral cavity. (**a**) An HIV-positive male patient with bilateral whitish to grayish mucous patches on the soft palate and oropharynx. (**b**) Similar mucous patches are observed across the entire lower lip. The presence of whitish lesions should be differentiated from oral leukoplakia

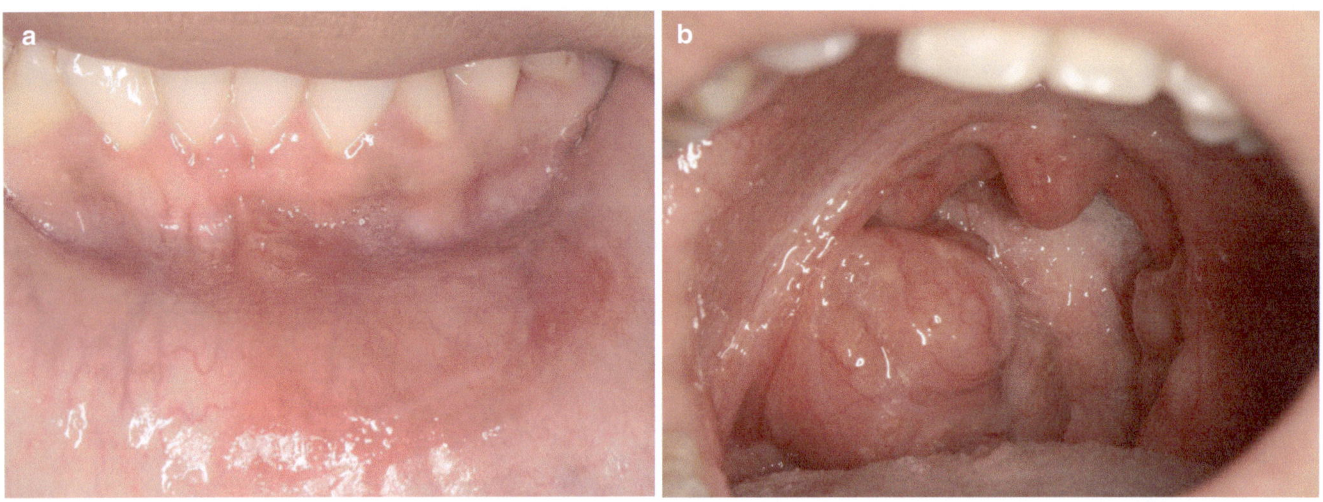

Fig. 3.4 Clinical presentation of syphilis in the oral cavity. (**a**) A female patient with an asymptomatic, irregular, reddish lesion on the lower lip. (**b**) The same patient also exhibited a large swelling in the right palatine tonsil, which resolved following treatment for syphilis

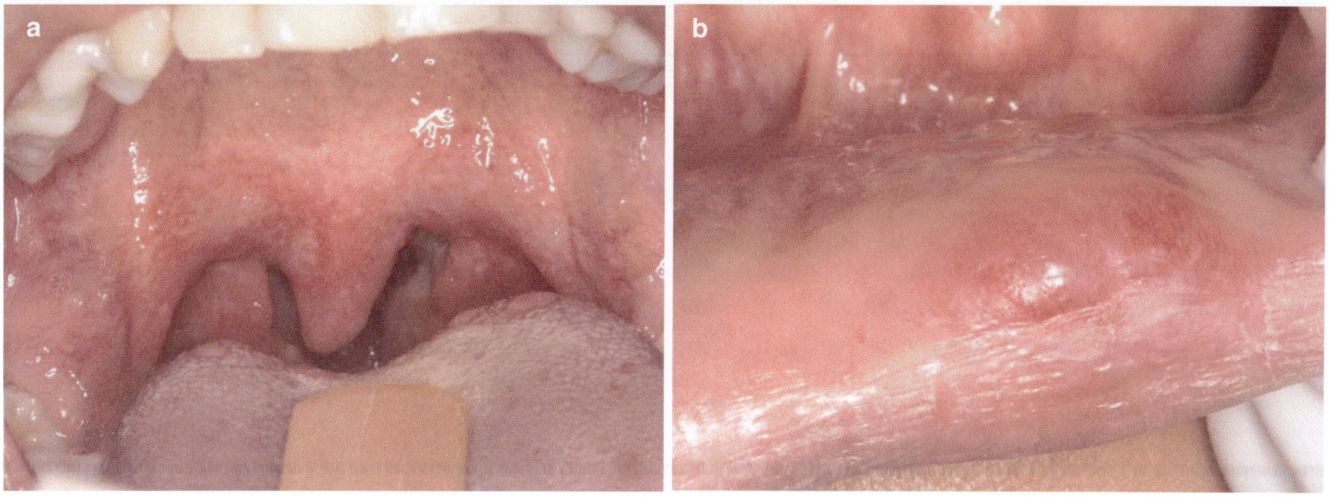

Fig. 3.5 Clinical presentation of syphilis in the oral cavity. (**a**) Reddish lesion affecting the soft palate in a male patient. (**b**) Lesion on the lower lip in the same patient

3.2 Microscopic Findings

- Microscopic findings in oral syphilis must be differentiated from lymphomas rich in plasma cells, such as MALT lymphoma or extramedullary plasmacytoma, especially in cases with pronounced and diffuse inflammatory infiltrates.
- Areas of epithelial ulceration.
- Elongated rete ridges, epithelial acanthosis, and exocytosis of neutrophils.
- Dense plasma cell infiltration beneath the overlying epithelium and deeper in the lamina propria.
- The inflammatory infiltrate in syphilis is a delayed hypersensitivity reaction to *T. pallidum*.
- A high concentration of plasma cells is predominantly located in the lamina propria, near the overlying epithelium.
- Plasma cells are also notably concentrated around blood vessels within the lamina propria.
- Lymphocytes and histiocytes are also found.
- In some tertiary syphilis, sensitized T-lymphocytes and macrophages can form gumma as a reaction (granulomatous inflammatory infiltrate) (Figs. 3.6, 3.7, 3.8, 3.9, and 3.10).

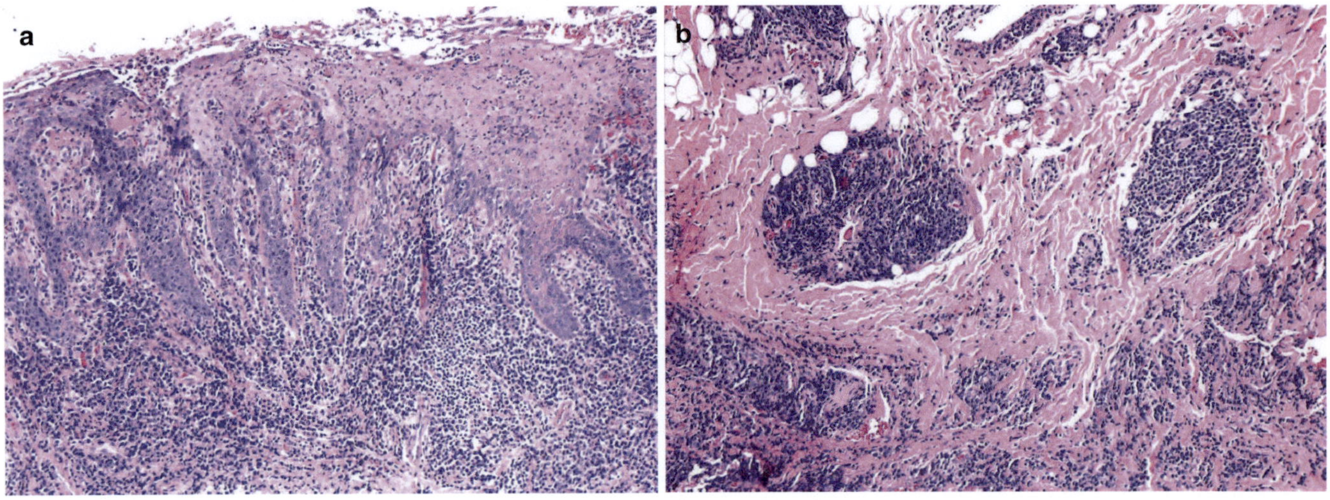

Fig. 3.6 Microscopic features of syphilis in the oral cavity. (**a**) A dense inflammatory infiltrate is typically observed, predominantly located near the overlying squamous epithelium. The presence of exocytosis in the overlying epithelium is a typical histologic finding (H&E; 25X). (**b**) Note the inflammatory infiltrate surrounding blood bessels (H&E; 100X)

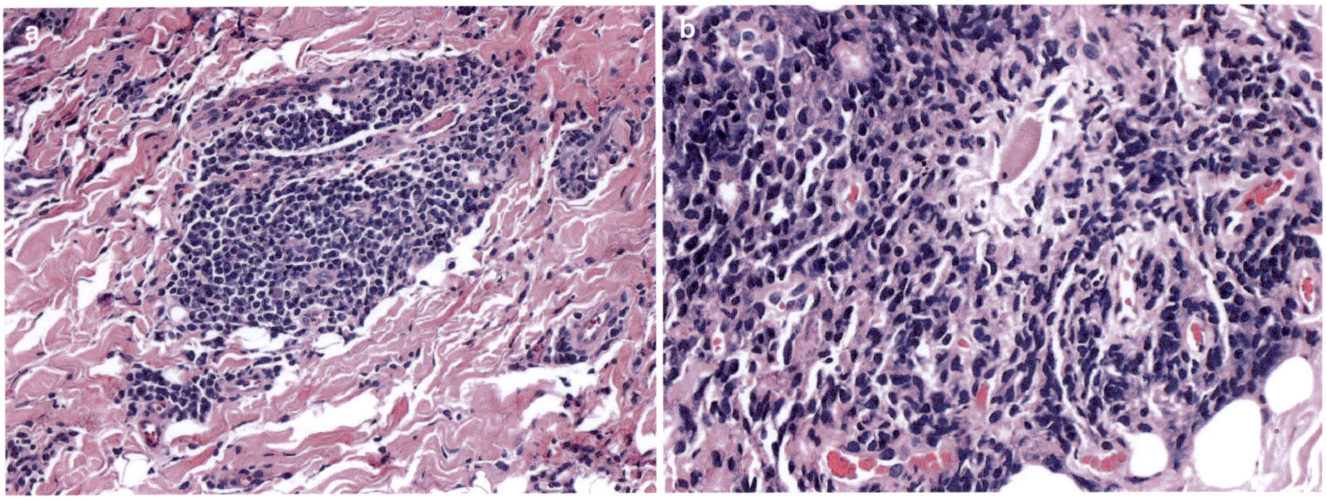

Fig. 3.7 Microscopic features of syphilis in the oral cavity. (**a**) Note the predominance of plasma cells in the inflammatory infiltrate (H&E; 200). (**b**) Areas containing a higher number of lymphocytes are also found in the lamina propria (H&E; 50X)

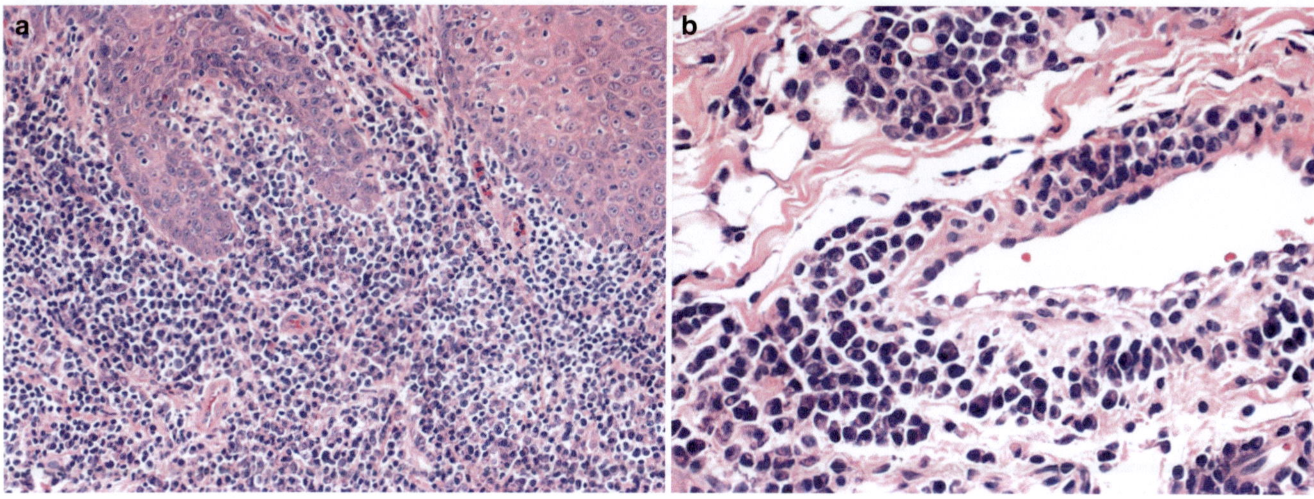

Fig. 3.8 Microscopic features of syphilis in the oral cavity. (**a**) The presence of a high number of plasma cells in the inflammatory infiltrate strongly indicates the need for investigation for syphilis, particularly when accompanied by neutrophilic exocytosis (H&E; 100×). (**b**) Perivascular plasma cell infiltration is also consistent with a diagnosis of syphilis (H&E; 200)

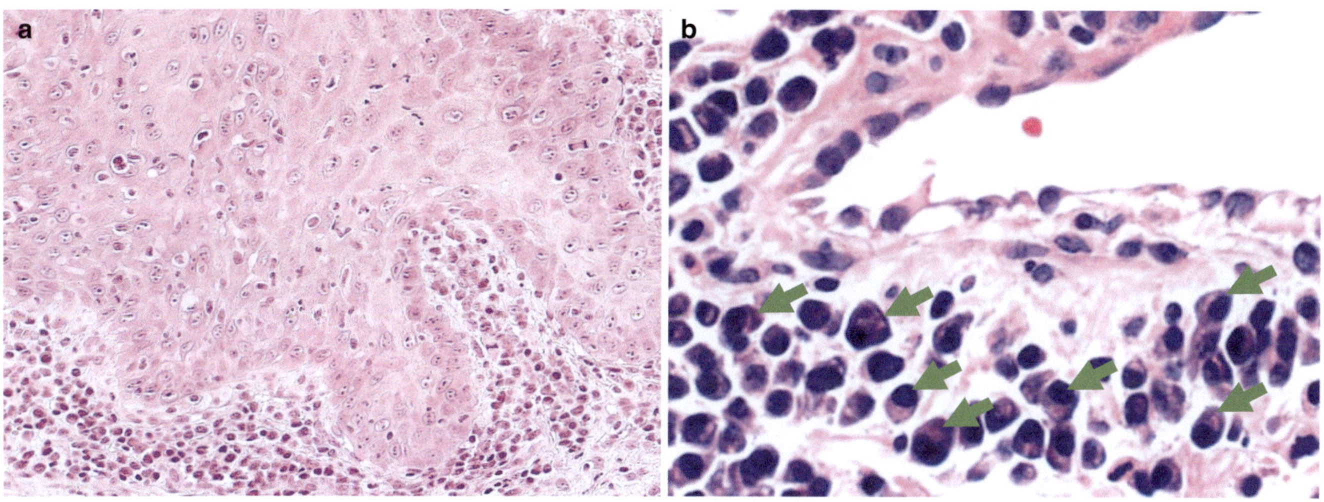

Fig. 3.9 Microscopic features of syphilis in the oral cavity. (**a**) Plasma cell infiltrate in the lamina propria and neutrophilic exocytosis in the epithelium are frequent histological findings in the oral manifestations of syphilis (H&E; 200×). (**b**) Note the presence of plasma cells (green arrows) distributed around the blood vessel (H&E; 400×)

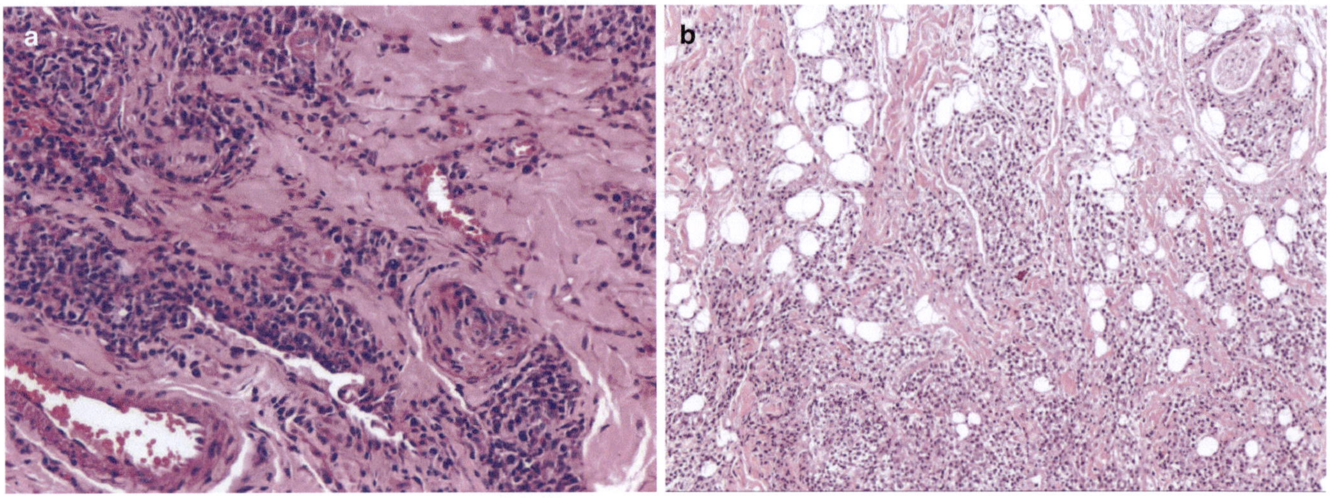

Fig. 3.10 Microscopic features of syphilis in the oral cavity. (**a**) The dense inflammatory infiltrate in syphilis can extend deeply into the lamina propria, surrounding different histological structures such as blood vessels, muscles, and nerves (H&E; 200X). (**b**) Infiltration of normal adipocytes and nerve bundles by reactive plasma cells and lymphocytes is often observed in syphilis (H&E; 100X)

Table 3.1 Summary of the main immunohistochemical reactions and histological stains that can be used for syphilis diagnosis

Antibody/stain	Most frequent results	Pattern	Objective
Treponema pallidum	Positive	Short filamentous structures	To demonstrate the presence of the bacteria
CD138	Positive	Membrane	To characterize the plasma cell infiltrate
MUM1	Positive	Nucleus	To characterize the plasma cell infiltrate
EMA	Positive	Membrane/cytoplasm	To characterize the plasma cell infiltrate
Plasma cell (VS38c)	Positive	Cytoplasm	To characterize the plasma cell infiltrate
Kappa/lambda	Polyclonal	Cytoplasm	To demonstrate the polyclonal nature of the infiltrate
Warthin-Starry[a]	Positive	Short filamentous structures	To demonstrate the presence of the bacteria

[a]Histological stain

3.3 Immunohistochemistry and/or Genetics

The diagnosis of syphilis is primarily based on correlating the results of treponemal and nontreponemal serological tests with clinical manifestations. Microscopic findings can also aid in diagnosis, and when necessary, immunohistochemistry can be employed to detect the presence of *T. pallidum* spirochetes. These microorganisms appear as small structures predominantly located in the epithelium, especially in the intercellular regions of keratinocytes, and in the lamina propria. Histochemical staining with Warthin-Starry is also a useful technique for visualizing the bacteria. The presence of plasma cells can be highlighted using antibodies such as CD138, EMA, MUM1, or plasma cell (VS38c). If necessary, the polyclonal nature of the plasma cells is demonstrated by immunoglobulin light chain reaction to Kappa and Lambda. RT-PCR has identified *T. pallidum* DNA in approximately 86.5% of oral syphilis cases, with negative results more commonly seen in the secondary stages (Table 3.1, Fig. 3.11).

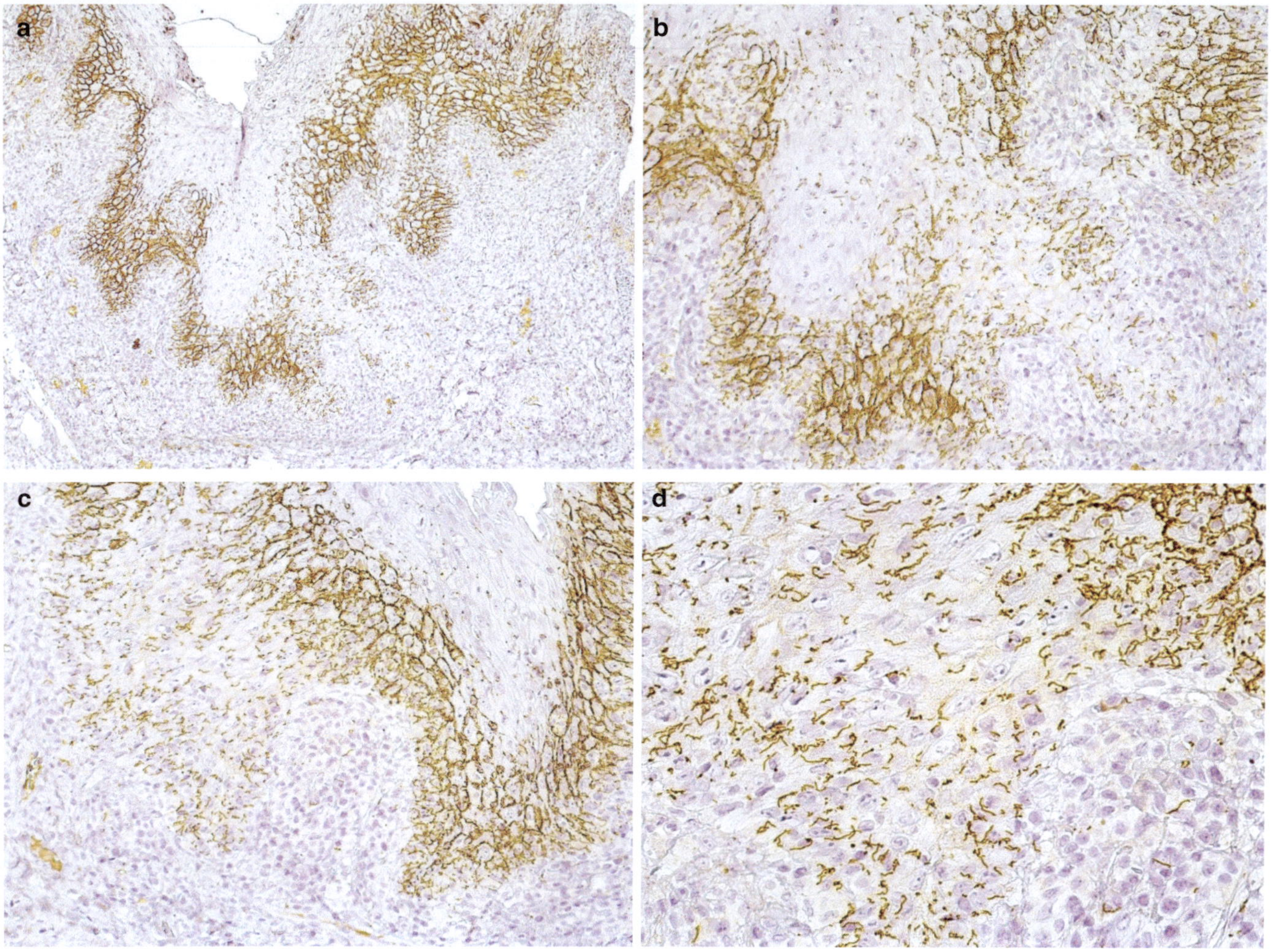

Fig. 3.11 Immunohistochemistry used to demonstrate *Treponema pallidum* in oral manifestations of syphilis. (**a**) A strong and diffuse immunohistochemical reaction is observed predominantly in the lower layers of the epithelium and adjacent regions of the lamina propria (DAB; 50×). (**b**) This expression pattern often exhibits accentuation in the intercellular spaces of keratinocytes, a common pattern when immunohistochemistry is used to detect the bacteria (DAB; 100×). (**c**) The bacteria can also be identified within the connective tissue (DAB; 100×). (**d**) At higher magnification, the bacteria appear as small, short, filamentous spirochetes both in the epithelium and connective tissue (DAB: 200×)

Sources

1. Barrett AW, Villarroel Dorrego M, Hodgson TA, Porter SR, Hopper C, Argiriadou AS, et al. The histopathology of syphilis of the oral mucosa. J Oral Pathol Med. 2004;33:286–91. https://doi.org/10.1111/j.0904-2512.2004.00099.x.
2. Tognotti E. The rise and fall of syphilis in renaissance Europe. J Med Humanities. 2009;30:99–113. https://doi.org/10.1007/s10912-009-9079-3.
3. Leuci S, Martina S, Adamo D, Ruoppo E, Santarelli A, Sorrentino R, et al. Oral syphilis: a retrospective analysis of 12 cases and a review of the literature. Oral Dis. 2013;19:738–46. https://doi.org/10.1111/odi.12058.
4. Kelner N, Rabelo GD, da Cruz Perez DE, Assunção JN Jr. Analysis of nonspecific oral mucosal and dermal lesions suggestive of syphilis: a report of 6 cases. Oral Surg Oral Med Oral Pathol Oral Radiol. 2014;117:1–7. https://doi.org/10.1016/j.oooo.2012.04.028.
5. Gama A, Carrillo-Casas EM, Hernández-Castro R, Vázquez-Aceituno VA, Toussaint-Caire S, Xicohtencatl-Cortes J, et al. Treponema pallidum ssp. pallidum identification by real-time PCR targetting the polA gene in paraffin-embedded samples positive by immunohistochemistry. Int J STD AIDS. 2017;28:1299–304. https://doi.org/10.1177/0956462417704123.
6. Schuch LF, da Silva KD, de Arruda JAA, Etges A, Gomes APN, Mesquita RA, et al. Forty cases of acquired oral syphilis and a review of the literature. Int J Oral Maxillofac Surg. 2019;48:635–43. https://doi.org/10.1016/j.ijom.2018.10.023.
7. de Andrade BAB, de Arruda JAA, Gilligan G, Piemonte E, Panico R, Molina Ávila I, et al. Acquired oral syphilis: a multicenter study of 339 patients from South America. Oral Dis. 2022;28:1561–72. https://doi.org/10.1111/odi.13963.
8. Delvaux T, Ouk V, Samreth S, Yos S, Tep R, Pall C, et al. Challenges and outcomes of implementing a national syphilis follow-up system for the elimination of congenital syphilis in Cambodia: a mixed-methods study. BMJ Open. 2023;13:e063261. https://doi.org/10.1136/bmjopen-2022-063261.

9. Ramchandani MS, Cannon CA, Marra CM. Syphilis: a modern resurgence. Infect Dis Clin N Am. 2023;S0891-5520:00016–8. https://doi.org/10.1016/j.idc.2023.02.006.
10. Gouk T, Nissanka-Jayasuriya E, Anushan Hiranya Jayasinghe L, Withanage S, Doumas S. Syphilitic ulcer mimicking oral cancer. Br Dent J. 2023;235:957–8. https://doi.org/10.1038/s41415-023-6696-6.
11. Ekselius L, Gerdin B, Vahlquist A. The syphilis pandemic prior to penicillin: origin, health issues, cultural representation and ethical challenges. Acta Derm Venereol. 2024;104:adv34879. https://doi.org/10.2340/actadv.v104.34879.
12. Barreto MEZ, Soares CD, de Andrade MMP, de Oliveira SA, Fonseca FP, Abreu LG, et al. Immunohistochemistry and RT-PCR as ancillary tools in the diagnosis of acquired oral syphilis. Oral Dis. 2025;31:890–8. https://doi.org/10.1111/odi.15107.
13. Papp JR, Park IU, Fakile Y, Pereira L, Pillay A, Bolan GA. CDC laboratory recommendations for syphilis testing, United States, 2024. MMWR Recomm Rep. 2024;73:1–32. https://doi.org/10.15585/mmwr.rr7301a1.
14. Dionne JA, Giacani L, Tamhane A, Workowski K, Lieberman NAP, Greninger AL, et al. Prevalence and predictors of Oral treponema pallidum detection by quantitative polymerase chain reaction in early syphilis. J Infect Dis. 2024;229:1628–36. https://doi.org/10.1093/infdis/jiad582.
15. Culbert AA, Israel AK, Ku J, Silver NL. The increasing problem of syphilis manifesting as head and neck cancer: a case series. Laryngoscope. 2024;134:236–9. https://doi.org/10.1002/lary.30765.

Leprosy

4

Mariana Villarroel-Dorrego, Aline Araujo Sampaio, Raquel Conceição Ferreira, Raghu Radhakrishnan, Juliana Diogo de Almeida Sampaio, and Felipe Paiva Fonseca

4.1 General Overview and Clinical Presentation

Leprosy is a chronic bacterial disease that has been known, since the historical discoveries of Gerhard Armauer Hansen more than 150 years ago in the nineteenth century, to be caused by the intracellular pathogen *Mycobacterium leprae*. In 2008, Han et al. described the pathogenic role played by another bacillus, termed *Mycobacterium lepromatosis*, which is implicated in a small number of cases, and its clinical characterization remains poorly investigated. These microorganisms are acid-fast bacilli that characteristically have a prolonged period of incubation, and cases containing simultaneous infection by both species have also been reported.

M. Villarroel-Dorrego (✉)
Instituto de Investigaciones Odontológicas, Universidad Central de Venezuela, Caracas, Venezuela
e-mail: mariana.villarroel@ucv.ve

A. A. Sampaio · F. P. Fonseca
Department of Oral Surgery and Pathology, School of Dentistry, Universidade Federal de Minas Gerais, Belo Horizonte, Brazil

R. C. Ferreira
Department of Social and Community Dentistry, School of Dentistry, Universidade Federal de Minas Gerais, Belo Horizonte, Brazil

R. Radhakrishnan
Department of Oral and Maxillofacial Pathology, Manipal College of Dental Sciences, Manipal Academy of Higher Education, Manipal, India

Unit of Oral Biology and Oral Pathology, Oman Dental College, Mina Al Fahal, Muscat, Oman

Oral and Maxillofacial Pathology, School of Clinical Dentistry, University of Sheffield, Sheffield, UK

Juliana Diogo de Almeida Sampaio
Prefeitura Municipal de Belo Horizonte – SMSA – Centro de Treinamento e Referência em Doenças Infecto-Parasitárias Orestes Diniz, Belo Horizonte, Brazil

Leprosy is a well-known infection that has a very long history that parallels that of humankind. It is believed that this infectious disease was not present in the New World in the pre-Columbian period, possibly being introduced to the Western Hemisphere after European colonization. It represents an important public health issue in many parts of the world and is associated with a strong and negative stigma for those individuals affected by this disease, who very frequently live isolated in colonies. Currently, approximately 200,000 cases are diagnosed each year in more than 100 endemic regions, and leprosy still represents a challenge for the public health systems of many developing countries, especially Indonesia, Brazil, and India. In these endemic regions, there is a presumed predominance of human-to-human transmission, whereas in the USA, this disease is mostly considered a zoonosis. In an attempt to minimize the historical stigma and discrimination associated with this condition and to dignify language and terminology, international recommendations for banning the term leprosy have been made, and in 1975, this term was officially banned in Brazil and replaced by hanseniase or Hansen's disease.

Affected patients are believed to be mainly infected through the upper airway after long and close contact with another infected person, and the nasal mucosa is thought to be the main route of transmission, although the presence of *Mycobacterium* DNA in the peripheral blood of some patients raises the possibility of other secondary routes of transmission for this disease, which also includes skin erosion, breast milk, and vertical transmission. Although bacillus usually originates from infected patients, it may also originate from the environment and animals, including armadillos, squirrels, soil, and water sources, and may act as important reservoirs for microorganisms.

Leprosy is associated with a wide spectrum of clinical manifestations that are directly associated with the immunological response of the host to microorganisms, and classification methods have evolved significantly over the years. In 1953, there was a recommendation for classifying leprosy

© The Author(s), under exclusive license to Springer Nature Switzerland AG 2025
F. P. Fonseca et al. (eds.), *Lymphoproliferative and Granulomatous Disorders of the Oral Cavity*,
https://doi.org/10.1007/978-3-031-98844-8_4

into malignant or benign forms, also referred to as stable polar types (lepromatous and tuberculoid categories), or as unstable groups, referred to as intermediate or midborderline categories. Some years later, Ridley and Jopling used the concept of spectral leprosy on the basis of clinical, immunological, and histopathological findings to classify patients into either lepromatous or tuberculoid subtypes (two extreme poles) and further proposed eliminating the intermediate type and introducing a borderline category that could assume either tuberculoid or lepromatous characteristics. The World Health Organization then recommended the use of the term paucibacillary when patients had fewer than five lesions without the presence of bacilli in skin smears or biopsies, and multibacillary disease when patients had more than five lesions or nerve involvement or the presence of bacilli in a slit-skin smear irrespective of the number of skin lesions.

Tuberculoid or paucibacillary leprosy is found in patients with a strong immune response against the pathogen, presenting a lower number of cutaneous lesions and a lower concentration of microorganisms in the morphologic exam. In contrast, lepromatous or multibacillary leprosy occurs in individuals who do not exhibit a strong immunological response against the bacillus, develop multiple lesions, and exhibit a relatively high concentration of pathogens according to histological analyses.

Leprosy typically affects the peripheral nerves, skin, and multiple internal organs. Cutaneous manifestations vary significantly, ranging from localized, well-defined, hypopigmented macules or plaques to multiple nodules coalescing in plaques on the forehead, ears, nose, and lips. In advanced stages, patients usually present loss of eyebrow hair and eyelashes, diffuse thickening of the facial skin, and deepening of natural facial lines characterizing the "leonine facies."

Oral mucosal involvement is considered uncommon, although it is well documented in the literature. It more often occurs in the lepromatous variant, although the tuberculoid type may also show oral involvement. It may result from hematogenous or lymphatic dissemination of the microorganism or from nasal lesions, which are present in approximately 95% of the cases, possibly due to the preference of the *Mycobacterium* for cooler sites. There are no specific findings in the oral manifestations of leprosy, which usually present as asymptomatic plaques, papules, or nodules, ranging from a normal color to a reddish to yellowish color. The nodules are sessile and firm on palpation. These lesions can evolve into ulcerations and necrosis, and hard and soft palates are the most affected locations, although any other site can also be affected. Hyperpigmentation of the oral mucosa from the palate, uvula, tonsils, gingiva, and tongue, as well as hypopigmentation of the oral mucosa, fissuring and loss of the papillae tongue, and retraction of the uvula, possibly as a result of scars or fibrosis in preexisting lesions, have been reported. The involvement of the facial nerve may impair mastication and speech, and atrophy of the anterior nasal spine is a common finding, which, together with recession of the alveolar process of the maxilla, may lead to tooth loss.

Scars and fibrosis from preexisting lesions usually do not require treatment unless they are associated with functional impairment, and prosthetic rehabilitation is necessary when there is tooth loss. Individuals with significant hand mutilations or deformities often demand made-to-measure grip aids to allow them to use toothbrushes to prevent dental caries and periodontal disease.

Standard leprosy treatment is based on multidrug therapy established by the World Health Organization, which consists of bacteriostatic (dapsone and clofazimine) and bactericidal (rifampicin) drugs. This therapeutic regimen led to a significant reduction in disabilities and deformities caused by the disease. The drugs used are usually well tolerated, but when they are contraindicated, ofloxacin and/or minocycline can be used (Figs. 4.1, 4.2, 4.3, and 4.4).

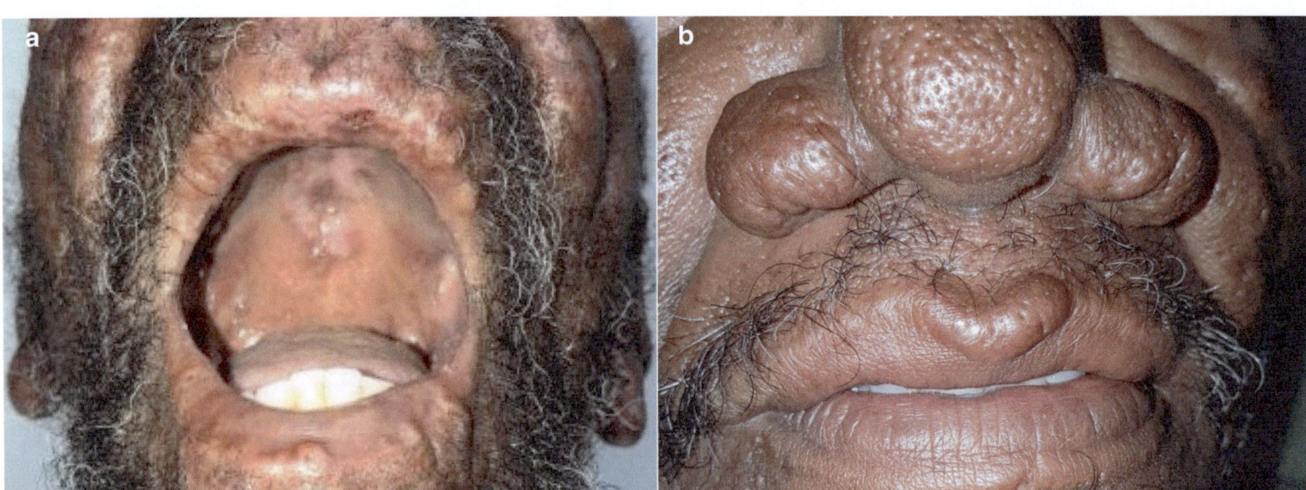

Fig. 4.1 Clinical presentation of leprosy. (**a**) The affected patient presented multiple nodules in the lips and a plaque in the palate with color ranging from whitish to reddish to melanotic. (**b**) Another patient showing the upper lip affected by the granulomatous reaction associated with leprosy infection

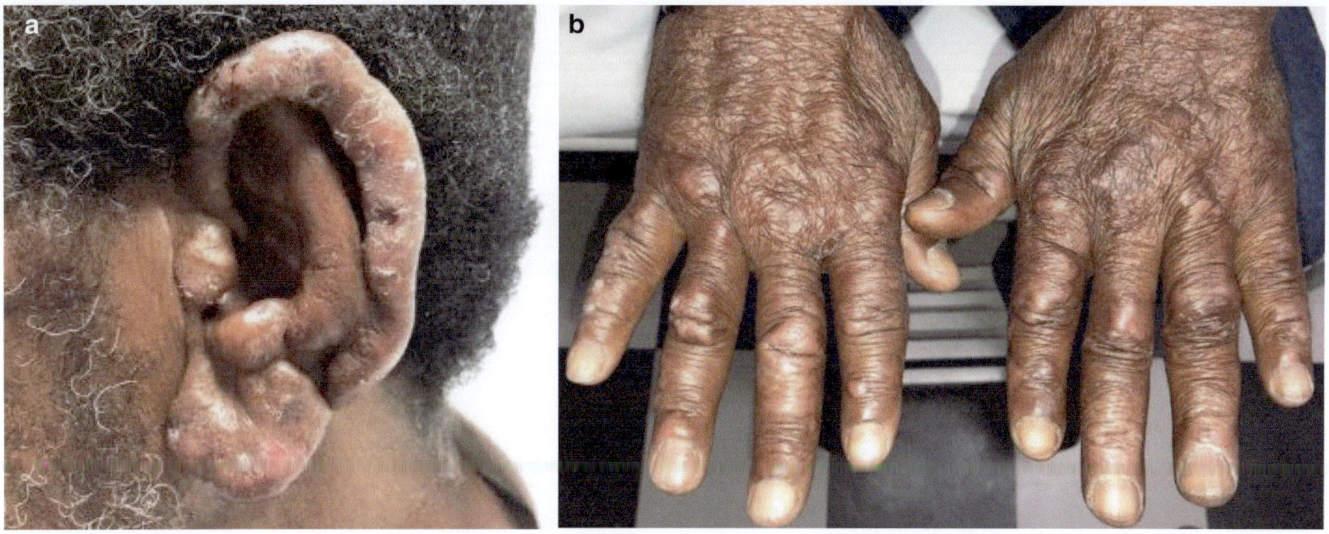

Fig. 4.2 Clinical presentation of a 70-year-old male patient. (**a**) The ears of the patient and (**b**) the hands of the patient presented multiple nodules of hardened consistency due to the underlying chronic granulomatous inflammatory process

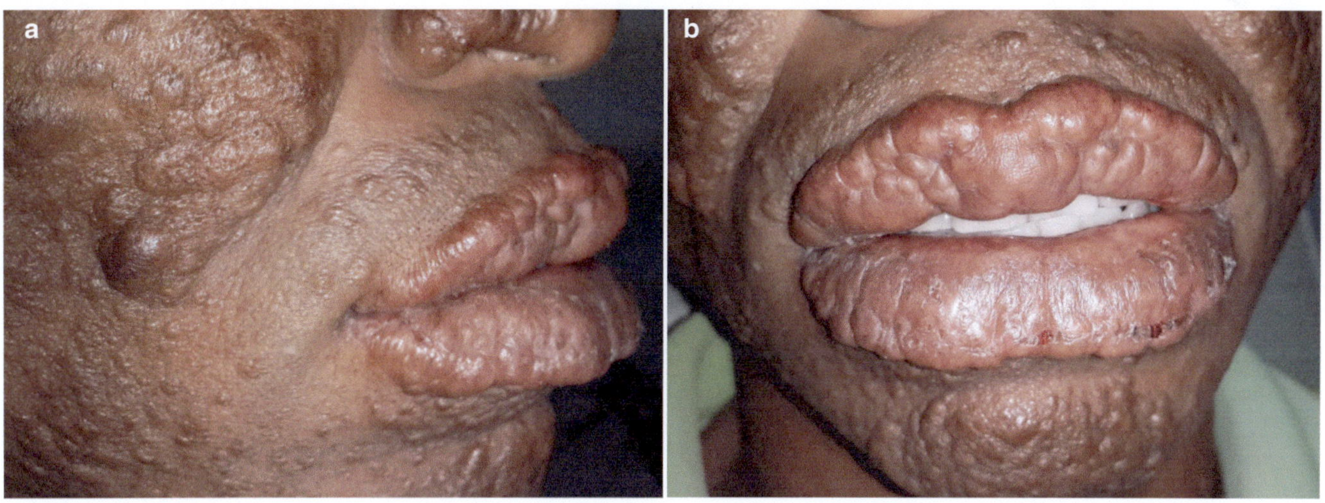

Fig. 4.3 Clinical presentation of lepromatous leprosy in an adult male patient. (**a**) Extraoral presentation of the patient depicts the presence of multiple nodular lesions (lepromas) in the face. (**b**) There was an extensive labial involvement. Upper and lower lips presented multiple nodules comprising a granulomatous reaction

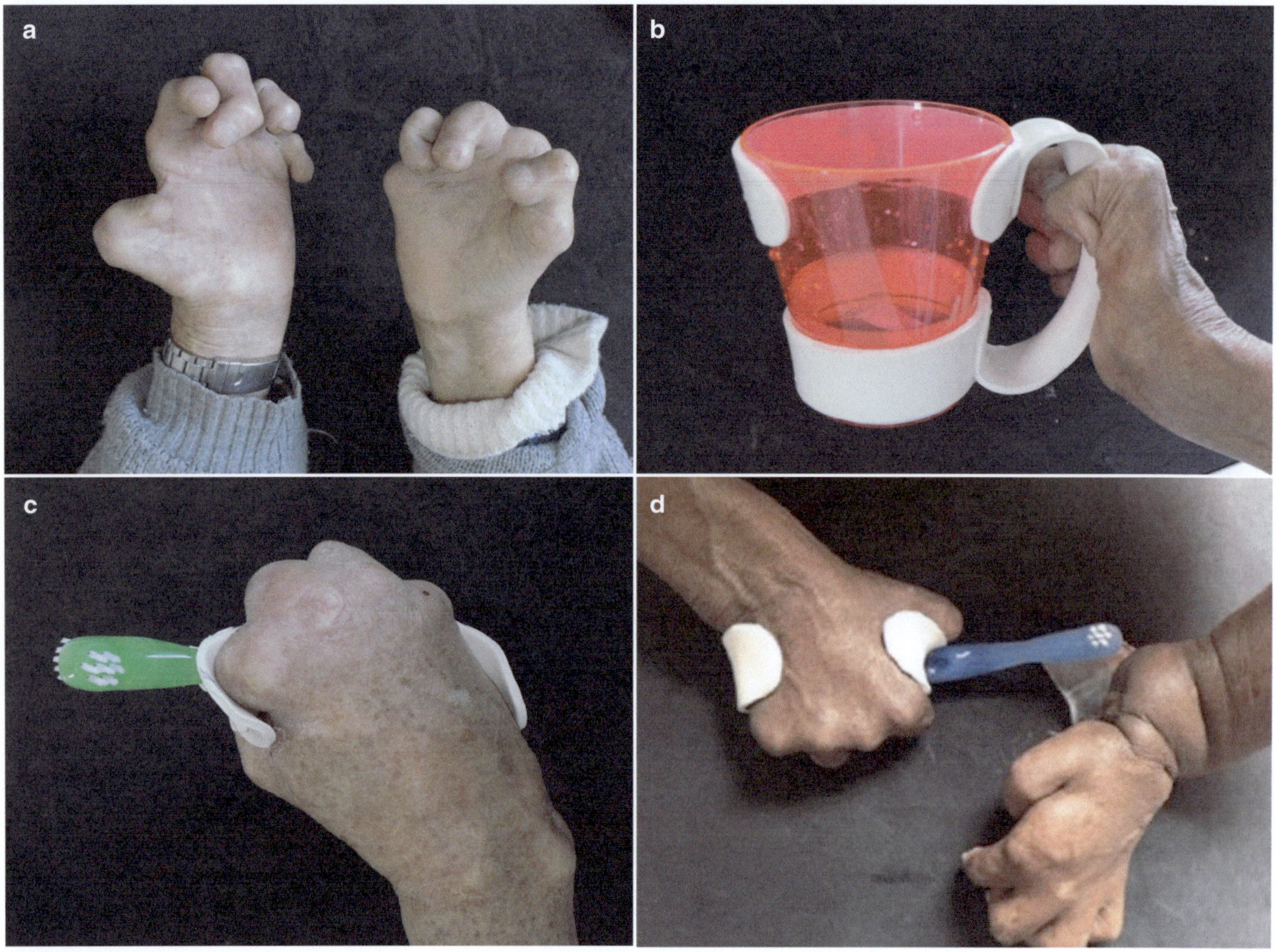

Fig. 4.4 Clinical presentation of patients affected by leprosy demonstrating significant hand deformities. (**a**) Important alterations in the hands and fingers were observed. (**b**) These patients often demand made-to-measure grip aids to allow them to use different instruments and tools. (**c**) In particular, for oral hygiene, these patients need made-to-measure toothbrushes to prevent dental caries and periodontal disease. (**d**) Observe the made-to-measure toothbrush to be used by this severely affected patient

4.2 Microscopic Findings

- Epithelial atrophy or epithelial hyperplasia with possible areas of ulceration.
- The presence of a free Grenz zone that represents a subepithelial layer of collagen and connective fibers is uncommon in the oral mucosa and is more often observed in cutaneous biopsies.
- The lamina propria usually has a dense chronic, lymphohistiocytic inflammatory infiltrate.
- Presence of well-formed or ill-formed granulomas in most of the cases.
- Predominance of histiocytes with abundant eosinophilic cytoplasm.
- Histiocytes with clear or foamy cytoplasm can also be present. They are often referred as Virchows cells and considered a hallmark of lepromatous leprosy.
- Lymphocytes and plasma cells are also found.
- Involvement of nerve bundles by the lymphohistiocytic infiltrate can be observed.
- The presence of Langhans-type multinucleated giant cells can be found.
- Acid-resistant bacilli are detected via special histological stains such as Fite-Faraco stain or Ziehl-Neelsen stain, and the concentration of pathogens in a given biopsy directly correlates with the cell-mediated immunity of the host against the pathogen, with more bacilli observed in

the lepromatous/multibacillary variant and fewer in the tuberculoid/paucibacillary subtype.

- Leprosy immunologic reactions can be clinically and histopathologically classified as Type 1 (delayed type of hypersensitivity), Type 2 (acute immune complex vasculitis, encompassing erythema nodosum leprosum), and Type 3 or Lucio's phenomenon (it is very rare and exhibits necrotizing vasculitis, ischemic necrosis, and the immune components in small vessels, more often in patients with diffuse lepromatous leprosy that can be life threatening) (Figs. 4.5, 4.6, 4.7, and 4.8).

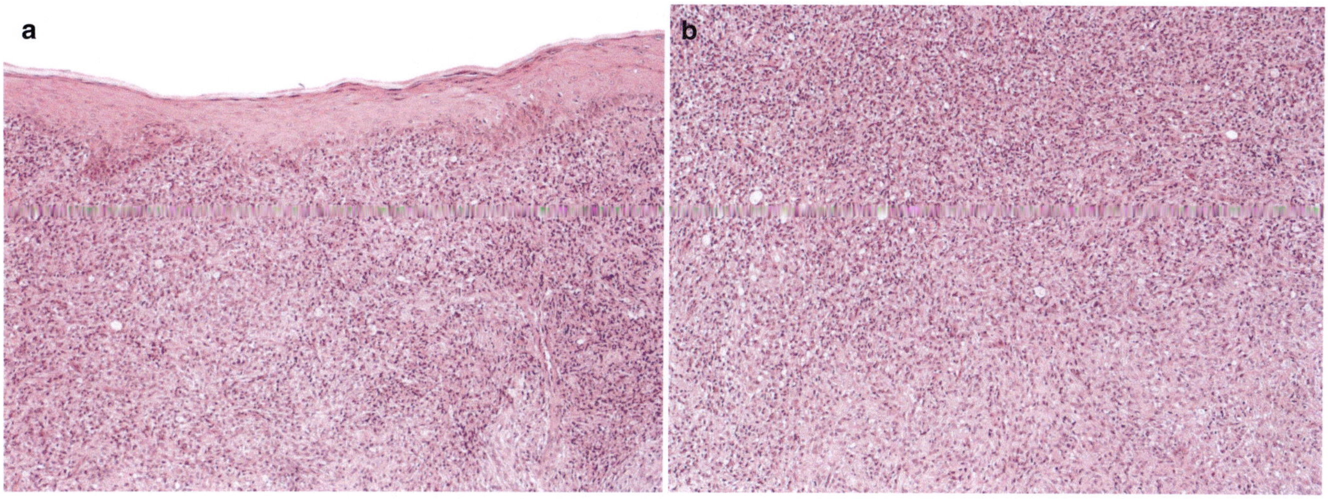

Fig. 4.5 Microscopic features of leprosy in the oral cavity. (**a**) The overlying squamous epithelium appeared atrophic in this case. In the lamina propria, there is a dense lymphohistiocytic infiltrate (H&E; 50×). (**b**) Dense infiltration in the lamina propria, which is predominantly composed of histiocytes, was observed (H&E; 50×)

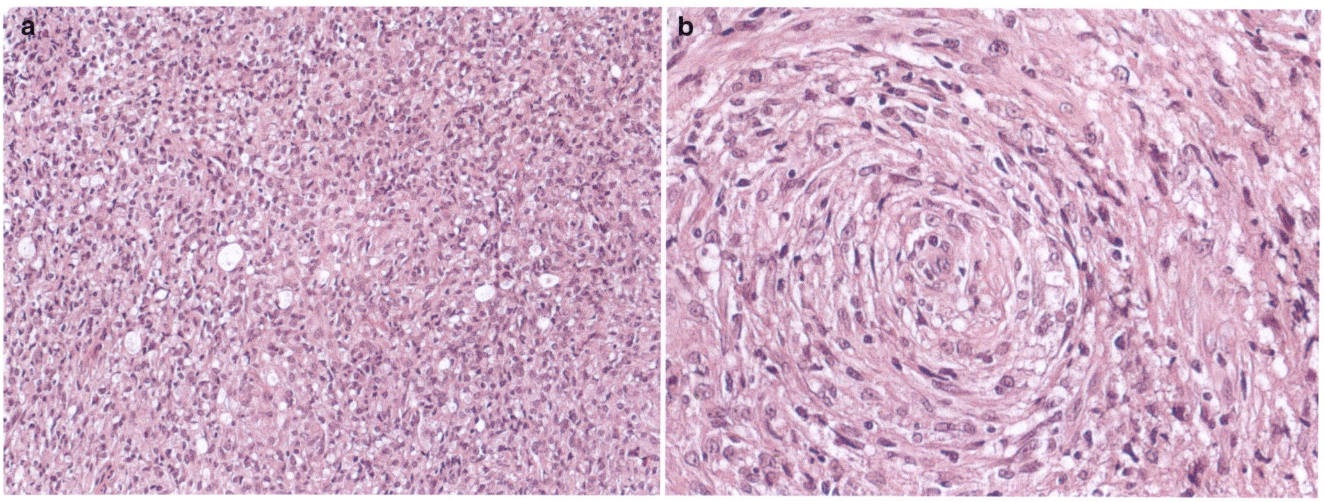

Fig. 4.6 Microscopic features of leprosy in the oral cavity. (**a**) In the lymphohistiocytic infiltrate, some foamy macrophages with a relatively clear cytoplasm can be found (H&E; 100×). (**b**) Perineural involvement with this targetoid pattern is one of the microscopic findings observed in many cases of leprosy (H&E; 200×)

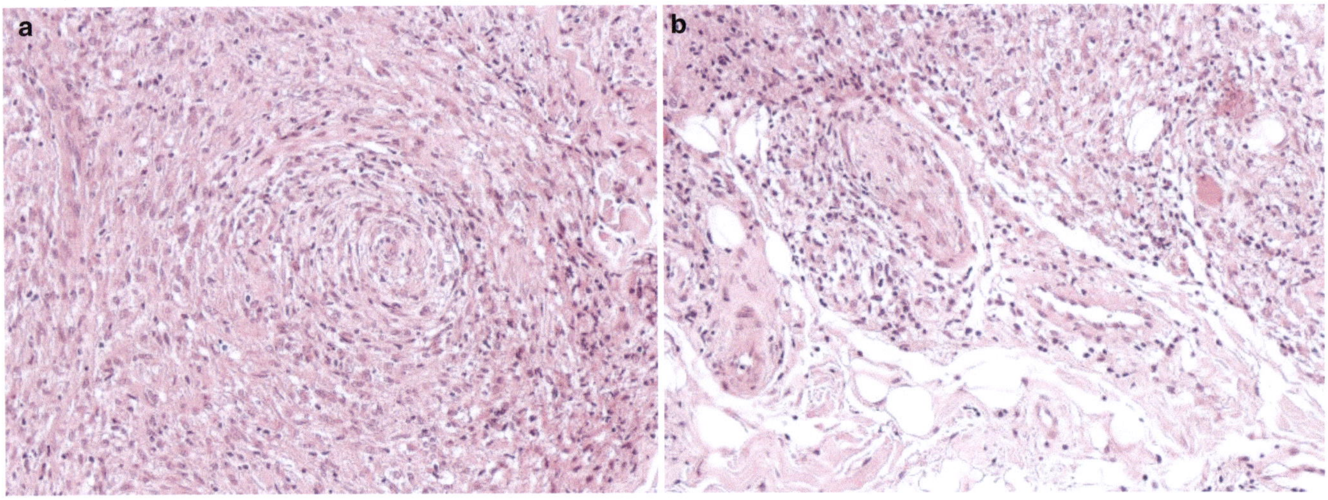

Fig. 4.7 Microscopic features of leprosy in the oral cavity. (**a**) Dense proliferation of macrophages in this case of oral leprosy. The target growth pattern of the cells was observed (H&E; 100×). (**b**) Example of perineural involvement in a patient with oral leprosy (H&E; 100×)

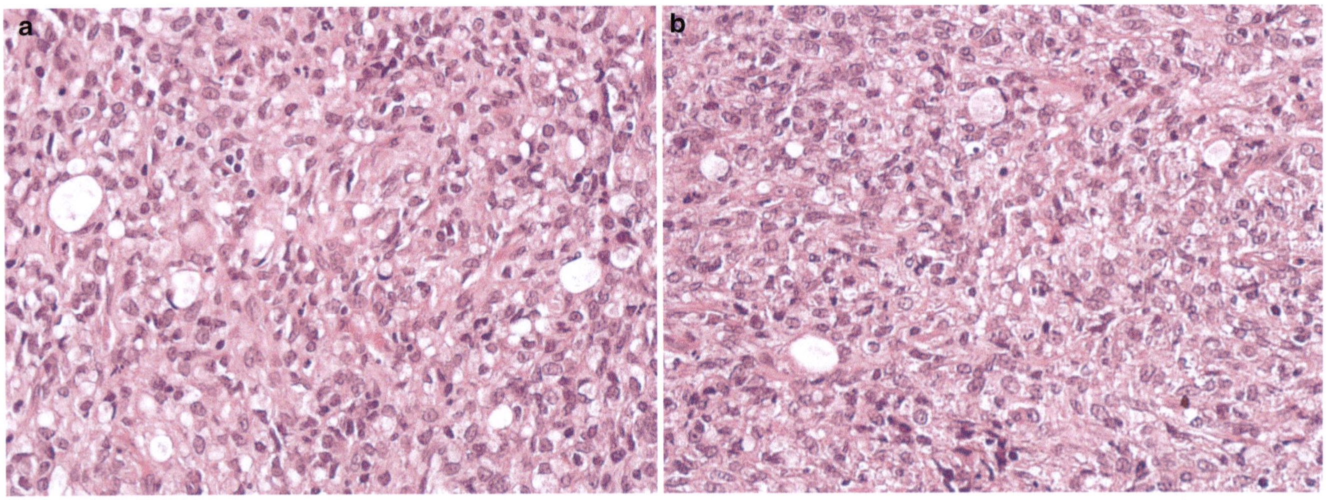

Fig. 4.8 Microscopic features of leprosy in the oral cavity. (**a**) Under higher magnification, we can observe that the histiocytes have an abundant eosinophilic cytoplasm and a round to oval, centrally located nucleus. There is no atypia, pleomorphism, or atypical mitosis (H&E; 200×). (**b**) The presence of foamy cells that also represent histiocytes was observed. Many macrophages have a granular cytoplasm (H&E; 200×)

4.3 Immunohistochemistry and/or Genetics

The histopathological diagnosis of leprosy more often comprises morphological analysis together with the use of special histological stains such as Fite-Faroco or Ziehl-Neelsen to demonstrate the presence of acid-fast bacilli. Immunohistochemistry can be helpful for demonstrating the histiocytic infiltrate present in the lesion with the positive expression of CD68 protein in the histiocytes (Table 4.1, Figs. 4.9, 4.10, and 4.11).

Table 4.1 Summary of the main immunohistochemical reactions and special histological stains used for leprosy diagnosis

Antibody/stain	Most frequent results	Pattern	Objective
CD20	Positive	Membrane	To characterize the B lymphocyte infiltrate
CD3	Positive	Membrane	To characterize the T lymphocyte infiltrate
CD138	Positive	Membrane	To characterize the plasma cell infiltrate
CD68	Positive	Cytoplasm	To demonstrate the presence of macrophages, multinucleated giant cells, and granulomas
Fite-Faroco[a]	Positive	In the bacillus	To show the presence of microorganisms
Ziehl-Neelsen[a]	Positive	In the bacillus	To show the presence of microorganisms

[a]Histological stain

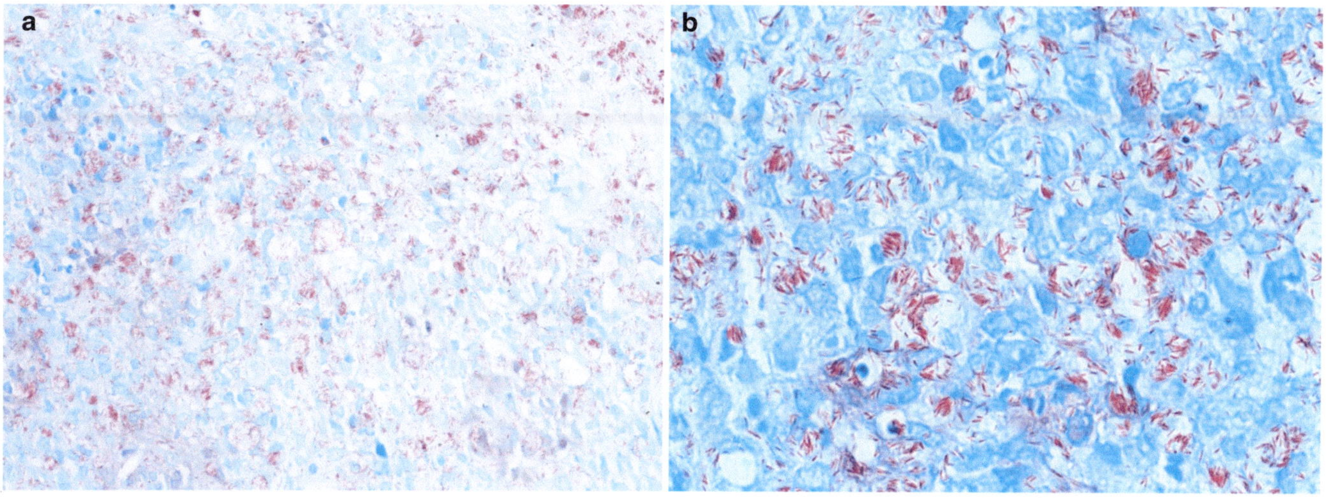

Fig. 4.9 Microscopic features of leprosy in the oral cavity. (**a**) Ziehl–Neelsen staining is very useful for demonstrating the presence of acid-fast bacilli. In this reaction, the background is blue, and the microorganisms present small reddish structures that may coalesce in some regions. In this example of lepromatous/multibacillary leprosy, there are many microorganisms, which makes their identification easier, whereas in tuberculoid/paucibacillary leprosy, the number of microorganisms is usually much lower, and their search frequently demands analysis under oil immersion (Ziehl-Neelsen; 100×). (**b**) Observe the high number of microorganisms (multiple, small reddish structures) present in this example of oral leprosy (Ziehl-Neelsen; 200×)

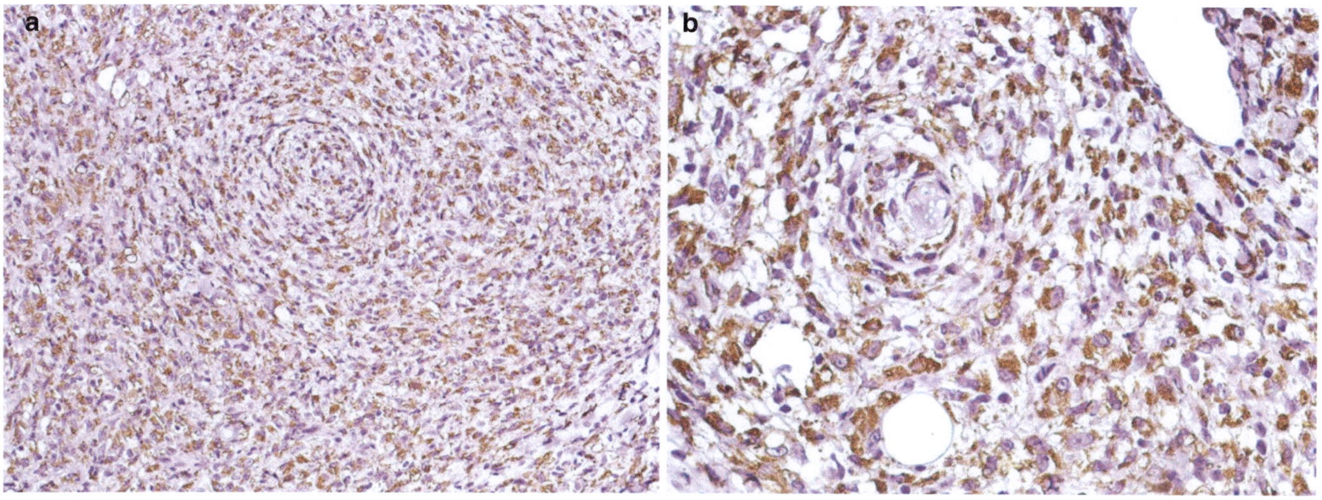

Fig. 4.10 Immunohistochemical features of leprosy in the oral cavity. (**a**) The presence of histiocytes can be demonstrated via CD68 staining (DAB; 100×). (**b**) A strong and diffuse staining pattern for CD68 was observed, demonstrating the large number of macrophages present in this infiltrate (DAB; 200×)

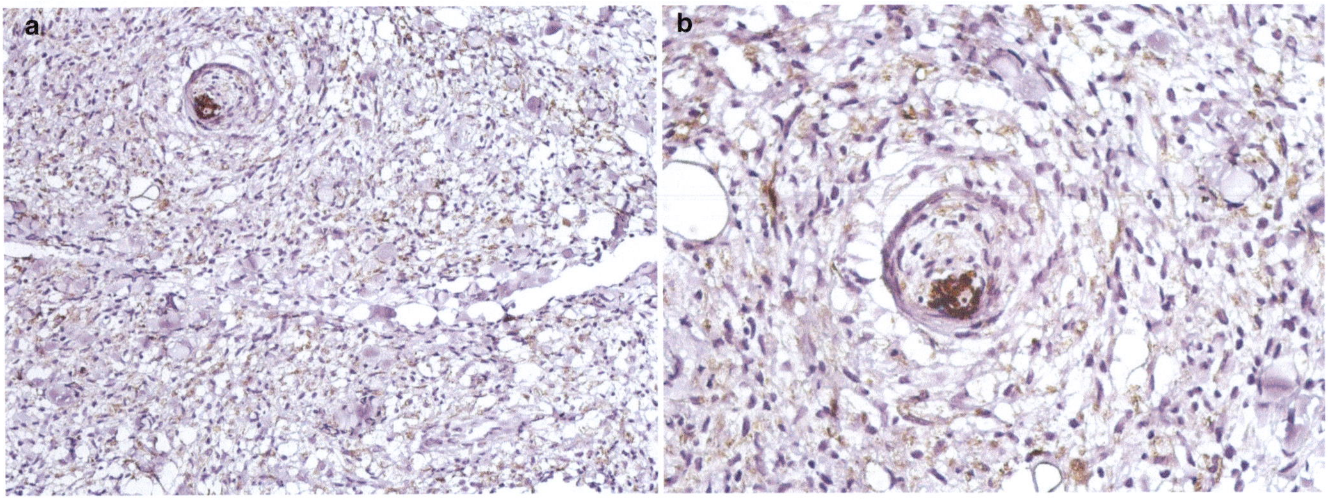

Fig. 4.11 Immunohistochemical features of leprosy in the oral cavity. (**a**) The presence of histiocytes can also be shown via S100 staining (DAB; 100×). (**b**) This reaction is also useful for revealing perineural involvement via the lymphohistiocytic infiltrate. The nerve centrally located in this image, surrounded by the histiocytic infiltrate, was observed (DAB; 200×)

Sources

1. Han XY, Seo YH, Sizer KC, Schoberle T, May GS, Spencer JS, et al. A new mycobacterium species causing diffuse lepromatous leprosy. Am J Clin Pathol. 2008;130:856–64. https://doi.org/10.1309/AJCPP72FJZZRRVMM.
2. Motta AC, Komesu MC, Silva CH. Leprosy-specific oral lesions: a report of three cases. Med Oral Patol Oral Cir Bucal. 2008;13:E479–82.
3. Benard G, Sakai-Valente NY, Bianconcini Trindade MA. Concomitant lucio phenomenon and erythema nodosum in a leprosy patient: clues for their distinct pathogeneses. Am J Dermatopathol. 2009;31:288–92. https://doi.org/10.1097/DAD.0b013e318193c74c.
4. Rodrigues LC, Lockwood DN. Leprosy now: epidemiology, progress, challenges, and research gaps. Lancet Infect Dis. 2011;11:464–70. https://doi.org/10.1016/S1473-3099(11)70006-8.
5. Taheri JB, Mortazavi H, Moshfeghi M, Bakhshi M, Bakhtiari S, Azari-Marhabi S, Alirezaei S. Oro-facial manifestations of 100 leprosy patients. Med Oral Patol Oral Cir Bucal. 2012;17:e728–32. https://doi.org/10.4317/medoral.17718.
6. Lastoria JC, Abreu MA. Leprosy: review of the epidemiological, clinical, and etiopathogenic aspects – part 1. An Bras Dermatol. 2014;89:205–18.
7. Massone C, Belachew WA, Schettini A. Histopathology of the lepromatous skin biopsy. Clin Dermatol. 2015;33:38–45.
8. Massone C, Belachew WA, Schettini A. Histopathology of the lepromatous skin biopsy. Clin Dermatol. 2015;33:38–45. https://doi.org/10.1016/j.clindermatol.2014.10.003.
9. Sharma R, Singh P, Loughry W, Lockhart J, Inman W, Duthie MS, et al. Zoonotic leprosy in the Southeastern United States. Emerg Infect Dis. 2015;21:2127–34. https://doi.org/10.3201/eid2112.150501.
10. Rodrigues GA, Qualio NP, de Macedo LD, Innocentini L, Ribeiro-Silva A, Foss NT. The oral cavity in leprosy: what clinicians need to know. Oral Dis. 2016;23:749–56. https://doi.org/10.1111/odi.12582.
11. Deps P, Cruz A. Why we should stop using the word leprosy. Lancet Infect Dis. 2020;20:e75–8. https://doi.org/10.1016/S1473-3099(20)30061-X.
12. Gupta B, Gupta S, Chaudhary M, Raj AT, Patil S. Oro-facial manifestations in lepromatous leprosy patients in Central India: clinical findings from a cross-sectional study. Clin Oral Investig. 2020;24:1981–6. https://doi.org/10.1007/s00784-019-03061-1.
13. Deps P, Collin SM. Mycobacterium lepromatosis as a second agent of Hansen's disease. Front Microbiol. 2021;12:698588. https://doi.org/10.3389/fmicb.2021.698588.
14. Juan C, Lledó L, Torralba M, Gómez JR, Giménez C. Leprosy in Spain: a descriptive study of admissions at Fontilles sanatorium between 1909 and 2020. Trop Med Infect Dis. 2024;9:130. https://doi.org/10.3390/tropicalmed9060130.
15. Moronta Castellano G, Villarroel-Dorrego M, Crespo LL. Characteristics of oral lesions in patients with Hansen disease. Actas Dermosifiliogr (Engl Ed). 2020;111:671–7. English, Spanish. https://doi.org/10.1016/j.ad.2020.05.007.
16. Magaña M, Vargas Bornacini MF, Landeta-Sa AP, Aguilar-Mena C. Lucio phenomenon: a review. Am J Dermatopathol. 2025;47:1–8. https://doi.org/10.1097/DAD.0000000000002833.

Tuberculosis

5

Leticia Ferreira Cabido, Mariana Villarroel-Dorrego,
Bruno Augusto Benevenuto de Andrade,
Igor Mesquita Lameira, and Felipe Paiva Fonseca

5.1 General Overview and Clinical Presentation

Tuberculosis is a chronic bacterial infection that has a very important, millennial history, being originally described many years before Christ, but it was only in 1882 that Dr. Robert Koch first isolated and cultivated the tuberculosis bacillus. Even though much of the biological basis of this disease is now well understood, it still represents a major public health issue worldwide, especially in developing countries where the incidence of this infection remains very high, with India representing the country with the highest incidence of the disease, accounting for approximately 26% of all cases diagnosed in the World. According to the World Health Organization, it is estimated that approximately 1.4 million deaths were recorded worldwide in 2019, and almost 10.0 million people were diagnosed with tuberculosis globally.

Although *Mycobacterium tuberculosis* and *Mycobacterium africanum* are recognized as the main etiologic agents of the disease, other bacteria that also belong to the *M. tuberculosis* complex like *Mycobacterium bovis* are also well known. The latter is more associated with a zoonotic manifestation of tuberculosis, and affected patients are more often those living in places close to cattle and in poor conditions and who usually drink unpasteurized milk products. *Mycobacterium caprae* and *Mycobacterium orygis* may also cause zoonotic tuberculosis.

In humans, tuberculosis transmission occurs through inhalation of infectious particles generated by aerosol from an infected individual. It usually primarily manifests as granulomatous lesions in the lungs, more often as small lesions in the pulmonary parenchyma that may heal by fibrosis or calcification. Extrapulmonary tuberculosis can be found in approximately 15% of the cases, affecting many other sites like the lymph nodes (scrofula or cervical tuberculous lymphadenitis), skin, pleura, peritoneum, central nervous system, muscle, and internal organs. These extrapulmonary manifestations may occur simultaneously with lung involvement or less commonly without lung involvement. Tuberculosis can manifest soon after the initial exposure when it is termed as the primary form of the disease, or after reactivation of a previous latent infection, which characterizes the secondary form and that can also occur by infection with another bacillus, representing the most common form of this disorder. Adult males are the most affected individuals, while HIV-seropositive patients and sociocultural determinants are the most common factors of a higher risk for tuberculosis development. The disease mainly presents as low-grade fever, persistent cough, fatigue, night sweats, and weight loss. Hemoptysis may occur when lung cavitations are present. Miliary tuberculosis represents a clinical scenario characterized by a disseminated disease, which is associated with an increased mortality rate.

Diagnosis of tuberculosis is made through different approaches and represents a very important topic of discussion that may impact epidemiological results. Sputum culture has a very high specificity for detecting mycobacteria, being currently considered the gold standard method for these patients. Immunologic tests such as the purified protein

L. F. Cabido (✉)
Department of Diagnostic Sciences, College of Dentistry, Texas A&M University (TAMU), Dallas, TX, USA
e-mail: lfcabido@exchange.tamu.edu

M. Villarroel-Dorrego
Instituto de Investigaciones Odontológicas, Universidad Central de Venezuela, Caracas, Venezuela
e-mail: mariana.villarroel@ucv.ve

B. A. B. de Andrade
Department of Oral Diagnosis and Pathology, School of Dentistry, Universidade Federal do Rio de Janeiro, Rio de Janeiro, Brazil

I. M. Lameira
Service of Oral Pathology, João de Barros Barreto University Hospital, Federal University of Pará, Belém, Brazil

F. P. Fonseca
Department of Oral Surgery and Pathology, School of Dentistry, Universidade Federal de Minas Gerais, Belo Horizonte, Brazil

© The Author(s), under exclusive license to Springer Nature Switzerland AG 2025

F. P. Fonseca et al. (eds.), *Lymphoproliferative and Granulomatous Disorders of the Oral Cavity*,
https://doi.org/10.1007/978-3-031-98844-8_5

derivative or tuberculin skin test (Mantoux test) are older techniques still used to detect tuberculosis exposure. However, they cannot distinguish active disease, and a positive result may also reflect prior Bacillus Calmette–Guérin (BCG) vaccination. Imaging exams of the chest and histologic analysis of biopsied tissue samples are other diagnostic alternatives, and routine H&E evaluation should be done together with the use of special histologic stains like Ziehl-Neelsen or Fite-Faroco stains; however, the sensitivity of these techniques is considered low and false-negative results are common; on the contrary, molecular tests by PCR has a higher level of sensitivity and accuracy, detecting the microorganism with up to 90% efficacy. Currently, the World Health Organization strongly recommends the use of effective tests for tuberculosis diagnosis, including bacilloscopy, culture, or rapid diagnostic tests such as the Xpert Assay MTB/RIF®.

In the head and neck region, tuberculosis more commonly manifests as cervical lymphadenopathy, accounting for 95% of the cases, either as single or bilateral neck masses. Cervical lymph node calcification may be found on panoramic radiographs. Oral and maxillofacial involvement is well described in the literature, although it is not considered a common finding in this group of patients, occurring isolated or associated with lung manifestations, and accounting for no more than 0.1%–5% of all cases of tuberculosis. Primary manifestation in the oral cavity is very rare, and it might occur due to a direct inoculation by the bacilli, but most cases are considered to represent the secondary form due to hematologic or lymphatic dissemination of the pathogen. In the oral cavity, any site can be affected by tuberculosis, but the tongue is usually the most frequently affected, followed by the palate and the buccal mucosa. The major salivary glands can also be affected, as well as the jawbones that usually present ill-defined, radiolucent images, predominantly affecting the mandible. The oral lesions more commonly manifest as painful, deep ulcers that can be solitary or multiple, with indurated, irregular, and ill-defined borders with a necrotic base strongly resembling oral cancer, one of its main clinical differential diagnoses. Other less common oral manifestations include large swellings, granulomatous gingival enlargement, confluent erosions, and macrocheilia.

The BCG vaccine was developed over a century ago by the French scientists Albert León Charles Calmette and Jean-Marie Camille Guérin, who announced the development of the vaccine in 1921 using an attenuated bacillus of *Mycobacterium bovis*. It is currently recommended to all newborns in high-incidence countries and more selectively in countries with low incidence of the disease. It is considered a very important tool for tuberculosis prevention, especially among infants, by reducing tuberculosis-related morbidity and preventing severe forms of the disease like tuberculosis meningitis and miliary tuberculosis, while the efficacy of the vaccine to prevent adult pulmonary disease varies across regions. Treatment strategy for patients affected by tuberculosis includes the use of a combination of antibiotic drugs, which has significantly changed the mortality rates. Isoniazid, rifampicin, pyrazinamide, and ethambutol are the drugs most frequently used for treating patients. However, the increasing occurrence of resistant strains to this first-line therapy has demanded the use of second-line approaches. One of the most important barriers to tuberculosis treatment relates to its long duration, ranging from 4 to 6 months, which leads many patients to leave the correct therapeutic scheme before it is concluded, while resistance to conventional drugs represents another important pitfall (Figs. 5.1, 5.2, and 5.3).

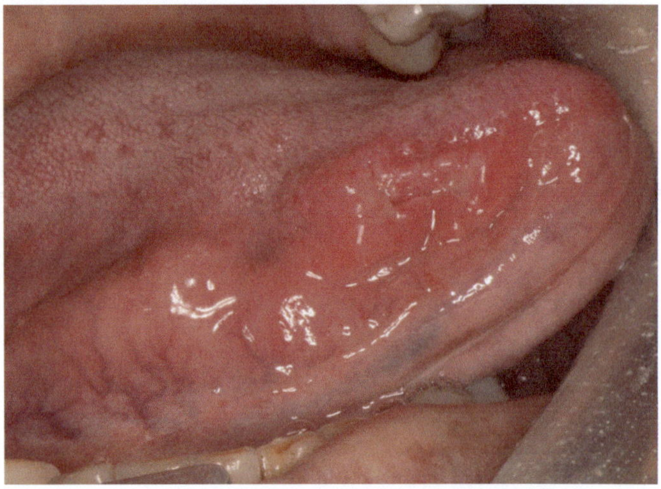

Fig. 5.1 Clinical presentation of tuberculosis in the oral cavity. Observe the painful ulcer with elevated borders affecting the right side of the lateral border of the tongue in a male patient

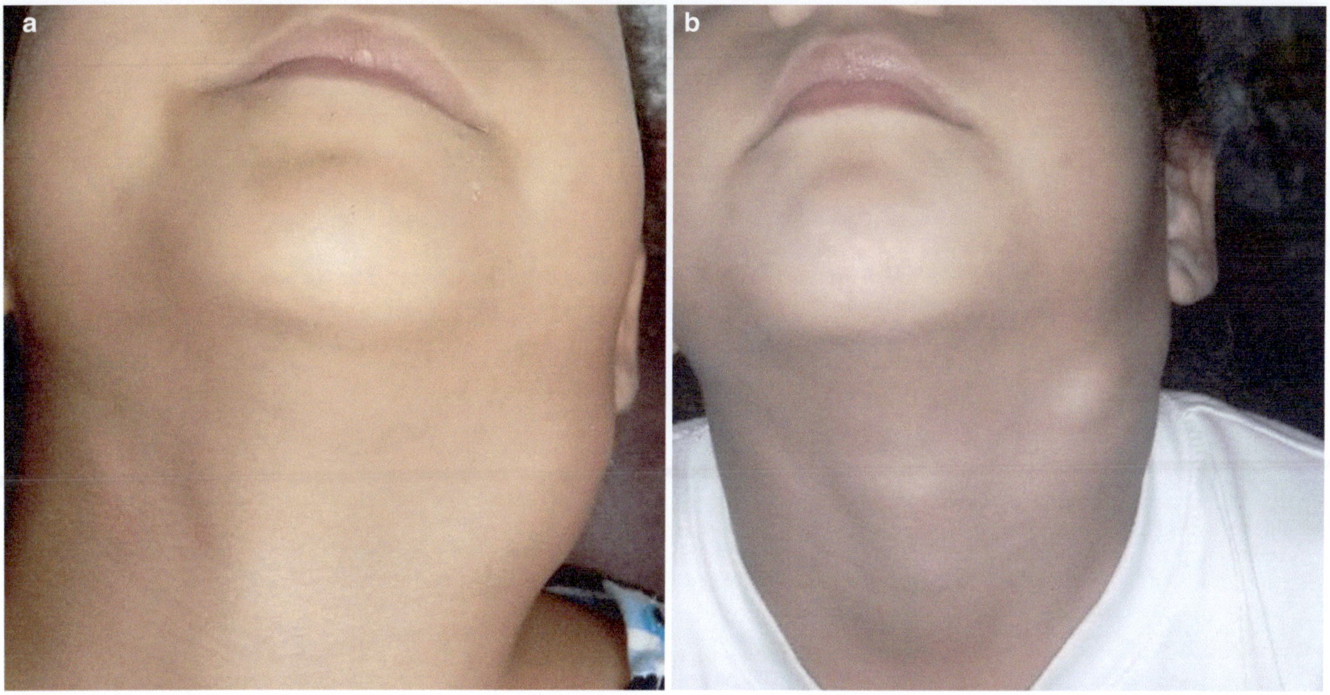

Fig. 5.2 Clinical presentation of tuberculosis affecting the lymph node. (**a**) Note the presence of a large swelling in the cervical lymph node of this female pediatric patient representing nodal manifestation of tuberculosis (scrofula). (**b**) Another view of the cervical lymph node. The patient did not have any focus of odontogenic infection

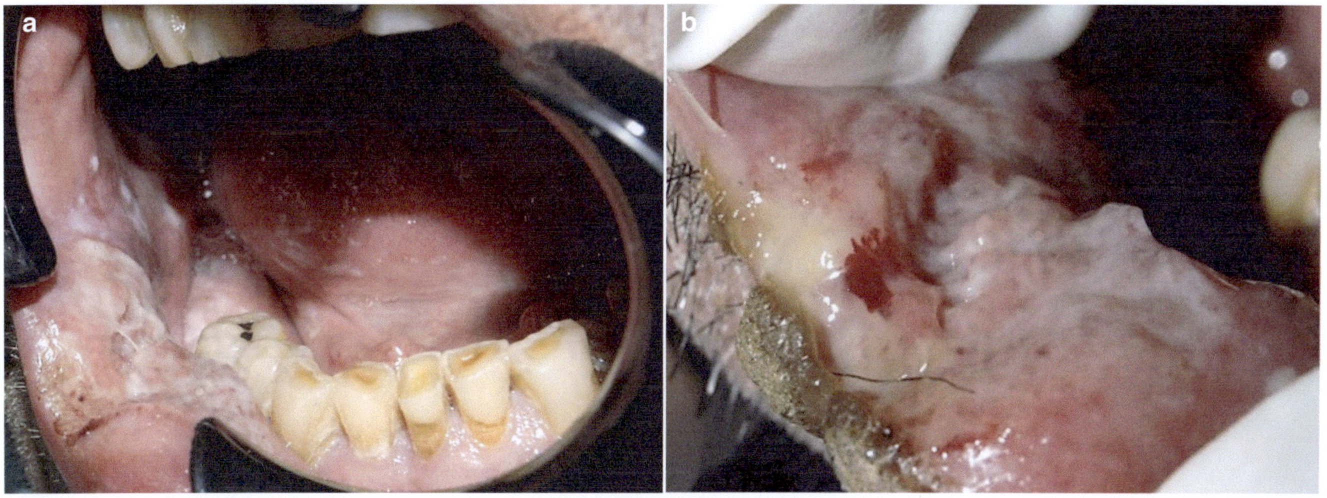

Fig. 5.3 Clinical presentation of tuberculosis in the oral cavity of a patient living with HIV. (**a**) Crateriform ulcer affecting the lower lip and extending to the vestibular mucosa. (**b**) Observe the necrotic regions and the yellowish membrane covering the ulcer

5.2 Microscopic Findings

- Presence of a dense lymphohistiocytic infiltrate in the lamina propria.
- Presence of granulomas in the lamina propria.
- Most of the granulomas exhibit caseous necrosis.
- Immunosuppressed patients usually show ill-formed granulomas or have no granuloma formation.
- Predominance of chronic inflammatory cells like histiocytes, lymphocytes, and plasma cells. Polymorphonuclear cells can also be found near ulcerated areas.
- Epithelioid histiocytes are typically present, represented by cells with large eosinophilic cytoplasm and round to oval nuclei.
- Langhans-type multinucleated giant cells are usually present (Figs. 5.4 and 5.5).

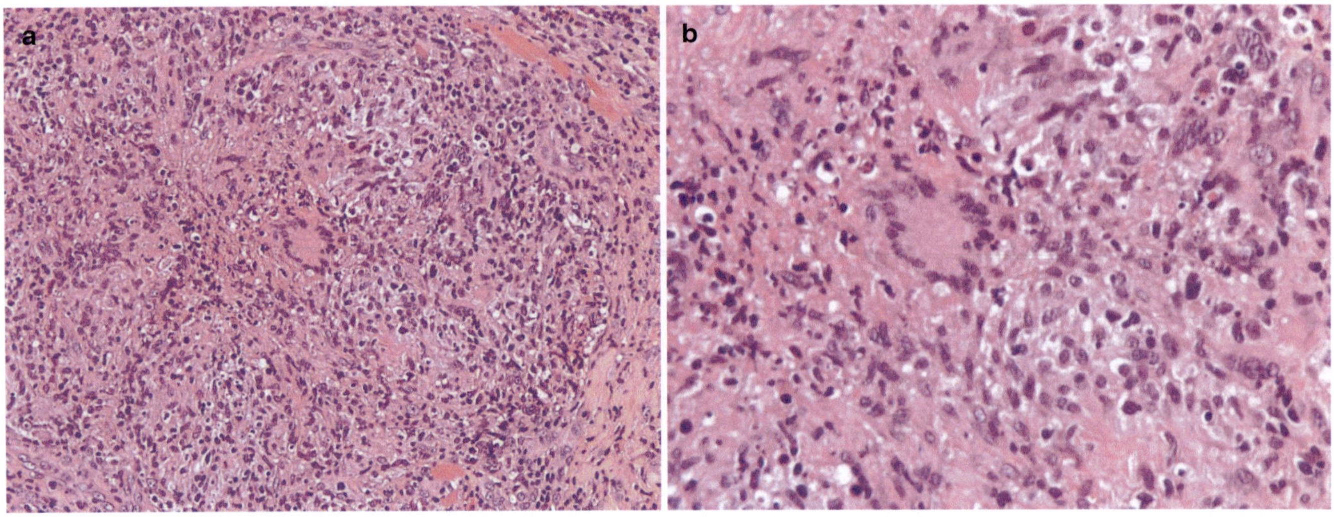

Fig. 5.4 Microscopic features compatible with tuberculosis affecting the oral cavity. (**a**) Lower magnification with the presence of a granuloma containing a more eosinophilic region in the center resembling tissue necrosis and the presence of a Langhans-type multinucleated giant cell (H&E; 100X). (**b**) Note the Langhans-type multinucleated giant cell in the center of the image. In the left side there is a more eosinophilic region suggestive of tissue necrosis, leading to the so-called caseous granuloma (H&E; 200X)

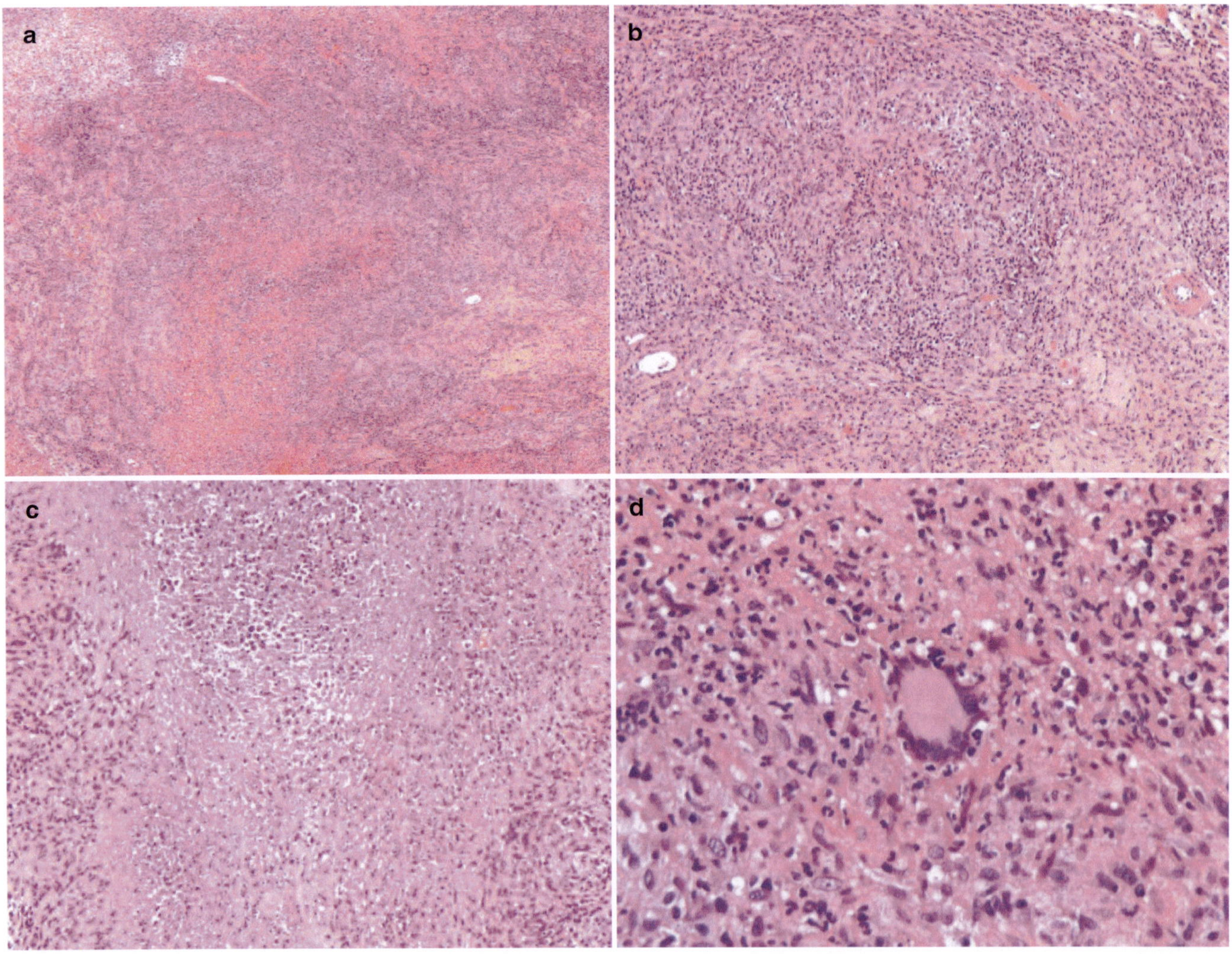

Fig. 5.5 Microscopic features compatible with the diagnosis of tuberculosis affecting the oral cavity. (**a**) Under lower magnification we observe a severe inflammatory infiltrate with eosinophilic regions consistent with tissue necrosis (H&E; 40X). (**b**) Note the presence of a granuloma in the center of the image a multinucleated giant cell. (**c**) Areas of tissue necrosis in the granulomatous infiltrate is characteristic of caseous granulomas. In this image the epithelioid macrophages are located in the periphery and the necrosis in the center of the image. (**d**) Higher magnification illustrating the granulomatous tissue with a necrotic background, a Langhans-type multinucleated giant cell and epithelioid macrophages (H&E; 400X)

5.3 Immunohistochemistry and/or Genetics

The microscopic findings of tuberculosis are usually very suggestive in the presence of caseous granulomas, but the diagnosis confirmation demands that the pathogens are demonstrated, which can be done through special histological stains like Fite-Faraco or Ziehl-Neelsen reactions, or using molecular approaches like PCR. Immunohistochemistry might be used to characterize the cellular populations that are present in the granulomatous infiltrate (Table 5.1, Fig. 5.6).

Table 5.1 Summary of the main immunohistochemical reactions and histological stains used for tuberculosis diagnosis

Antibody/stain	Most frequent results	Pattern	Objective
CD20	Positive	Membrane	To characterize the B lymphocyte infiltrate
CD3	Positive	Membrane	To characterize the T lymphocyte infiltrate
CD138	Positive	Membrane	To characterize the plasma cell infiltrate
CD68	Positive	Cytoplasm	To demonstrate the presence of macrophages, multinucleated giant cells, and granulomas
Fite-Faraco[a]	Positive	In the bacteria	To show the presence of the microorganisms
Ziehl-Neelsen[a]	Positive	In the bacteria	To show the presence of the microorganisms

[a]Histological stain

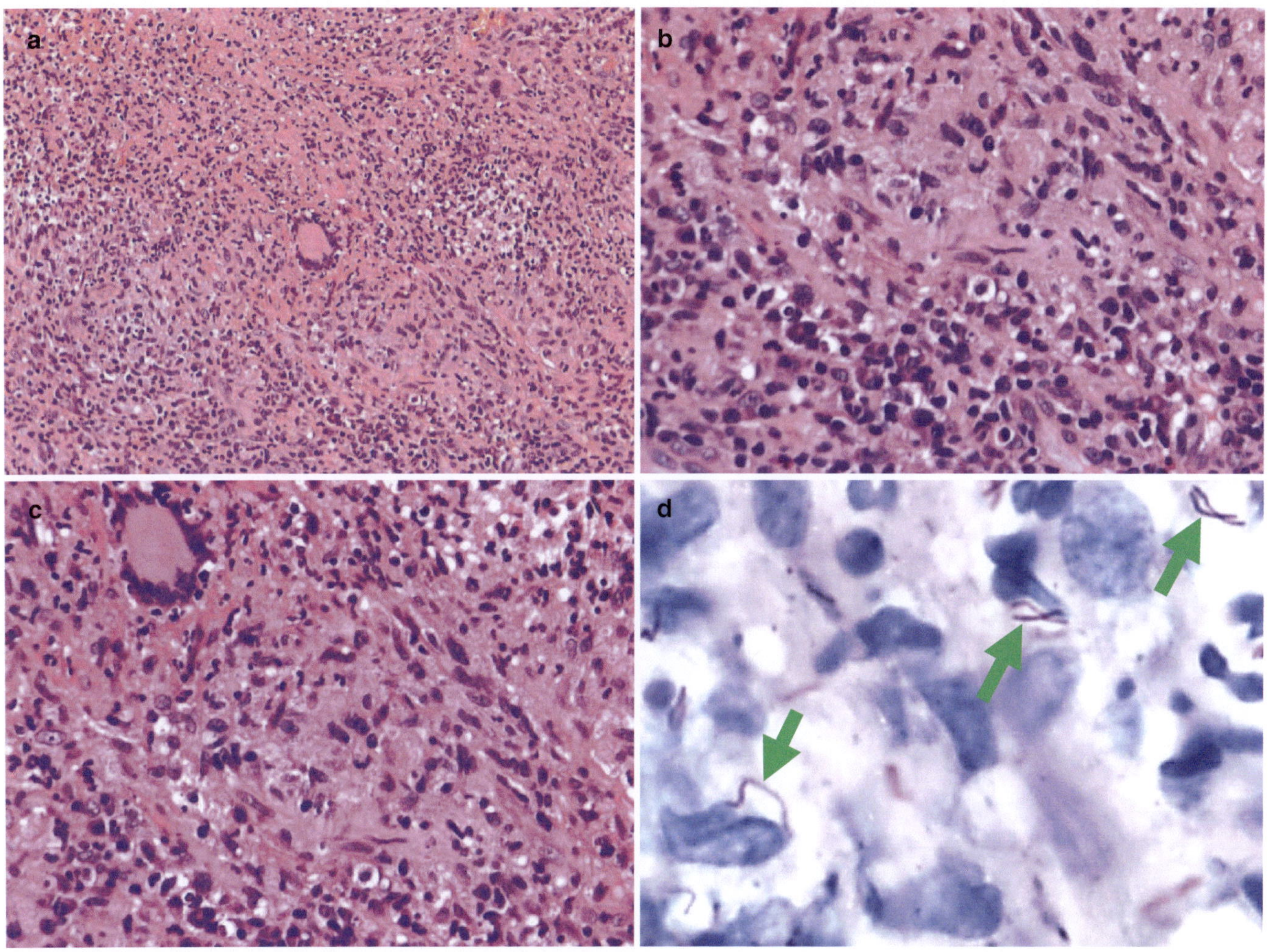

Fig. 5.6 Microscopic features compatible with tuberculosis affecting the oral cavity. (**a**) Strong granulomatous inflammation in the lamina propria. Note the presence of caseous granuloma and the Langhans-type multinucleated giant cell (H&E; 200X). (**b**) The inflammatory infiltrate is predominantly composed by macrophages, but plasma cells and lymphocyres are also present (H&E; 400). (**c**) Observe the epithelioid macrophages with their large eosinophilic cytoplasms and elongated nuclei, leading to a well-organized granuloma. A Langhans-type multinucleated giant cell is also present. (**d**) The microorganism is shown as small reddish structures (green arrows) (Zielh-Neelsen; 1000X)

Sources

1. Mignogna MD, Muzio LL, Favia G, Ruoppo E, Sammartino G, Zarrelli C, Bucci E. Oral tuberculosis: a clinical evaluation of 42 cases. Oral Dis. 2000;6:25–30. https://doi.org/10.1111/j.1601-0825.2000.tb00317.x.
2. Aydin U. Tuberculous lymph node calcification detected on routine panoramic radiography: a case report. Dentomaxillofac Radiol. 2003;32:252–4. https://doi.org/10.1259/dmfr/56579260.
3. Ito FA, de Andrade CR, Vargas PA, Jorge J, Lopes MA. Primary tuberculosis of the oral cavity. Oral Dis. 2005;11:50–3. https://doi.org/10.1111/j.1601-0825.2004.01055.x.
4. Menon K, Ben C, Gouldesbrough D, Strachan DR. A clinical review of 128 cases of head and neck tuberculosis presenting over a 10-year period in Bradford. UK J Laryngol Otol. 2007;121:362–8. https://doi.org/10.1017/S0022215106002507.
5. Kakisi OK, Kechagia AS, Kakisis IK, Rafailidis PI, Falagas ME. Tuberculosis of the oral cavity: a systematic review. Eur J Oral Sci. 2010;118:103–9.
6. Aoun N, El-Hajj G, El Toum S. Oral ulcer: an uncommon site in primary tuberculosis. Aust Dent J. 2015;60:119–22. https://doi.org/10.1111/adj.12263.
7. Wood RC, Luabeya AK, Weigel KM, Wilbur AK, Jones-Engel L, Hatherill M, Cangelosi GA. Detection of mycobacterium tuberculosis DNA on the oral mucosa of tuberculosis patients. Sci Rep. 2015;5:8668. https://doi.org/10.1038/srep08668.
8. Ju WT, Fu Y, Liu Y, Tan YR, Dong MJ, Wang LZ, Li J, et al. Clinical and pathologic analyses of tuberculosis in the oral cavity: report of 11 cases. Oral Surg Oral Med Oral Pathol Oral Radiol. 2018;125:44–51. https://doi.org/10.1016/j.oooo.2017.09.015.
9. Gupta S, Vats P, Jha A, Singh K, Ghosh S, Tandon S, et al. Gingival manifestations of tuberculosis in pediatric patients: series of 4 cases. Oral Surg Oral Med Oral Pathol Oral Radiol. 2019;128:508–14. https://doi.org/10.1016/j.oooo.2019.01.005.
10. Pontes HAR, de Souza LL, Costa AMPE, da Silva AA, Gonçalves FLN, Fonseca FP, et al. An ulcer on the ventral tip of tongue. Oral Surg Oral Med Oral Pathol Oral Radiol. 2019;127:92–6. https://doi.org/10.1016/j.oooo.2018.01.019.
11. de Farias Gabriel A, Kirschnick LB, Só BB, Schuch LF, Silveira FM, Martins MAT, et al. Oral and maxillofacial tuberculosis: a systematic review. Oral Dis. 2023;29:2483–92. https://doi.org/10.1111/odi.14290.
12. Kaye AD, Giles TP, O'Brien E, Zajac J, Upshaw WC, Jenks K, et al. Bacillus Calmette-Guerin (BCG) vaccine in America and overseas: a narrative review. Cureus. 2024;16:e73602. https://doi.org/10.7759/cureus.73602.
13. Sun Q, Li S, Gao M, Pang Y. Therapeutic strategies for tuberculosis: progress and lessons learned. Biomed Environ Sci. 2024;37:1310–23. https://doi.org/10.3967/bes2024.168.
14. Hasnaoui M, Chebil A, Masmoudi M, Ben Hammouda S, Jebahi S, Mighri K. Tongue ulceration as a first symptom of pulmonary tuberculosis: a case report. Ear Nose Throat J. 2024:1455613241271688. https://doi.org/10.1177/01455613241271688.
15. Shereen S, Manva MZ, Sheereen S, Patil NN. Exploring the oral manifestations of tuberculosis: a comprehensive analysis of prevalence and clinicopathological characteristics of oral lesions. Int J Mycobacteriol. 2024;13:53–7. https://doi.org/10.4103/ijmy.ijmy_224_23.

Infectious Mononucleosis

6

Alan Roger Santos-Silva, Liam Robinson, Márcio Ajudarte Lopes, Wilfredo Alejandro González-Arriagada, and Felipe Paiva Fonseca

6.1 General Overview and Clinical Presentation

Infectious mononucleosis is a benign, self-limited, lymphoproliferative disease caused by Epstein-Barr virus (EBV or HHV-4), a double-stranded DNA γ herpes virus that frequently manifests in adolescents and young adults between 15 and 24 years old. It is estimated that over 95% of the adult population worldwide has already been exposed to EBV, and seroprevalence increases with age, and tends to be higher among females, non-Caucasian ethnic groups, and people living in socio-economically deprived households. There seems to be a notable difference in the exposure rate of children depending on their geographic regions. The proportion of EBV-exposed children in developing countries is believed to be more than 90% between the ages of 5 and 9, with most becoming infected earlier in childhood. In contrast, this proportion in developed countries like Western Europe and North America is only 50% of the population in this age range.

Most of the infected individuals are usually asymptomatic, and the virus infection remains in the patient for a lifetime. Primary transmission occurs through personal contact with an infected person, particularly by saliva particles, with an incubation period estimated to vary from 2 to 5 weeks. Symptomatic patients are usually those not exposed to the virus early in life. They often present a clinical viral syndrome characterized by fever, pharyngitis, fatigue, and posterior cervical lymphadenopathy. Periorbital and/or palpebral edema, more usually bilaterally, is observed in approximately 33% of the patients. Evidence points out that some clinical manifestations of symptomatic infectious mononucleosis in children are associated with age. Younger infants (from 0 to 6 years old) present with nasal congestion more frequently, suggesting they have more manifestations of respiratory obstruction. In contrast, older infants (from 7 to 14 years old) more often present with fatigue and lymphadenopathy, combined with atypical lymphocytosis and elevated alanine aminotransferase.

Laboratory findings using serological analysis include the presence of leukocytosis in most of the patients, with lymphocytes accounting for approximately 50% of the total number of white blood cells and demonstrating an elevated number (10%) of atypical lymphocytes on peripheral smear. Serum testing for EBV-specific antibodies is considered the

A. R. Santos-Silva (✉) · M. A. Lopes
Department of Oral Diagnosis (Semiology), Piracicaba Dental School, University of Campinas (UNICAMP), Piracicaba, Brazil
e-mail: alan@unicamp.br; malopes@fop.unicamp.br

L. Robinson
Department of Oral and Maxillofacial Pathology, School of Dentistry, University of Pretoria, Pretoria, South Africa
e-mail: liam.robinson@up.ac.za

W. A. González-Arriagada
Facultad de Odontología, Universidad de Los Andes, Santiago, Chile
e-mail: wgonzalez@uandes.cl

F. P. Fonseca
Department of Oral Surgery and Pathology, School of Dentistry, Universidade Federal de Minas Gerais, Belo Horizonte, Brazil

© The Author(s), under exclusive license to Springer Nature Switzerland AG 2025
F. P. Fonseca et al. (eds.), *Lymphoproliferative and Granulomatous Disorders of the Oral Cavity*,
https://doi.org/10.1007/978-3-031-98844-8_6

gold standard for diagnosis, but results are usually not rapidly obtained. The most common diagnostic method is the mononuclear spot test or "monospot test" to demonstrate the presence of heterophilic antibodies (Paul–Bunnell heterophile antibody test) that represent antibodies that usually appear during the first week of symptom onset. However, despite its high specificity for a diagnosis of infectious mononucleosis, its sensitivity is considered low, ranging between 70% and 90%, and it is even lower among children younger than 4 years old, leading to a high number of false-negative results, especially in this younger group of patients. Other pathological conditions may also show heterophile antibodies, possibly causing false-positive results.

EBV is found in the throat of most patients with infectious mononucleosis, and during acute infection, the virus replicates in B cells. This is followed by a cellular immune response of the host to eliminate EBV-infected cells, although latent infection of memory B cells persists indefinitely. A smaller proportion of the patients with symptomatic infectious mononucleosis manifesting peritonsillar abscesses or acute tonsillitis may also have some bacterial co-infection, more often *Staphylococcus aureus*, but also Group A *streptococci*, *Fusobacteria nucleatum*, and *Prevotella intermedia*; however, any possible role played by these microorganisms in the pathogenesis of the disease remains to be demonstrated.

Patients often manifest with tonsillitis, including bilateral painful swelling of the palatine tonsils, frequently covered by an overlying yellowish pseudomembrane. Patients may also show the presence of palatine petechiae and enanthem. Most cases follow a benign, self-limiting course and a spontaneous recovery after 10–14 days. However, rare clinical complications may occur, including headache, splenic rupture, hemolytic anemia, aplastic anemia, skin rash, nephritis, jaundice, otitis media, and pneumonia, which is more frequently observed in immunosuppressed patients. Moreover, it has been reported that EBV infection may trigger hemophagocytic lymphohistiocytosis. Additionally, some neurologic conditions have also been associated with infectious mononucleosis, like Guillain-Barre syndrome, cranial nerve palsies, aseptic meningitis, and meningoencephalitis. Rare fatal infectious mononucleosis cases have also been reported.

Infectious mononucleosis is considered a benign, self-limiting condition in immunocompetent patients, with an excellent prognosis, requiring only supportive treatment. The efficacy of antibiotic usage is unclear, with divergent results reported in the literature. Complications may occur in immunosuppressed individuals, and antiviral treatments may be necessary in these individuals.

6.2 Microscopic Findings

- Tonsils show a diffuse proliferation of small- to medium-sized polymorphous lymphocytic infiltrate.
- Hyperplastic lymphoid follicles have prominent, irregularly shaped germinal centers.
- The occurrence of an interfollicular expansion, either as aggregates or as focal sheets of proliferating cells, is observed in many cases, consisting of large round to oval cells with vesicular nuclei and one or more prominent nucleoli (immunoblasts) in a background of smaller lymphocytes, as well as reactive plasma cells and histiocytes. Mitotic figures are present.
- Preserved areas of lymphoid tissue is usually found in the tonsillar biopsy.
- The lymphoproliferative nature of infectious mononucleosis must be differentiated from neoplastic lymphoid processes, both Hodgkin and non-Hodgkin lymphomas, which can be very challenging in some instances.
- A variable number of large EBV-infected cells are typically present.
- The EBV-positive cells are mononucleated or polynucleated, with prominent nucleoli.
- Reed-Sternberg-like cells may be found scattered in the tissue.
- Areas of tissue necrosis, mucosal ulceration, and neutrophilic abscess are common (Figs. 6.1, 6.2, and 6.3).

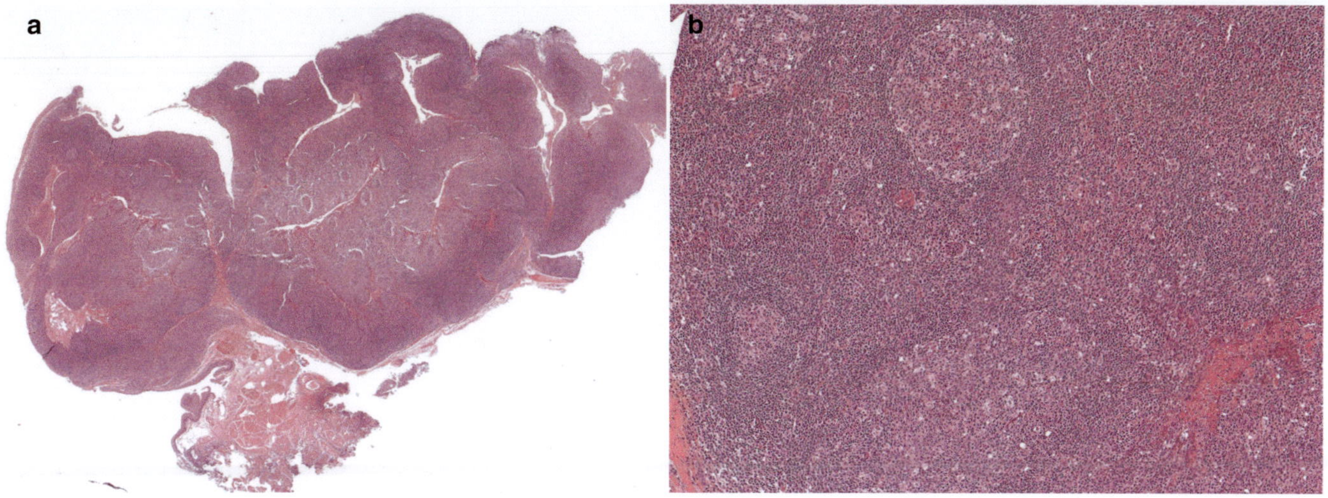

Fig. 6.1 Microscopic features of infectious mononucleosis affecting the tonsils. (**a**) Hyperplastic lymphoid tissue of the tonsil with the overlying epithelium and the lymphoid component in the lamina propria. There are many secondary follicles with reactive germinal centers (H&E; 10×). (**b**) Some of the reactive follicles contain tingible body macrophages in their germinal centers (H&E; 50×)

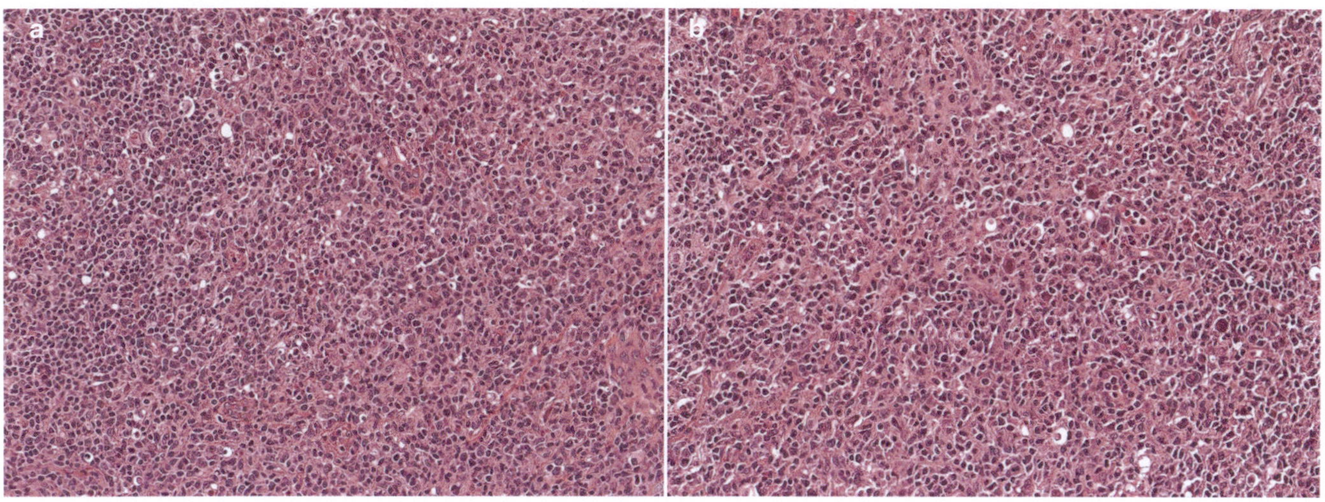

Fig. 6.2 Microscopic features of infectious mononucleosis affecting the tonsils. (**a**) Under high magnification, it is possible to find the predominance of small lymphocytes, but larger cells (centroblasts and immunoblasts) are also distributed in the tissue (H&E; 100×). (**b**) Scattered large binucleated cells with prominent nucleoli resembling Reed-Sternberg cells may be found (blue arrow) (H&E; 100×)

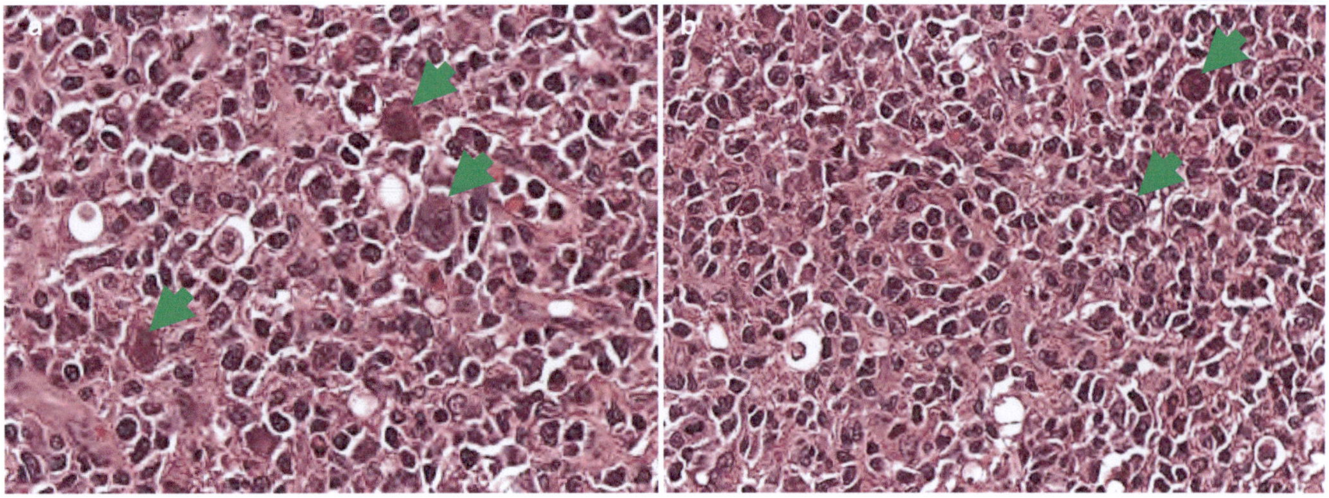

Fig. 6.3 Microscopic features of infectious mononucleosis affecting the tonsils. (**a**) Note the presence of large cells with atypia and often binucleated, resembling Reed-Sternberg cells (green arrows) (H&E; 400×). (**b**) Large binucleated cells scattered and distributed throughout the specimen (green arrows) (400×; 200×)

Table 6.1 Summary of the main immunohistochemical reactions used for infectious mononucleosis diagnosis

Antibody/probe	Most frequent results	Pattern	Objective
CD20	Positive	Membrane	To demonstrate the B lymphocyte population
CD3	Positive	Membrane	To demonstrate the T lymphocyte population
CD15	Negative	Membrane	To differentiate from Hodgkin lymphoma
CD30	Positive	Membrane	To differentiate from Hodgkin lymphoma
IFR4/MUM1	Positive	Nucleus	To differentiate from lymphomas[a]
CD10	Negative	Membrane	To differentiate from lymphomas[a]
BCL6	Negative	Nucleus	To differentiate from lymphomas[a]
Kappa/Lambda	Polyclonal	Cytoplasm	To demonstrate the polyclonal nature of the infiltrate
Ki67	Variable	Nucleus	To demonstrate the proliferative index of the lesion
LMP1[b]	Positive	Membrane	To demonstrate the presence of EBV
EBER[c]	Positive	Nucleus	To demonstrate the presence of EBV

Investigation of EBV is also described
EBV Epstein-Barr virus
[a]The expression pattern MUM1+/BCL6−/CD10− in the immunoblasts favors a diagnosis of infectious mononucleosis, but final diagnosis depends on overall morphological, clinical, and laboratory evaluation
[b]Although LMP1 expression can be found in infectious mononucleosis, the use of in situ hybridization is considered the gold standard for EBV identification
[c]Investigated by in situ hybridization

6.3 Immunohistochemistry and/or Genetics

Immunohistochemistry will show a polymorphic infiltrate with predominance of B and T cell populations in the hyperplastic lymphoid tissue, which demonstrates a polyclonal pattern investigated by immunoglobulin light chains kappa and lambda. The EBV-infected cells can be better demonstrated using in situ hybridization for EBER (Table 6.1, Fig. 6.4).

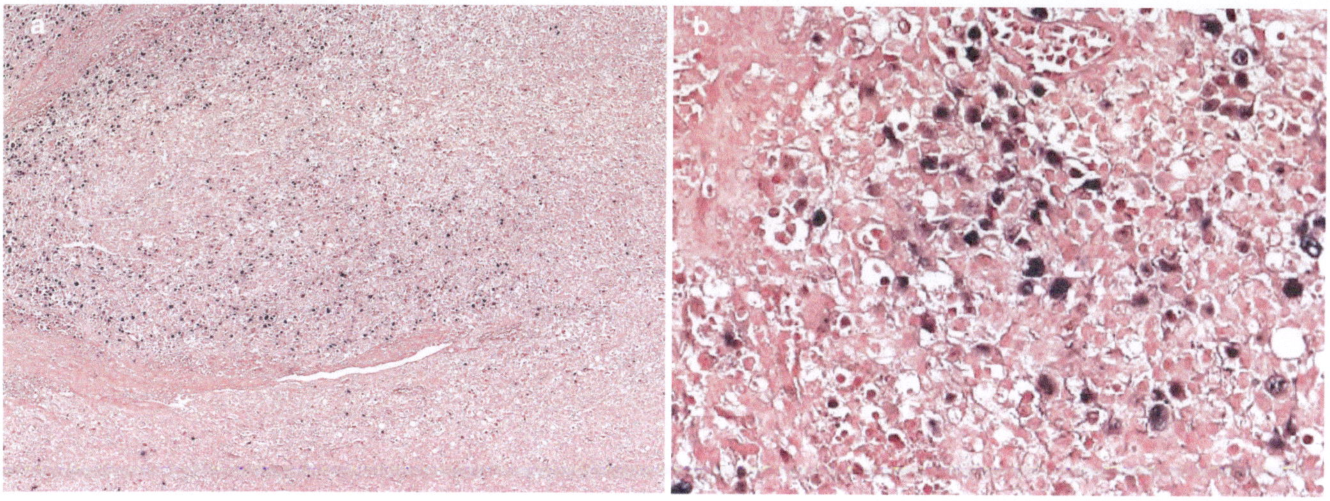

Fig. 6.4 Microscopic features of infectious mononucleosis affecting the tonsils. (**a**) The presence of EBV in the lesion is demonstrated by in situ hybridization, with positive cells stained dark blue (EBER; 50×). (**b**) Under high magnification, the EBV-positive cells demonstrating dark blue nuclei are better appreciated (EBER; 200×)

Sources

1. Ehsan A, Fan H, Eagan PA, Siddiqui HA, Gulley ML. Accumulation of p53 in infectious mononucleosis tissues. Hum Pathol. 2000;31:1397–403. https://doi.org/10.1053/hupa.2000.19447.
2. Kojima M, Nakamura S, Itoh H, Yamane Y, Miyawaki S, Masawa N. Lymph node lesion in infectious mononucleosis showing geographic necrosis containing cytologically atypically B-cells. A case report. Pathol Res Pract. 2004;200:53–7. https://doi.org/10.1016/j.prp.2003.12.006.
3. Kojima M, Kitamoto Y, Shimizu K, Matsuda H, Masawa N. Tonsillar lesions of infectious mononucleosis resembling MALT type lymphoma. A report of two cases. Pathol Oncol Res. 2008;14:489–92. https://doi.org/10.1007/s12253-008-9033-0.
4. Luzuriaga K, Sullivan JL. Infectious mononucleosis. N Engl J Med. 2010;362:1993–2000. https://doi.org/10.1056/NEJMcp1001116.
5. Kojima M, Nakamura N, Itoh H. Epstein–Barr virus-related atypical lymphoproliferative disorders in Waldeyer's ring: a clinicopathological study of 9 cases. Pathobiology. 2010;77:218–24.
6. Louissaint A Jr, Ferry JA, Soupir CP, Hasserjian RP, Harris NL, Zukerberg LR. Infectious mononucleosis mimicking lymphoma: distinguishing morphological and immunophenotypic features. Mod Pathol. 2012;25:1149–59. https://doi.org/10.1038/modpathol.2012.70.
7. Vouloumanou EK, Rafailidis PI, Falagas ME. Current diagnosis and management of infectious mononucleosis. Curr Opin Hematol. 2012;19:14–20. https://doi.org/10.1097/MOH.0b013e32834daa08.
8. Auerbach A, Aguilera NS. Epstein-Barr virus (EBV)-associated lymphoid lesions of the head and neck. Semin Diagn Pathol. 2015;32:12–22. https://doi.org/10.1053/j.semdp.2014.12.001.
9. Danstrup CS, Klug TE. Low rate of co-infection in complicated infectious mononucleosis. Dan Med J. 2019;166:A5564.
10. Kuri A, Jacobs BM, Vickaryous N, Pakpoor J, Middeldorp J, Giovannoni G, et al. Epidemiology of Epstein-Barr virus infection and infectious mononucleosis in the United Kingdom. BMC Public Health. 2020;20:912. https://doi.org/10.1186/s12889-020-09049-x.
11. Naughton P, Healy M, Enright F, Lucey B. Infectious mononucleosis: diagnosis and clinical interpretation. Br J Biomed Sci. 2021;78:107–16. https://doi.org/10.1080/09674845.2021.1903683.
12. Wu Y, Ma S, Zhang L, Zu D, Gu F, Ding X, Zhang L. Clinical manifestations and laboratory results of 61 children with infectious mononucleosis. J Int Med Res. 2020;48:300060520924550. https://doi.org/10.1177/0300060520924550.
13. Abidoye O, Raybon-Rojas E, Ogbuagu H. A rare case of Epstein-Barr virus: infectious mononucleosis complicated by Guillain-Barre syndrome. Cureus. 2022;14:e21085. https://doi.org/10.7759/cureus.21085.
14. Leung AKC, Lam JM, Barankin B. Infectious mononucleosis: an updated review. Curr Pediatr Rev. 2024;20:305–22. https://doi.org/10.2174/1573396320666230801091558.
15. Stuempfig ND, Seroy J. Monospot Test. StatPearls Publishing; 2024.
16. Anagnostopoulos I, Hummel M, Kreschel C, Stein H. Morphology, immunophenotype, and distribution of latently and/or productively Epstein-Barr virus-infected cells in acute infectious mononucleosis: implications for the interindividual infection route of Epstein-Barr virus. Blood. 1995;85:744–50.

Cytomegalovirus

7

Fábio Abreu Alves, Felipe Martins Silveira, Pablo Agustin Vargas, and Felipe Paiva Fonseca

7.1 General Overview and Clinical Presentation

Cytomegalovirus is a DNA virus that belongs to the β-herpesvirus family, also known as human herpesvirus-5 (HHV-5), representing the largest human virus with approximately 110–130 nm in diameter. The term cytomegalovirus comes from the Greek roots "*cyto*" and "*megalo*," meaning "big cell." It is estimated that approximately 90% of adults worldwide are infected with this virus at some point in their lives. The prevalence of cytomegalovirus-specific antibodies increases with age, ranging from 47% in children aged 10–12 years to 81% in adults aged 36–60 years. Seroprevalence rates among adults from developing countries are usually higher than in more industrialized regions, and other socioeconomic features like low family income and low educational levels may also be associated with a higher seroprevalence for this virus. Most of the infections are asymptomatic and persist for the whole life, being frequently considered harmless in healthy individuals. Primary symptomatic infection in immunocompetent individuals may occur most commonly among infants, more often as flulike symptoms with fever, malaise, lymphadenopathy, and mild hepatitis. The infection then becomes clinically occult, and the virus is undetectable by laboratory tests because its genome is integrated into host material and a latent status persists until the virus is reactivated under some immunosuppression state.

In immunosuppressed patients, cytomegalovirus infection represents a potential life-threatening opportunistic infection and it may affect multiple organs and be associated with pneumonia, peptic ulcers, retinitis, and/or encephalitis in this group of patients, representing one of the most common infections resulting in significant morbidity and mortality after solid organ transplantation and being used as criteria for AIDS diagnosis.

Transmission of cytomegalovirus may occur by different routes, including vertical transmission via the placenta, birth canal, and/or breast milk; horizontal transmission via the saliva, urine, semen, blood, and/or cervical and vaginal discharge; or organ transplantation. Diagnosis can be confirmed using different laboratory approaches like virus isolation, polymerase chain reaction, nucleic acid sequence-based amplification, and cytomegalovirus-specific immunoglobulin M antibody serological analysis. Enzyme-linked immunosorbent assay (ELISA) is the most common serological method used to detect cytomegalovirus antibodies; however, serology tests have limited utility in diagnosing cytomegalovirus clinical manifestations as a consequence of the high adult seroprevalence of the virus, only allowing clinicians to rule out cytomegalovirus infection in those individuals with a negative result for anti-cytomegalovirus antibodies.

The search for the viral protein using immunohistochemistry or for its genetic material by in situ hybridization on formalin-fixed paraffin-embedded tissue is the most frequently used methodology to confirm oral cavity manifestations, revealing the presence of the virus in the nuclei of infected cells. Cytomegalovirus shows a broad spectrum of cellular tropism, and following primary infection, it establishes latency in myeloid and lymphoid lineage cells, while the breast epithelium represents another important location

F. A. Alves (✉)
Department of Stomatology, A.C. Camargo Cancer Center, São Paulo, Brazil

Department of Stomatology, São Paulo University, São Paulo, Brazil
e-mail: faalves@usp.br

F. M. Silveira
Department of Diagnosis in Pathology and Oral Medicine, School of Dentistry, Universidad de la República, Montevideo, Uruguay

P. A. Vargas
Oral and Maxillofacial Division, Piracicaba Dental School, State University of Campinas (UNICAMP), Piracicaba, Brazil
e-mail: pavargas@fop.unicamp.br

F. P. Fonseca
Department of Oral Surgery and Pathology, School of Dentistry, Universidade Federal de Minas Gerais, Belo Horizonte, Brazil

© The Author(s), under exclusive license to Springer Nature Switzerland AG 2025

F. P. Fonseca et al. (eds.), *Lymphoproliferative and Granulomatous Disorders of the Oral Cavity*,
https://doi.org/10.1007/978-3-031-98844-8_7

of latent infection and viral reactivation. However, the endothelial cells of blood vessels represent the main site of cytomegalovirus infection.

It has been reported that cytomegalovirus infection may also be involved with the occurrence of ulcerations in the intestine, stomach, and esophagus. In the oral cavity, cytomegalovirus can be isolated from healthy mucosa and saliva; moreover, the presence of the virus has been demonstrated in dental pulpal and apical diseases, as well as in 63%–72% of aggressive periodontitis, but the pathogenetic role of the microorganism in these lesions is still being investigated. It has been shown that approximately 32.2% of patients who underwent allogeneic hematopoietic stem cell transplantation demonstrate oral shedding of cytomegalovirus in the oral cavity. Cytomegalovirus-associated oral mucosa lesions are very rare and more commonly reported in immunocompromised individuals, most often presenting as nonspecific ulcers in the lips, palate, tongue, and gingiva. These ulcers are usually shallow with well-defined borders and an overlying yellowish pseudomembrane; however, severely immunocompromised patients may show deeper and irregular ulcerations. Some oral ulcers may occasionally show histologic evidence of simultaneous coinfection by human herpes-simplex virus (HSV), which can be confirmed using immunohistochemistry reactions.

Symptomatic cytomegalovirus infection is considered a self-limited condition, but immunocompromised patients should have their immunological state corrected, and cytomegalovirus-associated ulcerations can be managed by antiviral drugs like ganciclovir. The prognosis is variable depending on the severity of the immunosuppression, but oral ulcers usually heal once treatment is initiated (Fig. 7.1).

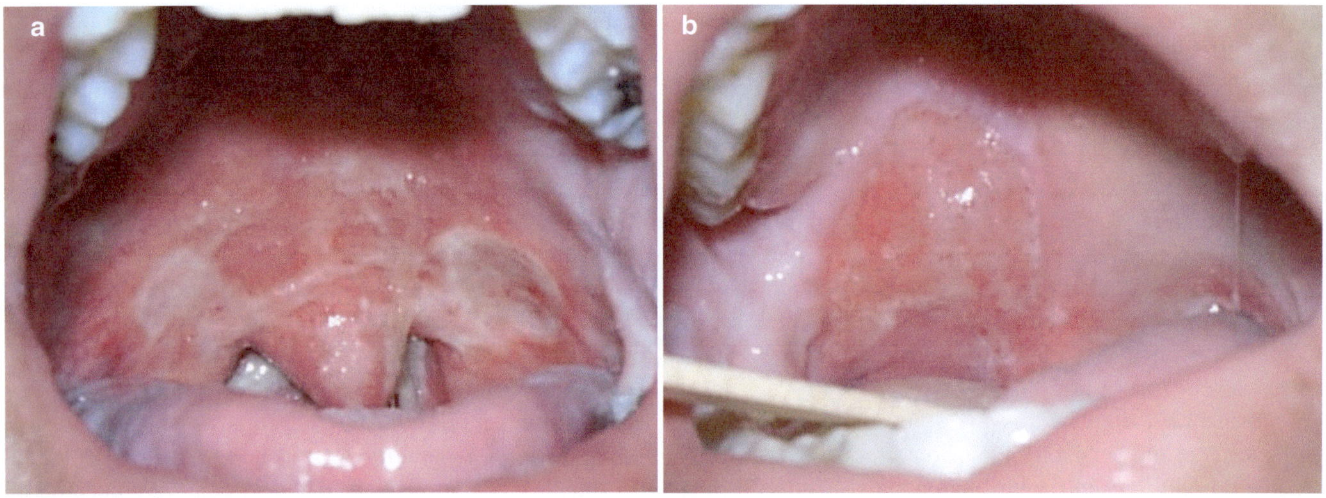

Fig. 7.1 Clinical presentation of cytomegalovirus-associated oral ulcers in bone marrow transplanted patients. (**a**) A male patient exhibiting a large ulcer affecting the palate bilaterally. (**b**) Ulcerative lesion affecting the right side of the palate. Observe the erythematous aspect of the lesion and the presence of yellowish pseudomembrane in some areas of the ulcer

7.2 Microscopic Findings

- Microscopic diagnosis of cytomegalovirus-associated oral lesions frequently demands from pathologists a high level of diagnostic suspicion due to its nonspecific inflammatory infiltrate and discrete viral features in the infected cells.
- There is an oral mucosa ulcer with infiltration of a moderate to severe nonspecific mixed inflammatory infiltrate.
- Presence of lymphocytes, plasma cells, histiocytes, and neutrophils.
- Infected cells are large (cytomegaly), with nuclei containing viral inclusions.
- This cellular aspect leads to the so-called "Owl's eye" characteristic.
- These inclusion viral bodies are the largest viral inclusions in humans (~15 μm).
- They are strongly acidophilic and surrounded by a clear vacuolar space.
- The presence of nucleoli in infected cells persists.
- Smaller viral inclusions in the cytoplasm may occur, but are very difficult to identify.
- Occasional large, atypical lymphoid cells with round, lobated nuclei and prominent nucleoli, resembling Hodgkin cells or Reed-Sternberg-like cells, can be found (Figs. 7.2 and 7.3).

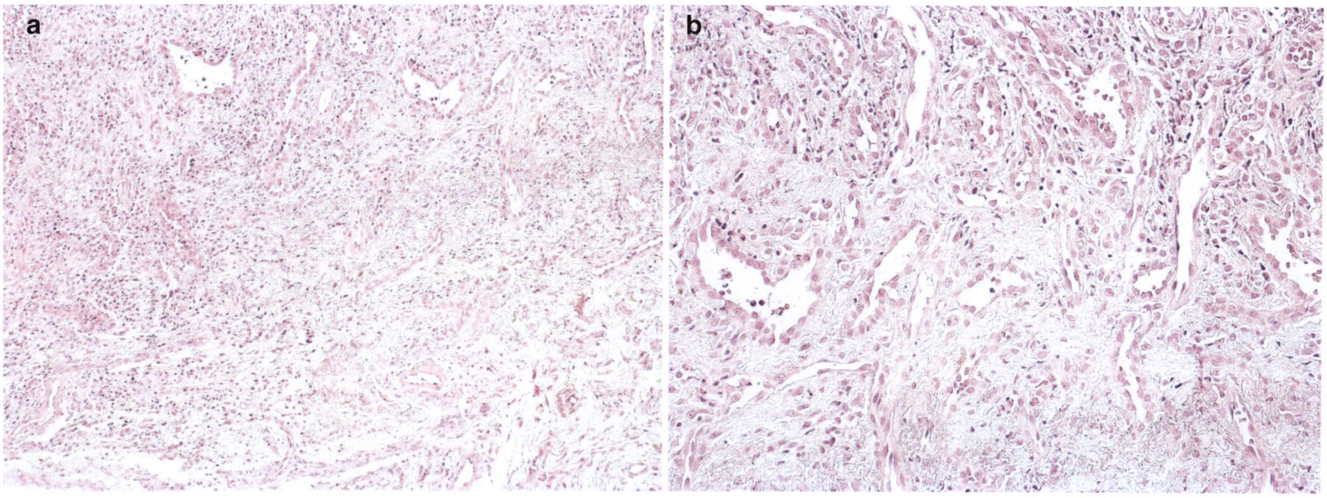

Fig. 7.2 Microscopic features of cytomegalovirus-associated oral ulcer. (**a**) The presence of chronic inflammatory infiltrate with predominance of lymphocytes, plasma cells, and macrophages surrounding blood vessels of variable size and shape in a fibrous stroma (H&E; 50×). (**b**) Observe that the endothelial cells of these blood vessels are more prominent (H&E; 100×)

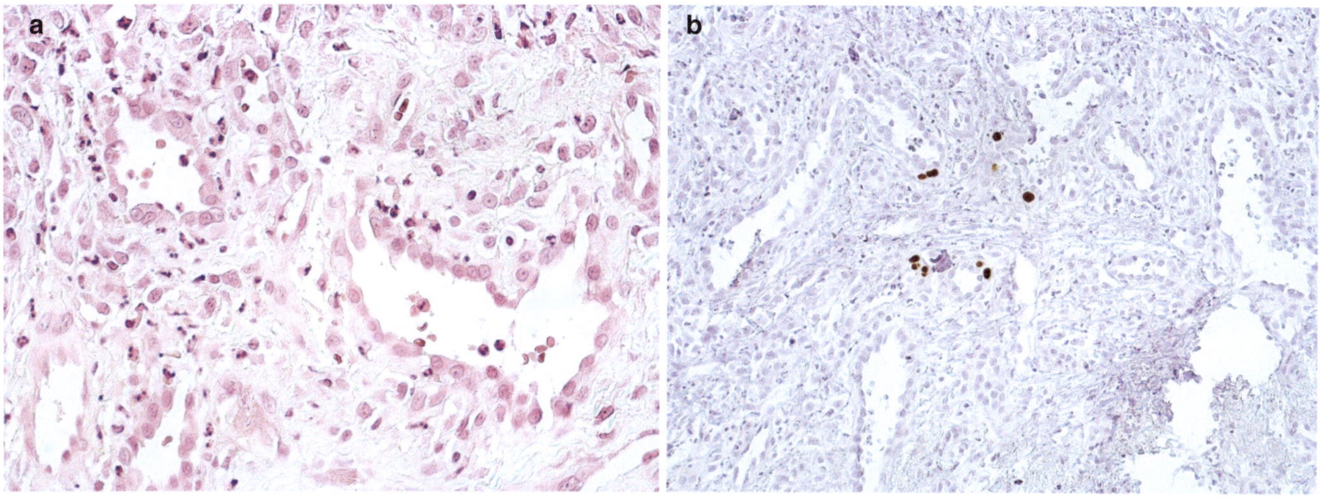

Fig. 7.3 Microscopic features of cytomegalovirus-associated oral ulcer. (**a**) Under higher magnification, it is possible to observe the blood vessels and the reactive lymphocytes (H&E; 200×). (**b**) The presence of the virus is demonstrated using immunohistochemistry for cytomegalovirus antigen. Observe the strong nuclear expression in a few infected cells (DAB; 100×)

7.3 Immunohistochemistry and/or Genetics

The identification of cytomegalovirus in the nuclei of infected cells can be demonstrated by immunohistochemistry or in situ hybridization. Moreover, viral inclusion can also stain positively for histochemical reactions like Feulgen and PAS (Table 7.1, Figs. 7.3 and 7.4).

Table 7.1 Summary of the main immunohistochemical reactions and histological stains used for cytomegalovirus-associated ulcers diagnosis

Antibody/stain	Most frequent results	Pattern	Objective
CD20	Positive	Membrane	To characterize the B lymphocyte infiltrate
CD3	Positive	Membrane	To characterize the T lymphocyte infiltrate
Cytomegalovirus	Positive	Nuclear	To demonstrate the presence of the virus
PAS[a]	Positive	Nuclear	To demonstrate the presence of the virus
Feulgen[a]	Positive	Nuclear	To demonstrate the presence of the virus

[a]Histological stain

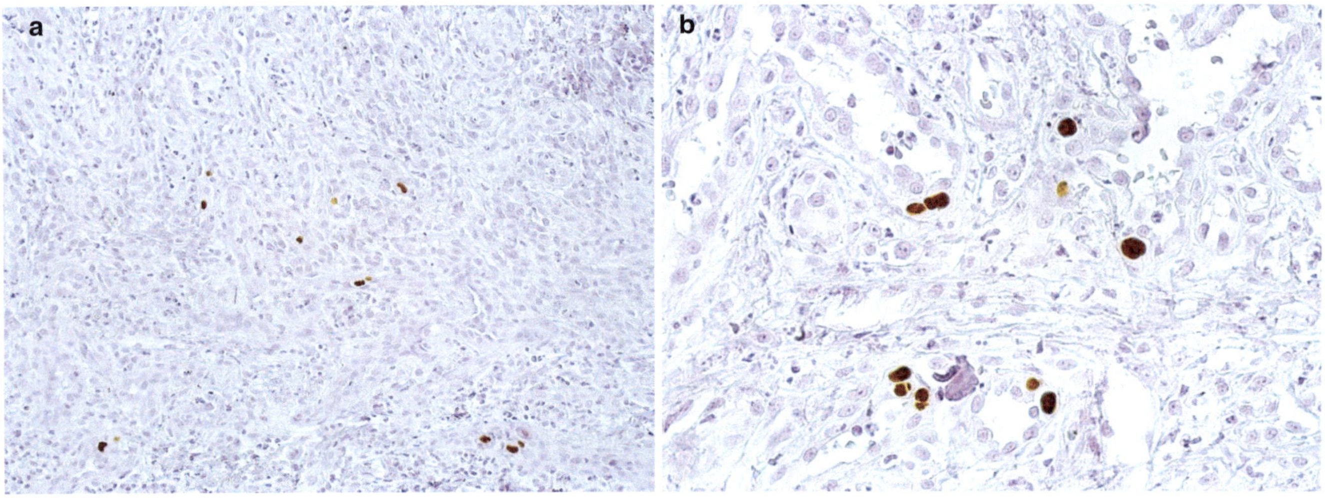

Fig. 7.4 Immunohistochemical findings in cytomegalovirus-associated oral ulcer. (**a**) In those areas containing a denser inflammatory infiltrate, the presence of cytomegalovirus-infected cells may be misinterpreted as nuclear pleomorphism in the context of a lymphoproliferative disorder, but the presence of the virus demonstrated by immunohistochemistry is supportive of the correct diagnosis, which should be confirmed by clinical manifestation and follow-up (DAB; 100×). (**b**) The presence of the virus can be seen in infected lymphocytes and endothelial cells (DAB; 200×)

Sources

1. Syrjänen S, Leimola-Virtanen R, Schmidt-Westhausen A, Reichart PA. Oral ulcers in AIDS patients frequently associated with cytomegalovirus (CMV) and Epstein-Barr virus (EBV) infections. J Oral Pathol Med. 1999;28:204–9. https://doi.org/10.1111/j.1600-0714.1999.tb02025.x.
2. López-Pintor RM, Hernández G, de Arriba L, Morales JM, Jiménez C, de Andrés A. Oral ulcers during the course of cytomegalovirus infection in renal transplant recipients. Transplant Proc. 2009;41:2419–21. https://doi.org/10.1016/j.transproceed.2009.06.053.
3. Mainville GN, Marsh WL, Allen CM. Oral ulceration associated with concurrent herpes simplex virus, cytomegalovirus, and Epstein-Barr virus infection in an immunocompromised patient. Oral Surg Oral Med Oral Pathol Oral Radiol. 2015;119:e306–14. https://doi.org/10.1016/j.oooo.2014.10.019.
4. Dittmer DP, Tamburro K, Chen H, Lee A, Sanders MK, Wade TA, et al. Oral shedding of herpesviruses in HIV-infected patients with varying degrees of immune status. AIDS. 2017;31:2077–84. https://doi.org/10.1097/QAD.0000000000001589.
5. Miranda-Silva W, Knebel FH, Tozetto-Mendozo TR, Palmieri M, Fonseca FP, Camargo AA, et al. Herpesviruses in the oral cavity of patients subjected to allogeneic hematopoietic stem cell transplantation and its relationship with oral mucositis. Clin Oral Investig. 2020;24:3597–608. https://doi.org/10.1007/s00784-020-03234-3.
6. Nishioka R, Kawano M. Tongue ulceration from cytomegalovirus infection. N Engl J Med. 2020;383:67. https://doi.org/10.1056/NEJMicm1914681.
7. Sato S, Takahashi M, Takahashi T. A case of cytomegalovirus-induced oral ulcer in an older adult patient with nephrotic syndrome due to membranous nephropathy. Case Rep Dent. 2020;2020:8843816. https://doi.org/10.1155/2020/8843816.
8. Costa ALF, Santos BA, Torregrossa VR, Miranda ECM, Vigorito AC, Palmieri M, et al. Oral shedding of CMV and HSV-1 in hematopoietic stem cell transplantation patients. Oral Dis. 2021;27:1572–9. https://doi.org/10.1111/odi.13690.
9. Maresca R, Varca S, Di Vincenzo F, Ainora ME, Mignini I, Papa A, et al. Cytomegalovirus infection: an underrated target in inflammatory bowel disease treatment. J Clin Med. 2023;13:130. https://doi.org/10.3390/jcm13010130.
10. Manabe M, Kondo T. Cytomegalovirus-induced stomatitis in a patient with refractory diffuse large B-cell lymphoma. Int J Hematol. 2023;117:629–30. https://doi.org/10.1007/s12185-023-03593-z.
11. Miranda-Silva W, de Molla VC, Knebel FH, Tozetto-Mendoza TR, Arrais-Rodrigues C, Camargo AA, et al. Oral shedding of herpesviruses and clinical outcomes in hematopoietic stem cell transplant patients. Oral Dis. 2023;29:815–26. https://doi.org/10.1111/odi.14022.
12. Touma J, Pantalone MR, Rahbar A, Liu Y, Vetvik K, Sauer T, et al. Human cytomegalovirus protein expression is correlated with shorter overall survival in breast cancer patients: a cohort study. Viruses. 2023;15:732. https://doi.org/10.3390/v15030732.
13. Hartsough EM, Nazarian RM, Cornejo KM, Stagner AM. Unusual isolated cytomegalovirus cutaneous infections: a subtle histopathologic diagnosis with review of the literature. J Cutan Pathol. 2024;51:565–71. https://doi.org/10.1111/cup.14608.
14. Dommisch H, Schmidt-Westhausen AM. The role of viruses in oral mucosal lesions. Periodontol. 2024;96:189–202. https://doi.org/10.1111/prd.12553.
15. Hermosilla Hermosilla K, Soto Cárdenas P, Donoso Zuñiga M, Pérez Ñanco C, Hernández-Vigueras S. The role of viruses in pulpal and apical disease: a systematic review. Viruses. 2024;16:1537. https://doi.org/10.3390/v16101537.

Histoplasmosis

8

Patrícia Carlos Caldeira, Elismauro Francisco de Mendonça, Flávia Sirotheau Correa Pontes, and Felipe Paiva Fonseca

8.1 General Overview and Clinical Presentation

Histoplasmosis is a systemic fungal infection caused by the dimorphic microorganism *Histoplasma capsulatum* that presents itself in the mold form when in the soil at ambient temperatures and as a yeast form when infecting human hosts. There are two varieties of *H. capsulatum* that are pathogenic to humans, *H. capsulatum var. capsulatum* and *H. capsulatum var. duboisii*, and a third variety that is considered an equine pathogen, *H. capsulatum var. farciminosum*. Histoplasmosis was first described in 1906 by the American physician Samuel Darling, who described a disseminated form of the disease while working in the Canal Zone in Panama.

It is currently known that this fungal infection is common in the United States especially in the Mississippi and Ohio rivers valleys where this disease is considered endemic due to their rich acidic soils very often contaminated by excreta of bat and birds, considered to be of high risk of infection and usually present in regions like chicken coops, attics, caves, abandoned buildings, trees, and roosting areas. Histoplasmosis can also be diagnosed in other parts of the World, like Central and South America, Africa, Asia, and Australia. Patients are usually infected by inhalation of the fungus's airborne spores, especially during activities that disrupt these contaminated environments, and clinical manifestations of the disease may take from a few days up to several weeks to develop, although most of the immunocompetent patients are asymptomatic and do not manifest any symptoms.

For those symptomatic individuals, three clinical presentations are well known for histoplasmosis and are believed to be directly associated with the number of spores to which the patients are exposed and also with their immunological status. Acute histoplasmosis is considered a self-limited pulmonary disease that occurs more often in immunocompetent individuals exposed to a small concentration of spores. It is characterized by clinical features resembling influenza with fever, malaise, headache, and anorexia, lasting for approximately 2 weeks. Chronic form of histoplasmosis resembles tuberculosis and is more often observed when immunosuppressed patients are exposed to a larger number of spores. The lungs are also affected, and these individuals present with a productive cough, weight loss, dyspnea, and weakness. Disseminated histoplasmosis is less common and is usually present in immunosuppressed patients. It is characterized by the dissemination of the disease to other extrapulmonary sites like the adrenal glands, spleen, liver, lymph nodes, kidneys, and the oral mucosa. The microorganism can also invade the central nervous system, potentially leading to fatal outcomes if not treated. The extrapulmonary form of the disease is more diagnosed in HIV seropositive patients, most of them not on appropriate antiretroviral treatment; therefore, this presentation of the disease was considered by the Centers for Disease Control and Prevention as an AIDS-defining illness and it has been considered one of the most frequent opportunistic infections and one of the main causes of mortality among this group of patients.

Oral manifestations of histoplasmosis are well documented in the literature and usually present in the disseminated form of the disease that more often occurs in immunosuppressed patients, many of them due to HIV infection. However, other immunosuppressive conditions such as

P. C. Caldeira (✉) · F. P. Fonseca
Department of Oral Surgery and Pathology, School of Dentistry, Universidade Federal de Minas Gerais, Belo Horizonte, Brazil

E. F. de Mendonça
School of Dentistry, Federal University of Goiás, Goiânia, Brazil
e-mail: elismaur@ufg.br

F. S. C. Pontes
Service of Oral Pathology, João de Barros Barreto University Hospital, Federal University of Pará, Belém, Brazil
e-mail: flaviapontes@ufpa.br

© The Author(s), under exclusive license to Springer Nature Switzerland AG 2025
F. P. Fonseca et al. (eds.), *Lymphoproliferative and Granulomatous Disorders of the Oral Cavity*,
https://doi.org/10.1007/978-3-031-98844-8_8

aging, uncontrolled diabetes and alcoholism, and post radiotherapy or organ transplantations may also account for some cases. Oral lesions commonly present as deep or superficial painful ulcerations or as granulomatous excrescences or as frequently indurated, necrotic, and possibly covered by a yellowish pseudo-membrane, which more often affect the palate, tongue, and buccal mucosa, although any region of the oral cavity can be affected. The involvement of the gingival tissue may simulate an aggressive periodontitis, leading to misdiagnoses and delaying the correct treatment. The lesions can be solitary or multiple, with variable size, possibly achieving large dimensions with several weeks of duration, strongly resembling oral cancer. Patients may also complain of hoarseness of voice, odynophagia, and dysphagia, while the occurrence of regional lymphadenopathy may also be frequently observed.

Diagnoses are usually well established on a clinical and microscopic basis, especially if a large number of microorganisms are present, but cell culture and serology are also complementary exams available for difficult cases, but sensitivity and specificity of serological exams are considered to be variable. For instance, serology tests are believed to result positively in almost 75% of infected patients 6 weeks after the onset of acute disease; however, antibodies can also be detected in up to 10% of asymptomatic individuals from endemic regions.

Although initial pulmonary infection may resolve spontaneously without intervention after the development of cellular immunity to the microorganism, early diagnosis of histoplasmosis is considered mandatory since this is a potentially fatal condition that demands prompt treatment, which is usually established with the use of systemic antifungals like intravenous amphotericin B, combined or not with other less toxic drugs like Itraconazole or Fluconazole depending on clinical parameters. Untreated disseminated infections may be associated with mortality rates that can reach up to 80%. Important to highlight that antifungal susceptibility of the affected patients varies, but resistance to amphotericin B and itraconazole remains low worldwide (Fig. 8.1).

8.2 Microscopic Findings

- The overlying squamous epithelium may be hyperplastic and acanthotic and may also show pseudoepitheliomatous proliferation in some cases.
- In the lamina propria, there is a dense and diffuse lymphohistiocytic infiltrate.
- Histiocytes predominate in the inflammatory infiltrate.
- Epithelioid histiocytes are characterized by large eosinophilic cytoplasm, although histiocytes presenting a clear cytoplasm are also frequently observed.
- Lymphocytes and plasma cells are also present.
- In some patients, histiocytes lead to well-formed granulomas, which, however, are not easily recognizable in all cases.
- In other patients, especially in immunosuppressed individuals, only ill-defined granulomas are present.
- Multinucleated giant cells of the Langhans type are frequently present.
- Microorganisms are considered to have 2–4 μm. They are small, round structures that are commonly found inside the cytoplasm of histiocytes or inside the multinucleated giant cells.
- The presence of microorganisms outside the histiocytes and dispersed in the lesion can also be observed in most of the cases.
- The microorganism is not encapsulated, but an "halo" appearance caused by cytoplasm retracting from the fungal cell wall is observed.
- Special histologic stains, such as Grocott-Gomori methenamine silver and Periodic acid-Schiff (PAS) methods, will highlight the fungal cell wall (Figs. 8.2, 8.3, 8.4, and 8.5).

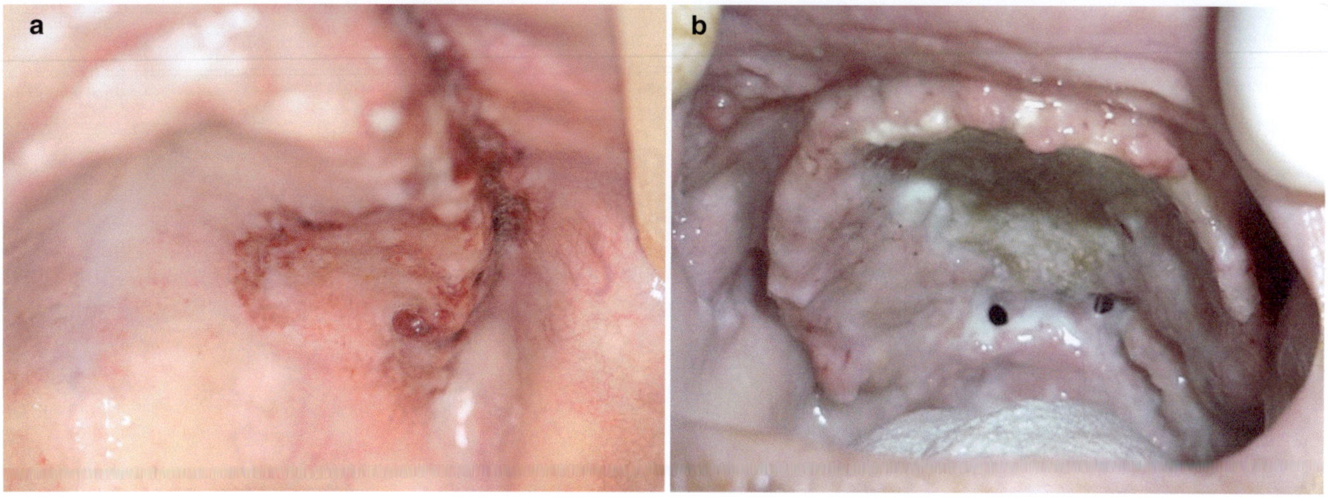

Fig. 8.1 Clinical presentation of histoplasmosis in the oral cavity. (**a**) A male patient exhibiting a painful ulceration in the palate and the alveolar ridge mucosa, extending toward the buccal mucosa. (**b**) Aggressive example of histoplasmosis affecting the palate of a female patient. Observe the extensive necrotic area in the palate

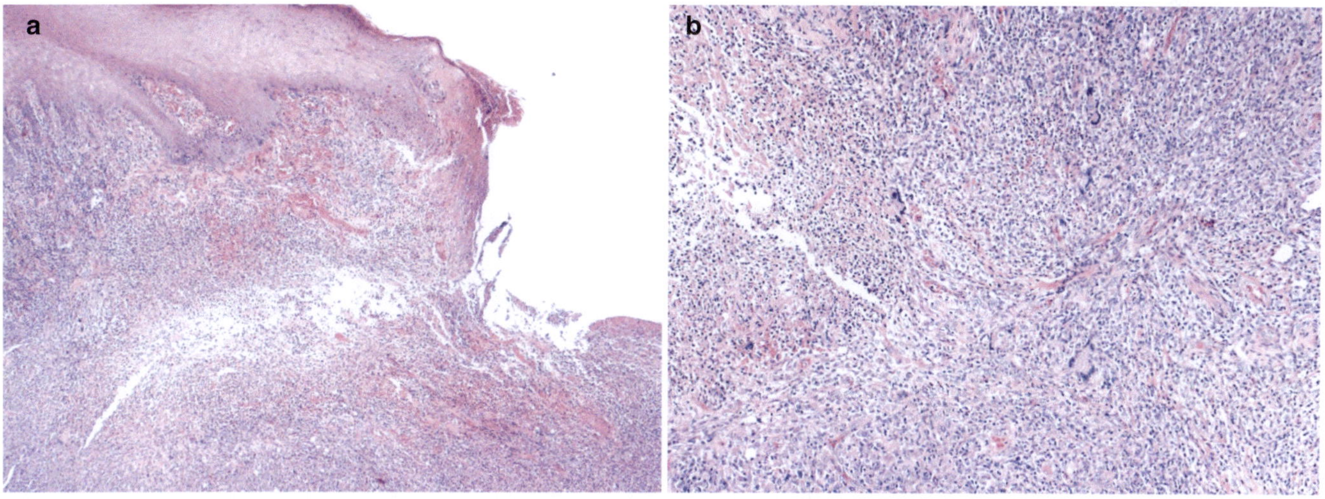

Fig. 8.2 Microscopic features of histoplasmosis in the oral cavity. (**a**) Ulcerated oral mucosa with the overlying squamous epithelium and a dense limphohistiocytic infiltrate in the lamina propria (H&E; 25×). (**b**) The dense infiltrate in the connective tissue of the lamina propria contains a predominance of chronic inflammatory cells like lymphocytes and histiocytes. Observe the presence of scattered multinucleated giant cells in this image (H&E; 50×)

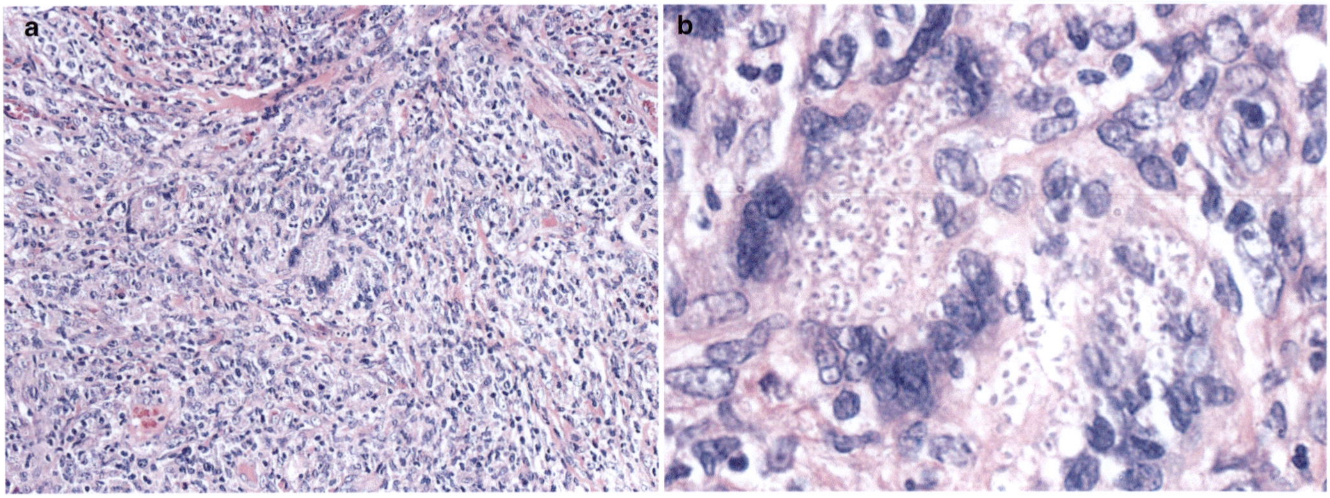

Fig. 8.3 Microscopic features of histoplasmosis in the oral cavity. (**a**) The presence of Langhans-type multinucleated giant cells in the specimen suggests an infectious origin for this process. Multiple small and round structures consistent with *Histoplasma capsulatun* can be observed in the cytoplasm of the histiocytes and multinucleated giant cells, but given their small size, these microorganisms are often difficult to observe under small or medium power (H&E; 100×). (**b**) The presence of the microorganisms can be better appreciated under higher power, as shown in this image. Observe the presence of *Histoplasma capsulatun* predominantly in the cytoplasm of the histiocytes (H&E; 400×)

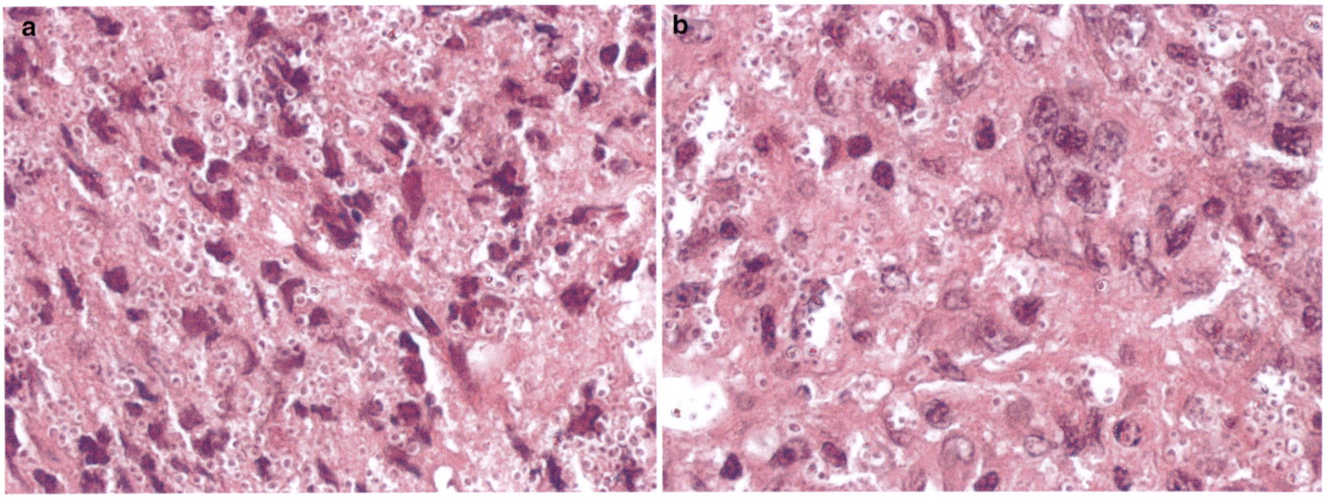

Fig. 8.4 Microscopic features of histoplasmosis in the oral cavity of an immunosuppressed patient. (**a**) Presence of epithelioid macrophages and a large number of round structures consistent with *Histoplasma capsulatun* (H&E; 400×). (**b**) The presence of the microorganisms can be observed with more detail in this image as small round structures surrounded by many macrophages (H&E; 400×)

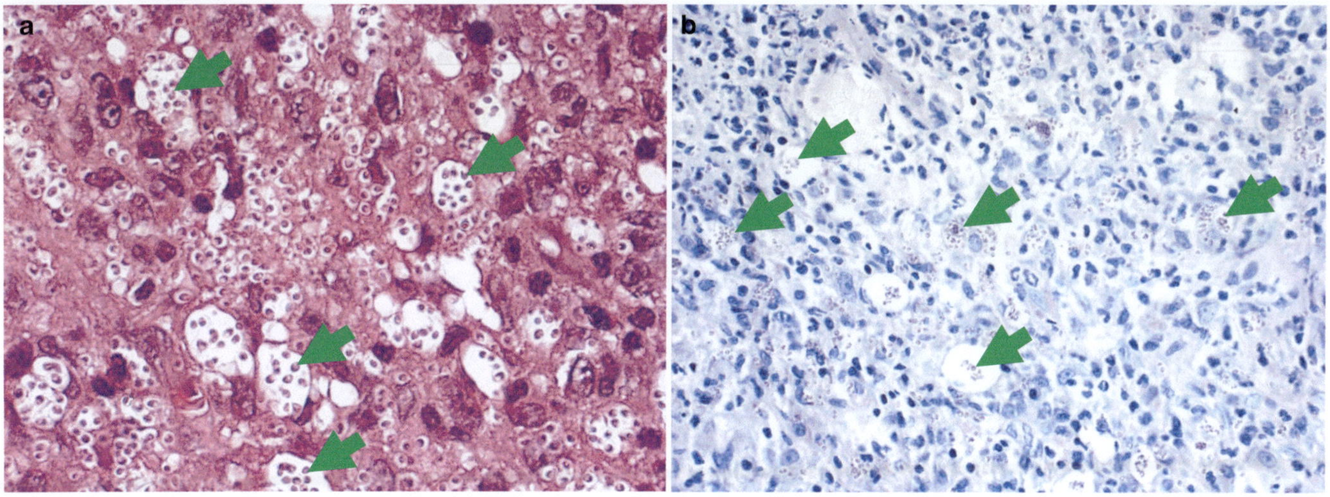

Fig. 8.5 Microscopic features of histoplasmosis in the oral cavity. (**a**) The presence of the microorganism can be easily observed in this high magnification image as small round structures disseminated in the tissue (green arrows) (H&E; 200×). (**b**) Using PAS reaction, note the presence of *Histoplasma capsulatun* predominantly in the cytoplasm of the histiocytes, but also distributed in the whole lesion, presenting as small, reddish structures (green arrows) (PAS; 100×)

8.3 Immunohistochemistry and/or Genetics

The microscopic diagnosis of histoplasmosis is usually established through conventional morphological analysis, with the support of special histological stains like Grocott-Gomori methenamine silver and PAS reactions. However, for pathologists not familiarized with this disease or in cases where the granulomatous features are not easily observed, immunohistochemistry can help demonstrate the reactive nature of the lymphohistiocytic infiltrate. The presence of histiocytes is evidenced using CD68 antibody, and the other chronic inflammatory cell populations, like lymphocytes (using CD20 and CD3, for B cells and T cells, respectively) and plasma cells (using CD138), can also be revealed (Table 8.1, Figs. 8.5 and 8.6).

Table 8.1 Summary of the main immunohistochemical reactions and histological stains that can be used for the diagnosis of histoplasmosis

Antibody/stain	Most frequent results	Pattern	Objective
CD20	Positive	Membrane	To demonstrate B lymphocyte infiltrates
CD3	Positive	Membrane	To demonstrate T lymphocyte infiltrates
CD138	Positive	Membrane	To demonstrate plasma cell infiltrates
CD68	Positive	Cytoplasm	To demonstrate the presence of histiocytes, multinucleated giant cells, and granulomas
PAS[a]	Positive	In the fungus	To show the presence of microorganisms
Grocott-Gomori[a]	Positive	In the fungus	To show the presence of microorganisms

PAS periodic acid-Schiff
[a]Histological stain

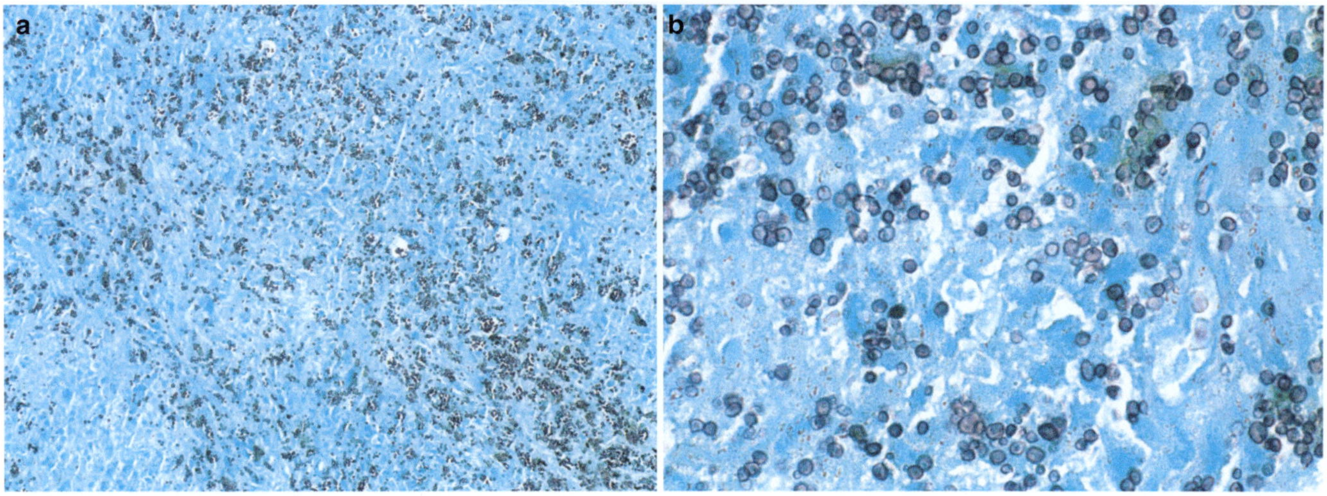

Fig. 8.6 Microscopic features of histoplasmosis in the oral cavity demonstrated by Grocott-Gomori staining. (**a**) The use of the Grocott-Gomori methenamine silver reaction is very useful to observe the microorganisms. Observe that even under medium power, it is possible to observe the fungus as small dark dots (Grocott-Gomori; 50×). (**b**) Under higher power, *Histoplasma capsulatun* can be even better appreciated as small dark dots in the cytoplasm of the histiocytes (Grocott-Gomori; 200×)

Sources

1. Darling ST. A protozoan general infection producing pseudotubercles in the lungs and focal necroses in the liver, spleen, and lymph nodes. JAMA. 1906;46:1283–5.
2. O'Sullivan MV, Whitby M, Chahoud C, Miller SM. Histoplasmosis in Australia: a report of a case with a review of the literature. Aust Dent J. 2004;49:94–7. https://doi.org/10.1111/j.1834-7819.2004.tb00057.x.
3. Hernández SL, López De Blanc SA, Sambuelli RH, Roland H, Cornelli C, Lattanzi V, et al. Oral histoplasmosis associated with HIV infection: a comparative study. J Oral Pathol Med. 2004;33:445–50. https://doi.org/10.1111/j.1600-0714.2004.00183.x.
4. Alcure ML, Di Hipólito JO, Almeida OP, Bonilha H, Lopes MA. Oral histoplasmosis in an HIV-negative patient. Oral Surg Oral Med Oral Pathol Oral Radiol Endod. 2006;101:e33–6. https://doi.org/10.1016/j.tripleo.2005.06.028.
5. Kaufmann CA. Histoplasmosis: a clinical and laboratory update. Clin Microbiol Rev. 2007;20:115–32. https://doi.org/10.1128/CMR.00027-06.
6. Viswanathan S, Chawla N, D'Cruz A, Kane SV. Head and neck histoplasmosis–a nightmare for clinicians and pathologists! Experience at a tertiary referral cancer centre. Head Neck Pathol. 2007;1:169–72. https://doi.org/10.1007/s12105-007-0034-1.
7. Muñante-Cárdenas JL, de Assis AF, Olate S, Lyrio MC, de Moraes M. Treating oral histoplasmosis in an immunocompetent patient. J Am Dent Assoc. 2009;140:1373–6. https://doi.org/10.14219/jada.archive.2009.0072.
8. Narayana N, Gifford R, Giannini P, Casey J. Oral histoplasmosis: an unusual presentation. Head Neck. 2009;31:274–7. https://doi.org/10.1002/hed.20882. Iqbal F, Schifter M, Coleman HG. Oral presentation of histoplasmosis in an immunocompetent patient: a diagnostic challenge. Aust Dent J. 2014;59:386–8. https://doi.org/10.1111/adj.12187
9. Folk GA, Nelson BL. Oral histoplasmosis. Head Neck Pathol. 2017;11:513–6. https://doi.org/10.1007/s12105-017-0797-y.
10. O'Connell Ferster AP, Jaworek A, Hu A. Histoplasmosis of the head and neck in the immunocompetent patient: report of 2 cases. Ear Nose Throat J. 2018;97:E28–31.
11. Pincelli T, Enzler M, Davis M, Tande AJ, Comfere N, Bruce A. Oropharyngeal histoplasmosis: a report of 10 cases. Clin Exp Dermatol. 2019;44:e181–8. https://doi.org/10.1111/ced.13927.
12. Singh A, Gauri M, Gautam P, Gautam D, Haq M, Handa AC, et al. Head and neck involvement with histoplasmosis; the great masquerader. Am J Otolaryngol. 2019;40:678–83. https://doi.org/10.1016/j.amjoto.2019.06.002.
13. Lv X, Jiang M, He R, Li M, Meng J. Clinical features and endemic trend of histoplasmosis in China: a retrospective analysis and literature review. Clin Respir J. 2020;14:307–13. https://doi.org/10.1111/crj.13125.
14. Alawi F, Shields BE, Omolehinwa T, Rosenbach M. Oral granulomatous disease. Dermatol Clin. 2020;38:429–39. https://doi.org/10.1016/j.det.2020.05.004.
15. Morote S, Nacher M, Blaizot R, Ntab B, Blanchet D, Drak Alsibai K, et al. Temporal trends of cutaneo-mucous histoplasmosis in persons living with HIV in French Guiana: early diagnosis defuses south American strain dermotropism. PLoS Negl Trop Dis. 2020;14:e0008663. https://doi.org/10.1371/journal.pntd.0008663.
16. Dao A, Kim HY, Halliday CL, Oladele R, Rickerts V, Govender MMed NP, et al. Histoplasmosis: a systematic review to inform the World Health Organization of a fungal priority pathogens list. Med Mycol. 2024;62:myae039. https://doi.org/10.1093/mmy/myae039.
17. Tello-Mercado AC, Martínez-Guerra BA, Román-Montes CM, Seoane-Hernandez L, Rangel-Cordero A, Martínez-Gamboa RA, et al. Histoplasmosis beyond human immunodeficiency virus (HIV): clinical characteristics and outcomes in a non-HIV population. Open Forum Infect Dis Ther. 2024;11:ofae079. https://doi.org/10.1093/ofid/ofae079.
18. Gandhi P, Hebert B, Yun A, Bradley J, Moldoveanu B. Histoplasmosis around the world: a global perspective on the presentation, virulence factors, and treatment of histoplasmosis. Am J Med Sci. 2024;368:287–99. https://doi.org/10.1016/j.amjms.2024.06.011.

Coccidioidomycosis and Paracoccidioidomycosis

9

Eduardo David Piemonte, Ricardo Martinez Pedraza, Ronell Bologna Molina, Leonardo Amaral dos Reis, João Adolfo Costa Hanemann, and Felipe Paiva Fonseca

9.1 General Overview and Clinical Presentation

Coccidioidomycosis, previously known as San Joaquin fever, Desert fever, or Valley fever, is a deep and invasive fungal infection first described in 1892 in Argentina and currently considered endemic and notifiable in some regions of the USA. The *Coccidioides immitis* occurs more often in the dry soil of the California central valley, portions of Arizona, Texas, New Mexico, and northern Mexico, whereas *Coccidioides posadasii* is more associated with cases diagnosed in the western USA and Latin America regions. *Coccidioides* spp. are dimorphic fungi that grow as mycelial strands that mature to infectious arthroconidia in the soil, and following the inhalation of the spores by mammals, it triggers a morpho-physiological change leading to pathogenic spherules in the lungs. The spherules develop thick walls and form endospores, which are eventually released and initiate a new spherule.

In some regions of the USA, there is a growing public health concern about coccidioidomycosis due to a rising number of cases and a possible influence of climate change on its increase. Different cycles of drought followed by wet winters allow the fungus to thrive and disperse, and when the soil is disturbed by wind or human activities, fungal spores become airborne and increase the risk of inhalation.

Most of the patients are asymptomatic or present as mild cases resembling community-acquired pneumonia, with cough, fever, and fatigue. In immunocompetent patients, the infection may resolve spontaneously. However, a minority of the infected individuals may present chronic and severe forms of the disease, demanding prompt antifungal treatment, especially in immunosuppressed individuals. The use of chest X-ray, PCR reactions, fungal culture, serology exams, and tissue biopsy can be used to aid in the correct diagnosis. Risk factors include exposure to contaminated dust such as archaeologists, military personnel, construction workers, hunters, and earthquake victims, among others. Males are more affected than females, and extrapulmonary coccidioidomycosis most often manifests in the cutaneous, skeletal, and meningeal regions. The clinical appearance of cutaneous lesions is widely variable, ranging from papules, nodules, gummas, ulcerated and verrucous plaques, to scars, abscesses, and fistulae. In the oral cavity, the infection more frequently affects the tongue, followed by the lips, more often as indurated ulcers with elevated borders that may mimic squamous cell carcinoma. Oral lesions may be painful or asymptomatic and can also present as solitary or multiple nodules in the oral mucosa.

Paracoccidioidomycosis is a deep fungal infection originally reported in 1908 in the city of São Paulo (Brazil) by the physician Adolpho Lutz, who reported it as American hyphoblastomycosis. In 1930, Floriano de Almeida first described the differences between *Coccidioides immitis* and the newly described fungus, demonstrating, therefore, that paracoccidioidomycosis and coccidioidomycosis were two distinct conditions. Paracoccidioidomycosis is a systemic and neglected tropical mycosis more frequently diagnosed in Latin America, where it represents the most common deep fungal disease, and Brazil accounts for approximately 80% of all

E. D. Piemonte (✉)
Department of Oral Medicine, Facultad de Odontología, Universidad Nacional de Córdoba, Córdoba, Argentina
e-mail: eduardo.piemonte@unc.edu.ar

R. M. Pedraza
School of Dentistry, Universidad Autónoma de Nuevo León, Nuevo León, Mexico

R. B. Molina
Department of Diagnostic in Pathology and Oral Medicine, Facultad de Odontología, Universidad de la República, Montevideo, Uruguay

L. A. dos Reis · J. A. C. Hanemann
School of Dentistry, Federal University of Alfenas, Alfenas, Brazil
e-mail: leonardo.reis@unifal-mg.edu.br

F. P. Fonseca
Department of Oral Surgery and Pathology, School of Dentistry, Universidade Federal de Minas Gerais, Belo Horizonte, Brazil

© The Author(s), under exclusive license to Springer Nature Switzerland AG 2025

F. P. Fonseca et al. (eds.), *Lymphoproliferative and Granulomatous Disorders of the Oral Cavity*,
https://doi.org/10.1007/978-3-031-98844-8_9

cases diagnosed in this region. It has been previously termed South American blastomycosis, and *Paracoccidioides brasiliensis* is considered the main etiologic agent of the disorder. It was once regarded as a monotypic taxon, but recent molecular taxonomy has demonstrated the existence of additional species, including *Paracoccidioides americana*, *Paracoccidioides restrepiensis*, *Paracoccidioides venezuelensis*, and *Paracoccidioides lutzii*.

Humans and the nine-banded armadillo (*Dasypus novemcinctus*) are the hosts of the dimorphic fungus *Paracoccidioides* spp., usually being infected in rural and peri-urban environments. Respiratory infection occurs via inhalation of conidia present in nature, which later reach the pulmonary alveoli. The acute or subacute ("juvenile") clinical form of the disease is less common and more prevalent among children and young adults. On the other hand, the chronic form of the disease accounts for 80–95% of all cases, more often diagnosed in individuals after the third decade of life, usually affecting the lungs, the oral mucosa, the nasal mucosa, skin in places adjacent to the mouth and nose, and cervical lymph nodes. The incubation period is uncertain, and the disease may manifest many months after the initial contact with the pathogenic agent. There is a striking male predominance due to occupational issues and the protective effect of female estrogen hormone that inhibits the fungal transformation to its pathogenic form, with a male-to-female ratio of approximately 10:1 in some studies. Diagnosis is usually based on clinical, radiographic, and histologic data, but serology, direct smear, fungal culture, and oral or pulmonary cytology are also described in the literature.

Oral lesions are commonly observed in paracoccidioidomycosis, reported in up to 60% of all cases. The oral manifestations of the disease usually present as "mulberry-like" ulcerations/moriform appearance, i.e., granular, erythematous, or ulcerated lesions surrounded by jagged edges with a thin hemorrhagic dotted edge, presenting as solitary or multiple lesions, with the gingiva and palate being the most affected regions, followed by the labial and buccal mucosae, but virtually any site of the oral mucosa can be involved. Affected mucosa presents a hardened consistency on palpation, and the lesions are usually painful. Squamous cell carcinoma and granulomatosis with polyangiitis are important differential diagnoses that should be ruled out using histopathological evaluation. The synchronous occurrence of oral paracoccidioidomycosis and oral squamous cell carcinoma is very rare, but it has already been described in the literature.

There is still no clinically useful vaccine to prevent coccidioidomycosis and paracoccidioidomycosis, and treatment more often comprises a combined use of different antifungal compounds, more commonly amphotericin B, itraconazole, and fluconazole (Figs. 9.1 and 9.2).

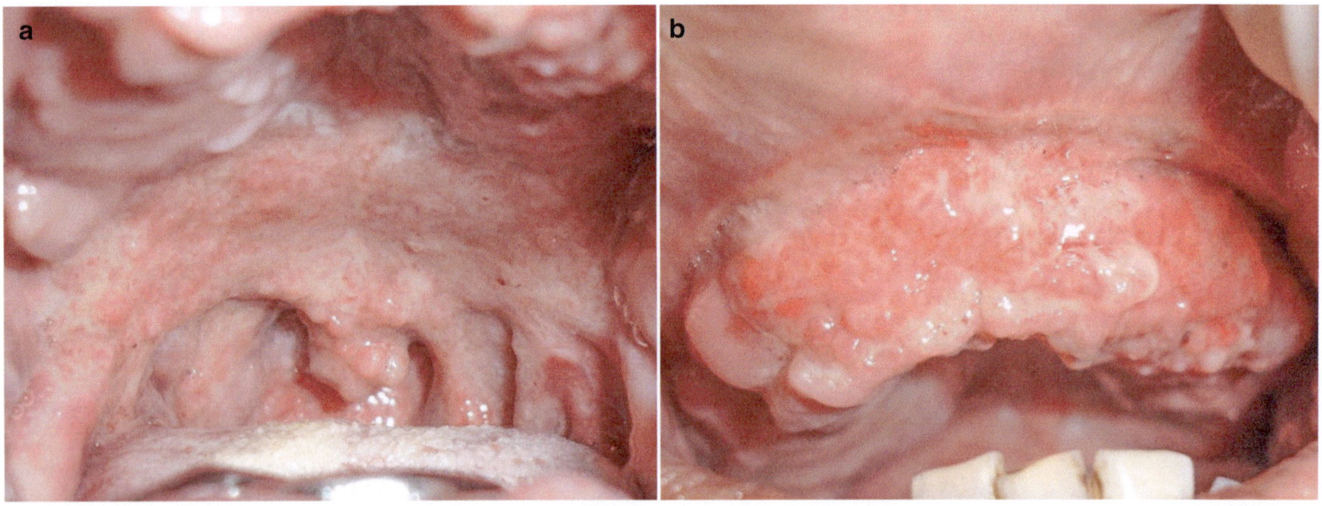

Fig. 9.1 Clinical presentation of paracoccidioidomycosis in the oral mucosa. (**a**) A male patient exhibiting a painful ulceration affecting the soft palate. Note the granular aspect of the ulcer. (**b**) The lesion also affected the maxillary alveolar mucosa. Observe the presence of a yellowish pseudo-membrane and the irregular, granular aspect of the ulcer that also contained small reddish dots characteristic of oral paracoccidioidomycosis

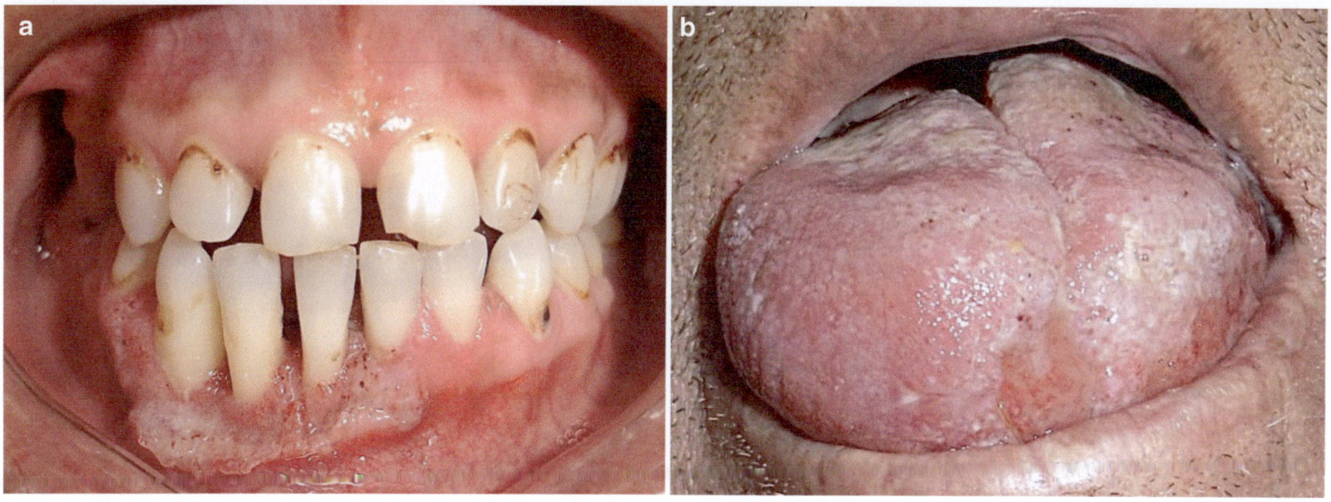

Fig. 9.2 Clinical presentation of paracoccidioidomycosis in the oral mucosa. (**a**) Patient exhibiting a painful ulceration affecting the lower gingival tissue. The presence of the reddish hemorrhagic dots leading to the so-called moriform ulcer is characteristic of paracoccidioidomycosis, but it can also be observed in other conditions like granulomatosis with polyangiitis. (**b**) A male patient exhibiting a diffuse involvement of the tongue by paracoccidioidomycosis. Note the moriform appearance on the tongue surface

9.2 Microscopic Findings

9.2.1 Coccidioidomycosis

- Overlying squamous epithelium may be hyperplastic and acanthotic, or ulcerated.
- The lamina propria typically shows a dense granulomatous inflammatory reaction.
- In addition to the presence of well-formed granulomas, there is an abundant lymphoplasmacytic chronic inflammatory infiltrate.
- Multinucleated giant cells, Langhans-type, are present.
- Neutrophils and necrosis may be present in some cases.
- Immunosuppressed patients more often show ill-formed granulomas or nonspecific chronic inflammatory infiltrate with a predominance of histiocytes, lymphocytes, and plasma cells.
- *Coccidioides* spp. are identified as large, round, spherical structures.
- The spheres stain positively with periodic acid-Schiff (PAS) and Grocott-Gomori methenamine silver histological stains.

9.2.2 Paracoccidioidomycosis

- Overlying squamous epithelium is usually hyperplastic, and pseudoepitheliomatous proliferation is a common finding. Ulcerated regions are also common, and intraepithelial neutrophilic microabscesses are usually present.
- In the lamina propria, there is a dense granulomatous inflammatory infiltrate.
- Well-formed granulomas are common, with the presence of epithelioid histiocytes and Langhans-type multinucleated giant cells.
- A dense lymphoplasmacytic infiltrate is observed, and eosinophils are also present.
- Only the yeast forms of the fungus are found in the tissues, frequently phagocytized by multinucleated giant cells or dispersed in the lamina propria.
- The microorganism is characterized by round structures ranging from 2 to 10 μm in diameter. The fungus cell walls are double refractile.
- The appearance of budding yeasts of *Paracoccidioides* spp. is usually comparable to "Mariner's wheel" or "Mickey Mouse ears."
- The microorganism stains positively with PAS and Grocott-Gomori methenamine silver histological stains (Figs. 9.3, 9.4, and 9.5).

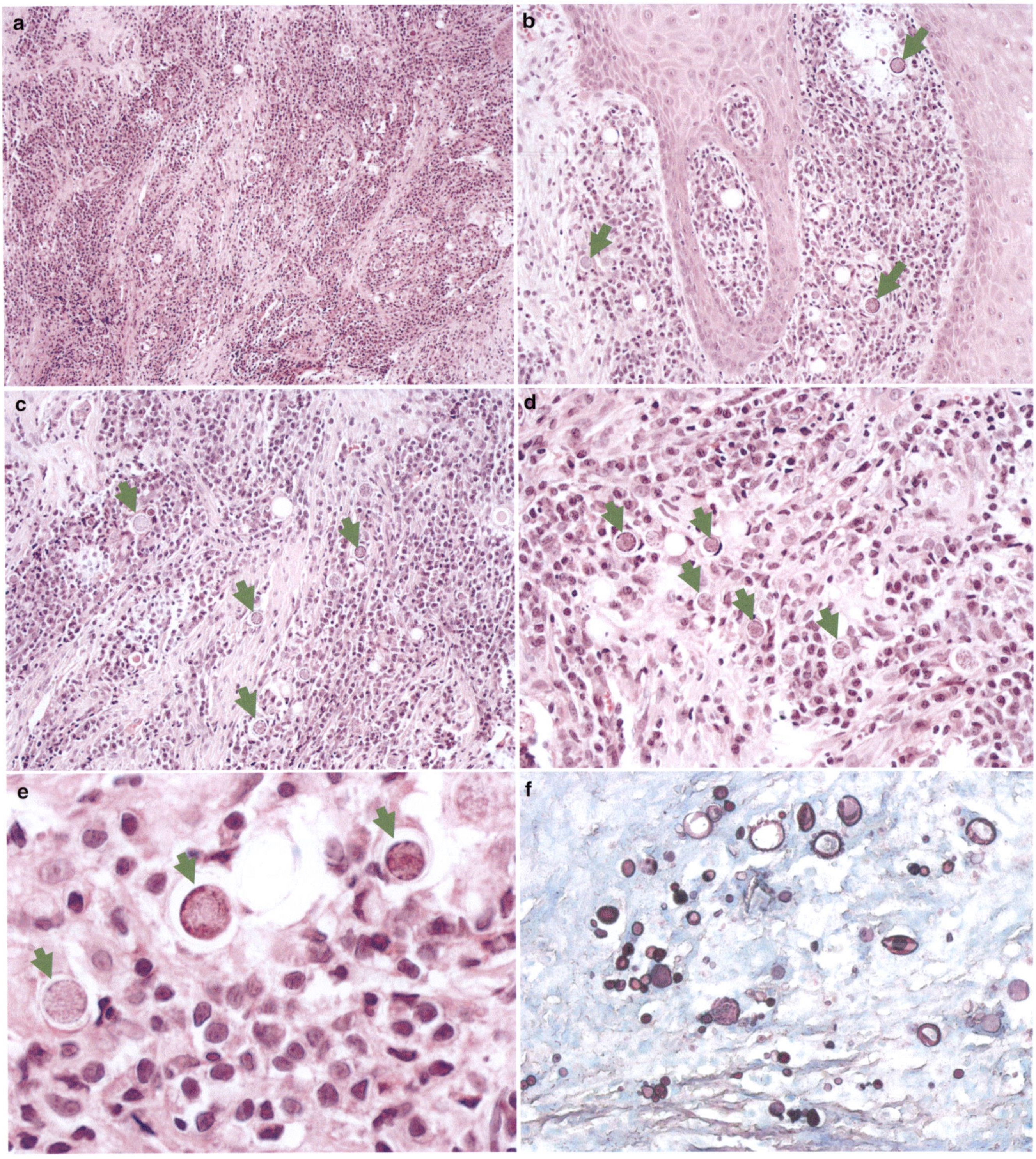

Fig. 9.3 Microscopic findings of coccidioidomycosis affecting the oral mucosa. (**a**) Granulomatous inflammatory process surrounded by diffuse lymphoplasmacytic infiltrate in the lamina propria (H&E; 100×). (**b**) The microorganisms (green arrows) are large, round structures surrounded by histocytes and plasma cells located near the overlying squamous epithelium (H&E; 100×). (**c**) Note the dense chronic inflammatory infiltrate associated with the fungus (green arrows) (H&E; 100×). (**d**) The microorganisms are round structures (green arrows) (H&E; 400×). (**e**) Under high magnification, it is possible to better appreciate the microscopic features of the microorganisms (green arrows). Observe that they are large, round structures (H&E; 1000×). (**f**) Methenamine silver Grocott-Gomory stain highlights the presence of the microorganisms by staining them in a black color pattern (Grocott-Gomory; 400×)

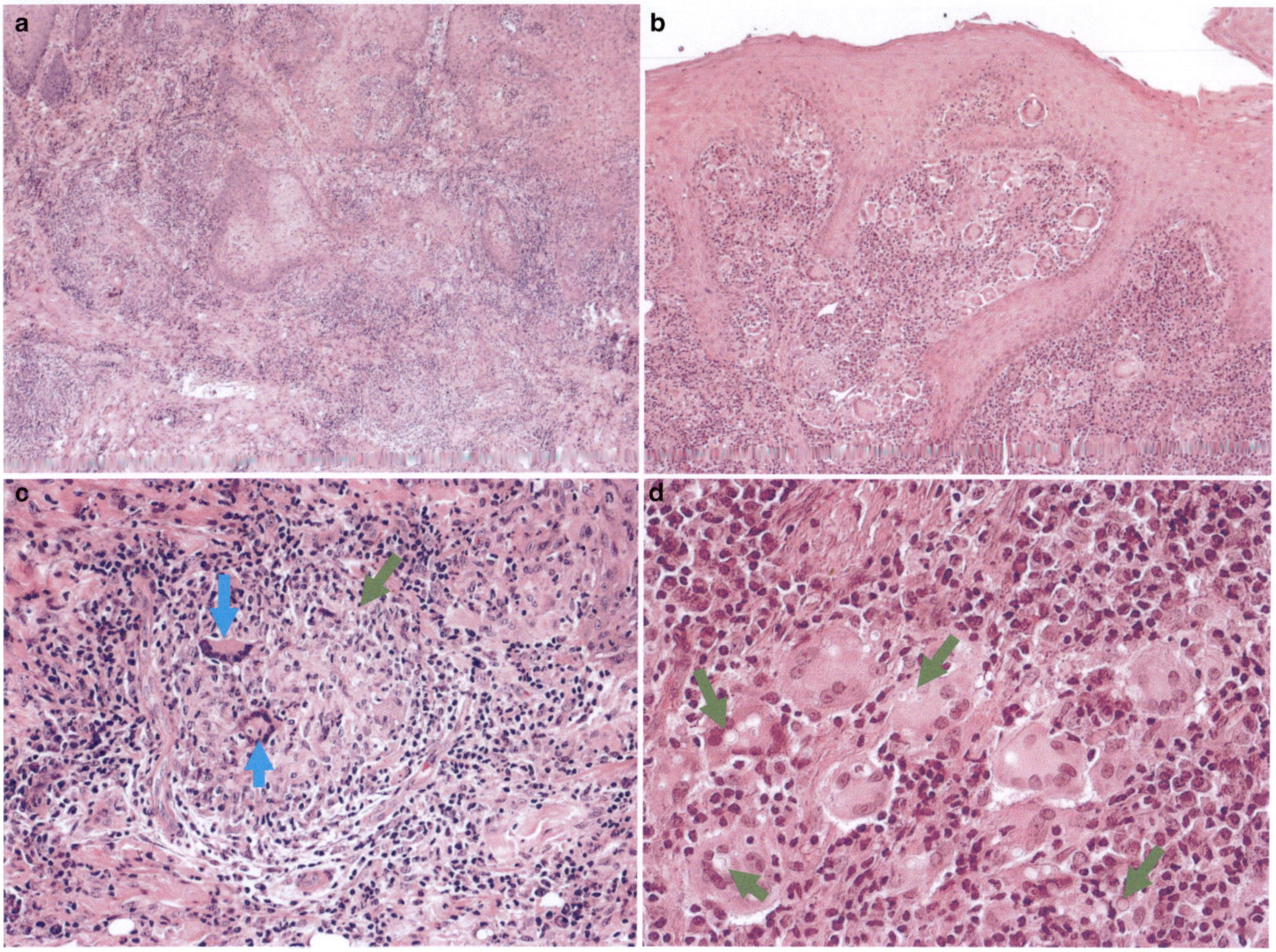

Fig. 9.4 Microscopic findings of paracoccidioidomycosis affecting the oral mucosa. (**a**) Hyperplastic squamous epithelium with pseudoepitheliomatous proliferation is a common finding in this infection (H&E; 50×). (**b**) In the lamina propria, it is possible to observe various Langhans-type multinucleated giant cells, surrounded by a histiocytic and lymphoplasmacytic inflammatory infiltrate (H&E; 100×). (**c**) The granulomatous inflammatory infiltrate is the hallmark of the disease, and it is characterized by the presence of well-formed granulomas (green arrow), most of them containing multinucleated giant cells (blue arrows) (H&E; 200×). (**d**) Langhans-type multinucleated giant cells containing multiple microorganisms (green arrows) in the cytoplasm. Note that the microorganisms are smaller than in coccidioidomycosis, and present as round structures that are also found outside the multinucleated giant cells, distributed through the lamina propria (H&E; 400×)

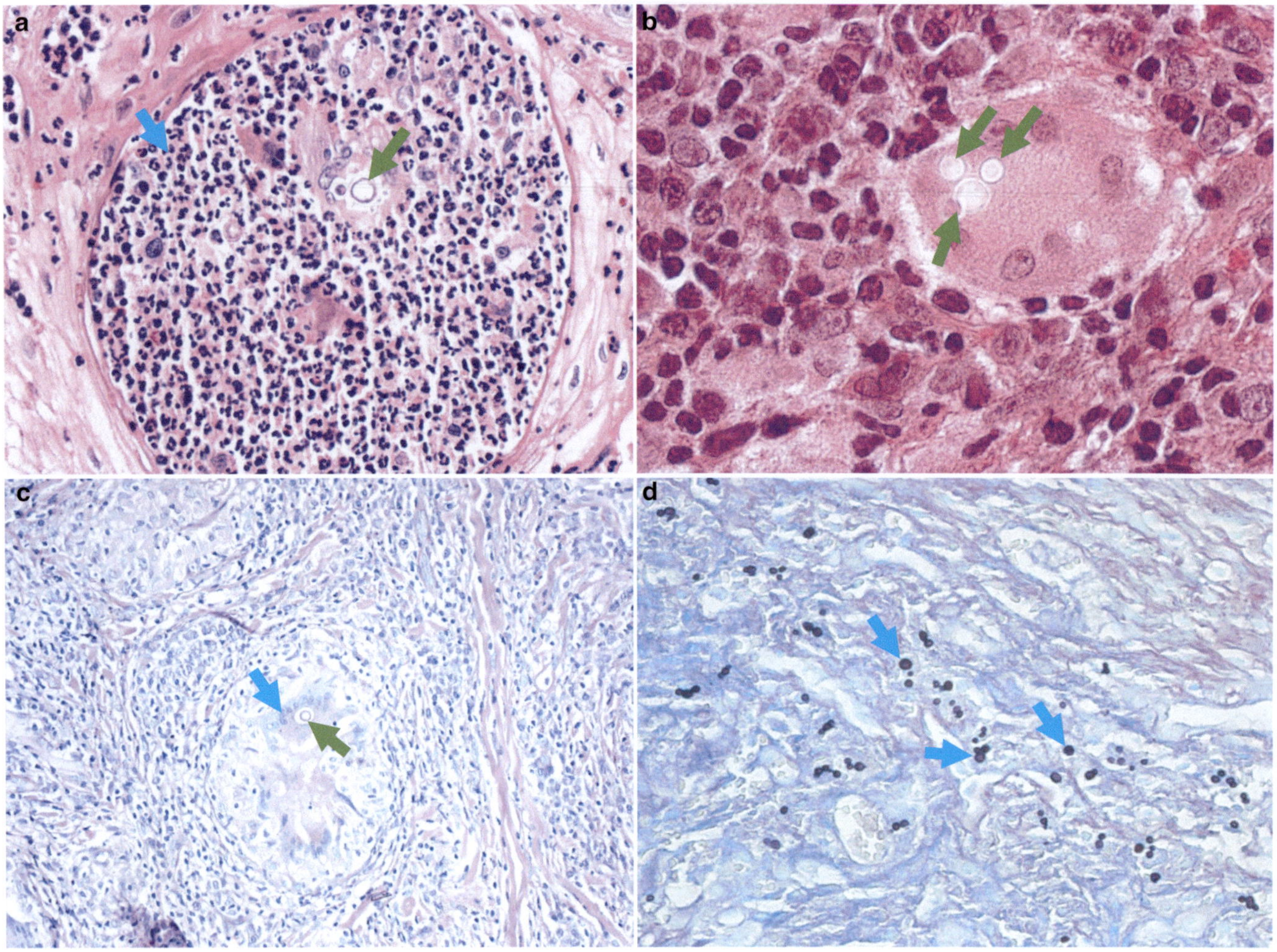

Fig. 9.5 Microscopic findings of paracoccidioidomycosis affecting the oral mucosa. (**a**) Neutrophilic abscesses (blue arrow) are commonly observed in paracoccidioidomycosis. Observe the presence of a microorganism inside the microabscess region (green arrow) (H&E; 400×). (**b**) Under high magnification, observe the presence of the round, birefringent microorganisms inside the Langhans-type multinucleated giant cell cytoplasm (green arrows) (H&E; 1000×). (**c**) Well-formed granuloma with multinucleated giant cells and the presence of a microorganism is highlighted by periodic acid-Schiff stain (PAS; 200×). (**d**) The microorganisms of paracoccidioidomycosis can also be better appreciated using methenamine silver Grocott-Gomori stain. Note the multiple round black colored structures that represent the microorganisms (green arrows) (H&E; 200×)

Table 9.1 Summary of the main immunohistochemical reactions and histological stains that can be used for the diagnosis of coccidioidomycosis and paracoccidioidomycosis

Antibody/stain	Most frequent results	Pattern	Objective
CD20	Positive	Membrane	To demonstrate B lymphocyte infiltrates
CD3	Positive	Membrane	To demonstrate T lymphocyte infiltrates
CD138	Positive	Membrane	To demonstrate plasma cell infiltrates
CD68	Positive	Cytoplasm	To demonstrate the presence of macrophages, multinucleated giant cells, and granulomas
PAS[a]	Positive	In the fungus	To show the presence of microorganisms
Grocott-Gomori[a]	Positive	In the fungus	To show the presence of microorganisms

PAS Periodic acid-Schiff
[a]Histological stain

9.3 Immunohistochemistry and/or Genetics

The microscopic diagnosis of coccidioidomycosis and paracoccidioidomycosis is usually established through conventional morphological analysis, with the support of special histological stains like Grocott-Gomori methenamine silver and PAS reactions. However, for pathologists not familiarized with this disease or in cases where the granulomatous features are not easily observed, immunohistochemistry can help demonstrate the reactive nature of the lymphohistiocytic infiltrate. The presence of macrophages is evidenced using the CD68 antibody, and other chronic inflammatory cell populations, like lymphocytes (using CD20 and CD3, for B cells and T cells, respectively) and plasma cells (using CD138), can also be revealed (Table 9.1, Figs. 9.3 and 9.5).

Sources

1. Almeida OP, Jacks J Jr, Scully C. Paracoccidioidomycosis of the mouth: an emerging deep mycosis. Crit Rev Oral Biol Med. 2003;14:377–83. https://doi.org/10.1177/154411130301400508.
2. Hirschmann JV. The early history of coccidioidomycosis: 1892–1945. Clin Infect Dis. 2007;44:1202–7. https://doi.org/10.1086/513202.
3. Azevedo RS, Gouvêa AF, Lopes MA, Corrêa MB, Jorge J. Synchronous oral paracoccidioidomycosis and oral squamous cell carcinomas with submandibular enlargement. Med Mycol. 2011;49:84–9. https://doi.org/10.3109/13693786.2010.496118.
4. Mendez LA, Flores SA, Martinez R, de Almeida OP. Ulcerated lesion of the tongue as manifestation of systemic coccidioidomycosis. Case Rep Med. 2017;2017:1489501. https://doi.org/10.1155/2017/1489501.
5. Trindade AH, Meira HC, Pereira IF, de Lacerda JCT, de Mesquita RA, Santos VR. Oral paracoccidioidomycosis: retrospective analysis of 55 Brazilian patients. Mycoses. 2017;60:521–5. https://doi.org/10.1111/myc.12622.
6. de Arruda JAA, Schuch LF, Abreu LG, Silva LVO, Mosconi C, Monteiro JLGC, et al. A multicentre study of oral paracoccidioidomycosis: analysis of 320 cases and literature review. Oral Dis. 2018;24:1492–502. https://doi.org/10.1111/odi.12925.
7. Dutra LM, Silva THM, Falqueto A, Peçanha PM, Souza LRM, Gonçalves SS, et al. Oral paracoccidioidomycosis in a single-center retrospective analysis from a Brazilian southeastern population. J Infect Public Health. 2018;11:530–3. https://doi.org/10.1016/j.jiph.2017.10.009.
8. Neves-Silva R, Fernandes PM, Santos-Silva AR, Vargas PA, de Souza Cavalcante R, Lopes MA. Unusual intestinal involvement by paracoccidioidomycosis diagnosed after oral manifestation. Mycopathologia. 2018;183:987–93. https://doi.org/10.1007/s11046-018-0250-0.
9. Hahn RC, Rodrigues AM, Della Terra PP, Nery AF, Hoffmann-Santos HD, Góis HM, et al. Clinical and epidemiological features of paracoccidioidomycosis due to Paracoccidioides lutzii. PLoS Negl Trop Dis. 2019;13:e0007437. https://doi.org/10.1371/journal.pntd.0007437.
10. Myers RA, Zmarlicka MT. Disseminated coccidioidomycosis. N Engl J Med. 2019;380:e44. https://doi.org/10.1056/NEJMicm1811100.
11. Gabriel A, Mu A. A 42-year-old man with lingual nodules and a headache. Clin Infect Dis. 2019;69:1827–9. https://doi.org/10.1093/cid/ciy1075.
12. Costa MC, de Carvalho MM, Sperandio FF, Ribeiro Junior NV, Hanemann JAC, Pigossi SC, et al. Oral Paracoccidioidomycosis affecting women: a systematic review. Mycoses. 2021;64:108–22. https://doi.org/10.1111/myc.13194.
13. Hahn RC, Hagen F, Mendes RP, Burger E, Nery AF, Siqueira NP, et al. Paracoccidioidomycosis: current status and future trends. Clin Microbiol Rev. 2022;35:e0023321. https://doi.org/10.1128/cmr.00233-21.
14. de Oliveira LLC, de Arruda JAA, Marinho MFP, Cavalcante IL, Abreu LG, Abrahão AC, et al. Oral paracoccidioidomycosis: a retrospective study of 95 cases from a single center and literature review. Med Oral Patol Oral Cir Bucal. 2023;28:e131–9. https://doi.org/10.4317/medoral.25613.
15. Heaney AK, Camponuri SK, Head JR, Collender P, Weaver A, Sondermeyer Cooksey G, et al. Coccidioidomycosis seasonality in California: a longitudinal surveillance study of the climate determinants and spatiotemporal variability of seasonal dynamics, 2000–2021. Lancet Reg Health Am. 2024;38:100864. https://doi.org/10.1016/j.lana.2024.100864.

Leishmaniasis

10

Gleyson Kleber do Amaral-Silva, Marianne de Vasconcelos Carvalho, Hélder Antônio Rebelo Pontes, Wilson Delgado-Azañero, and Felipe Paiva Fonseca

10.1 General Overview and Clinical Presentation

Leishmaniasis is a parasitic and noncontagious infection considered a neglected tropical disease by the World Health Organization, with a prevalence estimated at 12 million cases worldwide. Each year, approximately 700,000 to one million new cases are reported, and its incidence is believed to be increasing due to continuous urbanization, climate change, migration, and travel into endemic areas. It is caused by different species of the genus *Leishmania* spp., transmitted by the bite of infected female sandflies, and is considered endemic in many tropical and subtropical countries. There are at least 21 species of *Leishmania* that can cause human disease.

The genus *Leishmania* is believed to have evolved in the Mesozoic era, and the prehistoric existence of Leishmania-like species is documented in two fossils, one of them preserved in a 100-million-year-old Cretaceous Burmese amber. In the modern era, many reports are available from the sixteenth century onward regarding skin lesions consistent with the so-called "Oriental sore," and following the Spanish colonization process, reports provided by the conquistadors and missionaries describing diseases reminiscent of mucocutaneous leishmaniasis are known. One of the first reports of the disease in the Americas described cutaneous lesions in Brazil, referred to as "Bahia sore" or "Biskra sore." Years later, the Brazilian Physician Gaspar de Oliveira Vianna named the parasite *Leishmania braziliensis* and made significant contributions to the development of the treatment for this disease.

Leishmania species are usually separated into Old World and New World types according to their geographic location; the former is found in open semiarid areas or deserts in some parts of Asia, the Middle East, Africa (mainly in the northern and tropical regions), and southern Europe, whereas the latter is more common in the forests, specifically in Mexico and Central and South America. Old World leishmaniasis is caused primarily by *Leishmania major*, *Leishmania tropica*, and *Leishmania aethiopica*, whereas New World leishmaniasis is caused by *Leishmania mexicana*, *Leishmania venezuelensis*, *Leishmania amazonensis*, or the Viannia complex, such as *Leishmania brasiliensis*, *Leishmania panamensis*, *Leishmania guyanensis*, and *Leishmania peruviana*. Nonetheless, this traditional classification of *Leishmania* species (Old World × New World) is now regarded as imprecise, sparking ongoing discussions in contemporary research. It reflects a historical perspective that does not accurately represent the ecological and epidemiological complexities of the disease. In recognition of these limitations, the World Health Organization (WHO) adopts a region-specific approach, classifying leishmaniasis based on its predominant clinical forms and geographical distribution.

G. K. do Amaral-Silva (✉)
Department of Oral Pathology, School of Dentistry, Federal University of Mato Grosso do Sul, Campo Grande, Brazil
e-mail: gleyson.amaral@ufms.br

M. d. V. Carvalho
Department of Oral Pathology, School of Dentistry, Universidade de Pernambuco, Recife, Brazil

Integrated Center for Pathological Anatomy, Oswaldo Cruz University Hospital, Universidade de Pernambuco, Recife, Brazil
e-mail: marianne.carvalho@upe.br

H. A. R. Pontes
Service of Oral Pathology, João de Barros Barreto University Hospital, Federal University of Pará, Belém, Brazil
e-mail: harp@ufpa.br

W. Delgado-Azañero
Department of Oral Pathology, Oral Medicine and Oral Surgery, School of Dentistry, Universidad Peruana Cayetano Heredia, Lima, Peru
e-mail: wilson.delgado@upch.pe

F. P. Fonseca
Department of Oral Surgery and Pathology, School of Dentistry, Universidade Federal de Minas Gerais, Belo Horizonte, Brazil

© The Author(s), under exclusive license to Springer Nature Switzerland AG 2025
F. P. Fonseca et al. (eds.), *Lymphoproliferative and Granulomatous Disorders of the Oral Cavity*,
https://doi.org/10.1007/978-3-031-98844-8_10

Leishmania species exist as promastigotes (flagellated extracellular forms found in sandflies) and amastigotes (non-flagellated and obligate intracellular forms found in vertebral hosts). The life cycle of *Leishmania* begins when an infected female sandfly bites a human or other terrestrial mammal to take a blood meal, injecting promastigotes in the process. These promastigotes are then phagocytosed by macrophages, where they transform into amastigotes. Inside the macrophages, the amastigotes proliferate, infecting additional macrophages and spreading the infection throughout various tissues of the host. Subsequently, another female sandfly becomes infected by feeding on the host's blood, which contains macrophages filled with amastigotes. In the sandfly's gut, the amastigotes transform into extracellular promastigotes, which replicate and migrate to the mosquito's mouthparts. There, they await the opportunity to be transmitted to a new host.

The clinical manifestations of leishmaniasis are usually classified as cutaneous (localized or diffuse), mucocutaneous, and visceral and are determined by the parasite species and host immunological state. Cutaneous leishmaniasis is more often caused by *Leishmania mexicana*, *Leishmania braziliensis*, or *Leishmania panamensis* in the Americas, and *Leishmania major* or *Leishmania tropica* in all other countries. It usually begins with a painless papule or nodule at the site of microorganism inoculation and progresses to diffuse, non-ulcerating, erythematous to violaceous macules, nodules, and plaques heavily infiltrated with amastigotes. The most commonly affected sites are the face and the upper and lower extremities.

In contrast to cutaneous leishmaniasis, mucocutaneous leishmaniasis is a more potentially life-threatening disease, and mucosal manifestations occur in approximately 10% of the cases. The mucocutaneous variant is usually associated with *Leishmania braziliensis*, but also with *Leishmania panamensis*, *Leishmania guyanensis*, and *Leishmania amazonensis*. In these cases, the cutaneous lesions usually represent the first manifestation of the disease, but after the hematological and lymphatic spread of the microorganism, mucosal lesions may develop and the nasal, pharyngeal and the oral mucosas can be affected. In some cases, patients may show mucosal lesions from 1 to 5 years after the cutaneous lesion has healed, and most of the patients have scars from the prior cutaneous lesions. Anterior nasal septal granulomas can be appreciated using a light source and Thudicum's speculum. More advanced disease may show nasal septum perforation, which may eventually progress to destruction of the oronasopharyngeal mucosa and cartilaginous facial and upper airway structures, resulting in disfiguration, secondary infection, and airway obstruction. Lymphadenopathy is common and can be accompanied by fever and hepatomegaly.

In rare instances, oral lesions may represent the disease's first and only manifestation and may lead to a primary diagnosis. The palate is the most frequently affected location in the oral cavity, frequently secondary to palatine perforation and communication with the nasal cavity. In such cases, patients may already have nasal septum destruction, which can be used as a diagnostic finding for leishmaniasis, but that may also strongly simulate the clinical manifestation of extranodal NK/T cell lymphoma, and the differentiation between these two entities may be very difficult. Other oral mucosa sites like the tongue and cheek mucosa can also be affected, and the infection usually manifests as nonspecific deep and irregular, frequently indurated ulcerations. Moreover, erythema, erosions, and ulcers around the nares and lips are seen as the disease progresses.

Visceral leishmaniasis (also called "black fever" or "kala-azar" in India) is a disease usually caused by *Leishmania donovani* and *Leishmania infantum* (synonym for *Leishmania chagasi*) that more often demonstrates an insidious or subacute onset of clinical symptoms including malaise, fatigue, fever, moderate hepatomegaly, splenomegaly, lymphadenopathy, and gradually darkening discoloration of the skin. Diarrhea and malabsorption might occur, and anemia develops because of bone marrow suppression, while thrombocytopenia and hepatic dysfunction contribute to hemorrhagic complications. Neutropenia and eosinopenia are also observed. Late in the course of the disease, cachexia, hypoalbuminemia, jaundice, and ascites are observed due to severe hepatic dysfunction and hypoalbuminemia. Renal impairment and hemophagocytic lymphohistiocytosis are complications that may also occur, and if no treatment is administered, visceral leishmaniasis is lethal.

The diagnosis of leishmaniasis relies on a combination of clinical, laboratory, and molecular approaches to increase early detection and accurate disease recognition. Parasitological diagnosis remains the gold standard, with direct microscopic examination of Giemsa-stained smears, in vitro culture of the parasite in Novy–MacNeal–Nicolle (NNN) medium, or detection of amastigotes in tissue biopsies. The Montenegro skin test, a delayed-type hypersensitivity reaction, can indicate prior exposure but does not differentiate between active and past infections. Serological tests, including enzyme-linked immunosorbent assays (ELISA) and immunochromatographic rapid tests, are useful for visceral leishmaniasis but have limited sensitivity for cutaneous and mucocutaneous forms. Polymerase chain reaction (PCR) assays provide high sensitivity and specificity, enabling species identification and differentiation from other infections with similar clinical presentations. Emerging approaches such as loop-mediated isothermal amplification (LAMP) and next-generation sequencing (NGS) are being explored for improved diagnostic accuracy.

The treatment of leishmaniasis varies according to the clinical form of the disease and the Leishmania species involved. Pentavalent antimonials, such as meglumine antimoniate and sodium stibogluconate, remain the first-line treatment in most cases, with cure rates ranging from 60% to 90%. However, their toxicity and the need for prolonged parenteral administration limit their use. Liposomal amphotericin B is an effective alternative, particularly for patients with contraindications to antimonials, with cure rates exceeding 95%. Miltefosine, an oral agent, is increasingly used, especially for cutaneous and mucocutaneous leishmaniasis, due to its ease of administration and comparable efficacy to conventional treatments. Recent advances include combination therapies, immunomodulators, and targeted parasite inhibitors, aiming to improve efficacy and minimize resistance. The immunological state of the patient will significantly impact his/her prognosis, and despite various vaccines that are under clinical trials, no authorized/licensed vaccines are available to protect patients from leishmaniasis (Figs. 10.1, 10.2, and 10.3).

Leishmania–HIV coinfection represents a significant public health challenge, as HIV-positive individuals are at higher risk of developing disseminated leishmaniasis with atypical presentations, increased parasite burden, and poor treatment response. Co-infected individuals face higher relapse and mortality rates, with antiretroviral therapy playing a crucial role in delaying disease progression and improving survival outcomes.

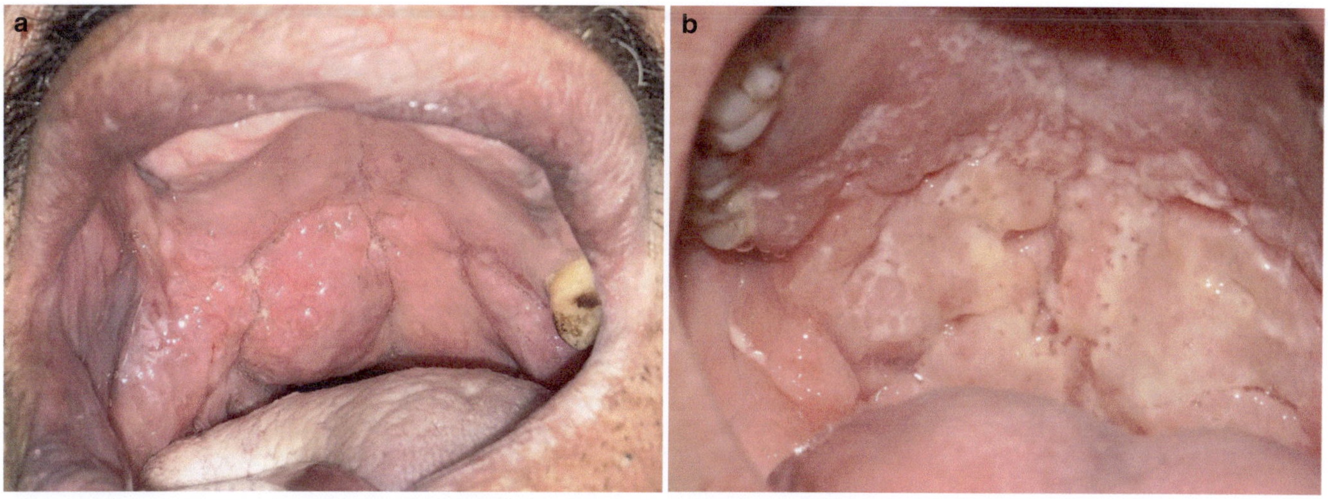

Fig. 10.1 Clinical presentation of leishmaniasis affecting the oral cavity. (**a**) A male patient presenting with a painful nodule with an irregular surface on the right side of the palate. The surrounding palatine mucosa is also affected, appearing erythematous with a granular and irregular surface. Therefore, the limits of the lesion are poorly defined. Small yellowish necrotic regions are seen. (**b**) The palatine mucosa is diffusely affected in this case. Observe extensive regions of tissue necrosis affecting the palate. In some instances, the distinction from an extranodal NK/T cell lymphoma is very difficult to accomplish

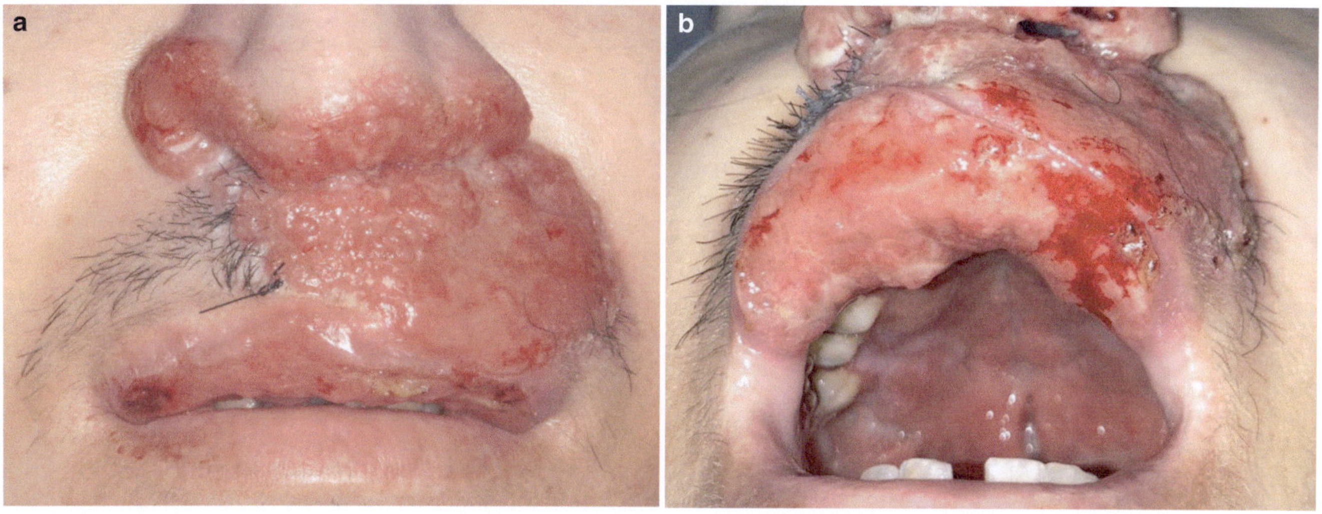

Fig. 10.2 Clinical presentation of leishmaniasis. (**a**) This male patient presented with the nasal cavity and the skin of the face extensively affected by leishmaniasis. The lesion extended toward the upper lip as multiple ulcers. The palate was also affected and ulcerated. (**b**) Observe that the upper lip of the patient is also affected, exhibiting a diffuse and irregular swelling, ulcerative regions, and a hard consistency on palpation. The hard and soft palates of the patient are also affected

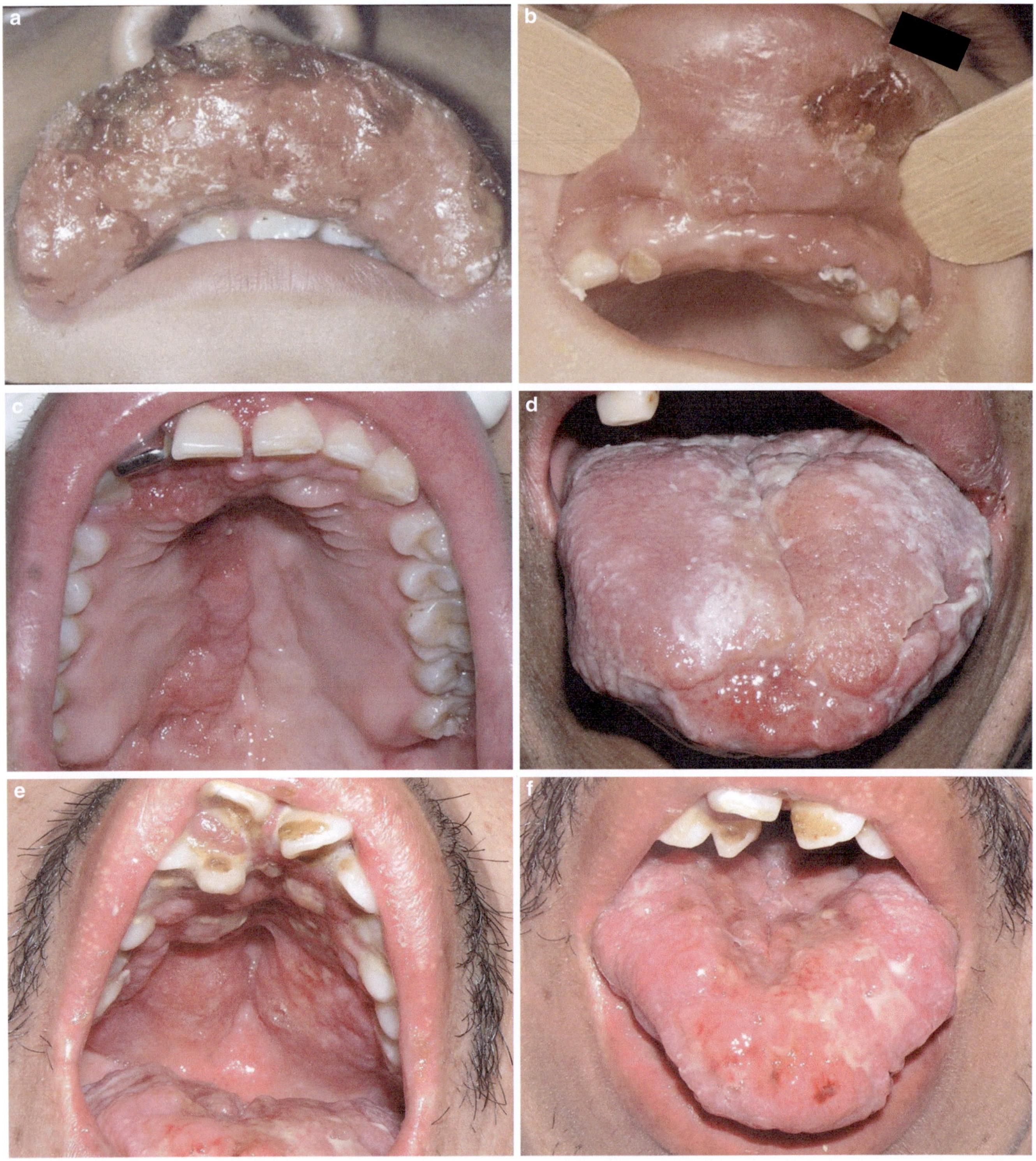

Fig. 10.3 Clinical presentation of leishmaniasis affecting Peruvian patients. (**a**) Diffuse enlargement of the upper lip of an infant patient affected by leishmaniasis. (**b**) Painful and indurated ulcer in the upper lip of a Peruvian child. (**c**) Oral leishmaniasis manifesting in the palate of a male patient. Note that the lesion extends toward the gingival mucosa. (**d**) A 50-year-old male patient presented with a painful ulcerated and indurated lesion in the tongue. (**e**) A male patient with extensive leishmaniasis manifestations in the oral cavity. The ulcerated lesion affected the hard and soft palates and extended to the oropharynx. (**f**) The same patient in *E* also presented an enlarged and ulcerated tongue, also affected by the infection

10.2 Microscopic Findings

- Hyperplastic or ulcerated squamous epithelium.
- Dense infiltration of chronic inflammatory infiltrate in the lamina propria.
- There is a predominance of lymphocytes and macrophages, but a variable number of neutrophils can also be seen, especially near ulcerated regions.
- Presence of non-necrotizing granulomatous inflammatory reaction is common.
- A background containing necrotic tissue is also common.
- Presence of numerous macrophages that present a clear or epithelioid aspect.
- Multinucleated giant cells may occur.
- Using Giemsa and H&E stains, microorganisms are observed in the form of amastigotes located within the cytoplasm of macrophages as pale blue oval bodies with a dark blue nucleus and a small rod-shaped kinetoplast (extranuclear structure containing mitochondrial DNA). The microorganisms are negative for Grocott-Gomori methenamine silver and PAS stains.
- Toxoplasmosis and histoplasmosis are important differential diagnoses that must be ruled out (Figs. 10.4, 10.5, 10.6, and 10.7).

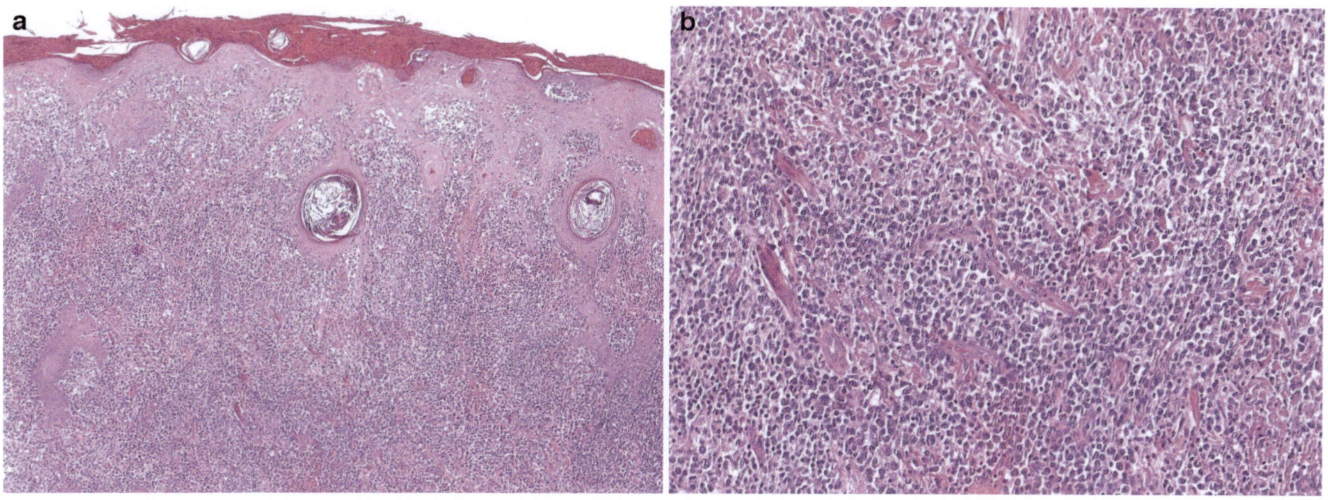

Fig. 10.4 Microscopic features of oral leishmaniasis. (**a**) Overlying squamous epithelium of the oral mucosa and a dense chronic inflammatory infiltrate in the lamina propria. Observe the predominance of lymphocytes and the presence of epithelioid macrophages (H&E; 50×). (**b**) The chronic inflammatory infiltrate is predominantly composed of lymphocytes, plasma cells, and macrophages (H&E; 100×)

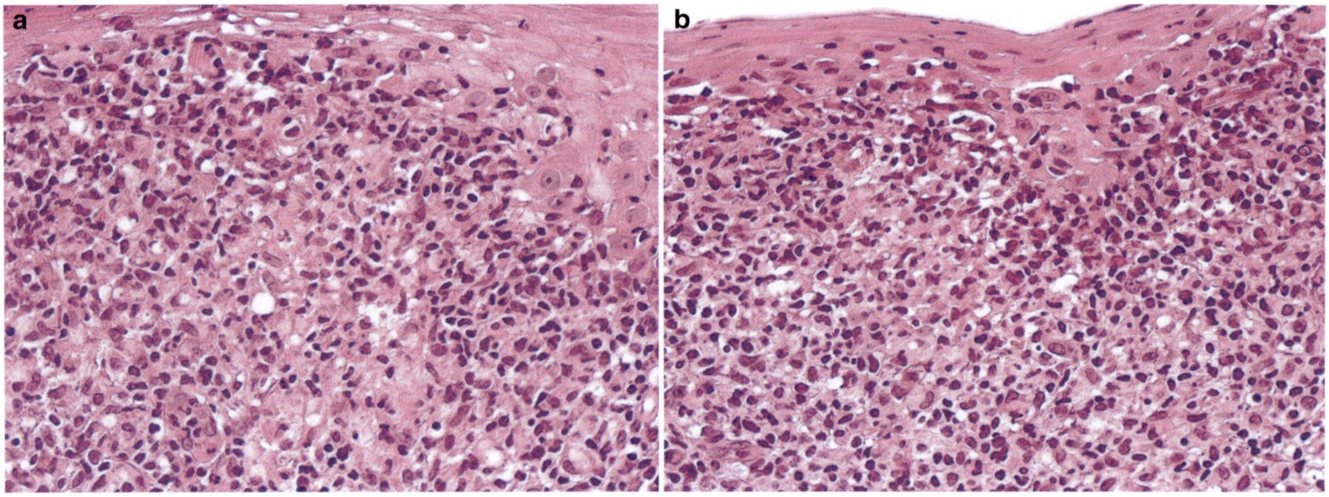

Fig. 10.5 Microscopic features of oral leishmaniasis. (**a**) A dense reactive inflammatory infiltrate is present in the lamina propria (H&E; 200×). (**b**) The chronic inflammatory infiltrate is predominantly composed of lymphocytes, plasma cells, and especially epithelioid macrophages. The presence of multinucleated giant cells and well or poorly formed granulomas can be found in some cases, although they are not present in this image (H&E; 200×)

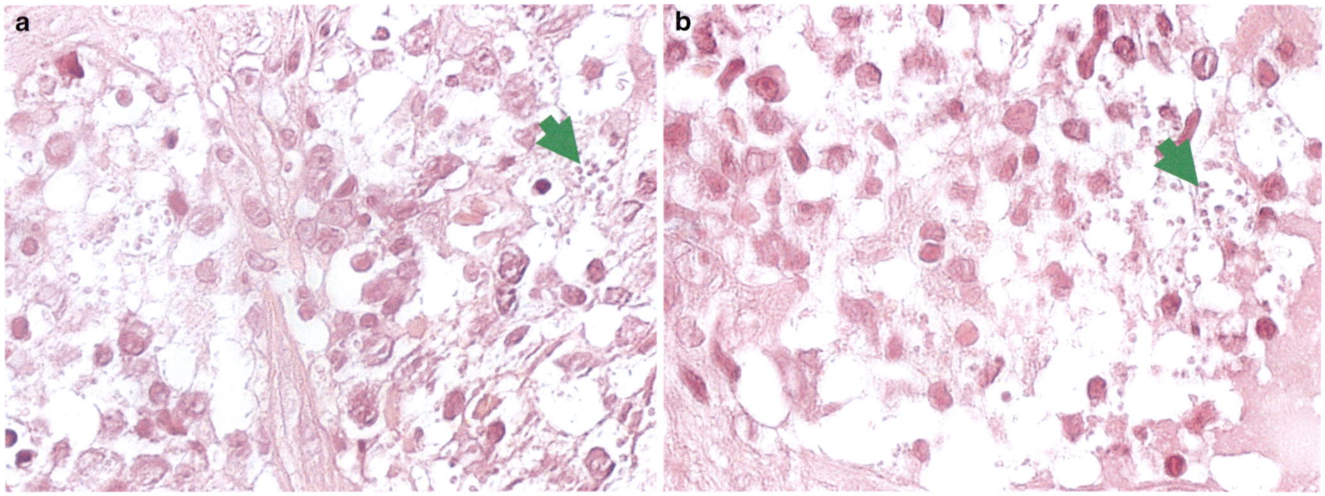

Fig. 10.6 Microscopic features of oral leishmaniasis. (**a**) Higher magnification showing the amastigotes in the biopsied tissue. Observe the small round structures near the green arrow and in other parts of the specimen, too (H&E; 400×). (**b**) Another example of amastigotes in a biopsied tissue of leishmaniasis. Observe the small round structures (green arrow) (H&E; 400×)

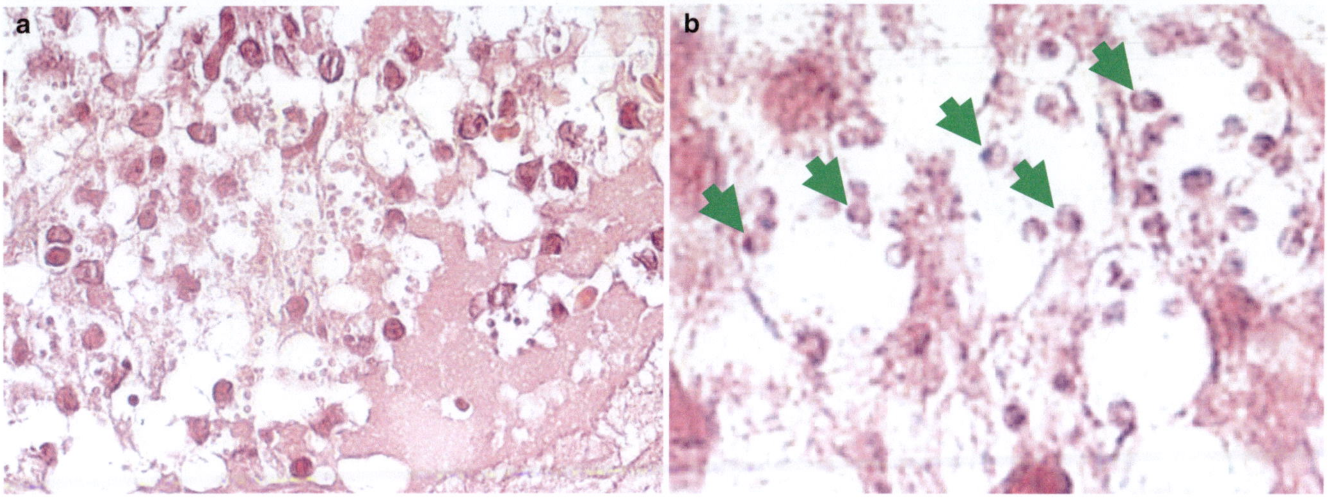

Fig. 10.7 Microscopic features of oral leishmaniasis. (**a**) Higher magnification showing innumerable amastigotes in the biopsied tissue (H&E; 400×). (**b**) Observe that amastigotes have a darker structure located in the periphery representing the kinetoplast (green arrow) (H&E; 1000×)

Table 10.1 Summary of the main immunohistochemical reactions and histological stains used for leishmaniasis diagnosis

Antibody/stain	Most frequent results	Pattern	Objective
CD20	Positive	Membrane	To characterize the inflammatory infiltrate (B lymphocytes)
CD3	Positive	Membrane	To characterize the inflammatory infiltrate (T lymphocytes)
CD68	Positive	Cytoplasm	To characterize the inflammatory infiltrate (macrophages)
Leishmaniasis antigen	Positive	In the microorganisms	To demonstrate the presence of the microorganism
Giemsa[a]	Positive	Nonspecific	To facilitate the identification of the microorganism

[a]Histological stain

10.3 Immunohistochemistry and/or Genetics

The identification of the parasite is mandatory to establish the diagnosis of Leishmaniasis in a tissue biopsy. Although in immunosuppressed patients, a high number of microorganisms might become easily identifiable using routine staining or Giemsa stain; however, in many cases, the number of microorganisms is scarce, and the chronic inflammatory infiltrate becomes very nonspecific. Brown-Hopps, Gram, or Leishman stains are other, less-used stains useful for diagnosing leishmaniasis. In these circumstances, the identification of the leishmania will demand the use of immunohistochemistry, which, however, may reveal a false-negative result in many instances, or even a PCR reaction to demonstrate the DNA content of the parasite (Table 10.1, Figs. 10.8 and 10.9).

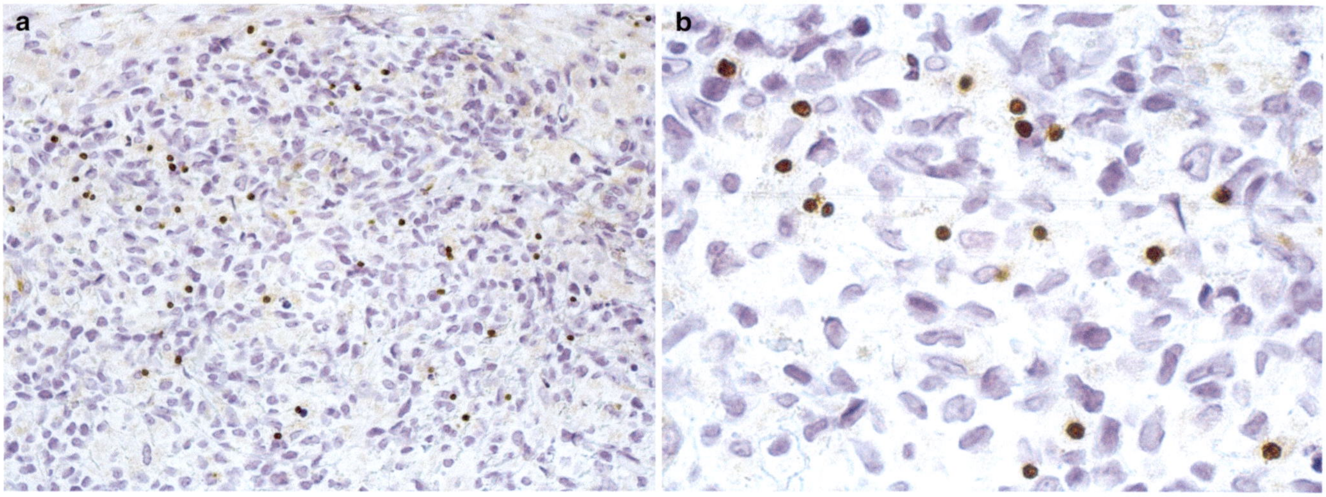

Fig. 10.8 Immunohistochemistry applied to oral leishmaniasis diagnosis. (**a**) The microorganism is distributed in the tissue (DAB; 200×). (**b**) Observe the dot-like pattern highlighting the presence of the microorganisms (DAB; 400×)

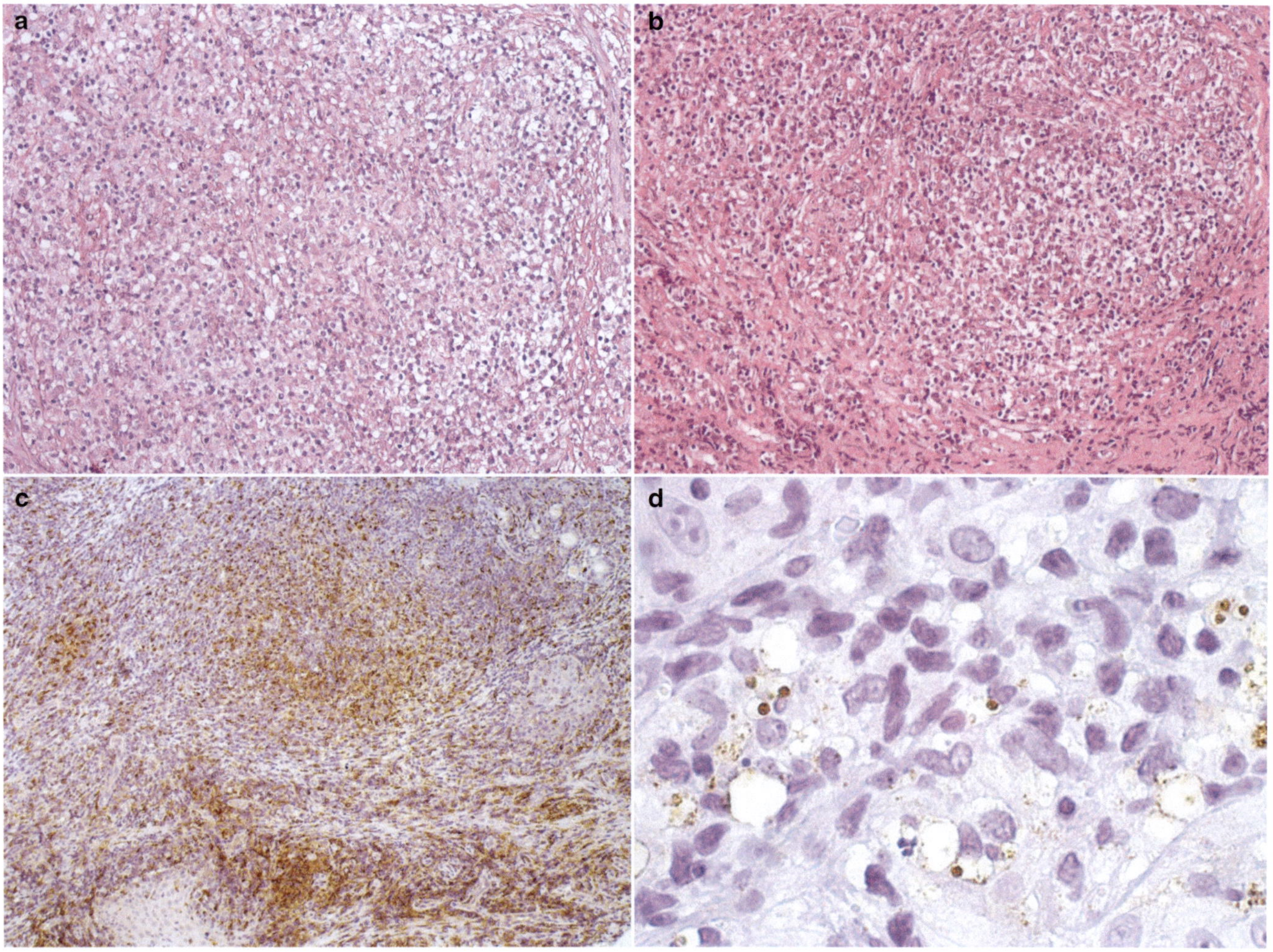

Fig. 10.9 Microscopic features of oral leishmaniasis. (**a**) Dense chronic inflammatory infiltrate predominantly composed of macrophages and lymphocytes (H&E; 100×). (**b**) Note the presence of clear cells in some regions consistent with macrophages (H&E; 100×). (**c**) The use of CD68 immunohistochemical staining can be useful to confirm the macrophagic nature of the inflammatory infiltrate, highlighting the presence of granulomas (DAB; 50×). (**d**) The microorganisms can also be demonstrated by immunohistochemistry (DAB; 400×)

Sources

1. Motta AC, Lopes MA, Ito FA, Carlos-Bregni R, de Almeida OP, Roselino AM. Oral leishmaniasis: a clinicopathological study of 11 cases. Oral Dis. 2007;13:335–40. https://doi.org/10.1111/j.1601-0825.2006.01296.x.
2. David CV, Craft N. Cutaneous and mucocutaneous leishmaniasis. Dermatol Ther. 2009;22:491–502. https://doi.org/10.1111/j.1529-8019.2009.01272.x.
3. Nadler C, Enk CD, Leon GT. Diagnosis and management of oral leishmaniasis-case series and literature review. J Oral Maxillofac Surg. 2014;72:927–34. https://doi.org/10.1016/j.joms.2013.10.021.
4. Crovetto-Martínez R, Aguirre-Urizar JM, Orte-Aldea C, Araluce-Iturbe I, Whyte-Orozco J, Crovetto-de la Torre MA. Mucocutaneous leishmaniasis must be included in the differential diagnosis of midline destructive disease: two case reports. Oral Surg Oral Med Oral Pathol Oral Radiol. 2015;119:e20–6. https://doi.org/10.1016/j.oooo.2014.09.008.
5. Mignogna MD, Celentano A, Leuci S, Cascone M, Adamo D, Ruoppo E, et al. Mucosal leishmaniasis with primary oral involvement: a case series and a review of the literature. Oral Dis. 2015;21:e70–8. https://doi.org/10.1111/odi.12268.
6. Almeida TF, da Silveira EM, Santos CR. Exclusive primary lesion of oral leishmaniasis with immunohistochemical diagnosis. Head Neck Pathol. 2016;10:533–7. https://doi.org/10.1007/s12105-016-0732-7.
7. Cruz AF, Resende RG, Albuquerque DR, de Lacerda JC, Leite CF, Aguiar MCF. Mucosal leishmaniasis in Brazilian patients: two case reports with similar clinical presentation and different approaches. Oral Surg Oral Med Oral Pathol Oral Radiol. 2016;122:e199–203. https://doi.org/10.1016/j.oooo.2016.02.017.
8. Ponte-Sucre A, Gamarro F, Dujardin JC, Barrett MP, López-Vélez R, García-Hernández R, Pountain AW, Mwenechanya R, Papadopoulou B. Drug resistance and treatment failure in leishmaniasis: a 21st century challenge. PLoS Negl Trop Dis. 2017;11:e0006052. https://doi.org/10.1371/journal.pntd.0006052.
9. Steverding D. The history of leishmaniasis. Parasit Vectors. 2017;10:82. https://doi.org/10.1186/s13071-017-2028-5.
10. Maia-Elkhoury ANS, Sierra Romero GA, Valadas SYOB, Sousa-Gomes ML, Lindoso JAL, Cupolillo E, et al. Premature deaths by visceral leishmaniasis in Brazil investigated through a cohort study: a challenging opportunity? PLoS Negl Trop Dis. 2019;13:e0007841. https://doi.org/10.1371/journal.pntd.0007841.
11. Mariz BALA, Sánchez-Romero C, Alvarado NAP, Campos EMM, Almeida OP, Martínez-Pedraza R. Diffuse cutaneous leishmaniasis with oral involvement in a patient of northern Mexico. Trop Dr. 2019;49:303–6. https://doi.org/10.1177/0049475519852207.
12. Sánchez-Romero C, Júnior HM, Matta VLRD. Immunohistochemical and molecular diagnosis of mucocutaneous and mucosal leishmaniasis. Int J Surg Pathol. 2020;28:138–45. https://doi.org/10.1177/1066896919876706.
13. Chong GM, Ong DSY, de Mendonça MM, van Hellemond JJ. Painful and swollen tongue: mucosal leishmaniasis due to leishmania infantum. Int J Infect Dis. 2021;113:109–12. https://doi.org/10.1016/j.ijid.2021.09.071.
14. de Arruda JAA, Tomo S, Cunha JLS, Guevara JR, Martínez I, Reyes O, et al. Mucosal leishmaniasis of the lip: report of an exuberant case in a young man. Head Neck Pathol. 2023;17:540–5. https://doi.org/10.1007/s12105-022-01497-8.
15. Karampas G, Koulouraki S, Daikos GL, Nanou C, Aravantinos L, Eleftheriades M, et al. Visceral leishmaniasis in a twin pregnancy: a case report and review of the literature. J Clin Med. 2024;13:2400. https://doi.org/10.3390/jcm13082400.
16. Rosa ACG, de Senna AM, Santos FP, Soares AB, de Araújo VC. Oral leishmaniasis in HIV-positive and HIV-negative patients: a comparative analysis with two new case reports. Head Neck Pathol. 2024;18:69. https://doi.org/10.1007/s12105-024-01674-x.
17. van Dijk NJ, Hagos DG, Huggins DM, Carrillo E, Ajala S, Chicharro C, Kiptanui D, Solana JC, Abner E, Wolday D, Schallig HDFH. Simplified molecular diagnosis of visceral leishmaniasis: laboratory evaluation of miniature direct-on-blood PCR nucleic acid lateral flow immunoassay. PLoS Negl Trop Dis. 2024;18:e0011637. https://doi.org/10.1371/journal.pntd.0011637.
18. Yizengaw E, Gashaw B, Yimer M, Takele Y, Nibret E, Yismaw G, et al. Demographic characteristics and clinical features of patients presenting with different forms of cutaneous leishmaniasis, in lay Gayint, northern Ethiopia. PLoS Negl Trop Dis. 2024;18:e0012409. https://doi.org/10.1371/journal.pntd.0012409.
19. Mehrotra S, Tiwari R, Kumar R, Sundar S. Advances and challenges in the diagnosis of leishmaniasis. Mol Diagn Ther. 2025;29:195–212. https://doi.org/10.1007/s40291-024-00762-6.
20. World Health Organization. Leishmaniasis [Internet]. Geneva: World Health Organization; 2023 Jan 12 [cited 2024 Feb 19]. Available from: https://www.who.int/news-room/fact-sheets/detail/leishmaniasis.

Part III

Non-neoplastic Lesions

Lymphoid Hyperplasias in the Oral Cavity

11

Vivian Petersen Wagner, Victor Zanetti Drumond, Ricardo Alves Mesquita, and Felipe Paiva Fonseca

11.1 General Overview and Clinical Presentation

Reactive lymphoid proliferations are frequently found in the oral and maxillofacial region under different presentations. They may appear as part of the microscopic presentation of non-lymphoid conditions, such as lymphoepithelial cysts or mucosal diseases, including leukoplakia and lichenoid reactions. Additionally, they can manifest as lymphoproliferative disorders, such as follicular lymphoid hyperplasia, which often pose diagnostic difficulties to pathologists not familiarized with these entities.

Currently, literature does not propose any classification scheme for lymphoid hyperplasias in the oral cavity, and they are randomly described in manuscripts dealing with different entities. However, to better appreciate the biological importance and significance of these lymphoid aggregates in the oral cavity, it is possible to organize them under five different clinicopathological scenarios, which are summarized in Fig. 11.1. The dental and periodontal inflammatory infiltrates associated with biofilm accumulation and other specific dental and gingival conditions will be discussed in Chap. 12.

Intra-oral biopsies might reveal a (1) *reactive lymph node*, which is considered a benign idiopathic proliferation of small lymph nodes located in the face. It is an uncommon finding, but when present, it is characterized by an asymptomatic, well-defined, and mobile nodule, more often in the buccal mucosa or upper lip. Occasionally, a subset of these lymph nodes demonstrates the occurrence of progressive transformation of germinal centers (PTGC), a benign reactive process with a poorly understood pathogenesis. This condition is characterized by the proliferation the mantle zone cells toward the germinal center, which, in some instances, becomes atrophic and poorly defined. PTGC is often identified during occasional microscopic evaluation of lymph nodes, as most cases are asymptomatic, though a few may present as painless swellings. It has been hypothesized that the presence of PTGC may increase the risk for lymphoma development, especially nodular lymphocyte predominant Hodgkin Lymphoma (NLPHL), an uncommon type of B-cell lymphoma characterized by large neoplastic germinal center-derived lymphocyte predominant cells within a vaguely nodular reactive background of small, mature lymphocytes and histiocytes. This theory, however, still lacks full validation (Fig. 11.2).

The (2) Waldeyer's ring consists of non-contiguous *mucosa-associated lymphoid tissues (MALT)*. It includes four main tonsillar structures: the pharyngeal, tubal, palatine, and lingual tonsils, along with small collections of lymphoid tissue dispersed throughout the mucosal lining. These lymphoid tissues may also proliferate under a myriad of unspecific antigenic stimuli, requiring pathologists to carefully evaluate them microscopically to rule out other conditions, especially low-grade lymphomas. Palatine tonsils are the most frequently affected and usually manifest as painful or asymptomatic bilateral swellings (Figs. 11.3, 11.4, and 11.5). Another very commonly affected site by lymphoid hyperplastic growths in the oral cavity comprises the lingual tonsils located in the postero-lateral region of the tongue (Fig. 11.6). This site also represents the most commonly affected location by (3) *lymphoepithelial cysts* that typically carry a dense lymphoid component in their fibrous capsule and that in some circumstances can be misdiagnosed as a lymphoid hyperplasia or as a low-grade lymphoma due to the lack of a visible epithelial component lining the cystic cavity (Fig. 11.7).

Different (4) *mucosal diseases* affecting the oral cavity and the lips, such as lichen planus, lichenoid reactions, actinic cheilitis, leukoplakia, and oral squamous cell

V. P. Wagner (✉)
Department of Oral Medicine, School of Dentistry, University of São Paulo, São Paulo, Brazil

V. Z. Drumond · R. A. Mesquita · F. P. Fonseca
Department of Oral Surgery and Pathology, School of Dentistry, Universidade Federal de Minas Gerais, Belo Horizonte, Brazil
e-mail: ramesquita@ufmg.br

© The Author(s), under exclusive license to Springer Nature Switzerland AG 2025

F. P. Fonseca et al. (eds.), *Lymphoproliferative and Granulomatous Disorders of the Oral Cavity*,
https://doi.org/10.1007/978-3-031-98844-8_11

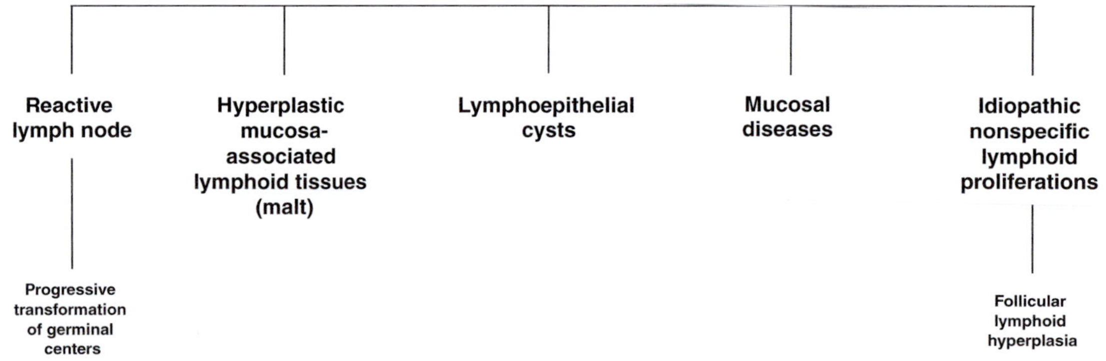

Fig. 11.1 Schematic summary of oral lesions containing reactive lymphoid aggregates

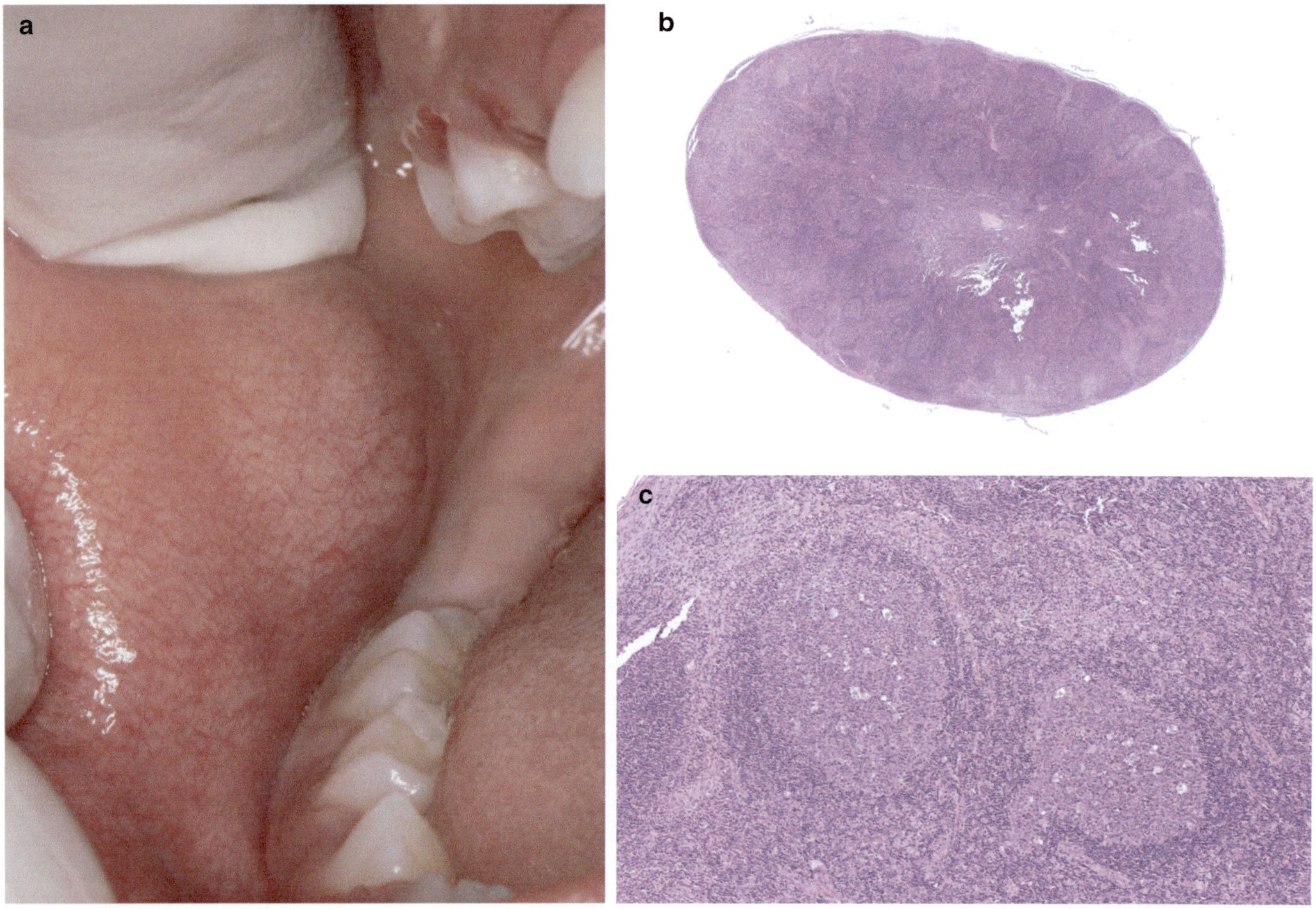

Fig. 11.2 Reactive hyperplastic lymph node with intra-oral manifestation. (**a**) Clinical appearance of a reactive hyperplastic lymph node causing an asymptomatic swelling intra-orally in the buccal mucosa. (Courtesy image: Dr. Manoela Domingues Martins). (**b**) Microscopic features of the resected specimen revealed the presence of a reactive lymph node (H&E; 10×). (**c**) Normal follicles were observed, with the germinal centers containing tingible body macrophages and a surrounding mantle zone (H&E; 50×)

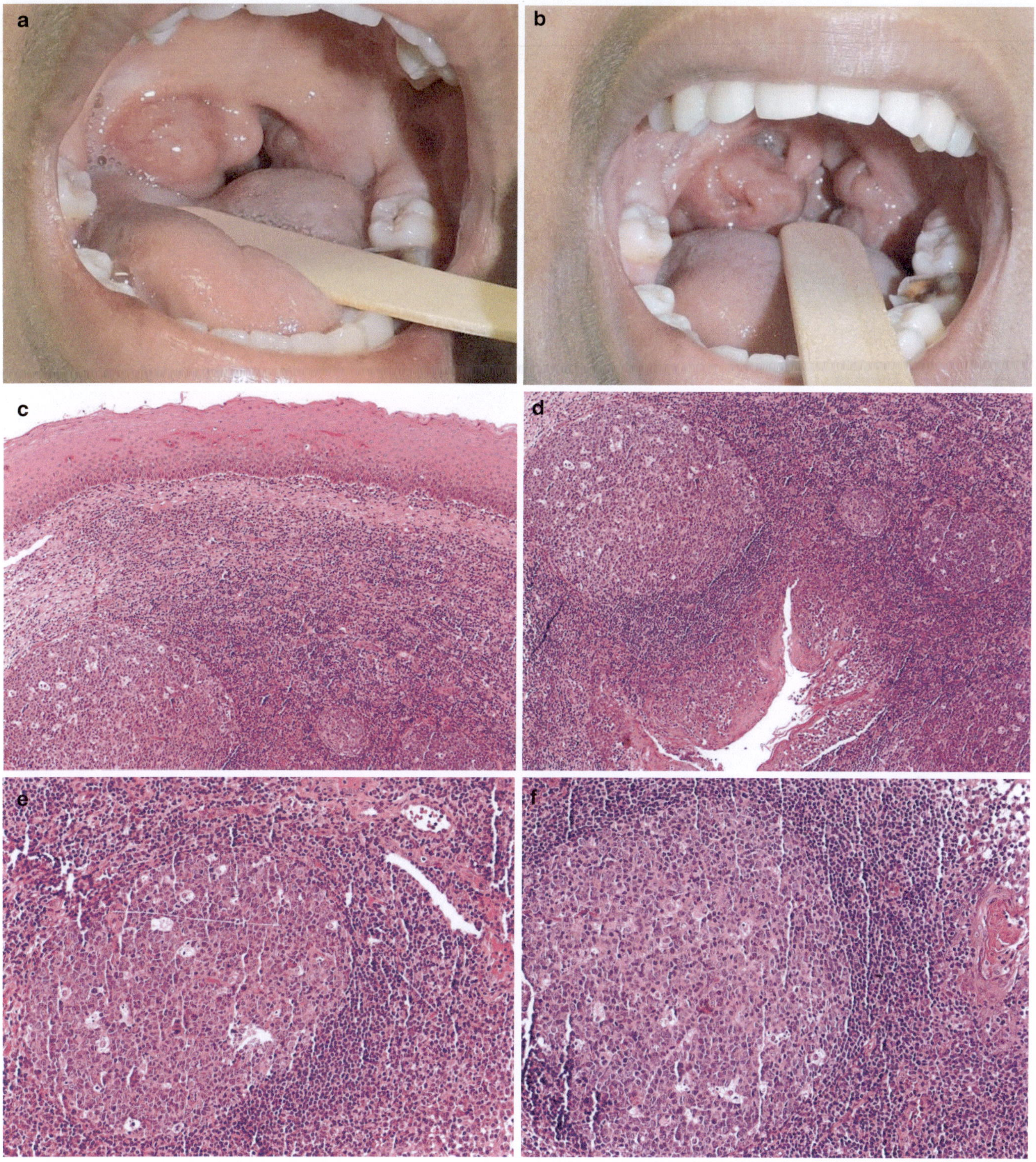

Fig. 11.3 Clinical and microscopic features of reactive hyperplastic palatine tonsils. (**a**) Large bilateral hyperplastic palatine tonsils in a 12-year-old male patient who complained of continuous mild pain. (**b**) The reactive hyperplasia was bilateral. (**c**) Overlying squamous epithelium and the presence of the reactive lymphoid tissue in the lamina propria of the biopsied tonsil. Note the prominent reactive germinal center in the lower left region (H&E; 100×). (**d**) The presence of secondary follicles throughout the specimen is a common finding. The reactive nature of these follicles is indicated by the presence of a normal mantle zone, the tingible body macrophages in the germinal center, the zonation pattern of the germinal center, and the variability in the shape and size of the secondary follicles. Observe the presence of the normal epithelium of the tonsillar crypts in the lower portion of the image (H&E; 100×). (**e**) Secondary reactive lymphoid follicle containing a germinal center. Observe the presence of tingible body macrophages, which is suggestive of the reactive nature of the disorder (H&E; 200×). (**f**) The secondary follicle also has a prominent mantle zone at the periphery of the lymphoid follicle. It is also possible to observe the zonation pattern of the germinal center (H&E; 200×)

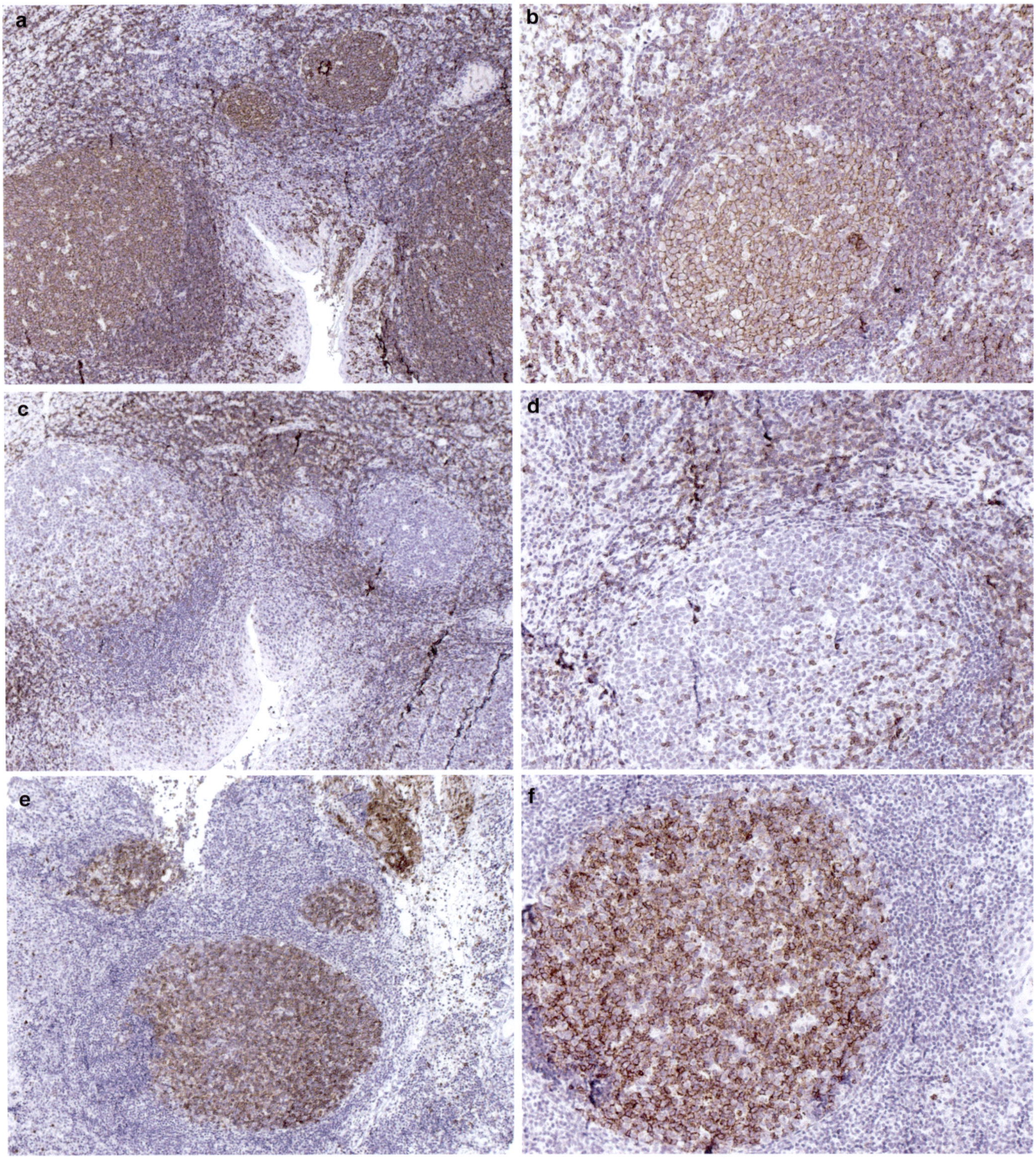

Fig. 11.4 Immunohistochemical features of the hyperplastic palatine tonsils. (**a**) The lymphoid follicles present in the lesion are consistently positive for CD20, revealing the presence of B lymphocytes in this compartment (DAB; 50×). (**b**) Observe the predominance of B lymphocytes highlighted by CD20 expression in the follicles and the germinal centers (DAB; 100×). (**c**) CD3 protein highlights the presence of T lymphocytes predominantly in the interfollicular region (DAB; 50×). (**d**) Observe the presence of reactive helper T cells positively staining for CD3 inside the germinal center. This finding is important to understand the expression of BCL2 in scattered cells in the reactive germinal center (DAB; 100×). (**e**) Using the CD23 antibody, it is possible to demonstrate the presence of a well-organized follicular dendritic cell network, confirming the presence of a germinal center (DAB; 50×). (**f**) The germinal center can also be demonstrated by observing the expression of CD10 protein (DAB; 100×)

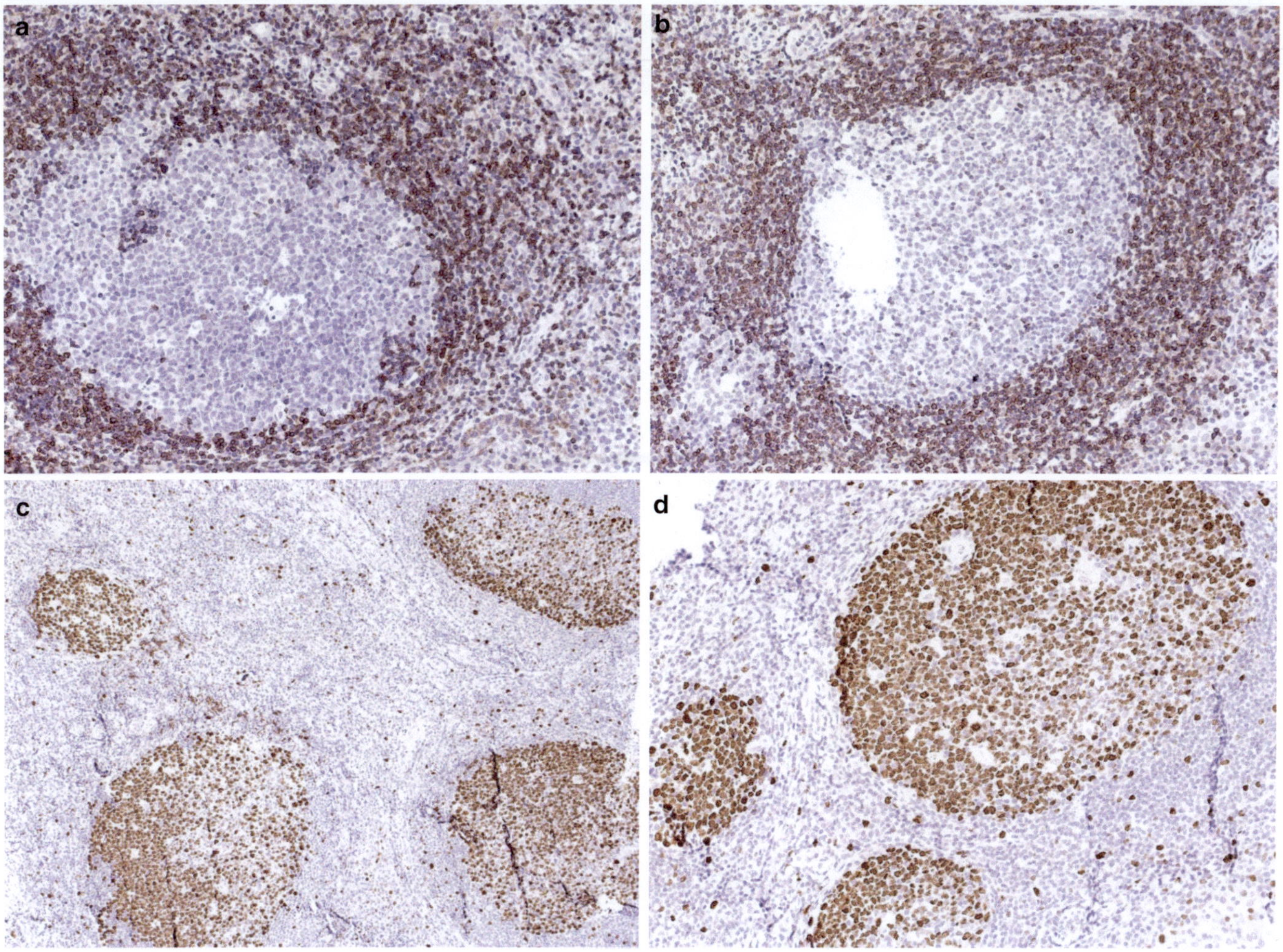

Fig. 11.5 Immunohistochemical features of the hyperplastic palatine tonsils (cont.). (**a**) In addition to the histological features, the reactive nature of the secondary follicles in hyperplastic tonsils can be demonstrated by the expression of BCL2 protein in the outer region of the lymphoid follicle and in the interfollicular region (DAB; 100×). (**b**) Observe that the germinal center cells are negative for BCL2 protein in this reactive follicle, except for the scattered helper T cells that are present inside the germinal center (DAB; 100×). (**c**) The germinal centers present a high proliferative index, which can be demonstrated by Ki67 expression. Observe the presence of a slight zonation pattern with an even higher expression of Ki67 in the dark zone of the germinal center compared to the light zone. This zonation pattern of cellular proliferation is consistent with a reactive process, which is often lost in follicular lymphomas (DAB; 100×). (**d**) Under high magnification, it is possible to observe the high proliferative index of germinal center by Ki67 expression and the zonation pattern consistent with a reactive process (DAB; 200×)

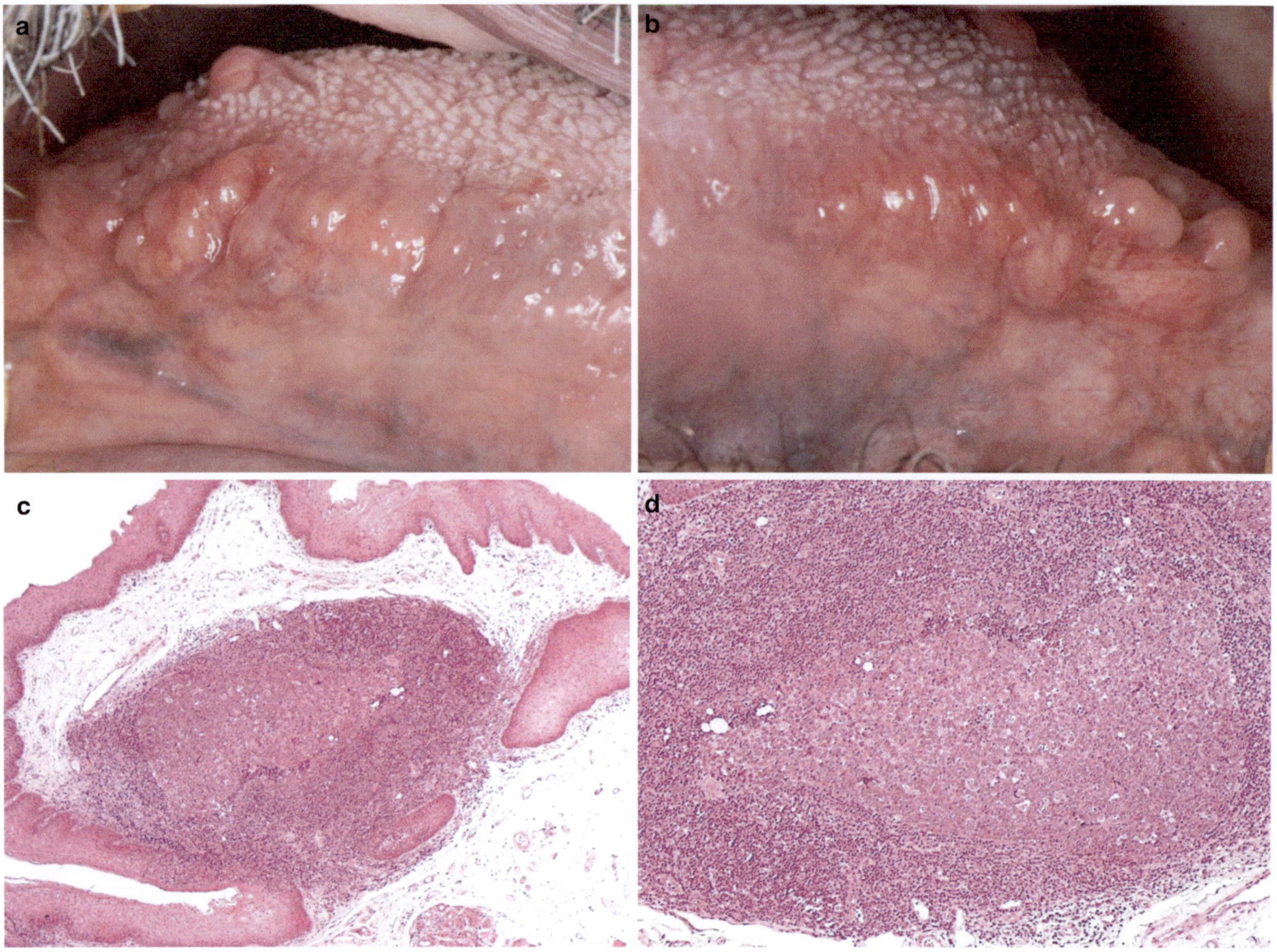

Fig. 11.6 Clinical and microscopic features of a hyperplastic lingual tonsil in an adult male patient. (**a**) The presence of a slightly painful, enlarged tissue in the right posterior lateral border of the tongue. This site is common for tongue cancer, and caution should be taken to avoid misdiagnosis. (**b**) On the left side, the patient also demonstrated an enlarged lingual tonsil. This reactive condition is frequently observed on both sides simultaneously. (**c**) Observe the presence of the overlying squamous epithelium of the tongue and, in the lamina propria, the presence of a hyperplastic lymphoid aggregate exhibiting the formation of a secondary follicle (H&E; 25×). (**d**) The reactive germinal center exhibits tingible body macrophages and a zonation pattern with the dark zone on the right side and the light zone on the left side of the germinal center (H&E; 100×)

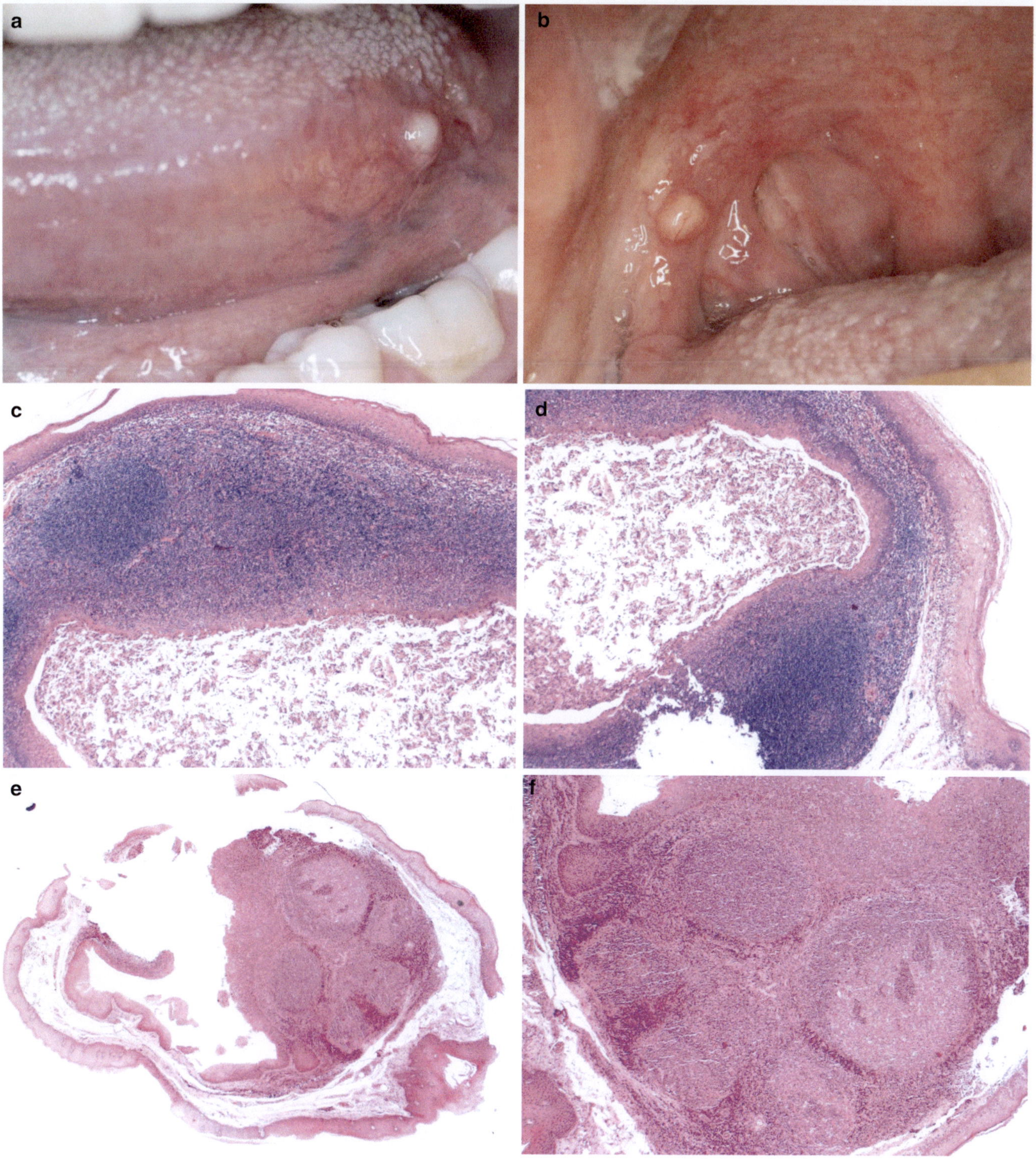

Fig. 11.7 Clinical and microscopic features of lymphoepithelial cysts. (**a**) This lesion is commonly observed in the oral cavity, more often in the latero-posterior border of the tongue, or (**b**) in the tonsillar pillar as asymptomatic, yellowish, small nodules. (**c**) This disorder exhibits a prominent lymphoid component in its capsule, with the formation of primary or secondary lymphoid follicles in many cases. Observe the overlying squamous epithelium of the oral mucosa and, lower in the image, the presence of the cystic epithelium, which in some cases can be very small and difficult to identify. In such cases, the presence of the lymphoid infiltrate may cause some concern for oral pathologists (H&E; 100×). (**d**) The cystic cavity is filled with keratin, and the cystic wall contains a dense, reactive lymphoid infiltrate (H&E; 100×). (**e**) An example of a lymphoepithelial cyst with an exuberant lymphoid aggregate in the capsule. Observe the presence of several secondary follicles containing reactive germinal centers (H&E; 25×). (**f**) In one of the secondary follicles located on the right side of the image, there is an invasion of mantle cells (darker cells) toward the central region of the germinal center (lighter region), resembling a progressive transformation of germinal centers (H&E; 50×)

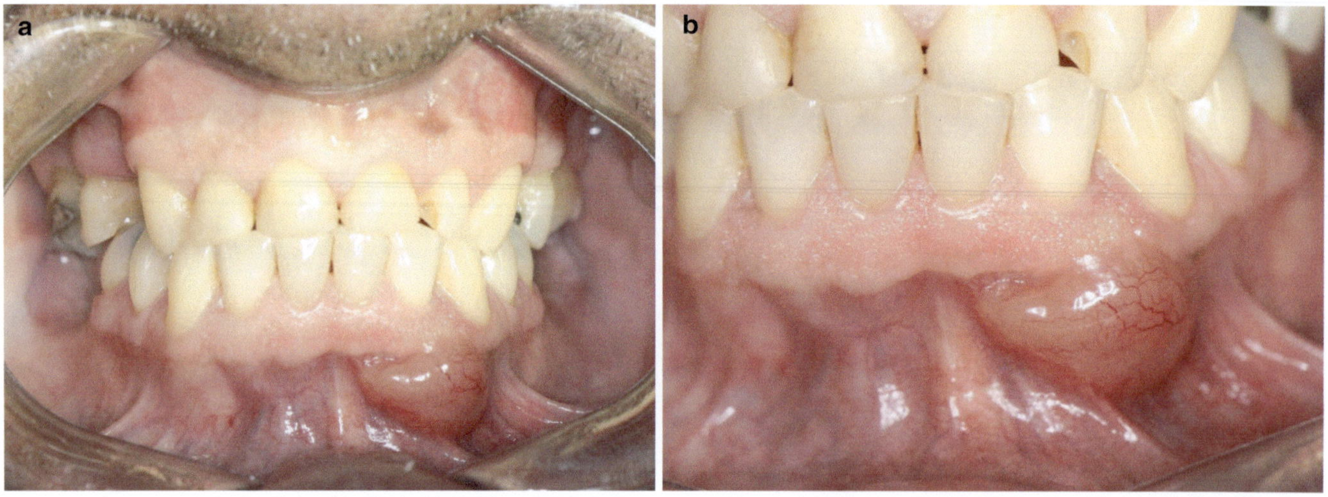

Fig. 11.8 Clinical manifestation of follicular lymphoid hyperplasia in the oral cavity. (**a**) An asymptomatic nodule affecting the lower alveolar mucosa of a 68-year-old male patient. (**b**) The nodule was normal-colored, well-defined, and non-ulcerated. No other lesions were present in the mouth or in other anatomical regions. After surgical removal, no recurrence was observed during the 6 years of follow-up

carcinoma, frequently show the presence of dense lymphoid aggregates in the connective tissue, sometimes accompanied by reactive germinal center formation. A careful clinicopathological correlation is mandatory to achieve the correct diagnosis.

The occurrence of (5) *idiopathic nonspecific lymphoid proliferations* in the oral and maxillofacial region can also be found and requires a careful clinical evaluation to confirm the diagnosis of a reactive condition, which typically exhibits a polymorphous nature and indolent clinical behavior, with no recurrences after surgical removal. Many of these reactive lymphoid proliferations demonstrate a specific histological feature characterized by the presence of follicular proliferations, and it is more specifically termed as follicular lymphoid hyperplasia, which has also been reported as florid follicular lymphoid hyperplasia, atypical follicular lymphoid hyperplasia, or reactive follicular hyperplasia. It is defined as a benign lymphoproliferative disorder whose etiology and pathogenesis are poorly understood, but that may clinically and microscopically strongly resemble a lymphoma, especially follicular lymphoma. In the oral cavity, follicular lymphoid hyperplasia is more often diagnosed in female patients as a painless, firm, well-demarcated, usually nonulcerated, slow-growing swelling, in the majority of cases affecting the palate, but the tongue, buccal mucosa, and the lips may also be affected (Fig. 11.8). This diagnosis demands a careful microscopic and immunohistochemical analysis, preferably followed by systemic evaluation of the patient and a long clinical follow-up to confirm its benign nature.

Because of the presence of normal lymphoid structures (lymph nodes and MALT) and due to many lesions containing a dense reactive lymphoid tissue, it is mandatory for pathologists to be familiarized with the normal distribution of the lymphoid tissues in the oral cavity and neighboring structures, and with their cellular composition.

Regarding therapeutic management of these benign conditions, hyperplastic reactive lymph nodes are more often treated by excisional biopsies, which is usually done with the aim of diagnosing an unspecific asymptomatic nodule in the oral mucosa, and recurrences are usually not observed, even in the presence of PTGC. Clinical follow-up is recommended for hyperplastic lingual tonsil, but conservative surgical removal is done when the clinical diagnosis is not convincing. Similarly, conservative removal of lymphoepithelial cysts is also the most recommended approach. Treatment of mucosal diseases associated with the presence of lymphoid aggregates in their microscopic component will depend on each specific diagnosis. Follicular lymphoid hyperplasia also has a favorable prognosis, although local recurrences have already been reported and patients demand a long clinical follow-up. Most of the cases are treated by surgical removal, but the use of intralesional steroids has also been described.

11.2 Microscopic Findings

11.2.1 Lymph Nodes and Progressive Transformation of Germinal Centers (PTGC)

- Proliferation of a dense lymphoid tissue with an outer layer representing the cortex and an inner zone representing the medulla.

- A peripheral fibrous capsule surrounding the lymph node is observed.
- The cortex typically contains many lymphoid follicles, some appearing as dense aggregates of lymphocytes (primary follicles), while most display a paler central area called the germinal center (secondary follicles).
- The lymphoid follicles are predominantly composed of B lymphocytes, whereas interfollicular regions are predominantly composed of T lymphocytes.
- Secondary follicles exhibit, in addition to the germinal center, the mantle zone, a darker region around the follicle.
- The germinal center has a more condensed, darker pole and an opposite, less condensed lighter pole (zonation pattern).
- In the reactive germinal centers, the presence of tingible body macrophages is common.
- An increased number of blood vessels are found in the medullary zone of the lymph node, alongside proliferation of lymphocytes and plasma cells, but with no lymphoid follicles (Fig. 11.2).
- In some cases, a proliferation of B lymphocytes is seen in the mantle zone toward the germinal center region, representing the PTGC.
- The proliferation of the mantle zone can be focal or more diffuse and efface the germinal center partially or entirely.
- The reactive B and T lymphocytes that are found in their respective compartments in a hyperplastic lymph node present as a hyperchromatic, small, round cell, with scant cytoplasm and inconspicuous nucleoli.
- Plasma cells also show typical features with a displaced nucleus and abundant eosinophilic cytoplasm. Nucleoli are multiple and peripherally located. The perinuclear hof zone is present.
- Tingible body macrophages are typically found in the germinal centers of the lymphoid follicles in hyperplastic lymph nodes. These cells present abundant and clear cytoplasm and a pale, round to oval nucleus. They actively phagocyte apoptotic lymphoid cells, and the apoptotic bodies can be seen as dark (tingible) structures dispersed in the clear cytoplasm.
- The presence of cells in the germinal centers exhibiting pale, multilobated nuclei and a small nucleolus is consistent with follicular dendritic cells.
- Mitotic figures are common in the germinal center, especially in the dark zone, where the proliferative index is higher.
- The cells present in the PTGC are hyperchromatic, small, normal appearing B lymphocytes from the mantle zone and stain positively for BCL2 and IgD proteins by immunohistochemistry (Figs. 11.9, 11.10, and 11.11).

11.2.2 Mucosa-Associated Lymphoid Tissue (MALT) in the Lingual Tonsils

- Proliferation of a dense lymphoid tissue that surrounds the normal adjacent structures like salivary glands, muscular bundles, and nerve fibers, approaching the overlying epithelium.
- The presence of von Ebner glands is usually used as an indicator of the anatomical location.
- The presence of reactive germinal centers, as described previously, is frequently found.
- The reactive B and T lymphocytes exhibit the normal morphological aspects as described earlier.
- Plasma cells are variably present.
- The presence of neural fibers surrounded by the lymphoid aggregate may mislead to an erroneous interpretation of neural invasion (Fig. 11.6).

11.2.3 Lymphoepithelial Cyst

- The cyst contains an epithelial and a lymphoid component.
- The epithelium invaginates from the surface toward the adjacent lamina propria, giving rise to a cystic cavity surrounded by a keratinized squamous epithelium.
- The presence of keratin layers inside the cystic cavity is very common.
- In some cases, the epithelial component is very small and difficult to observe, demanding serial sections to be adequately appreciated.
- The lymphoid compartment of the cyst is located in the fibrous capsule/lamina propria.
- The lymphoid tissue is frequently very dense, but cases exhibiting smaller lymphoid aggregates can also occur.
- The cellular composition of the lymphoid tissue is similar to that found in normal lymph nodes, with B lymphocytes present in lymphoid follicles and T lymphocytes in the interfollicular regions. Plasma cells and a few macrophages are also present.
- The occurrence of reactive germinal centers is common and exhibits the same morphological features described for hyperplastic lymph nodes.
- The morphological features of the lymphoid cells present in the lymphoepithelial cysts are similar to those described earlier for hyperplastic lymph nodes.

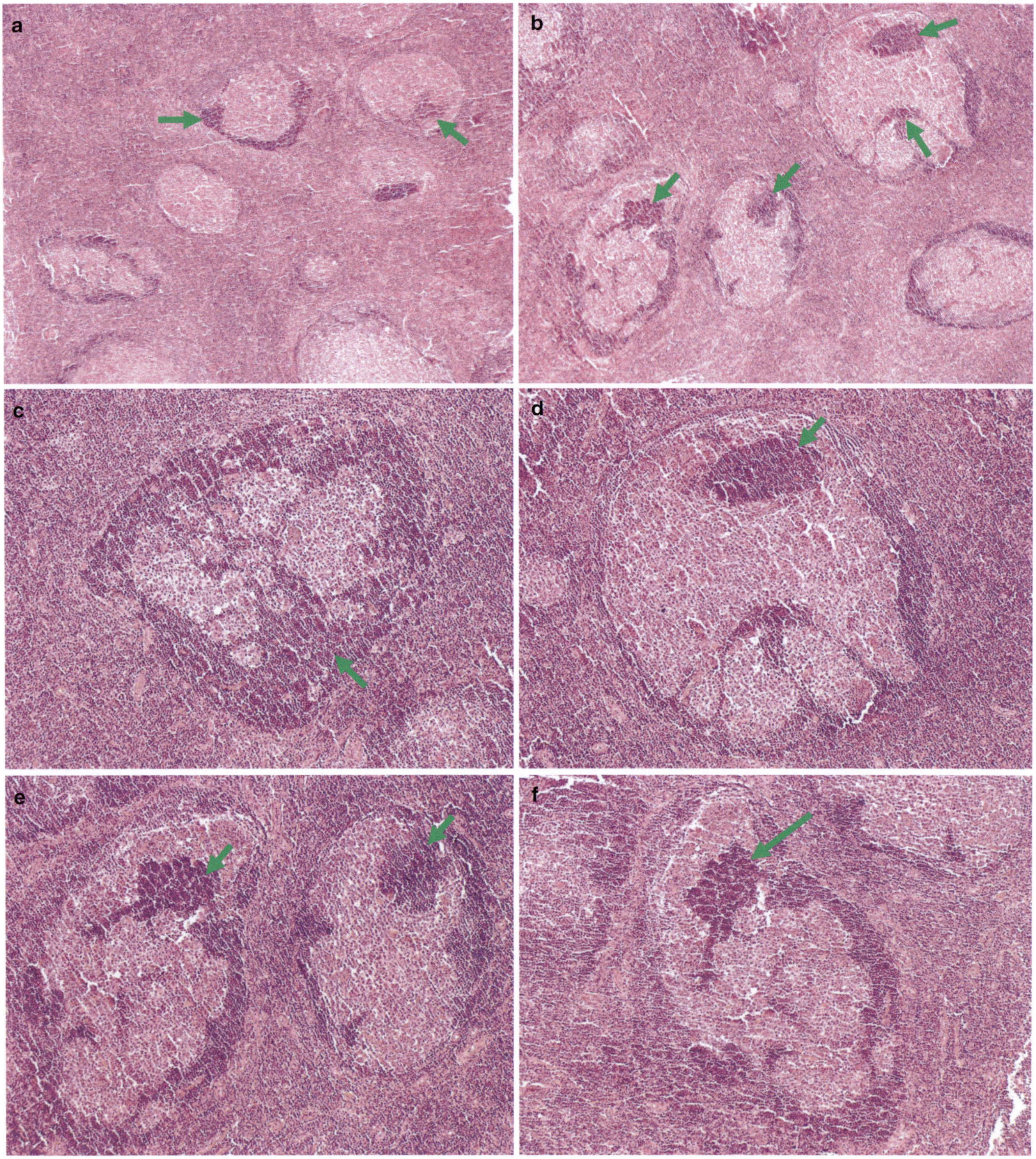

Fig. 11.9 Microscopic features of progressive transformation of germinal centers. (**a**) Although very unusual, some hyperplastic follicular hyperplasias in the oral cavity may demonstrate a proliferation of the mantle zone of secondary follicles toward the germinal center area (green arrows), which characterizes a progressive transformation of the germinal center (H&E; 50×). (**b**) Observe the proliferation of the mantle zone of the secondary follicles as an irregular darker region toward the central region of the germinal centers that present as a lighter region (green arrows) (H&E; 50×). (**c**) The mantle zone proliferation toward the germinal center can present as different patterns, and as in this example, it may infiltrate a large area of the germinal center (green arrow) (H&E; 100×). (**d**) In this example, there are smaller areas of mantle zone cells infiltrating the germinal center (green arrow) if compared to the previous example (H&E; 100×). (**e**) Observe the presence of mantle zone cells (dark regions) (green arrows) infiltrating the germinal center (light region) (H&E; 100×). (**f**) Another example of a secondary lymphoid follicle exhibiting a progressive transformation of the germinal center with the presence of mantle zone cells (dark areas) (green arrow) infiltrating the germinal center (light region) (H&E; 100×)

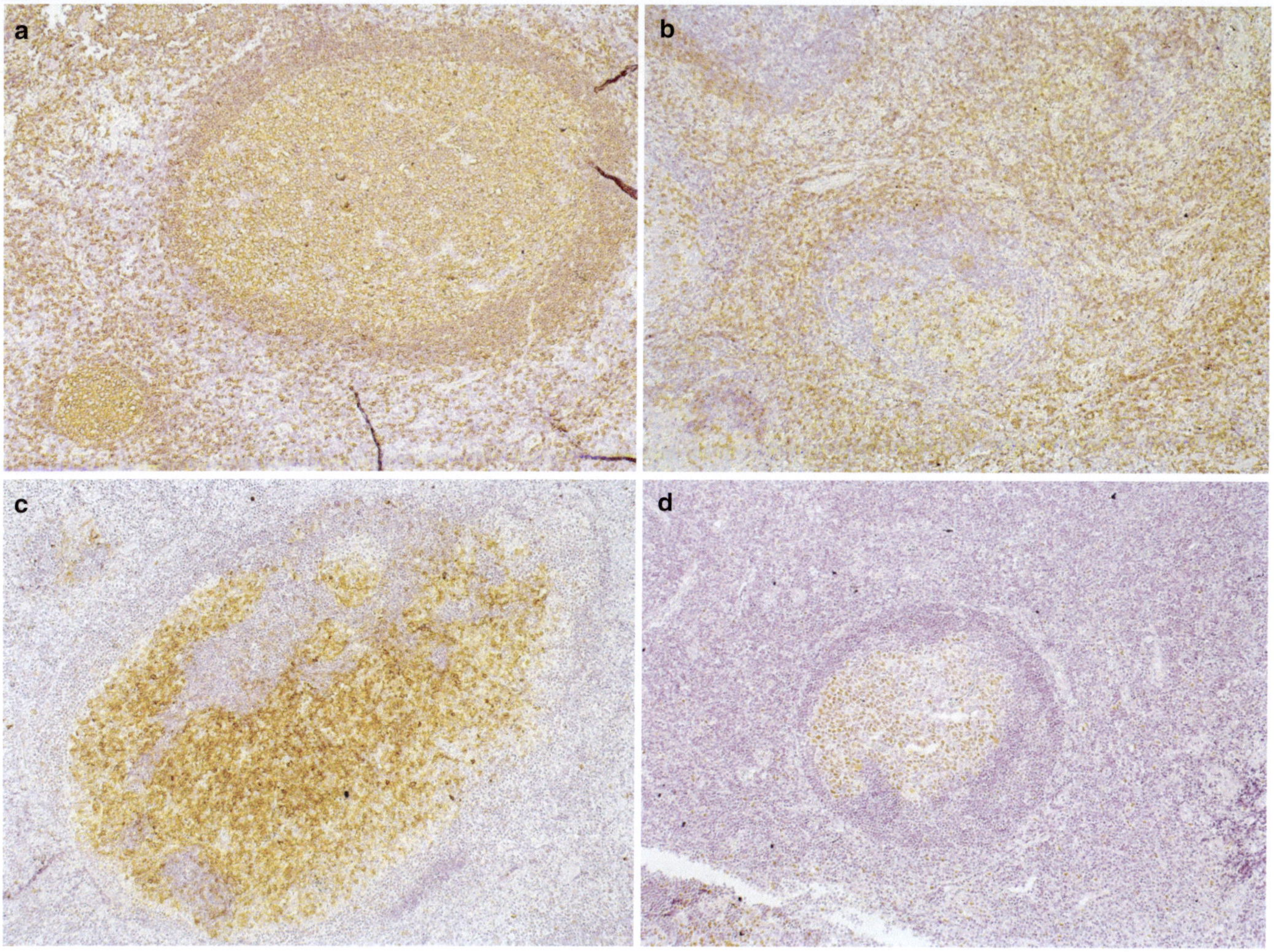

Fig. 11.10 Immunohistochemical features of progressive transformation of germinal centers. (**a**) The cells of the secondary lymphoid follicle, both the mantle zone cells and the germinal center cells, are positive for CD20 expression (DAB; 100×). (**b**) The T lymphocytes, expressing CD3, are predominantly distributed in the interfollicular regions. These expression patterns of CD20 and CD3 are consistent with the distribution of B and T lymphocytes, respectively, in normal lymph nodes (DAB; 100×). (**c**) The germinal center cells (equivalent to those cells in the light regions previously exemplified in the H&E-stained photos) are strongly positive for CD10 protein in the cell membrane and cytoplasm (DAB; 100×), (**d**) and they also exhibit a nuclear expression for BCL6 protein. These markers are useful to confirm the germinal center origin of these cells (DAB; 100×)

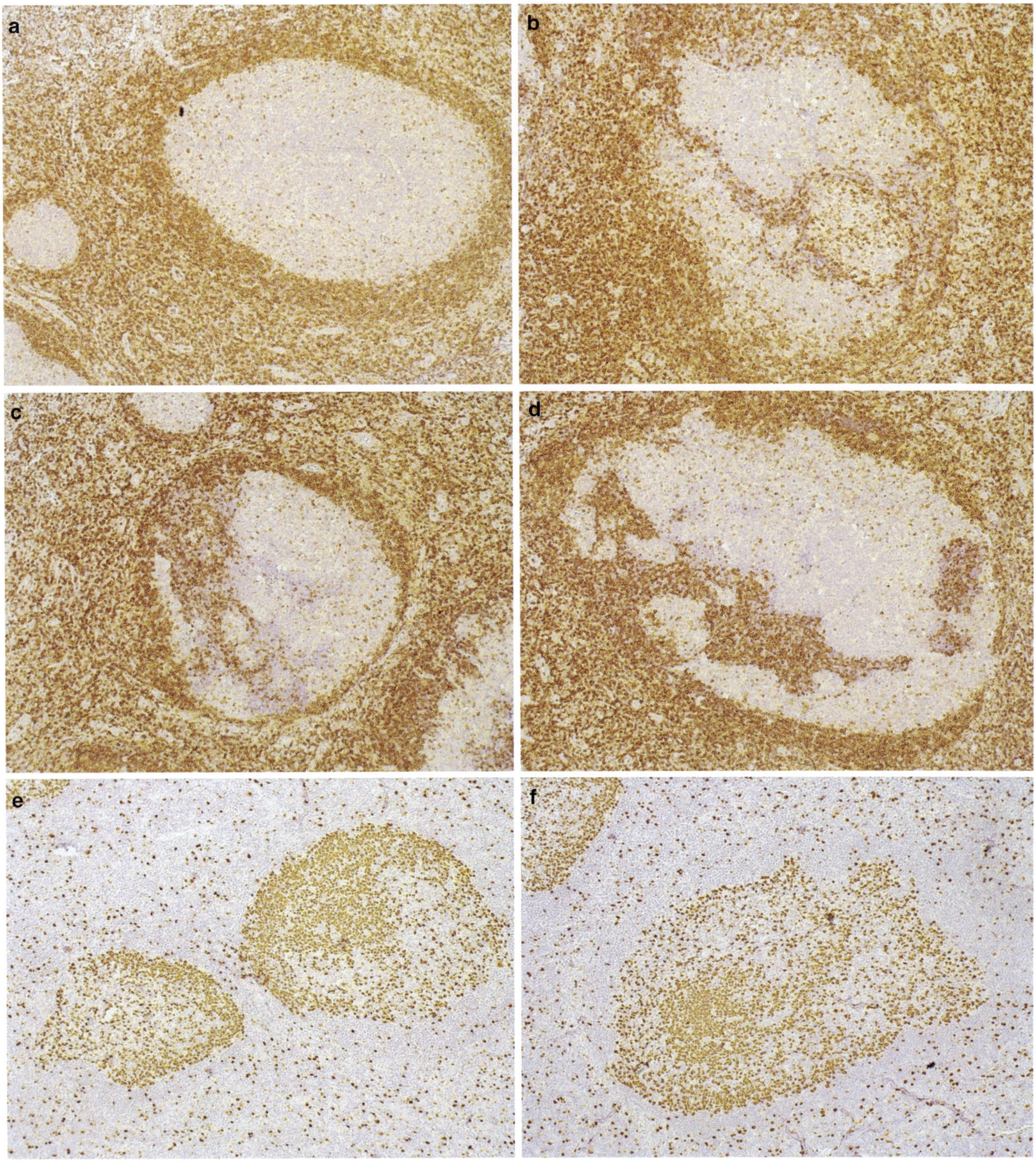

Fig. 11.11 Immunohistochemical features of progressive transformation of germinal centers. (**a**) The reactive nature of this microscopic phenomenon is also demonstrated by BCL2 expression in the interfollicular regions and the absence of BCL2 in the germinal center, except for scattered normal helper T cells that are typically positive for BCL2 (DAB; 100×). (**b**) Mantle zone cells are normally positive for BCL2; we can observe in this image that those regions where the mantle zone cells invade the germinal center are also typically positive for this protein (DAB; 100×). (**c**) The presence of progressive transformation of germinal center can be better observed using BCL2 staining since the mantle zone cells are typically strongly positive and the invaded germinal center is negative (DAB; 100×). (**d**) Another example of progressive transformation of the germinal center with BCL2-positive mantle zone cells invading the germinal center (DAB; 100×). (**e**) The proliferative pattern (Ki67 positive cells) of progressive transformation of germinal center is higher in the mantle zone and lower in the germinal center, although in both areas, positive cells are frequently found (DAB; 100×). (**f**) Observe in this example a higher proliferative index in the mantle zone cells than in the surrounding germinal center cells, although a very high proliferation index is observed in the whole secondary lymphoid follicle structure if compared to the interfollicular region that also shows the expression of Ki67 but in a much lower proportion (DAB; 100×)

11.2.4 Oral Mucosa Diseases with Reactive Lymphoid Component

- In addition to specific morphological features of each mucosal disease, proliferation of lymphoid aggregates can also be observed in the lamina propria.
- The lymphoid tissue can be predominantly located near the overlying squamous epithelium or may proliferate toward deeper portions of the mucosa.
- There may be different degrees of exocytosis in the epithelium.
- The presence of reactive germinal centers with similar morphological aspects to those described earlier for hyperplastic lymph nodes can also be found in some cases.
- Presence of lymphocytes, plasma cells, and macrophages in variable distribution and proportion, always exhibiting the normal morphological features expected for these populations (Fig. 11.12).

11.2.5 Idiopathic Nonspecific Lymphoid Proliferations (Follicular Lymphoid Hyperplasia)

- These unspecific conditions are characterized by the presence of dense proliferations of lymphoid tissue.
- There are no germinal centers or follicular proliferations.
- Mitoses are uncommon, and the cells exhibit few or minimal atypia.
- Confirmation of polymorphic lymphoid infiltrate is crucial to characterize the condition as a reactive process rather than a neoplastic proliferation. The presence of B and T lymphocytes, alongside a variable amount of plasma cells, and macrophages, favors the diagnosis of a reactive lymphoid process.
- Other more specific conditions should be ruled out.
- If ulcerated areas are present, polymorphonuclear cells may be present;
- In follicular lymphoid hyperplasia, there is a proliferation of dense lymphoid tissue with a follicular growth pattern.
- The follicles vary in number, shape, and size.
- A well-defined mantle zone similar to follicular hyperplasia in the lymph nodes is usually present.
- The presence of tingible body macrophages in the germinal centers leads to a focal starry sky pattern and suggests a reactive nature.
- In some follicles, it is possible to observe the difference between the light and dark zones inside the germinal centers.
- The lymphoid follicles exhibit the development of germinal centers that contain a mixture of small and large lymphocytes.
- Tingible body macrophages have a large, clear cytoplasm with a variable number of small apoptotic bodies (Fig. 11.13).

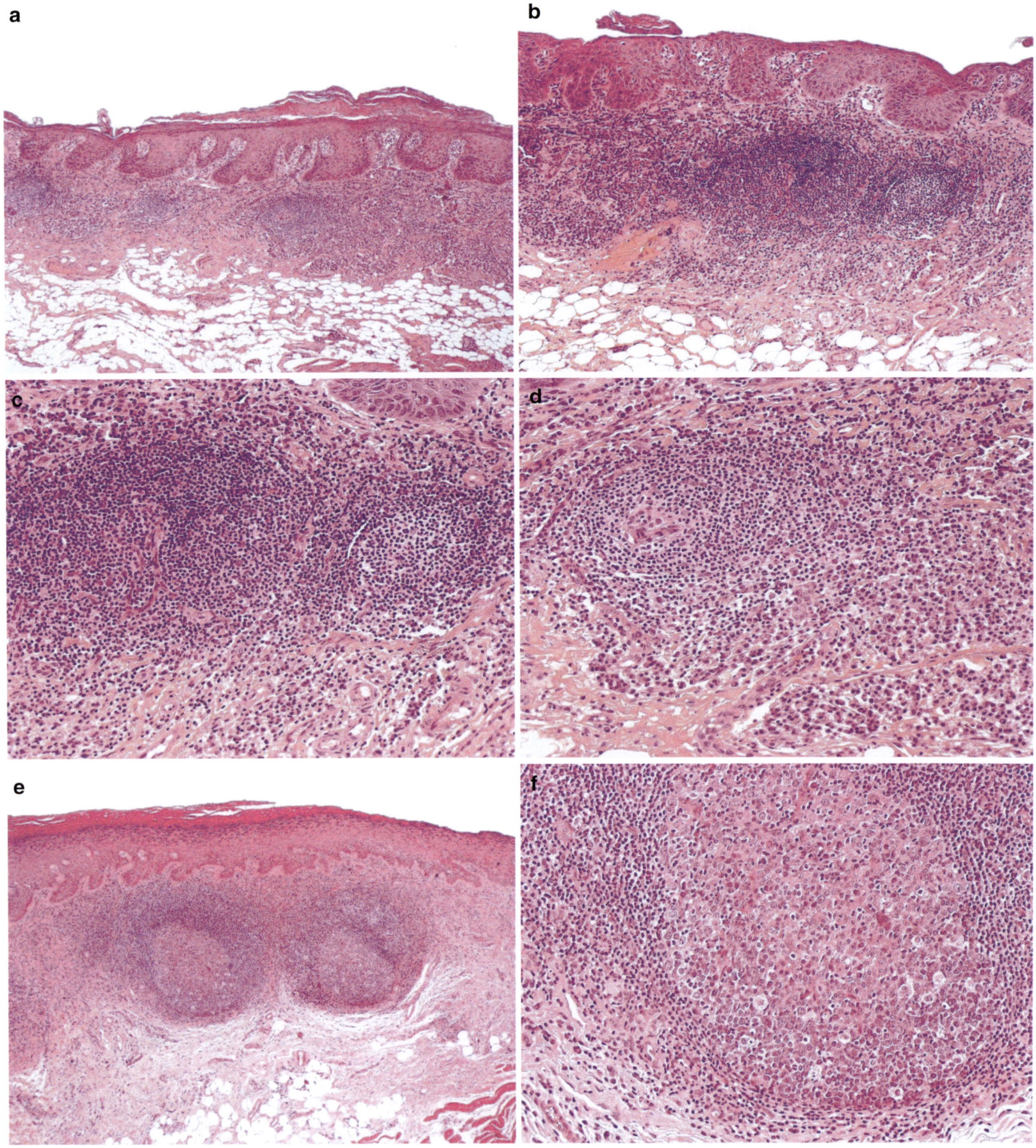

Fig. 11.12 Several oral mucosa diseases may demonstrate the presence of reactive lymphoid infiltrates near the overlying squamous epithelium or deeper in the lamina propria. These infiltrates should not be interpreted as neoplastic conditions, but clinical data are often necessary to correctly understand their biological significance. (**a**) This is an oral leukoplakia affecting the lateral border of the tongue that, in the microscopic analysis, in addition to the epithelial alterations containing a moderate degree of cellular atypia, also exhibited a lymphoid infiltrate in the lamina propria (H&E; 50×). (**b**) In some regions of the lesion, the lymphoid infiltrate was more prominent and a secondary lymphoid follicle could be observed (H&E; 100×). (**c**) The presence of lymphoid follicles near the overlying epithelium (H&E; 100×). (**d**) Observe that lymphocytes are the predominant lymphoid cells in this reactive infiltrate present in the oral leukoplakia. In the follicles, there is a predominance of B lymphocytes, while in the interfollicular regions or in the outer regions of the follicles, an increased amount of T lymphocytes will be possible to be observed using immunohistochemistry. Plasma cells are also present in this reactive infiltrate (H&E; 100×). (**e**) Severe inflammatory infiltrate in the lamina propria presenting secondary lymphoid follicles in a verrucous proliferative leukoplakia affecting a female patient (H&E; 25×). (**f**) Observe the presence of germinal centers with histological features consistent with a reactive origin, like the presence of tingible body macrophages (H&E; 200×)

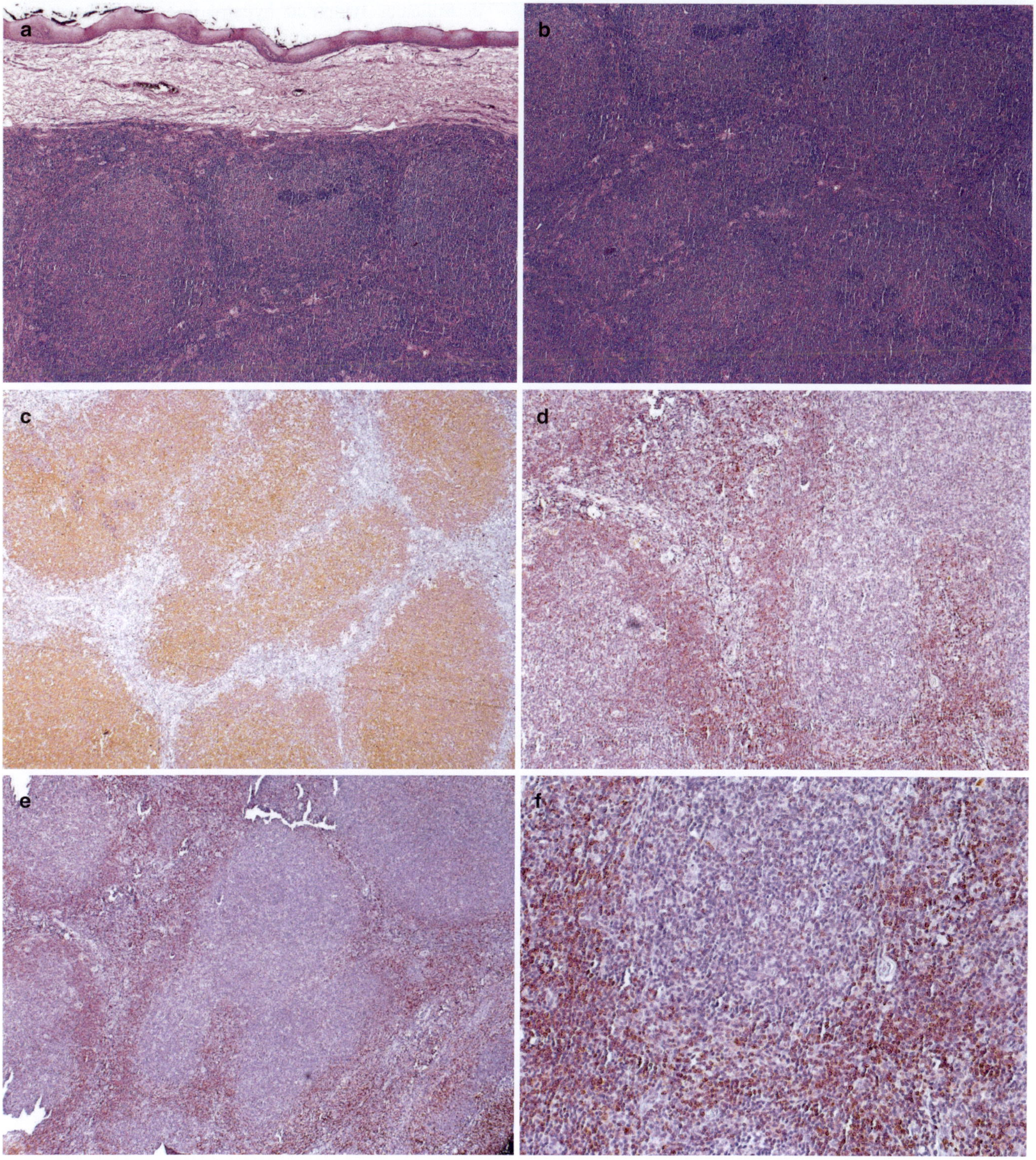

Fig. 11.13 Microscopic features of the follicular lymphoid hyperplasia affecting the adult male patient previously described. (**A**) Lymphoid tissue exhibiting a nodular/follicular growth pattern (H&E; 100×). (**B**) The follicles have different sizes and shapes (H&E; 100×). (**C**) The lymphoid follicles are strongly positive for CD20 (DAB; 50×). (**D**) The expression of CD3 demonstrates T lymphocytes predominantly located in the interfollicular zone (DAB; 100×). (**E**) The lack of BCL2 expression in the germinal center of the follicular proliferations supports a reactive nature, which should be in accordance with other microscopic, immunohistochemical, and clinical findings for the final diagnosis (DAB; 50×). (**F**) BCL2 shows a strong expression in the interfollicular one and in several helper T cells located in the germinal center (DAB; 100×)

11.3 Immunohistochemistry and/or Genetics

The most important objective of immunohistochemical reactions in diagnosing reactive lymphoid processes is to differentiate them from neoplasms, particularly follicular lymphoma and MALT lymphoma. It is important to carefully observe the distribution pattern of the cellular subtypes present in each lesion, which very often will have both B and T lymphocytes, and varying amounts of plasma cells, and macrophages. These findings should be correlated with microscopic features and clinical data.

Reactive lymph nodes will demonstrate the normal cellular distribution with B lymphocytes predominantly located in the follicles and T lymphocytes in the interfollicular area. The germinal centers are negative for BCL2 expression, which is predominantly located in the interfollicular region and in scattered helper T lymphocytes in the germinal center. The lymphoid component of the lymphoepithelial cysts and the lymphoid follicles present in the lingual tonsils demonstrate the same distribution pattern observed in the reactive lymph nodes.

In follicular lymphoid hyperplasia, it is important to assess whether the presence and organization of different cell types align with the distribution typically observed in reactive lymph nodes. In follicular lymphoid hyperplasia, B lymphocytes are located in the lymphoid follicles, indicated by CD20 expression, while CD3-positive T lymphocytes are mainly located in the interfollicular region. Germinal centers are B cell structures that express CD10 and BCL6, and the presence of follicular dendritic cells, revealed by CD21, CD23, or CD35 expression, helps identify these structures. Tingible body macrophages express the histiocytic marker CD68, and reactive plasma cells are demonstrated by CD138/plasma cell/EMA/MUM1 antibodies. The antiapoptotic protein BCL2 should be limited to a few helper T lymphocytes in the germinal centers and is strongly expressed in the interfollicular zone to support the diagnosis of a reactive process. Zonation of germinal centers can also be illustrated by Ki67, which shows higher expression in the dark zone compared to the light zone. In those infiltrates containing a large number of plasma cells, the polyclonal nature can be confirmed by kappa and lambda light chain expression. The staining patterns, in conjunction with the morphological findings, support a benign nature for the disease (Table 11.1).

Table 11.1 Summary of the main immunohistochemical reactions used for the diagnosis of reactive lymphoid proliferations

Antibody	Most frequent results	Pattern	Objective
CD20	Positive	Membrane	To reveal B lymphocytes
CD3	Positive	Membrane	To reveal T lymphocytes
CD138	Positive	Membrane	To reveal plasma cells
CD68	Positive	Cytoplasm	To reveal macrophages
Kappa/lambda	Polyclonal	Cytoplasm	To show the polyclonal nature of the disease in cases with the presence of plasma cells
CD21/CD23/CD35	Positive	Membrane	To reveal the presence of FDC in the reactive follicles
BCL2	Positive	Cytoplasm	Predominantly expressed in the interfollicular regions in reactive lymphoid proliferations
CD10	Positive	Membrane	To demonstrate the presence of germinal centers
BCL6	Positive	Nuclear	To demonstrate the presence of germinal centers
Ki67	Variable	Nucleus	To illustrate the proliferative index of the lesion

FDC follicular dendritic cells

Sources

1. Larsson A, Warfvinge G. Immunohistochemistry of 'tertiary lymphoid follicles' in oral amalgam-associated lichenoid lesions. Oral Dis. 1998;4:187–93. https://doi.org/10.1111/j.1601-0825.1998.tb00277.x.
2. Menasce LP, Shanks JH, Banerjee SS, Harris M. Follicular lymphoid hyperplasia of the hard palate and oral mucosa: report of three cases and a review of the literature. Histopathology. 2001;39:353–8. https://doi.org/10.1046/j.1365-2559.2001.01210.x.
3. Hicks J, Flaitz C. Progressive transformation of germinal centers: review of histopathologic and clinical features. Int J Pediatr Otorhinolaryngol. 2002;65:195–202. https://doi.org/10.1016/s0165-5876(02)00176-3.
4. Kolokotronis A, Dimitrakopoulos I, Asimaki A. Follicular lymphoid hyperplasia of the palate: report of a case and review of the literature. Oral Surg Oral Med Oral Pathol Oral Radiol Endod. 2003;96:172–5. https://doi.org/10.1016/s1079-2104(03)00095-7.
5. Kojima M, Nakamura S, Iijima M, Yoshizumi T, Sakata N, Masawa N. Follicular lymphoid hyperplasia of the oral cavity representing progressive transformation of germinal center. APMIS. 2005;113:221–4. https://doi.org/10.1111/j.1600-0463.2005.apm1130311.x.
6. Jham BC, Binmadi NO, Scheper MA, Zhao XF, Koterwas GE, Kashyap A, Levy BA. Follicular lymphoid hyperplasia of the palate: case report and literature review. J Craniomaxillofac Surg. 2009;37:79–82. https://doi.org/10.1016/j.jcms.2008.11.007.
7. Yamakawa PE, Andrade EH, Watanabe-Silva CH, Dos Santos Neto LL. Lingual tonsil pseudolymphoma and obstructive sleep apnea. Braz J Otorhinolaryngol. 2009;75:469. https://doi.org/10.1016/s1808-8694(15)30670-4.
8. Kojima M, Nakamura N, Sakamoto K, Sakurai S, Tsukamoto N, Itoh H, et al. Progressive transformation of the germinal center of extranodal organs: a clinicopathological, immunohistochemical, and genotypic study of 14 cases. Pathol Res Pract. 2010;206:235–40. https://doi.org/10.1016/j.prp.2009.12.001.
9. Lima MDM, Artico G, Soares FA, Martins MT, Alves FA. Follicular lymphoma in the palate with clinical appearance similar to salivary gland tumors. Quintessence Int. 2010;41:661–3.
10. Sands NB, Tewfik M. Benign lymphoid hyperplasia of the tongue base causing upper airway obstruction. Case Rep Otolaryngol. 2011;2011:625185. https://doi.org/10.1155/2011/625185.
11. Anjomshoaa I, Bulford LA, Dym H, Woo SB. Florid follicular lymphoid hyperplasia of the hard palatal mucosa managed with intralesional steroids: a case report and review of the literature. J Oral Maxillofac Surg. 2013;71:1202–8. https://doi.org/10.1016/j.joms.2013.01.015.
12. Almeida LKY, Silveira HA, Ferrisse TM, Silva EV, Almeida LY, Bufalino A, León JE. Unilateral enlargement of the lateral lingual tonsil: an immunohistochemical study and literature review. Oral Oncol. 2020;109:104857. https://doi.org/10.1016/j.oraloncology.2020.104857.
13. da Silva KD, Coelho LV, do Couto AM, de Aguiar MCF, Tarquínio SBC, Gomes APN, et al. Clinicopathological and immunohistochemical features of the oral lymphoepithelial cyst: a multicenter study. J Oral Pathol Med. 2020;49:219–26. https://doi.org/10.1111/jop.12978.
14. Lafuente-Ibáñez de Mendoza I, Vigarios E, Herbault-Barres B, Alberdi-Navarro J, Sibaud V, Maret D, Aguirre-Urizar JM. Non-infectious granulomatous disorders of the upper lip: clinicopathological analysis of 11 patients. BMC Oral Health. 2022;22:173. https://doi.org/10.1186/s12903-022-02189-z.
15. Brooks JK, Alajaji S, Sultan AS, Parraguirre YE, Cerrito JF, Gupta R, et al. Florid follicular lymphoid hyperplasia of the palate: review of the literature and report of an illustrative case. Quintessence Int. 2024;55:494–502. https://doi.org/10.3290/j.qi.b5316965.

Dental and Periodontal Inflammatory Diseases

12

Rafael Paschoal Esteves Lima,
Cinthia Veronica Bardalez Lopez de Caceres,
Omar Kujan, and Felipe Paiva Fonseca

12.1 General Overview and Clinical Presentation

Radicular periapical abscesses, granulomas, and *cysts* are common inflammatory endodontic disorders associated with a necrotic dental pulp. These lesions affect patients across a broad age range, more frequently adults with poor oral hygiene conditions. They are typically linked to dental caries or dental trauma and require endodontic treatment, which is often followed by local surgical approaches to remove the lesions that do not spontaneously heal after endodontic management. There is no sex predilection, and any tooth can be associated with periapical inflammatory lesions. These disorders are more often asymptomatic, but may present with tissue swelling and fistulae formation. Accurate assessment of dental pulp vitality is crucial to support microscopic diagnosis and ensure a correct clinical diagnosis. Radiographically, these lesions present as radiolucent areas at the apex of the dental roots, or less commonly, in the lateral region of the radicular surface. Clinicopathological correlation becomes particularly important for accurate diagnosis in patients with a history of hematolymphoid neoplasms, as the reactive inflammatory infiltrate may mimic neoplastic infiltration at the apex of the teeth (Figs. 12.1 and 12.2).

The periodontal tissues are frequently affected by innumerous non-neoplastic inflammatory or immunologic processes. The biological heterogeneity and varied clinical manifestations of these conditions require pathologists to perform a careful and detailed clinicopathological correlation to ensure an accurate diagnosis and to avoid misinterpreting the reactive lymphoplasmacytic infiltrates as a potential neoplastic condition. Simultaneously, certain cases of oral lymphomas, leukemic infiltrations, and other lymphoproliferative disorders affecting the gingiva can closely mimic reactive periodontal inflammatory disease in its first stages. Any delay in correctly identifying these disorders may adversely affect the patients' prognosis.

The current classification of periodontal and peri-implant diseases and conditions is comprehensive. In addition to the more common biofilm-induced inflammatory processes, it includes many other pathological entities that can primarily develop in the gingiva or that may represent secondary manifestation of systemic disorders, including auto-immune processes such as lichen planus, pemphigus vulgaris, and membranous pemphigoid, as well as hypersensitivity reactions, granulomatous disorders, neoplastic conditions, and more.

Biofilm-induced gingivitis and *periodontitis* are very common and significant oral diseases, most frequently observed among adult patients with a wide age range, with no sex predilection. Biofilm-induced gingivitis is a nonspecific, chronic inflammatory response to biofilm, which may present as either painful or asymptomatic. Clinically, it manifests as diffuse or localized gingival swelling with a reddish, smooth surface, often exhibiting spontaneous bleeding while maintaining a stable level of periodontal attachment. If left untreated, this inflammatory process may progress to periodontitis, characterized by the destruction of periodontal collagen fibers and alveolar bone, which constitute the supportive framework for teeth. This progression can ultimately lead to dental mobility and tooth loss. The clinical hallmark of periodontitis is the presence of periodontal pockets, identified and measured by periodontal probes, in the absence of non-periodontal causes. *Periodontitis* is associated with irreversible tissue changes, even after the removal

R. P. E. Lima
Department of Oral Surgery and Pathology (Periodontics), School of Dentistry, Universidade Federal de Minas Gerais, Belo Horizonte, Brazil

C. V. B. L. de Caceres · F. P. Fonseca
Department of Oral Surgery and Pathology, School of Dentistry, Universidade Federal de Minas Gerais, Belo Horizonte, Brazil

O. Kujan (✉)
UWA Dental School, The University of Western Australia, Nedlands, WA, Australia
e-mail: omar.kujan@uwa.edu.au

© The Author(s), under exclusive license to Springer Nature Switzerland AG 2025
F. P. Fonseca et al. (eds.), *Lymphoproliferative and Granulomatous Disorders of the Oral Cavity*,
https://doi.org/10.1007/978-3-031-98844-8_12

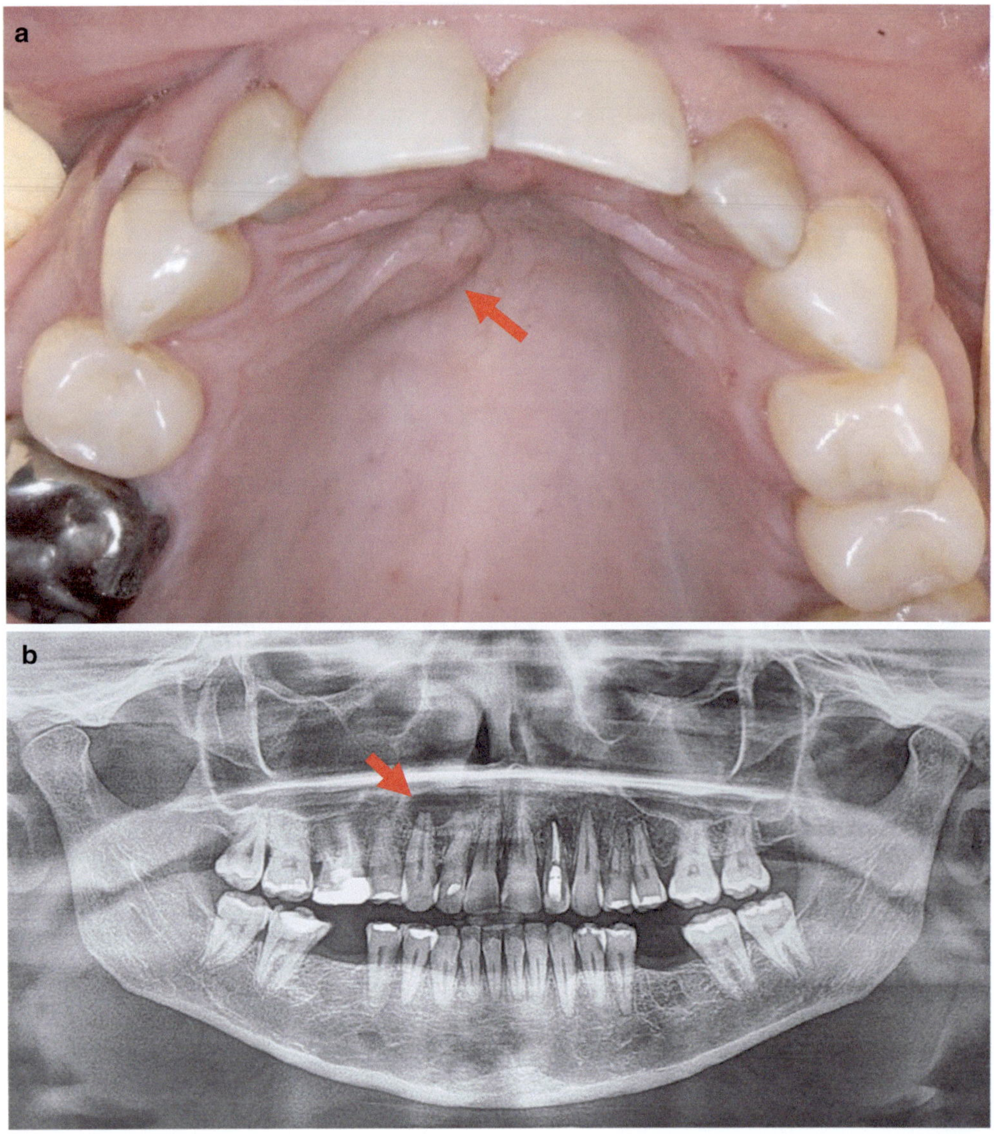

Fig. 12.1 Clinical and radiographic features of radicular periapical cyst. (**a**) Clinical manifestation of a male patient exhibiting an asymptomatic swelling in the palate (red arrow). (**b**) Panoramic radiograph showing the radicular periapical cyst associated with tooth apex (red arrow)

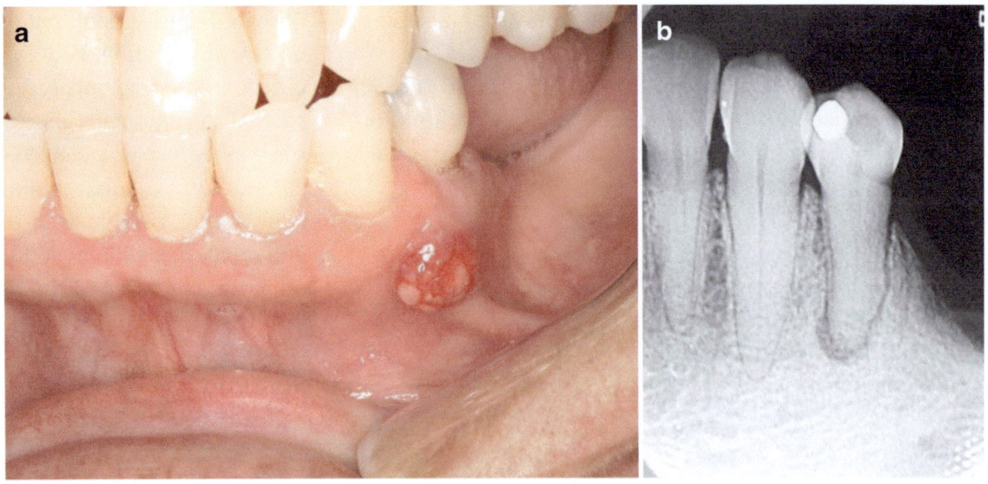

Fig. 12.2 Clinical and radiographic features of radicular periapical abscess. (**a**) Clinical presentation of gingival fistulae associated with a periapical abscess. (**b**) Periapical radiograph showing a small radiolucent ill-defined image in the periapical region of the lower premolar

of the dental biofilm. With the advent of dental implants and the establishment of osseointegration principles, *peri-implantitis* has gained significant attention. It is currently defined as a pathological condition affecting tissues surrounding dental implants, characterized by inflammation in the peri-implant connective tissue and progressive loss of supporting bone. *Localized juvenile spongiotic gingival hyperplasia* is a rare and recently described entity distinct from biofilm-induced gingivitis. It does not respond to biofilm removal. This condition primarily affects children and young adults, with no sex predilection. Clinically, it presents as a solitary, red, and papillated lesion, which may be ulcerated or prone to bleeding, most commonly occurring in the anterior maxillary gingiva.

Plasma cell gingivitis is a rare, benign inflammatory condition affecting the marginal and attached gingiva, for which a definitive diagnosis requires ruling out other more specific conditions. This disorder is typically associated with allergic processes due to various antigens, including dental materials, toothpastes, oral rinses, chewing gums, and spices. Consequently, an accurate diagnostic workup heavily relies on patients' history. Similar conditions that affect other regions of the oral mucosa, such as the lips, buccal mucosa, palate, and tongue have been reported and termed as *plasma cell mucositis*; however, the exact biological significance of this polyclonal idiopathic nonspecific condition remains debatable and poorly understood. Plasma cell gingivitis commonly presents as erythematous regions in the anterior vestibular gingiva of intense red color, confluent, and delimited from the healthy neighboring gingival tissue. The affected areas may also exhibit ulceration or hyperplasia. The maxillary gingiva is more affected than mandibular gingiva, although both jaws can be simultaneously affected in some cases. Although the condition is usually asymptomatic, patients may report burning sensation or a feeling of local tension. Unlike biofilm-related gingivitis, plasma cell gingivitis often extends beyond the marginal gingiva. A distinguishing feature from bullous disorders is the negative Nikolsky sign. A thorough clinical and microscopic differential diagnosis is essential for plasma cell gingivitis and plasma cell mucositis. Considerations should include immune-related oral mucosal conditions, such as oral lichen planus and foreign-body gingivitis; systemic conditions, including Crohn's disease and IgG4-related disease; and plasma cell malignancies.

The presence of local traumatic agents that cause a continuous and low-intensity irritative stimulus in the oral mucosa, in the gingiva, such as biofilm or calculus accumulation, often leads to non-neoplastic proliferative processes like *pyogenic granuloma* or *gingival inflammatory hyperplasia.* These conditions are characterized by a nonspecific chronic inflammatory infiltrate with a variable degree of blood vessel proliferation. Clinically, they present symptomatic nodules of varying size and shape in the gingival tissue, typically exhibiting an ulcerated surface and a color spectrum ranging from normal to reddish to purple, reflecting the vascular component of each lesion.

Treatment of these reactive dental and periodontal inflammatory processes is usually localized and involves the removal of the irritative agent responsible for chronic aggression to the gingival tissue. The elimination of the biofilm is essential for managing biofilm-induced gingivitis and periodontitis. In contrast, localized juvenile spongiotic gingival hyperplasia does not respond to conventional oral hygiene like brushing and flossing and this disorder carries potential for recurrence after biopsy. The use of localized ablative procedures such as cryotherapy has also been recommended. Although there is no consensus on the optimal treatment for plasma cell gingivitis and plasma cell mucositis, these conditions are frequently associated with hypersensitivity to certain antigens. Therefore, identifying and removing the etiologic agent is considered mandatory step in treatment. Pyogenic granuloma requires surgical removal along with periodontal treatment. The prognosis for patients is generally excellent, provided that the etiologic agents are effectively eliminated.

12.2 Microscopic Findings

12.2.1 Radicular Periapical Abscess, Granuloma, and Cyst

- Periapical abscesses are characterized by the presence of many neutrophils in an edematous stroma.
- There may be simultaneous chronic and acute inflammatory infiltrates within the same lesion.
- Periapical granuloma is defined by a dense chronic inflammatory infiltrate containing histiocytes, lymphocytes, and plasma cells (granulation tissue).
- The presence of Russel bodies is frequently observed, especially in cases with a large number of plasma cells. In patients with a medical history of multiple myeloma, dental periapical granulomas rich in plasma cells should be differentiated from infiltration by neoplastic plasma cells. The absence of light chain immunoglobulin (kappa/lambda) restriction can help distinguish a reactive infiltrate from a neoplasm.
- Foamy macrophages are commonly seen.
- Dystrophic calcifications are common.
- Despite its terminology, true granuloma formation does not occur; instead, granulation tissue is present.
- Blood vessels are abundant and fibrotic stroma is variable.

- The inflammatory infiltrate observed in the capsule of radicular periapical cysts is similar to that of periapical granulomas, with the presence of a non-keratinized epithelial lining often serving as a distinguishing feature between the two entities (Figs. 12.3, 12.4, and 12.5).

12.2.2 Biofilm-Induced Gingivitis, Periodontitis, and Peri-implantitis

- Acanthosis and exocytosis of the overlying stratified and keratinized squamous epithelium.
- The non-keratinized epithelium of the gingival sulcus presents hyperplastic and with exocytosis.
- The lamina propria is edematous and with chronic inflammatory infiltrate.
- The inflammatory infiltrate contains lymphocytes and a large number of plasma cells.
- Vascular blood proliferation (Fig. 12.6).

12.2.3 Localized Juvenile Spongiotic Gingival Hyperplasia

- The overlying gingival stratified squamous epithelium exhibits spongiotic and acanthotic features.
- There is the presence of elongated rete ridges.
- The epithelium shows areas of both atrophy and hyperplasia.
- A dense reactive inflammatory infiltrate is frequently observed in the connective tissue.
- An abrupt transition is evident between the disordered epithelium and the adjacent normal mucosa.
- The inflammatory infiltrate is predominantly neutrophilic.
- Plasma cell infiltration in the connective tissue is also common, with scattered eosinophils (Fig. 12.7).

12.2.4 Plasma Cell Gingivitis and Plasma Cell Mucositis

- Acanthosis and exocytosis of the overlying stratified squamous epithelium are present.
- The lamina propria is edematous and contains a dense plasmacytic infiltrate.
- Inflammatory lichenoid features are present in some cases.
- Superficial and deep perivascular inflammation is also frequently observed.
- The inflammatory infiltrate is densely populated with plasma cells.
- Vascular blood proliferation is noted.
- Russel bodies are commonly found.
- These pathological processes are polyclonal, with plasma cells demonstrating a normal immunoglobulin light chain kappa/lambda ratio (Fig. 12.8).

12.2.5 Pyogenic Granuloma

- Acanthosis and exocytosis of the overlying stratified and keratinized squamous epithelium are present.
- Areas of ulceration are covered by a fibrinous pseudo-membrane.
- The lamina propria is edematous and contains dense chronic inflammation.
- Proliferation of numerous blood vessels.
- The inflammatory infiltrate contains lymphocytes and plasma cells.
- Scattered macrophages are also present.
- The region adjacent to the ulcer contains a high number of neutrophils.
- The ulcerated area is covered by an eosinophilic fibrinous exudate.
- Numerous blood vessels of varying size and shape are found (Fig. 12.9).

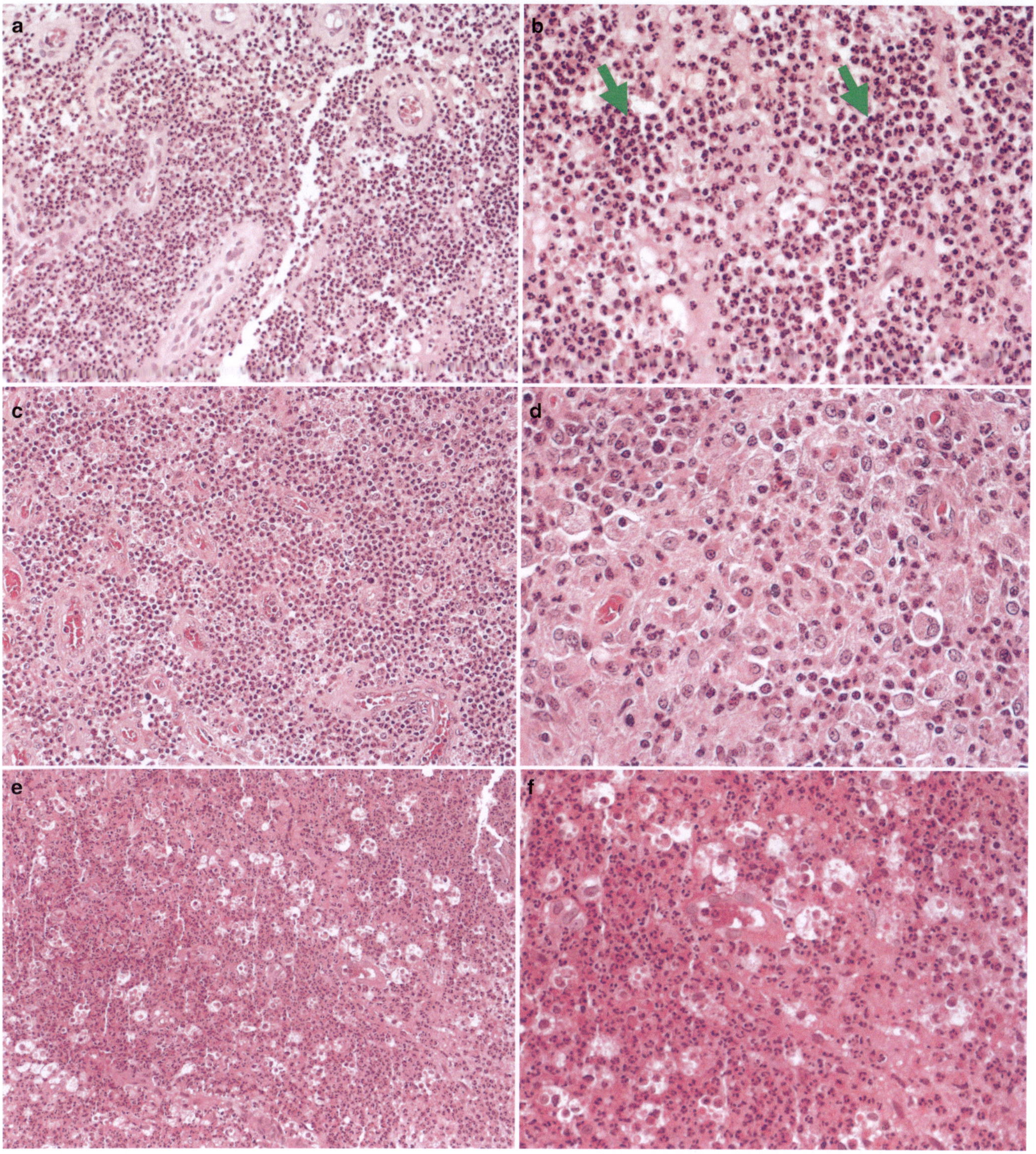

Fig. 12.3 Microscopic findings of radicular periapical abscess. (**a**) Diffuse distribution of neutrophils (H&E; 50×). (**b**) Note the large number of polymorphonuclear cells (neutrophils) (green arrows) in an edematous stroma with several blood vessels (H&E; 200×). (**c**) Periapical abscess exhibiting areas of chronic inflammatory infiltrate with proliferation of blood vessels and mononuclear inflammatory cells (H&E; 100×). (**d**) In these areas where periapical abscess exhibits a changing to a more chronic inflammatory infiltrate, there is an increased number of histiocytes and plasma cells, although neutrophils are still easily observed (H&E; 400×). (**e**) In some instances, there may be the presence of scattered histiocytes with clear cytoplasm (H&E; 100×). (**f**) Note that the presence of clear cell histiocytes impart a starry-sky-like pattern (H&E; 200×)

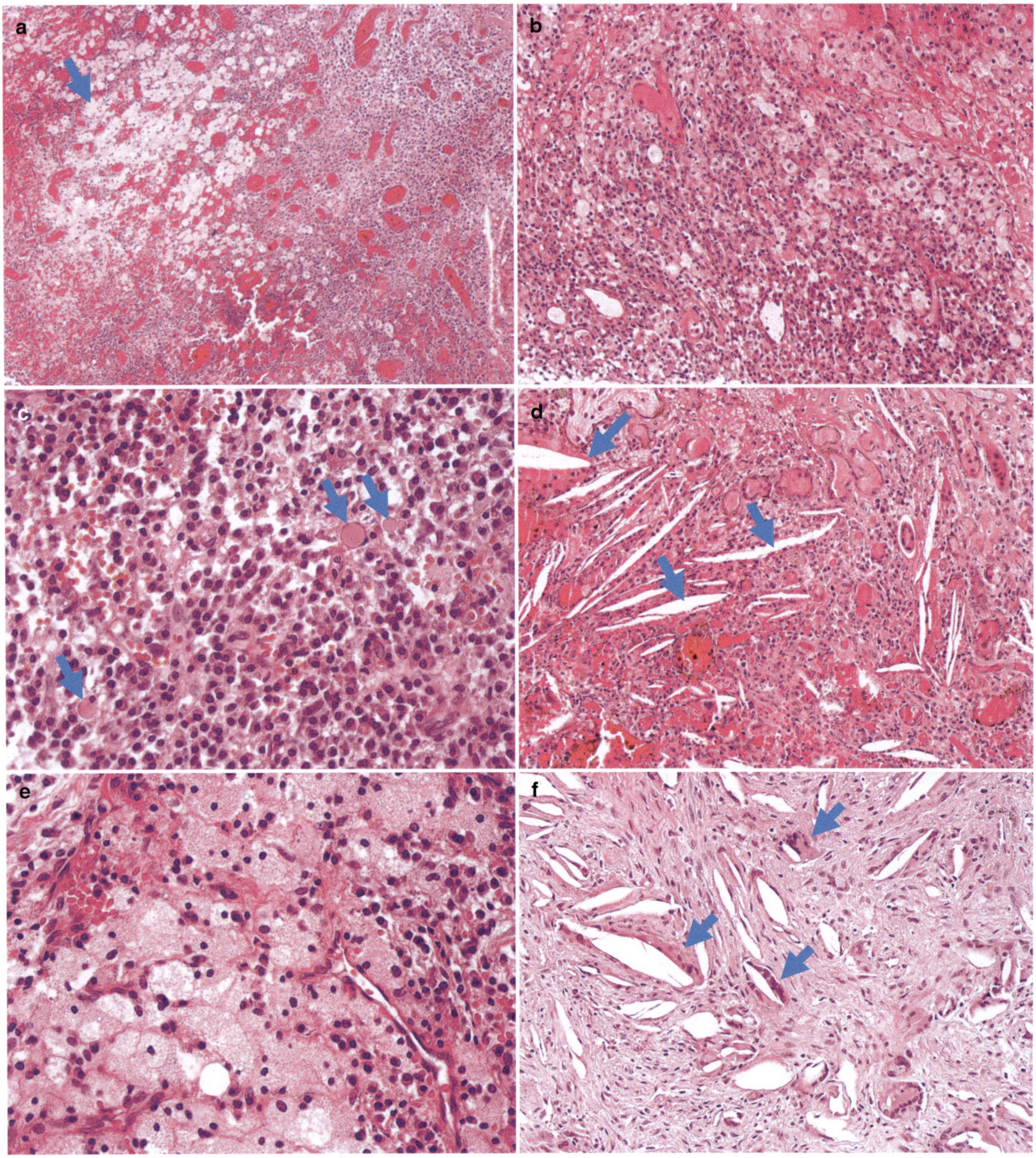

Fig. 12.4 Microscopic findings of radicular periapical granuloma. (**a**) Chronic inflammatory infiltrate with blood vessel proliferation and the presence of foamy histiocytes (blue arrow) (H&E; 50×). (**b**) The chronic inflammatory infiltrate contains a predominance of lymphocytes and plasma cells, with a variable number of histiocytes (H&E; 100×). (**c**) Russel bodies (blue arrow) are commonly found surrounded by many reactive plasma cells. Despite its terminology, there is no granulomatous inflammatory tissue or granuloma formation, but rather, a nonspecific granulation tissue (H&E; 200×). (**d**) The presence of cholesterol crystals (blue arrow) may be associated with foreign body-type multinucleated giant cells (H&E; 200×). (**e**) Histiocytes are frequently observed in radicular periapical granulomas, very often as foamy cells (H&E; 200×). (**f**) There is an increased number of blood vessels and a variable degree of fibrosis in the stroma. Note in this image the presence of cholesterol crystal surrounded by multinucleated giant cells (blue arrow) (H&E; 200×)

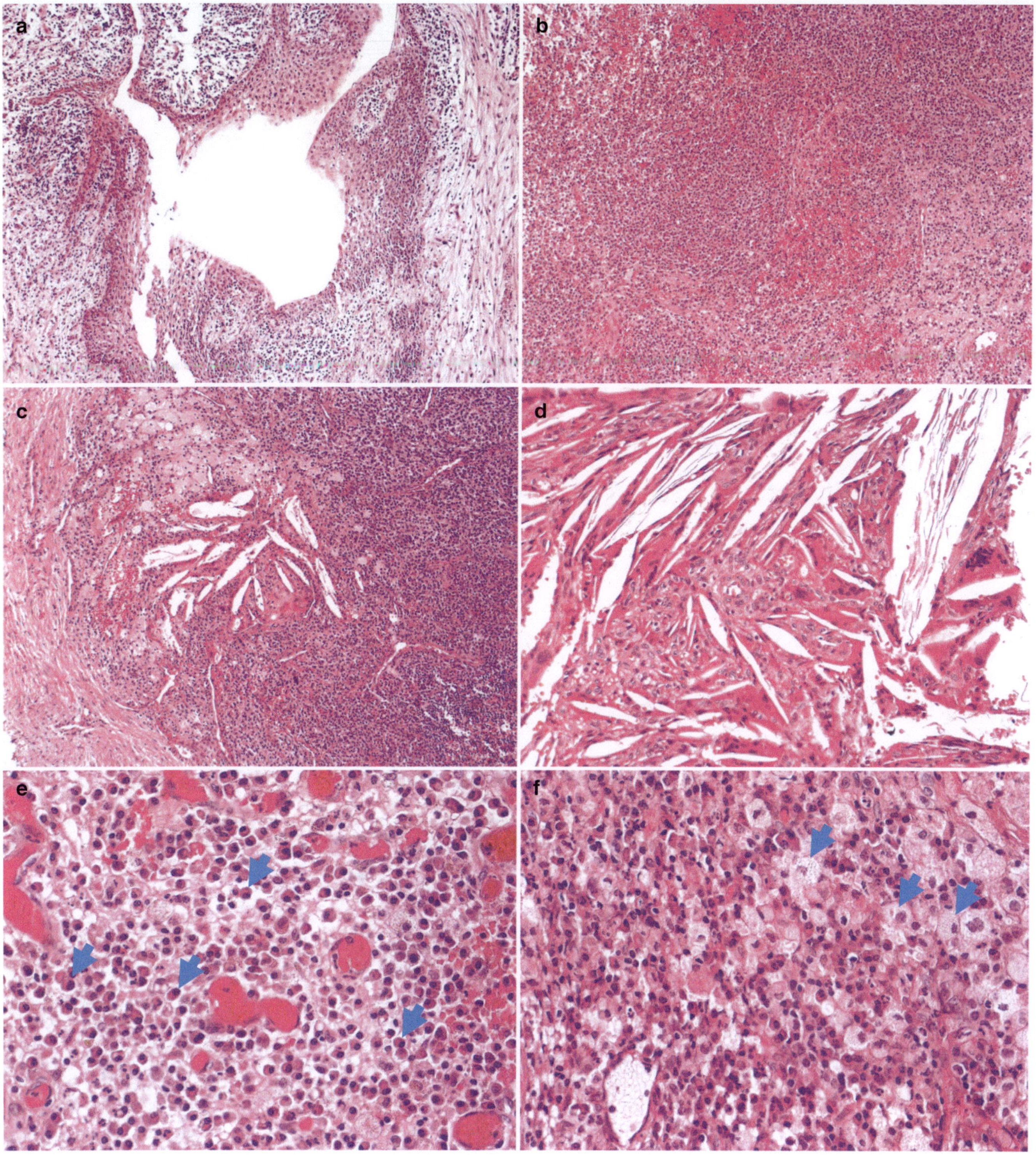

Fig. 12.5 Microscopic features of radicular periapical cysts. (**a**) The epithelium lining usually present as non-keratinized with exocytosis and hyperplastic features (H&E; 100×). (**b**) The fibrous capsule of the cyst contains a chronic inflammatory infiltrate with lymphocytes, histiocytes, and plasma cells (H&E; 100×). (**c**) Cholesterol crystals are commonly observed in the capsule or in the lumen of the inflammatory periapical cysts (H&E; 100×). (**d**) Note the presence of foreign body-type multinucleated giant cells surrounding the cholesterol crystals (H&E; 200×). (**e**) Note the presence of plasma cells (blue arrows) and blood vessels (H&E; 100×). (**f**) The presence of foamy histiocytes is also common (blue arrows) (H&E; 200×)

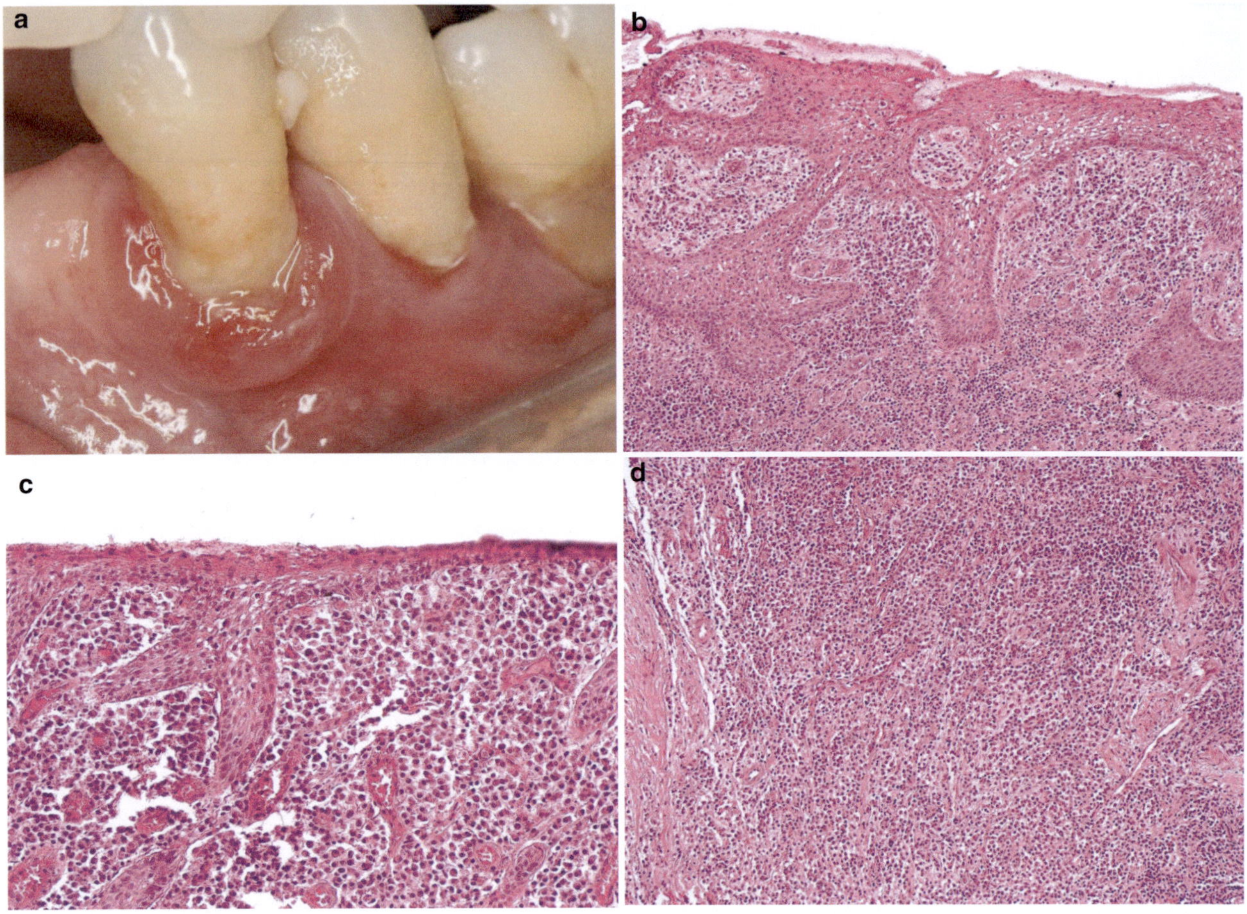

Fig. 12.6 Clinical and microscopic presentation of biofilm-induced gingivitis and periodontitis. (**a**) Erythematous and swollen gingival tissue. The inflammatory process in this case is more advanced and caused supportive periodontal tissue loss and tooth mobility, characterizing a periodontitis. Observe the presence of biofilm accumulated in the gingival margin. (**b**) Non-keratinized squamous epithelium of the gingival sulcus exhibiting exocytosis. Observe the severe chronic inflammatory infiltrate in the lamina propria (H&E; 50×). (**c**) Atrophic epithelium of the gingival sulcus and severe chronic inflammatory infiltrate with predominance of plasma cells, a characteristic of this reactive process (H&E; 100×). (**d**) The inflammatory infiltrate extends toward deeper regions of the lamina propria (H&E; 100×)

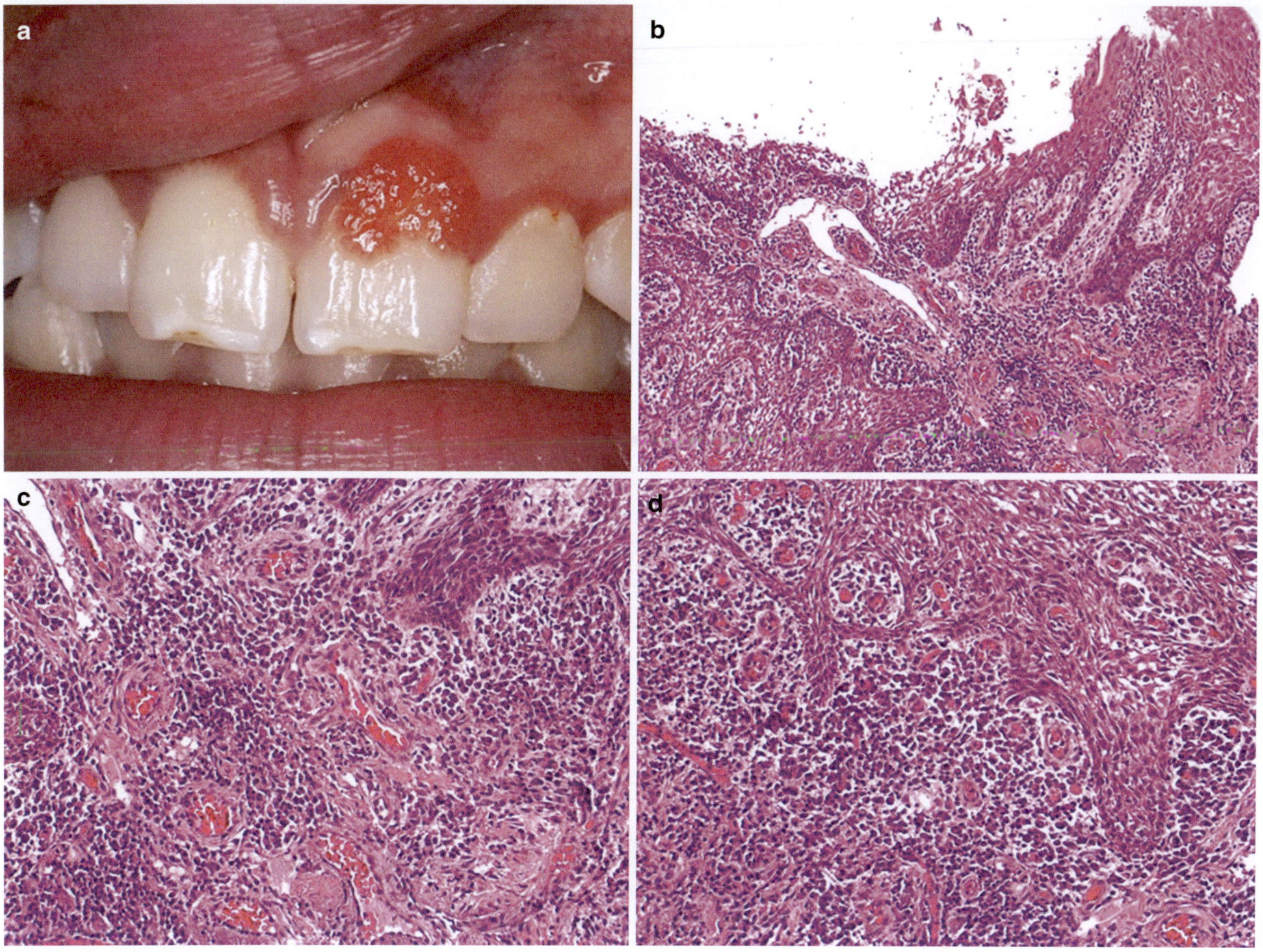

Fig. 12.7 Clinical and microscopic features of localized juvenile spongiotic gingival hyperplasia. (**a**) Observe the lesion affecting the anterior maxillary tooth of a 28-years-old female patient. The lesion presented as a reddish nodule in the gingival margin. (**b**) Microscopically, there was epithelial spongiosis, acanthosis, and hyperplasia (H&E; 50×). (**c**) Presence of chronic inflammatory cells in the epithelium (H&E; 100×). (**d**) Presence of plasma cells and lymphocytes in the lamina propria (H&E; 100×)

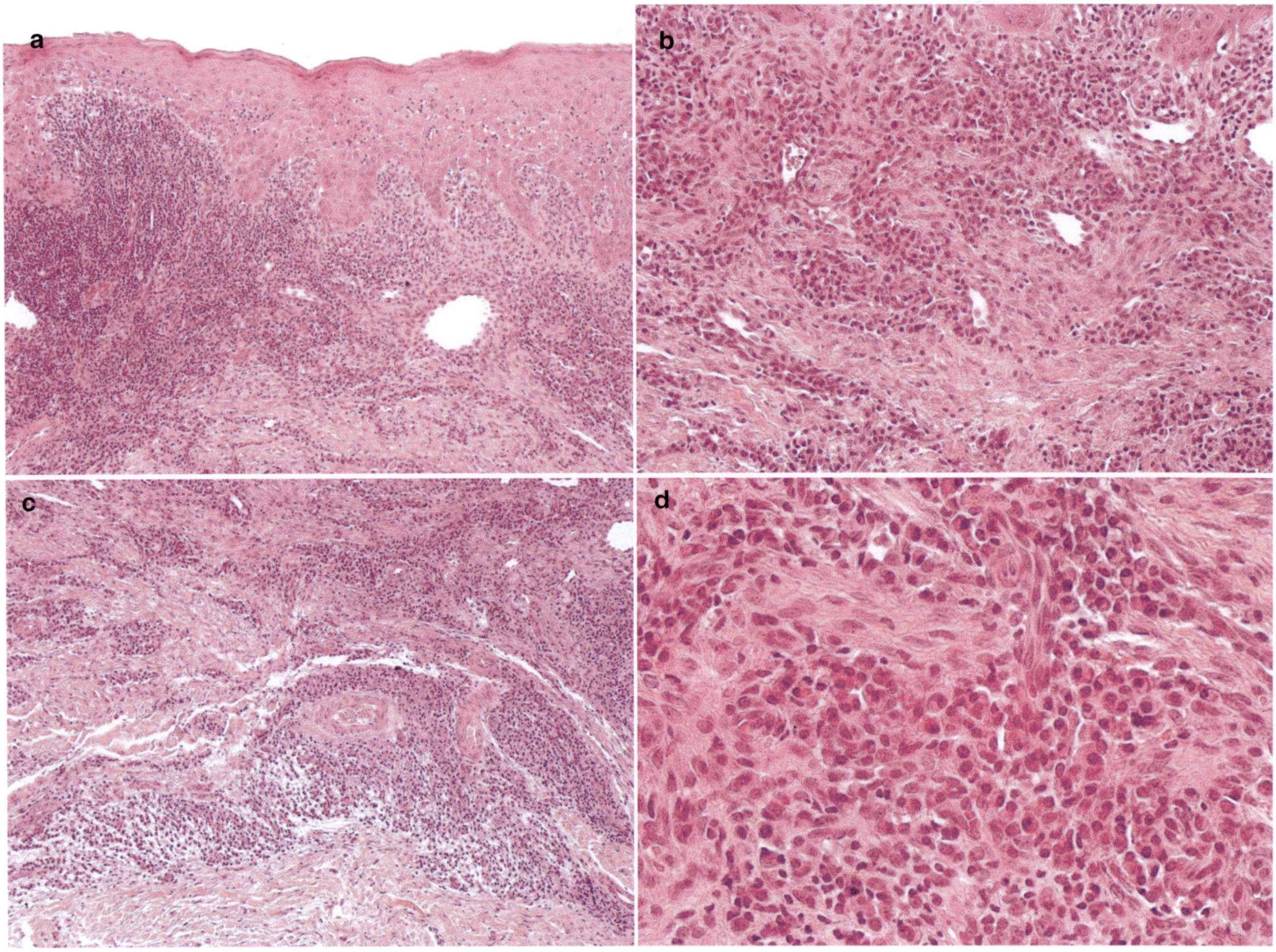

Fig. 12.8 Microscopic features of plasma cell gingivitis. (**a**) Overlying squamous epithelium exhibiting a moderate degree of exocytosis. Observe a dense inflammatory infiltrate in the lamina propria (H&E; 50×). (**b**) In the connective tissue, the inflammatory infiltrate is composed predominantly by plasma cells (H&E; 100×). (**c**) This infiltrate is also located deeper in the connective tissue and surrounds blood vessels (H&E; 100×). (**d**) Under higher magnification, it is possible to observe with more details the plasma cells that are present in this inflammatory infiltrate (H&E; 200×)

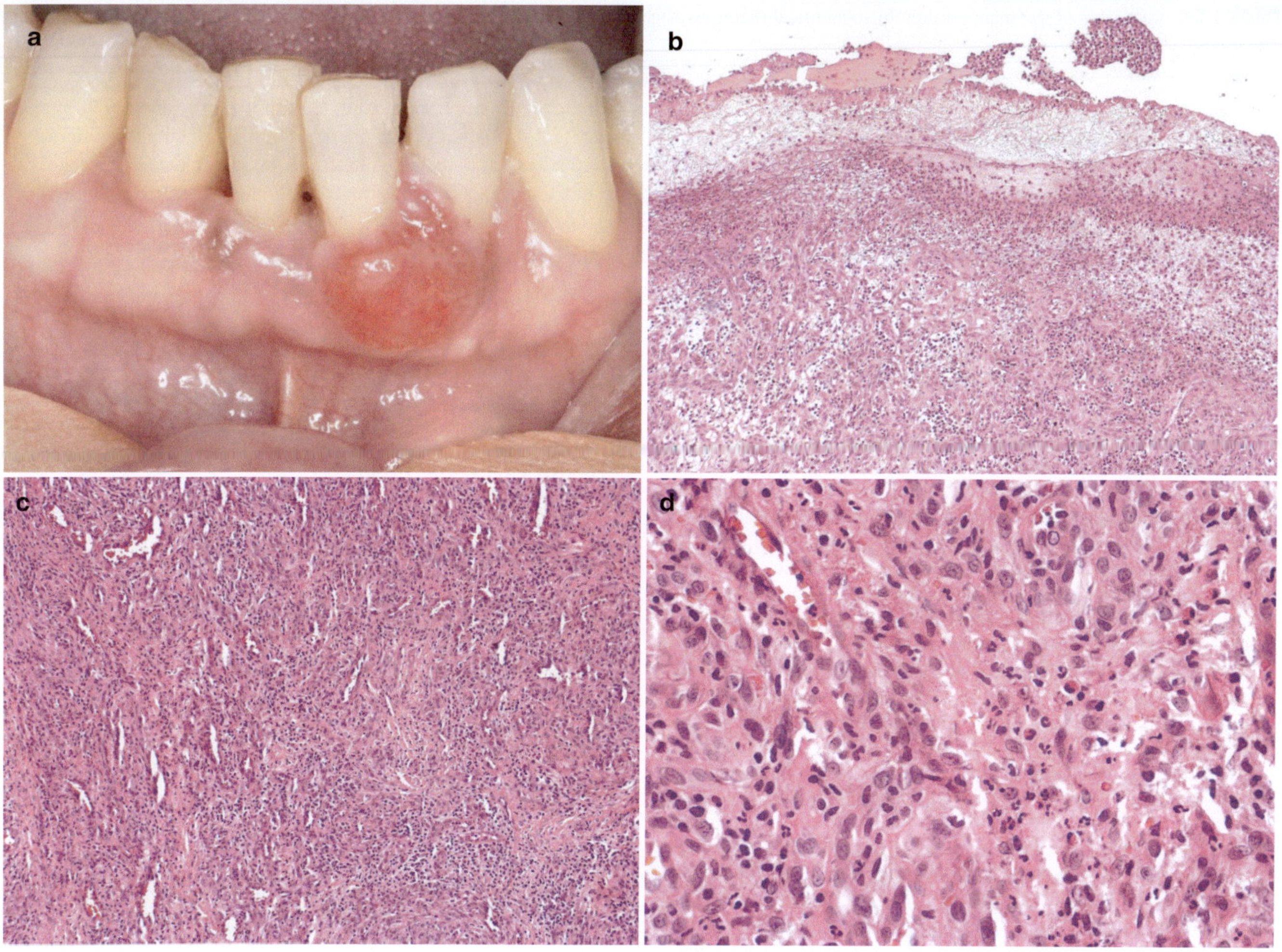

Fig. 12.9 Clinical and microscopic features of pyogenic granuloma in the gingival tissue. (**a**) The presence of a reddish nodule in the lower gingiva. (**b**) The ulcerated region of this lesion is covered by a fibrinous pseudomembrane (H&E; 50×). (**c**) In the connective tissue, there is a dense chronic inflammatory infiltrate predominantly composed of lymphocytes and plasma cells, with a strong blood vessel proliferation (H&E; 100×). (**d**) Under higher magnification, it is possible to observe with more details the lymphocytes and plasma cells, as well as the blood vessels and neutrophils (H&E; 200×)

12.3 Immunohistochemistry and/or Genetics

Radicular periapical inflammatory lesions are typically diagnosed using hematoxylin and eosin (H&E)-stained slides in conjunction with clinical and radiographic data, while immunohistochemistry has limited applicability for these diagnoses. However, demonstrating the polyclonal nature of the plasma cell infiltrate in radicular periapical granulomas can be helpful in ruling out potential neoplastic infiltration in patients with multiple myeloma. In cases where differentiating reactive gingival disease from a neoplastic process is necessary, immunohistochemistry can also demonstrate the presence of a polyclonal inflammatory infiltrate. This infiltrate contains B and T lymphocytes, which are stained by CD20 and CD3, respectively, along with scattered macrophages (CD68). Plasma cells (CD138/MUM1/EMA) are often abundant and do not exhibit immunoglobulin light chain restriction, as these lesions are polyclonal with normal kappa and lambda ratio. The proliferative index is variable, but typically low (Table 12.1).

Table 12.1 Summary of the main immunohistochemical reactions used for characterizing the reactive periapical and periodontal inflammatory processes

Antibody	Most frequent results	Pattern	Objective
CD20	Positive	Membrane	To demonstrate the B lymphocyte component of the inflammatory infiltrate
CD3	Positive	Membrane	To demonstrate the T lymphocyte component of the inflammatory infiltrate
CD138	Positive	Membrane	To demonstrate the plasma cell component of the inflammatory infiltrate
CD68	Positive	Cytoplasm	To demonstrate the presence of macrophages in the inflammatory infiltrate
Kappa/lambda	Polyclonal	Cytoplasm	To demonstrate the polyclonal nature of the plasma cell infiltrate
Ki67	Variable	Nucleus	To demonstrate the proliferative index of the inflammatory infiltrate

Sources

1. León JE, Takahama Júnior A, Vassallo J, Soares FA, de Almeida OP, Lopes MA. EBV-associated polymorphic posttransplant lymphoproliferative disorder presenting as gingival ulcers. Int J Surg Pathol. 2011;19:241–6. https://doi.org/10.1177/1066896909353599.
2. Thorbert-Mros S, Larsson L, Berglundh T. Cellular composition of long-standing gingivitis and periodontitis lesions. J Periodontal Res. 2015;50:535–43. https://doi.org/10.1111/jre.12236.
3. Tavares DP, Rodrigues JT, Dos Santos TC, Armada L, Pires FR. Clinical and radiological analysis of a series of periapical cysts and periapical granulomas diagnosed in a Brazilian population. J Clin Exp Dent. 2017;9:e129–35. https://doi.org/10.4317/jced.53196.
4. Holmstrup P, Plemons J, Meyle J. Non–plaque-induced gingival diseases. J Clin Periodontol. 2018;45:S28–43. https://doi.org/10.1111/jcpe.12938.
5. Schwarz F, Derks J, Monje A, Wang H-L. Peri-implantitis. J Clin Periodontol. 2018;45:S246–66. https://doi.org/10.1111/jcpe.12954.
6. Trombelli L, Farina R, Silva CO, Tatakis DN. Plaque-induced gingivitis: case definition and diagnostic considerations. J Clin Periodontol. 2018;45:S44–67. https://doi.org/10.1111/jcpe.12939.
7. Wang MZ, Jordan RC. Localized juvenile spongiotic gingival hyperplasia: a report of 27 cases. J Cutan Pathol. 2019;46:839–43. https://doi.org/10.1111/cup.13549.
8. Couto AMD, Meirelles DP, Valeriano AT, Almeida DS, Moraes Ê, Tarquinio SBC, et al. Chronic inflammatory periapical diseases: a Brazilian multicenter study of 10,381 cases and literature review. Braz Oral Res. 2021;35:e033. https://doi.org/10.1590/1807-3107bor-2021.vol35.0033.
9. Coppola N, Cantile T, Canfora F, Adamo D, Bucci P, Mignogna MD, Leuci S. Pitfalls and challenges in oral plasma cell mucositis: a systematic review. J Clin Med. 2022;11:6550. https://doi.org/10.3390/jcm11216550.
10. Younis RH, Georgaki M, Nikitakis NG. Plasma cell gingivitis and its mimics. Oral Maxillofac Surg Clin North Am. 2023;35:261–70. https://doi.org/10.1016/j.coms.2022.10.003.
11. Baesso RC, Azevedo RS, Picciani BL, Pires FR. Gingival and alveolar mucosal reactive hyperplastic lesions: a retrospective clinical and histological study of 996 cases. Med Oral Patol Oral Cir Bucal. 2023;28:e347–54. https://doi.org/10.4317/medoral.25766.
12. Fitzpatrick SG, Alramadhan S, Islam MN, Bhattacharyya I. Increased frequency of oral plasma cell mucositis/plasma cell gingivitis after the COVID-19 pandemic: a 23-year retrospective analysis and review of diagnostic challenges relating to this condition. Oral Surg Oral Med Oral Pathol Oral Radiol. 2024;137:153–60. https://doi.org/10.1016/j.oooo.2023.08.010.
13. Visarnta S, Ratisoontorn C, Panichuttra A, Sinpitaksakul P, Chantarangsu S, Dhanuthai K. Macrophage polarization in human periapical lesions in relation to histopathological diagnosis, clinical features and lesion volume: an ex vivo study. Int Endod J. 2024;57:1829–47. https://doi.org/10.1111/iej.14138.
14. Immanuel J, Pandiar D, Krishnan RP. Clinicopathological comparison of periapical cyst and periapical granuloma in a cohort of Tamil population. J Conserv Dent Endod. 2024;27:524–8. https://doi.org/10.4103/JCDE.JCDE_160_24.
15. Wongpattaraworakul W, Krongbaramee T, Lanzel EA, Hellstein JW, Teixeira FB. Hematolymphoid neoplasm mimicking endodontic lesions: case series and review of the literature. Oral Surg Oral Med Oral Pathol Oral Radiol. 2025;139:e1–e12. https://doi.org/10.1016/j.oooo.2024.07.011.

Lichenoid Granulomatous Reaction

13

Cinthia Veronica Bardalez Lopez de Caceres,
Pablo Agustin Vargas, Hélder Antônio Rebelo Pontes,
and Felipe Paiva Fonseca

13.1 General Overview and Clinical Presentation

Lichenoid granulomatous reaction is a very rare and controversial entity, microscopically characterized by the presence of histiocytes and granulomatous infiltrate together with a justaepithelial band-like lymphocytic process. It may be under-reported and frequently misdiagnosed by pathologists not familiarized with this condition. Depending on the anatomical location affected by this disorder, it can be named as lichenoid granulomatous dermatitis when the skin is primarily affected, or lichenoid granulomatous stomatitis when the oral mucosa is the affected tissue. It is believed that lichenoid granulomatous reactions were first described by Gonzalez et al. in 1986, and were more detailed and characterized by Magro and Crowson in 2000, who proposed a classification scheme based on the degree of histiocytic and granulomatous components in the microscopic features of the disorder.

The etiology and pathogenesis of this condition are largely unknown, but different authors claim that it can be associated with medications, microorganisms, and foreign materials. However, such hypotheses further contribute to making the understanding of this entity very difficult, and its recognition as an independent entity is also challenged by the possible inability to find small foreign materials or the lack of clinical data on medication use that could more specifically explain the granulomatous reaction.

C. V. B. L. de Caceres (✉) · F. P. Fonseca
Department of Oral Surgery and Pathology, School of Dentistry, Universidade Federal de Minas Gerais, Belo Horizonte, Brazil

P. A. Vargas
Oral and Maxillofacial Division, Piracicaba Dental School, State University of Campinas (UNICAMP), Piracicaba, Brazil
e-mail: pavargas@fop.unicamp.br

H. A. R. Pontes
Service of Oral Pathology, João de Barros Barreto University Hospital, Federal University of Pará, Belém, Brazil
e-mail: harp@ufpa.br

Lichenoid granulomatous dermatitis is more common in adult females between 40 and 55 years old, and clinical manifestations range from erythematous to maculopapular to desquamative cutaneous processes that more often occur in the trunk, arms, and legs. In the oral cavity, lichenoid granulomatous stomatitis was initially described in 2006 by Robinson et al. who described a series of six patients presenting erythematous patches or swellings in the upper lip mucosa. In a large series published by Hakeen et al. in 2019, the authors described 47 new cases, with a mean age of 59 years, a female predominance (64%), and more often affecting the gingiva, buccal mucosa, vestibule, tongue, lip, and palate. Desquamative gingivitis and multifocal involvement of the oral mucosa have also been described. The lesions can be painful or completely asymptomatic. First clinical impression varied significantly, ranging from leukoplakia, squamous cell carcinoma, lichen planus, vesiculobullous disease, trauma, and allergy.

Affected patients are usually treated with steroids; however, Robinson et al. demonstrated that all their patients submitted to steroid medications were persistent and refractory to treatment, showing phases of active disease followed by periods of quiescence.

13.2 Microscopic Findings

- Cases typically demonstrate a lichenoid inflammatory infiltrate, characterized by hyperkeratosis of the overlying squamous epithelium, with the presence of basal cell damage, occasional apoptotic bodies, and a band-like lymphohistiocytic infiltrate located in the lamina propria near the epithelium.
- The band-like lymphohistiocytic infiltrate also extends toward deeper areas of the connective tissue, which is a useful finding to differentiate this entity from oral lichen planus.

© The Author(s), under exclusive license to Springer Nature Switzerland AG 2025
F. P. Fonseca et al. (eds.), *Lymphoproliferative and Granulomatous Disorders of the Oral Cavity*,
https://doi.org/10.1007/978-3-031-98844-8_13

- There is a variable degree of granulomatous inflammation, typically containing epithelioid macrophages, but only a few or no multinucleated giant cells. The occurrence of more organized granulomas is reported in 42% of the patients, ranging from well-formed to ill-formed granulomas.
- Necrosis is not observed.
- Plasma cells can be found.
- Many cases characteristically demonstrate the presence of lymphoid nodules composed of monotonous, medium-sized lymphocytes that infiltrate the connective tissue.
- Perineural and perivascular distribution has been reported.
- The histological search for foreign material using polarized microscopy, and acid-alcohol-fast bacilli or any other microorganisms using special histologic stains should result in negative.
- Hakeen et al. (2019) proposed a modified histological classification for lichenoid granulomatous stomatitis based on the Magro and Crowson Classification for lichenoid granulomatous stomatitis. According to the authors, the lesions can be classified according to four types, as follows:

  Type 1: Band-like lymphocytic infiltration with superficially loose or aggregates of histiocytes and perivascular inflammatory infiltrate.

  Type 2: Band-like lymphocytic infiltration with superficially loose or aggregates of histiocytes and no perivascular inflammatory infiltrate.

  Type 3: Lichenoid infiltration with epithelioid giant cell granuloma and perivasculitis.

  Type 4: Lichenoid infiltration with epithelioid giant cell granuloma and no perivasculitis (Figs. 13.1, 13.2, 13.3, 13.4, 13.5, and 13.6).

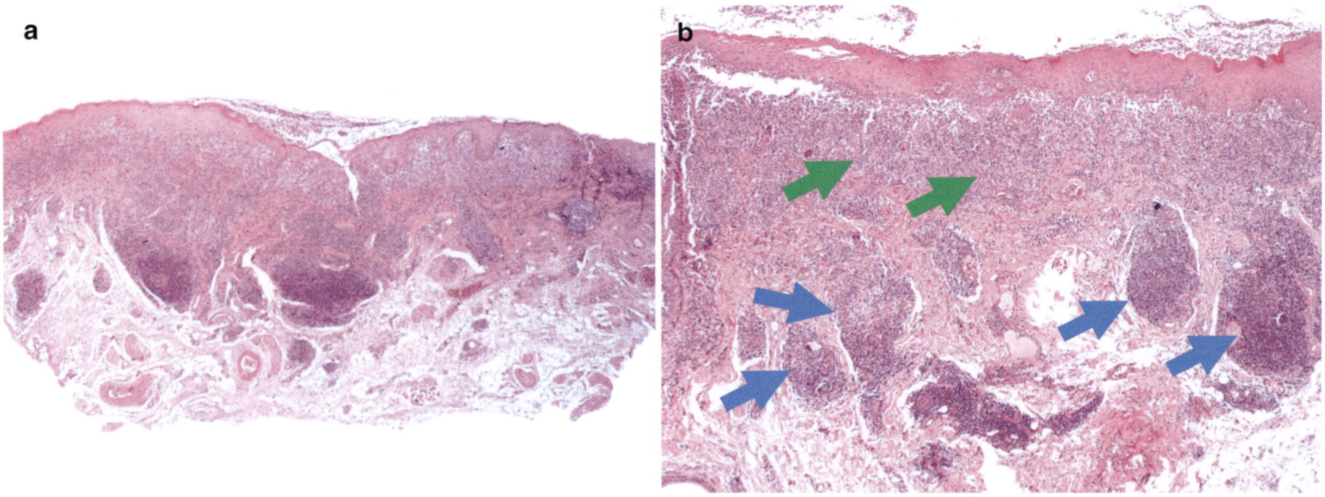

Fig. 13.1 Microscopic features of lichenoid granulomatous stomatitis affecting the upper lip of a young adult male patient. (**a**) Presence of a justa-epithelial band-like inflammatory infiltrate with lymphoid nodules proliferating deeper in the lamina propria (H&E; 25×). (**b**) Note the lymphoid nodules in the lamina propria (blue arrows) and the lichenoid pattern beneath the epithelium (green arrows) (H&E; 100×)

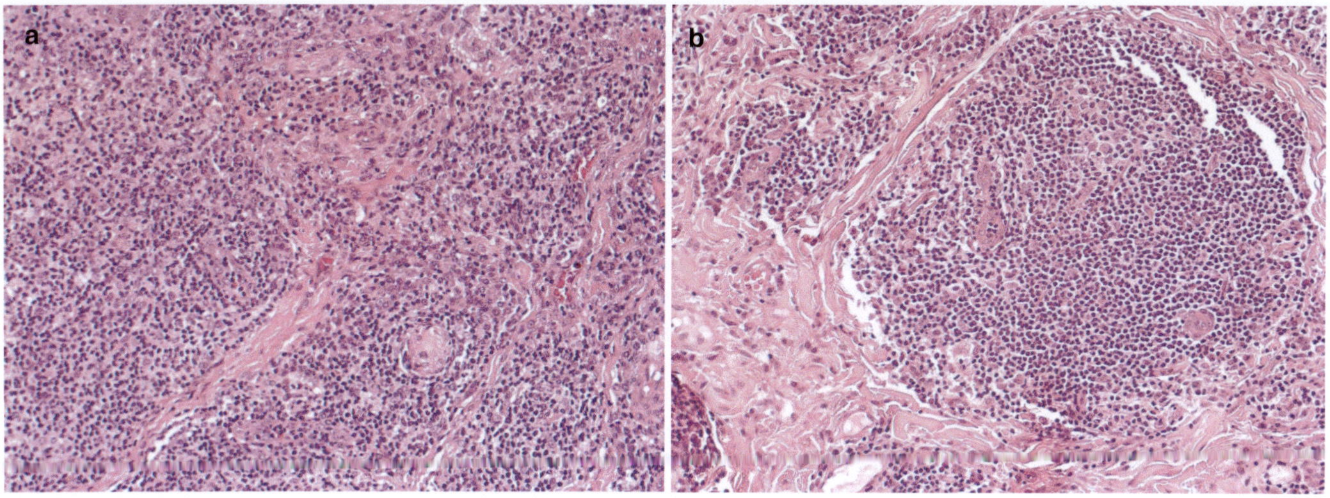

Fig. 13.2 Microscopic features of lichenoid granulomatous stomatitis affecting the upper lip of a young adult male patient. (**a**) Predominance of lymphoid cells in the nodules (H&E; 200×). (**b**) Note the lymphoid nodule in the lamina propria (H&E; 200)

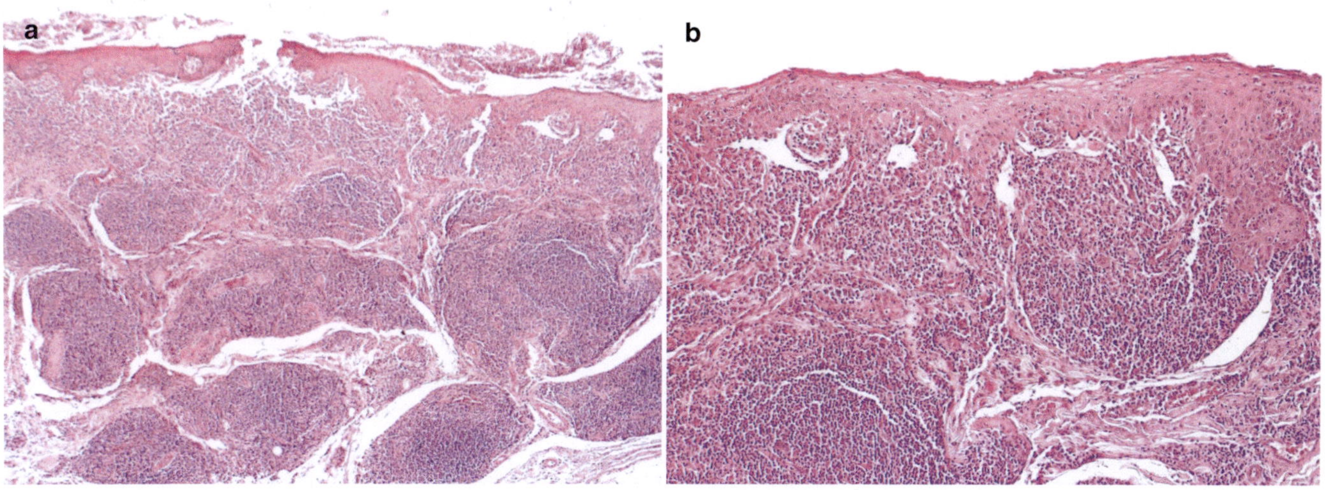

Fig. 13.3 Microscopic features of lichenoid granulomatous stomatitis. (**a**) The disease is typically characterized by the presence of a justa-epithelial band-like inflammatory infiltrate and the presence of lymphoid nodules that proliferate toward a deeper portion of the lamina propria (H&E; 50×). (**b**) The overlying epithelium is atrophic, with some areas showing basal layer degeneration (H&E; 100×)

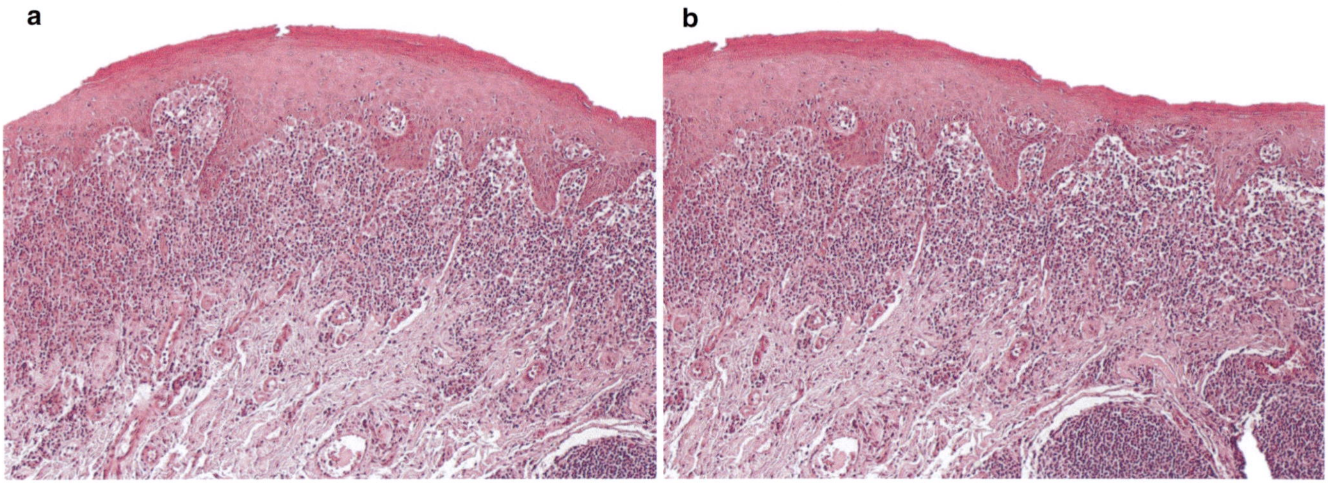

Fig. 13.4 Microscopic features of lichenoid granulomatous stomatitis. (**a**) Observe the presence of a dense inflammatory infiltrate distributed as a band-like process in a justa-epithelial location (H&E; 100×). The infiltrate contains a predominance of T lymphocytes, but it also has other reactive populations like plasma cells and B lymphocytes. Histiocytes are typically present; however, well-formed granulomas can be absent in some cases. (**b**) The band-like inflammatory infiltrate is located near the overlying epithelium (H&E; 100×)

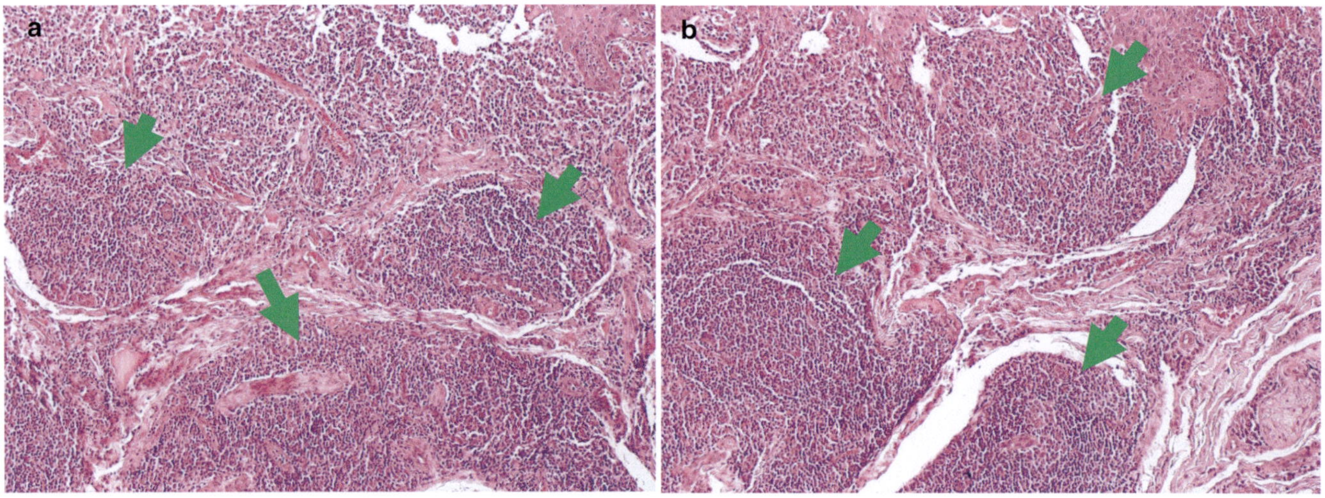

Fig. 13.5 Microscopic features of lichenoid granulomatous stomatitis. (**a**) The inflammatory infiltrate is also located in deeper areas of the lamina propria, exhibiting the formation of nodular structures (green arrows) predominantly composed of lymphocytes (H&E; 100×). (**b**) In this image, the presence of lymphoid nodules can also be observed (green arrows) (H&E; 100×)

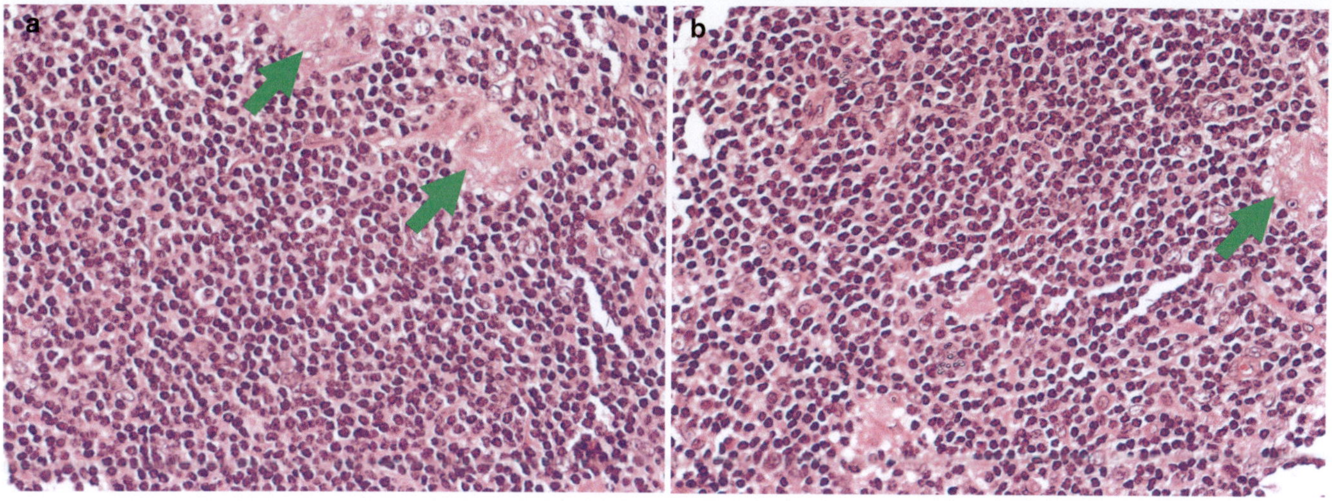

Fig. 13.6 Microscopic features of lichenoid granulomatous stomatitis. (**a**) In the inflammatory infiltrate, there is a predominance of lymphocytes, with scattered plasma cells and aggregates of epithelioid histiocytes (green arrows). The presence of well-formed granulomas is not considered mandatory for the final diagnosis (H&E; 200×). (**b**) Note the cellular distribution with predominance of lymphocytes, presence of plasma cells, and some epithelioid histiocytes (green arrow) (H&E; 200×)

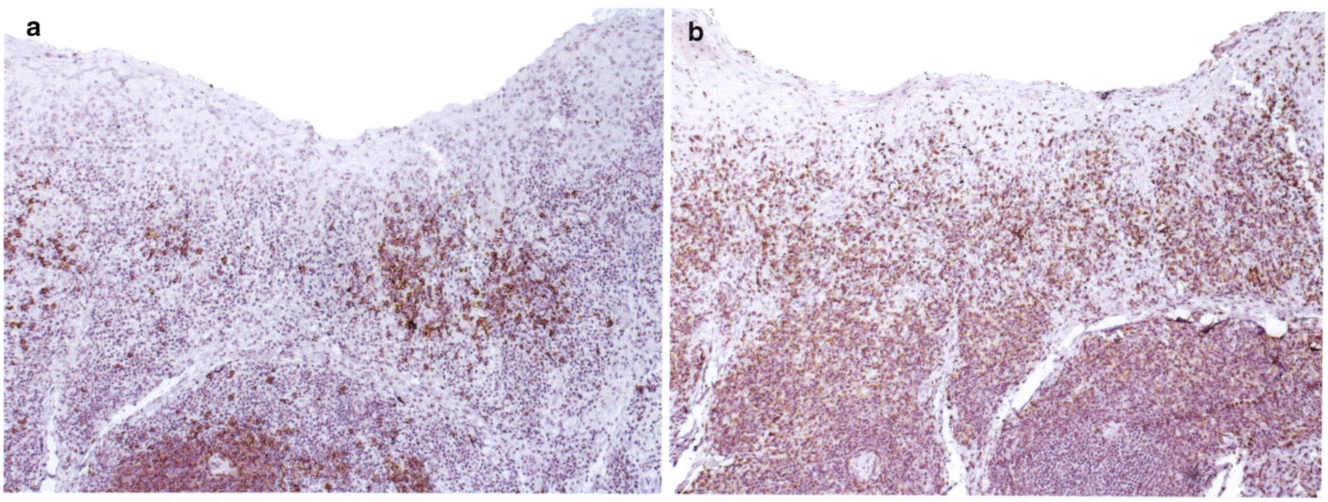

Fig. 13.7 Immunohistochemical features of lichenoid granulomatous stomatitis. (**a**) Presence of B lymphocytes distributed by the lesion can be demonstrated by CD20 expression, revealing a lower number of cells (DAB; 100×), (**b**) if compared to T lymphocytes demonstrated by CD3 expression. Note the predominance of this cell population over B lymphocytes (DAB; 100×)

13.3 Immunohistochemistry and/or Genetics

The diagnosis of lichenoid granulomatous stomatitis is challenging, but it is usually based on clinical presentation associated with the microscopic findings observed using routine H&E-stained sections. Immunohistochemistry has a limited value for the diagnostic approach of this disorder but can be used to characterize the cellular components. There is a predominance of CD3-positive T lymphocytes compared to CD20-positive B lymphocytes. The histiocytes and the granulomas can be highlighted by investigating CD68 expression. The absence of microorganisms should be determined using special histological reactions like PAS, Grocott-Gomori, and Ziehl-Neesen stains (Figs. 13.7, 13.8, and 13.9, Table 13.1).

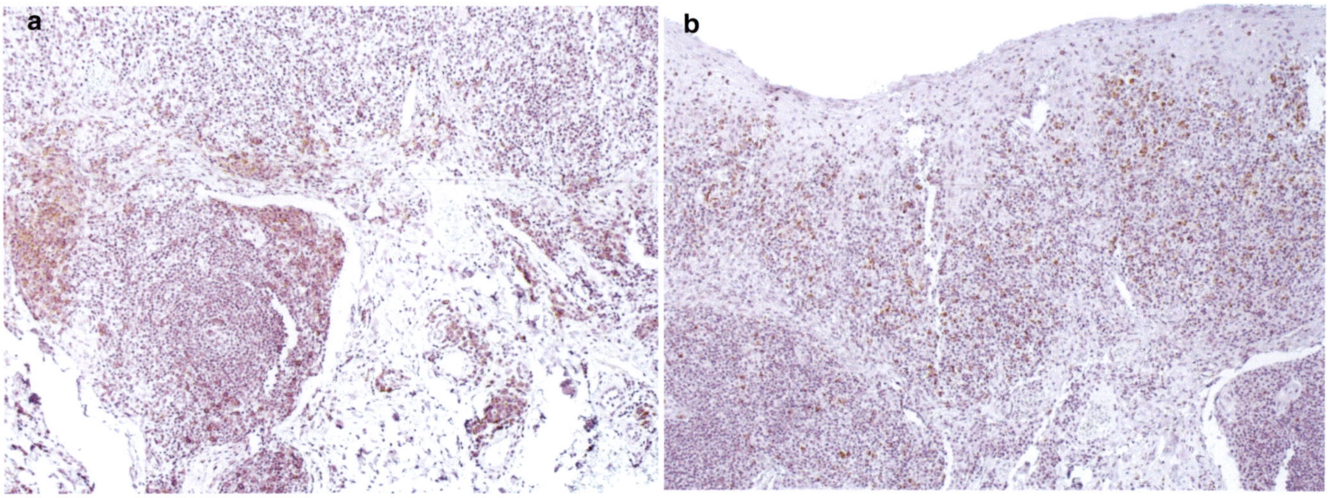

Fig. 13.8 Immunohistochemical features of lichenoid granulomatous stomatitis. (**a**) The expression of CD138 is useful to show the presence of plasma cells (DAB; 100×). (**b**) Proliferating cells that express Ki67 protein are predominantly located in the lichenoid component of the disease (DAB; 100×)

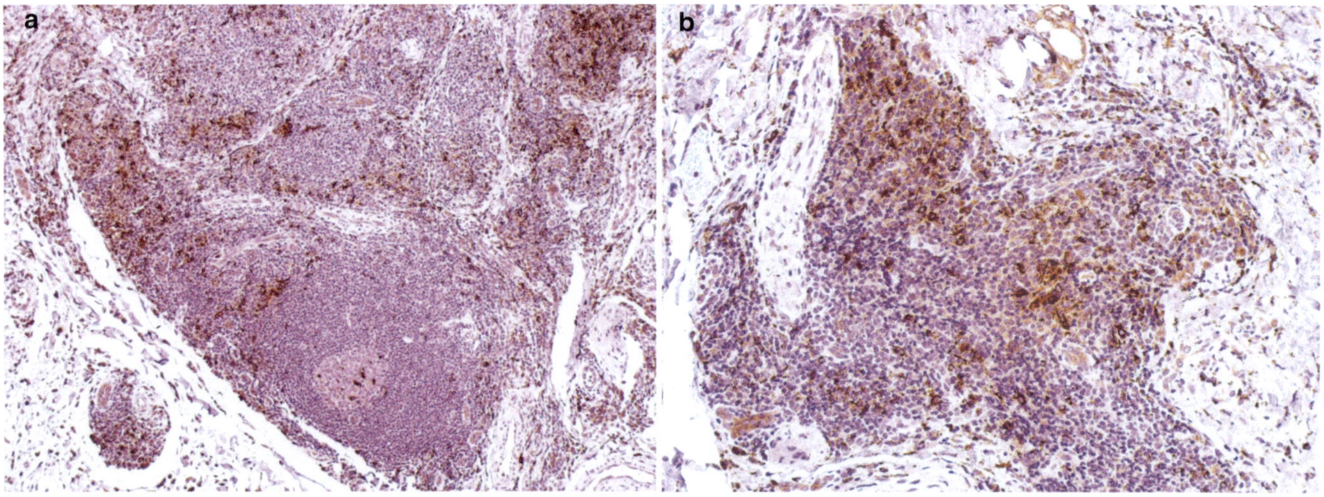

Fig. 13.9 Immunohistochemical features of lichenoid granulomatous stomatitis. (**a**) The expression of CD68 was used to show the presence of histiocytes (DAB; 100×). (**b**) Note the diffuse distribution of the histiocytes, not forming a well-organized granuloma in this example (DAB; 200×)

Table 13.1 Summary of the main immunohistochemical reactions that can be used to characterize the inflammatory infiltrate of lichenoid granulomatous reaction. The results of histological stains are also described

Antibody/stain	Most frequent results	Pattern	Objective
CD20	Positive	Membrane	To demonstrate the presence of B lymphocytes
CD3	Positive	Membrane	To demonstrate the presence of T lymphocytes
CD138	Positive	Membrane	To demonstrate the presence of plasma cells
CD68	Positive	Cytoplasm	To demonstrate the presence of macrophages, multinucleated giant cells, and granulomas
PAS[a]	Negative	–	To show the absence of microorganisms
Grocott-Gomori[a]	Negative	–	To show the absence of microorganisms
Ziehl-Neelsen[a]	Negative	–	To show the absence of microorganisms

PAS Periodic-acid Schiff
[a]Histological stains

Sources

1. Gonzalez JG, Marcus MD, Cruz DJ. Giant cell lichenoid dermatitis. J Am Acad Dermatol. 1986;15:87–92.
2. Magro CM, Crowson AN. Lichenoid and granulomatous dermatitis. Int J Dermatol. 2000;39:126–33.
3. Robinson CM, Oxley JD, Weir J, Eveson JW. Lichenoid and granulomatous stomatitis: an entity or a non-specific inflammatory process? J Oral Pathol Med. 2006;35:262–7. https://doi.org/10.1111/j.1600-0714.2006.00419.x.
4. Braswell DS, Hakeem A, Walker A, Sokumbi O, Kapil J, Motaparthi K. Lichenoid granulomatous dermatitis revisited: a retrospective case series. J Am Acad Dermatol. 2019;81:1157–64. https://doi.org/10.1016/j.jaad.2019.05.100.
5. Hakeem A, Bhattacharyya I, Aljabri M, Bindakhil M, Pachigar K, Islam MN, et al. Lichenoid reaction with granulomatous stomatitis: a retrospective histologic study of 47 patients. J Oral Pathol Med. 2019;48:846–54. https://doi.org/10.1111/jop.12918.
6. Lafuente-Ibáñez de Mendoza I, Vigarios E, Herbault-Barres B, Alberdi-Navarro J, Sibaud V, Maret D, et al. Non-infectious granulomatous disorders of the upper lip: clinicopathological analysis of 11 patients. BMC Oral Health. 2022;22:173. https://doi.org/10.1186/s12903-022-02189-z.
7. Alamoudi WA, Abdelsayed RA, Sollecito TP, Alhassan GA, Kulkarni R, Bindakhil MA. Causes of oral granulomatous disorders: an update and narrative review of the literature. Head Neck Pathol. 2024;18:72. https://doi.org/10.1007/s12105-024-01678-7.

Granulomatous Foreign Body Reaction

14

Hélen Kaline Farias Bezerra,
Cinthia Veronica Bardalez Lopez de Caceres,
Daniel Galera Bernabé, and Felipe Paiva Fonseca

14.1 General Overview and Clinical Presentation

Foreign bodies are responsible for the majority of the granulomatous inflammatory disorders that affect the oral cavity, and numerous foreign materials causing oral lesions have been described in the literature. They are frequently classified as either endogenous substances that include, for instance, hair fibers, keratin clusters, cholesterol crystals, fatty substances, or exogenous substances that comprise a myriad of examples, including dental materials, glass, sutures, and dermal fillers, among others. All these foreign bodies may lead to a localized inflammatory granulomatous reaction whose intensity varies significantly. The microscopic examination is very important to confirm the presence of foreign bodies as etiologic factors for a granulomatous process and, therefore, a biopsy is considered essential in making the final diagnosis. However, the evidence of foreign substances in the biopsied sample may be very difficult to demonstrate because of their very small microscopic aspect or due to the very severe inflammatory infiltrate that may impair the correct histological identification of these substances. Therefore, it is important to consider that the inability to recognize a foreign material under routine histology evaluation does not rule out an exogenous substance as a possible etiological factor for an unexplained inflammatory infiltrate, while the simple presence of a foreign body does not exclude a possible systemic condition occurring simultaneously. A rigorous clinicopathological correlation is always mandatory to achieve the most correct diagnosis.

The clinical manifestation of oral lesions associated with foreign bodies is highly variable and frequently considered nonspecific, affecting both males and females of a wide age range, which may lead to a broad list of differential diagnoses. The presence of teeth polishing materials in the gingiva may cause a chronically inflamed tissue that does not resolve after conventional periodontal therapy, demonstrating a localized or diffuse reddish and swollen aspect that may bleed easily, often resembling a desquamative gingivitis. Other iatrogenically introduced substances may manifest as plaques, swellings, or ulcerations in the traumatized regions, more often affecting the lips, nasolabial fold, tongue, buccal mucosa, and gingiva. In some patients, the filler substance can migrate from its primary injected location to other regions of the oral cavity. Most of the cases are painless and present a normal-colored aspect, but in some cases, a reddish or a yellowish aspect may be observed; moreover, the presence of a large amount of foreign body material associated with the granulomatous reaction leads to a hardened consistency in the affected oral mucosa.

The use of cosmetic dermal fillers for esthetic purposes in the perioral regions has significantly increased in the last years, and a number of granulomatous foreign body reactions associated with these products have also become more common. They are frequently classified as degradable/resorbable fillers like collagen and hyaluronic acid or as permanent/nonresorbable fillers exemplified by silicone. The intensity and type of inflammatory or immunological reaction are believed to depend on the characteristics of each filler, including its particle size and biocompatibility. Females are more frequently affected by granulomatous reactions to dermal fillers than males, representing approximately 90% of all cases. A careful anamnesis may be highly

H. K. F. Bezerra (✉)
Department of Oral Diagnosis (Pathology), Piracicaba Dental School, University of Campinas (UNICAMP), Piracicaba, Brazil

Department of Oral Diagnosis (Semiology), Piracicaba Dental School, University of Campinas (UNICAMP), Piracicaba, Brazil

C. V. B. L. de Caceres · F. P. Fonseca
Department of Oral Surgery and Pathology, School of Dentistry, Universidade Federal de Minas Gerais, Belo Horizonte, Brazil

D. G. Bernabé
Oral Oncology Center and Department of Diagnosis and Surgery, São Paulo State University (Unesp), School of Dentistry, Araçatuba, São Paulo, Brazil
e-mail: daniel.bernabe@unesp.br

© The Author(s), under exclusive license to Springer Nature Switzerland AG 2025
F. P. Fonseca et al. (eds.), *Lymphoproliferative and Granulomatous Disorders of the Oral Cavity*,
https://doi.org/10.1007/978-3-031-98844-8_14

contributory to the diagnosis, but some patients may deny the use of esthetic products, or the granulomatous inflammatory response may develop years after the time of exposure to the foreign body and patients may not recall exposure to the substance, making the correct diagnosis more difficult. There is a large number of dermal fillers that can be found associated with granulomatous reactions in the oral or perioral regions, including hyaluronic acid, silicone, poly-l-lactic acid, polymethyl methacrylate, and calcium hydroxyapatite.

Granulomatous reactions secondary to the use of graft materials may also occur in the jaws, which can be detected by radiographs or computed tomography exams as nonspecific radiopacities associated with radiolucent regions. Many cases are asymptomatic, but some patients may develop secondary infections, and clinical information is important to the correct interpretation of the biopsied tissue. Dental materials such as endodontic fillers and sealers, impression materials, suture threads, and restorative materials have also been associated with the occurrence of adverse inflammatory reactions.

Foreign body reactions in the gnathic bones and oral cavity may also be caused by food debris in several stages of breakdown. It may be found in the posterior region of an edentulous mandible in patients with full or partial dentures, in the periapex of decayed teeth and retained dental roots, in teeth receiving endodontic treatment, and in post-extraction sockets. This material may also be found in the gingival tissue of impacted third molars with pericoronitis and in the cystic wall of odontogenic cysts communicating with the oral cavity. Traumatic implantation of food particles may also be present in the soft tissues of the oral mucosa.

Treatment of granulomatous foreign-body reactions in the oral cavity and gnathic bones usually comprises the conservative surgical removal of the etiologic substances, which often leads to complete resolution of the signs and symptoms. However, extensive lesions may be associated with scars and localized anatomical deformities. The administration of topical or intralesional corticosteroids has also been reported in the literature (Fig. 14.1).

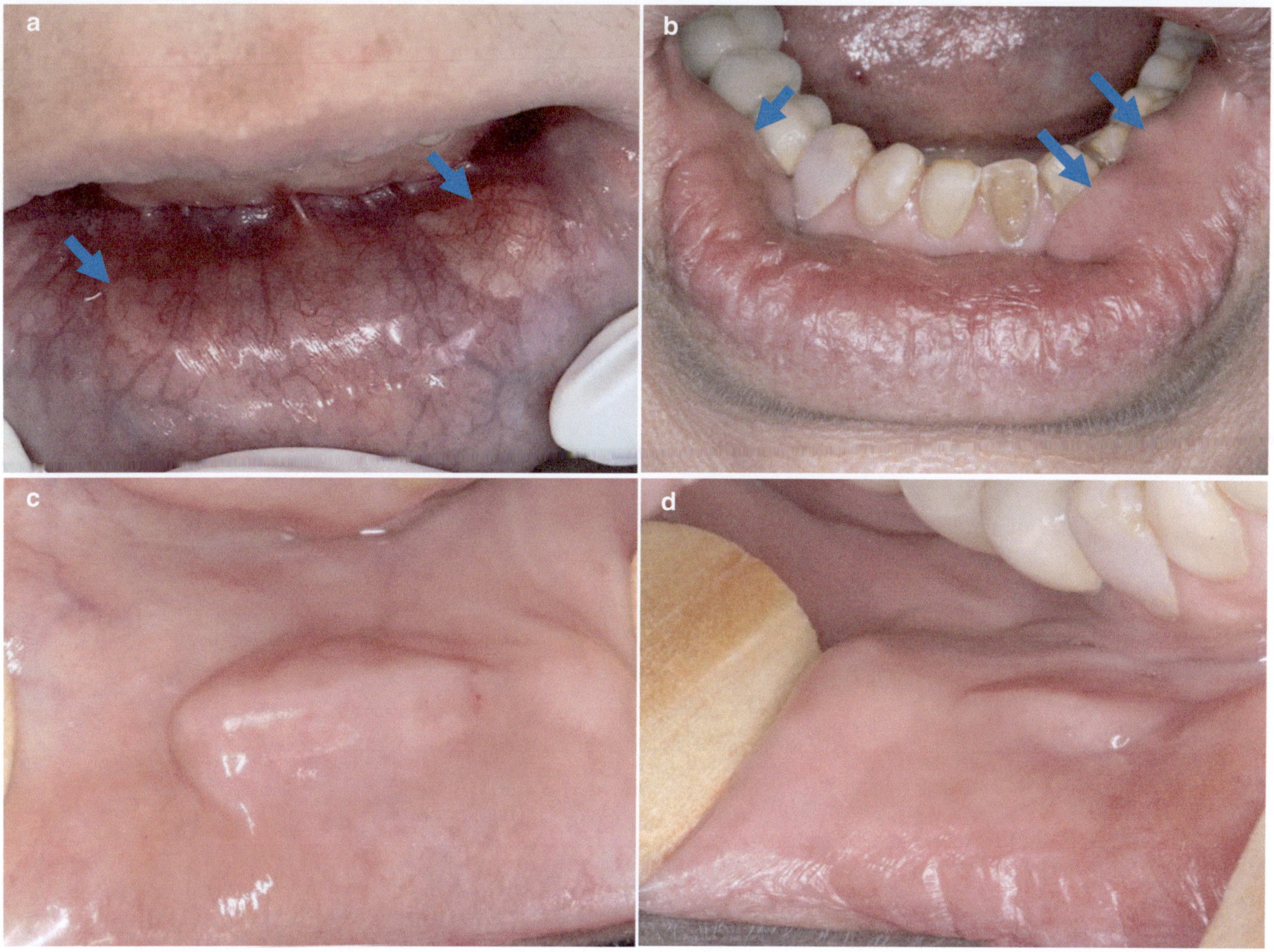

Fig. 14.1 Clinical presentation of granulomatous foreign body reaction due to cosmetic fillers. (**a**) A 37-year-old female patient submitted to an esthetic procedure developed a granulomatous foreign body reaction in the lower lip. Observe the asymptomatic, yellowish plaques (blue arrows) affecting both sides of the lower lip mucosa (Courtesy image: Dr. Gabriela Ribeiro de Araujo). (**b**) A 46-year-old female patient submitted to a cosmetic procedure using polymethylmethacrylate developed a granulomatous foreign body reaction in the lower lip. Note the bilateral swellings in the lower lip (blue arrows). (**c**) On the left side of the lower lip, there was a painless, normal colored nodule. (**d**) On the right side of the lower lip, an asymptomatic, ill-defined nodule was also present

14.2 Microscopic Findings

- Overlying squamous epithelium may demonstrate variable degrees of acanthosis.
- The lamina propria exhibits a non-encapsulated, variable inflammatory infiltrate typically consistent with foreign body granulomatous reaction, which varies from mild to severe.
- The granulomatous infiltrate is characterized by multiple histiocytes that may present epithelioid, clear cell, and/or foamy aspects.
- Other reactive inflammatory cells are also present, including neutrophils, lymphocytes, and plasma cells.
- Foreign body-type multinucleated giant cells are commonly observed. Some of them can be found strictly associated with the foreign body and surrounding the exogenous substances.
- Asteroid bodies can be found in multinucleated giant cells in some cases.
- The presence of well-formed granulomas is very common, but it is possible that only ill-formed granulomas or an unspecific chronic inflammatory infiltrate rich in histiocytes can be observed in a few cases.
- Variable fibrosis is usually described, and tissue necrosis is not a common finding.

- The microscopic features of the foreign substance vary significantly, and pathologists should be familiarized with their histological features to make the most precise diagnosis.
- Some reports describing the use of fine needle aspiration cytology as an auxiliary tool for the diagnosis of some foreign body materials have already been published.
- The use of polarized light can be useful to demonstrate the presence of some foreign bodies that present birefringence features.
- Histological features observed in some of the most common cosmetic injectable soft tissue fillers are the following:
  - Silicone: Empty round to oval vacuoles of varying size.
  - Poly-l-lactic acid: Small translucent but birefringent particles of different sizes and forms, some with spindle shape and others as microspheres of 30–40 μm.
  - Hyaluronic acid: nonbirefringent, nontranslucent basophile flakes without any particles.
  - Polymethylmethacrylate: uniform vacuoles, with a homogeneous shape and different sizes, resembling mature adipocytes. Lobules of the exogenous material if formed and separated by connective tissue septa.
- Graft materials used for bone surgery are frequently represented by Bio-Oss®, Bio-Gran®, and Hydroxyapatite, usually presenting as amorphous basophilic aggregates under microscopic examination.
- Dental amalgam tattoo may also elicit a foreign body giant cell reaction (Figs. 14.2, 14.3, 14.4, 14.5, and 14.6).

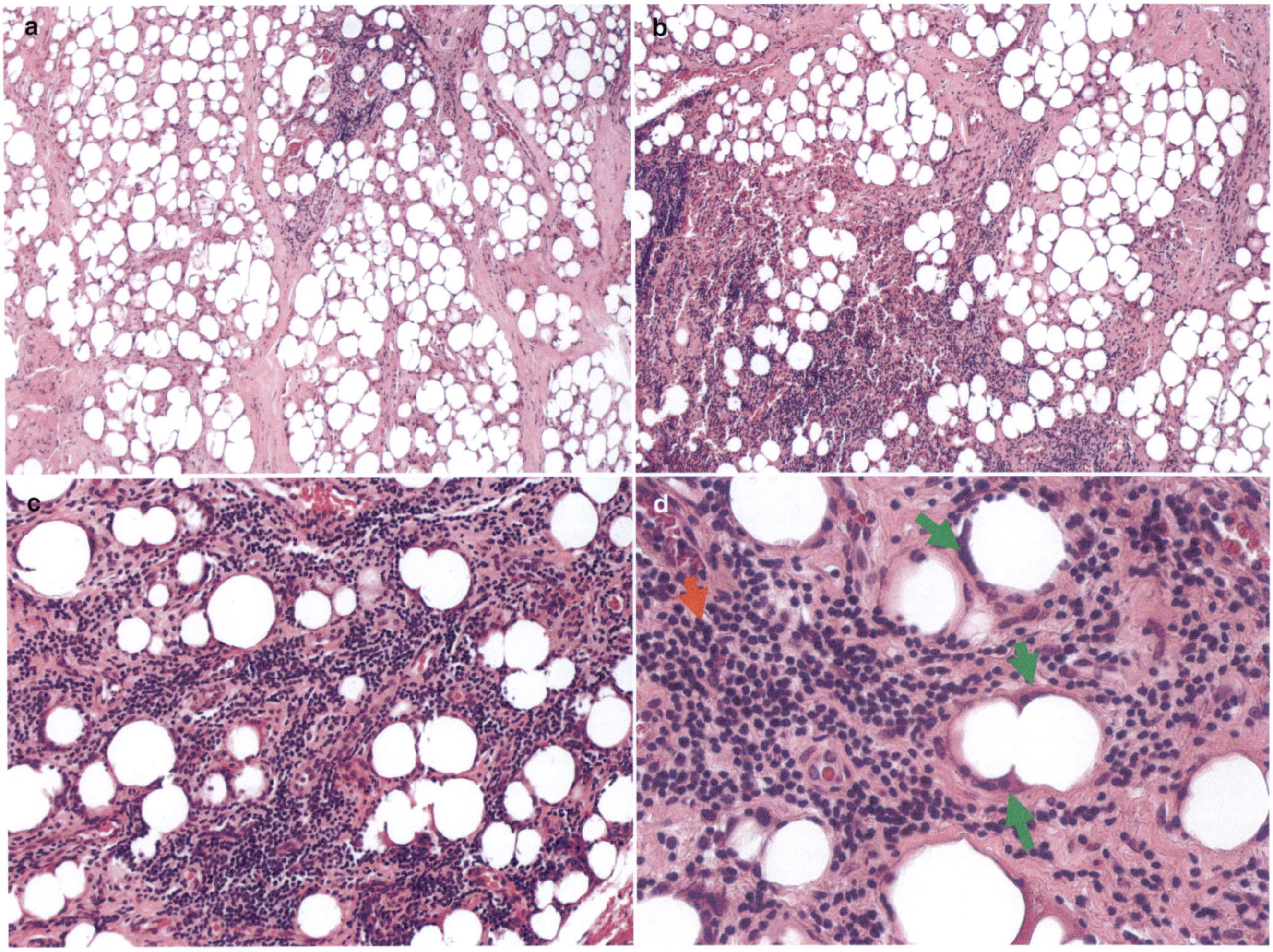

Fig. 14.2 Microscopic features of oral granulomatous foreign body reaction due to cosmetic fillers. (**a**) The negative image of polymethylmethacrylate is diffusely distributed in the lamina propria (H&E; 50×). (**b**) Note the typical white, round to oval characteristic of the foreign body material that strongly resembles mature adipocytes. A reactive chronic inflammatory infiltrate is located in the lower left side of the image (H&E; 50×). (**c**) Observe the strong chronic inflammatory infiltrate surrounding the foreign material. In this image, there is a predominance of lymphocytes (H&E; 100×). (**d**) Lymphocytes are present as small round hyperchromatic cells (red arrow), and the multinucleated giant cells are surrounding the cosmetic material. Note the nuclei and the cytoplasm around the whitish round structures (green arrows) (H&E; 100×)

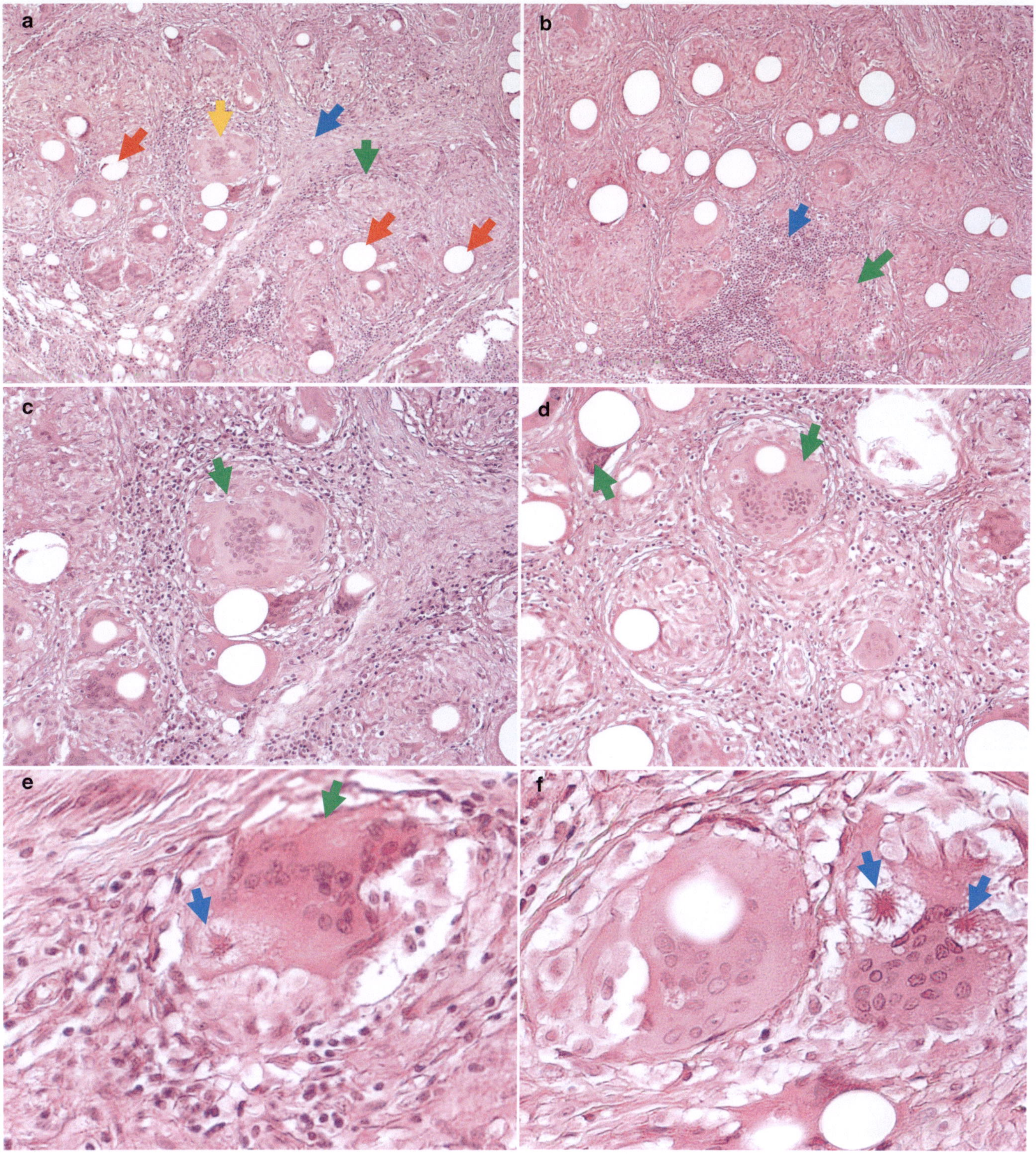

Fig. 14.3 Microscopic features of oral granulomatous foreign body reaction due to cosmetic fillers. (**a**) A typical granulomatous process due to the presence of foreign material. Observe the diffuse inflammatory infiltrate in the lamina propria. Negative images of polymethylmethacrylate structures are round to oval in shape (red arrows), and foreign body-type multinucleated giant cells are diffusely present in the tissue (yellow arrow). The histiocytic component of the inflammatory infiltrate is eosinophilic and diffusely distributed (green arrow). Observe the eosinophilic fibrotic bands in the lesion (blue arrow) (H&E; 50×). (**b**) In some regions of the lesion, there is a predominance of lymphocytes with a more basophilic aspect (blue arrow), while in most of the tissue, there is a predominance of histiocytes with a more eosinophilic appearance (granulomatous process) (green arrow) (H&E; 50×). (**c**) The presence of foreign body-type multinucleated giant cells containing multiple nuclei randomly distributed is characteristically found (green arrow) (H&E; 100×). (**d**) Observe the foreign body-type multinucleated giant cells surrounding the cosmetic material (green arrows) (H&E; 100×). (**e**) A foreign body-type multinucleated giant cell (green arrow) containing an asteroid body in the cytoplasm (blue arrow) (H&E; 400×). (**f**) Another example of a foreign body-type multinucleated giant cell containing two asteroid bodies in the cytoplasm (blue arrows) (H&E; 400×)

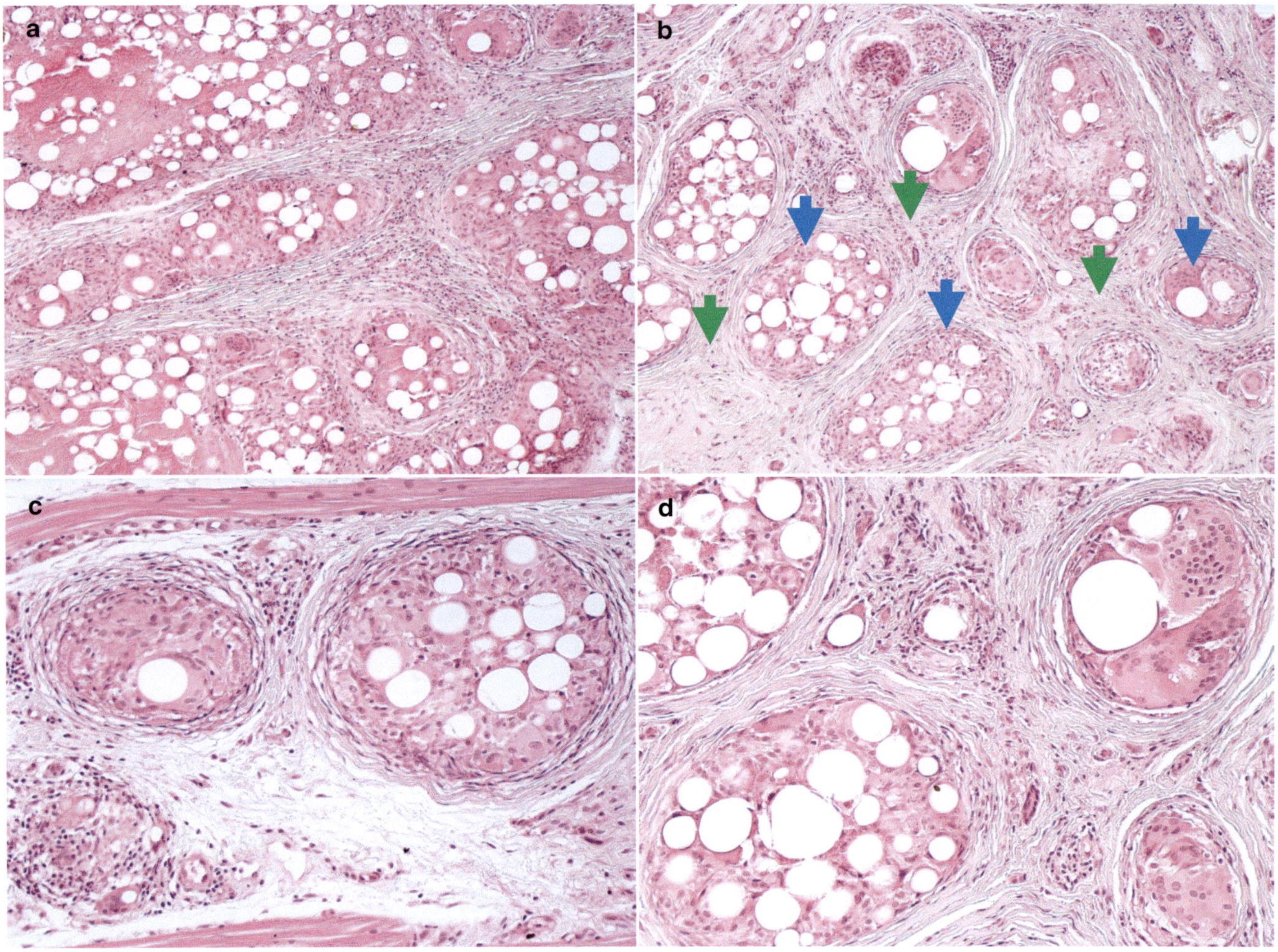

Fig. 14.4 Microscopic features of oral granulomatous foreign body reaction due to cosmetic fillers. (**a**) Diffuse granulomatous process associated with esthetic foreign material. The cosmetic material strongly resembles mature adipocytes (H&E; 50×). (**b**) The histiocytic reaction surrounds the foreign bodies (blue arrows). Note the presence of fibrotic bands (green arrows) between the granulomatous processes (H&E; 50×). (**c**) The presence of granulomatous inflammatory infiltrate surrounding the foreign body material and presenting as multiple nodules in the connective tissue (H&E; 100×). (**d**) Observe the foreign body-type multinucleated giant cells surrounding the cosmetic material and the nodular aspect of the inflammatory infiltrate (H&E; 100×)

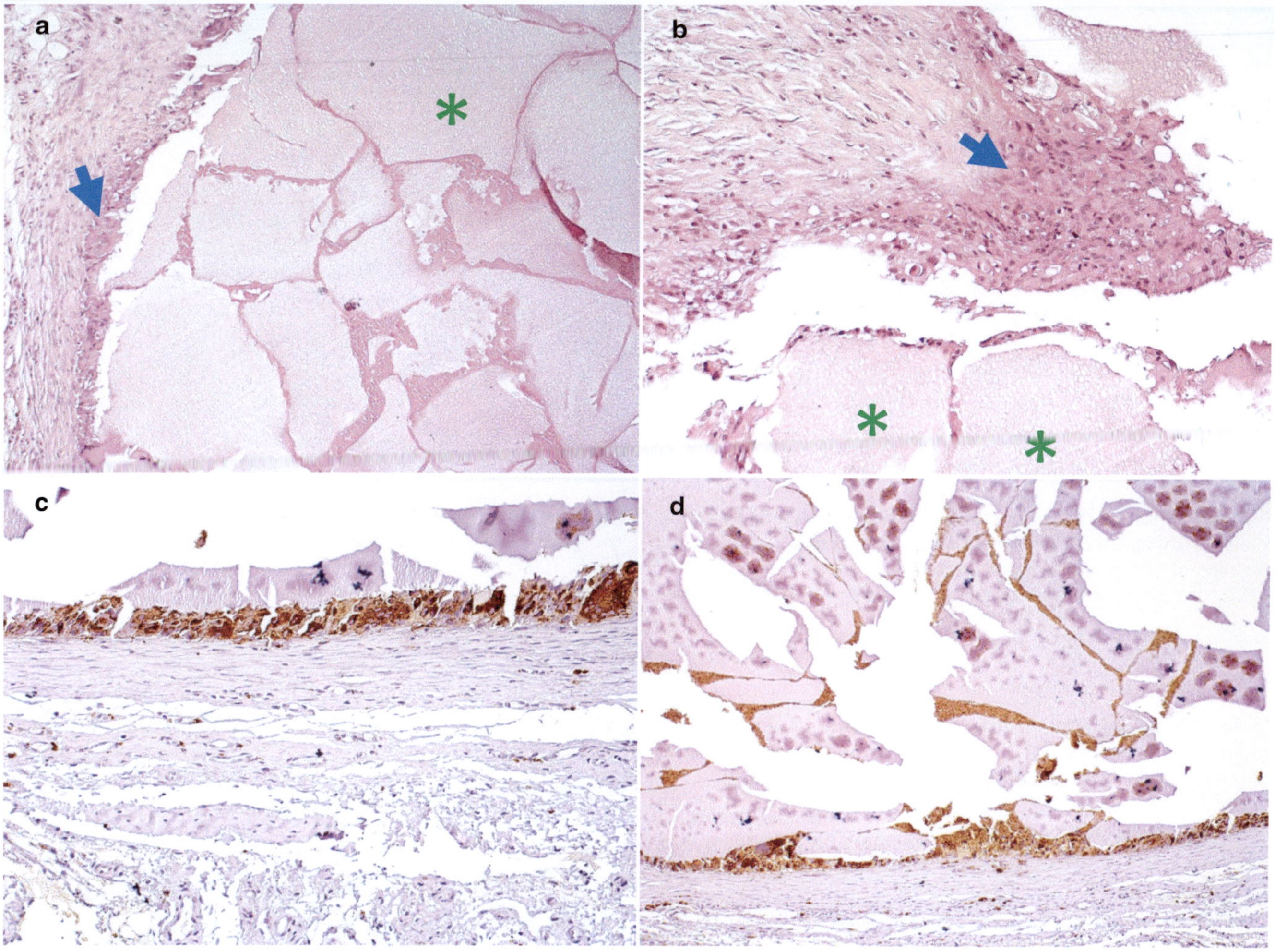

Fig. 14.5 Microscopic features of oral granulomatous reaction due to foreign body material. (**a**) Granulomatous reaction (blue arrow) surrounding the foreign body material (asterisks) (H&E; 50×). (**b**) Note a stronger chronic inflammatory infiltrate (green arrows) and the presence of a basophilic foreign body (asterisks) (H&E; 100×). (**c**) The presence of the histiocytic infiltrate surrounding the foreign material can be better appreciated by immunohistochemistry using the CD68 antibody. Observe the strong cytoplasmic reaction that confirms the presence of histiocytes (DAB; 100×). (**d**) Note the presence of multiple histiocytes in the granulomatous infiltrate around the foreign body material (H&E; 200×)

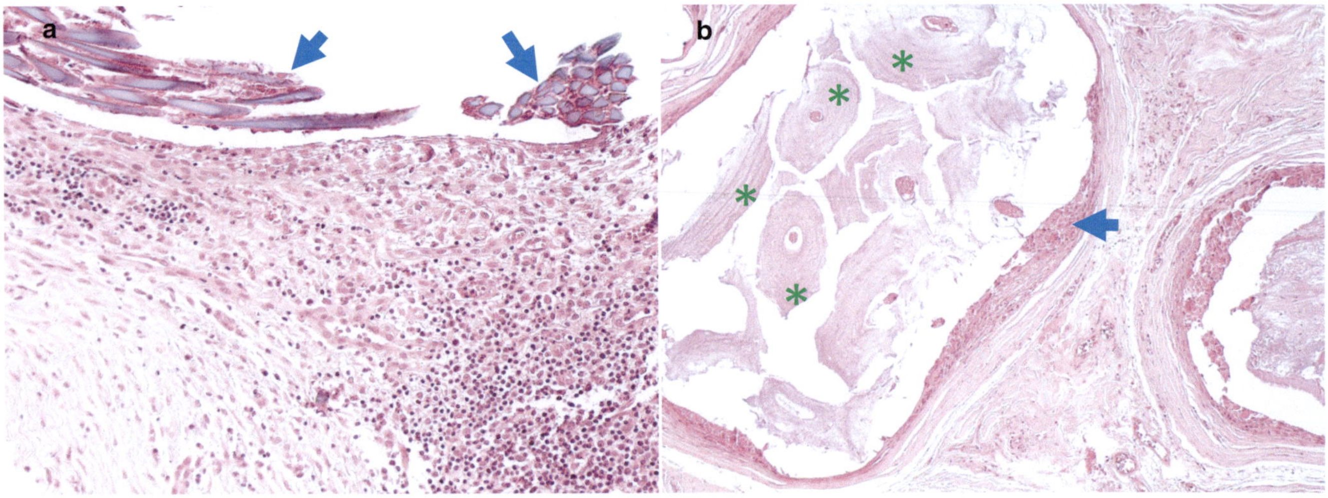

Fig. 14.6 Microscopic features of oral granulomatous reaction due to foreign body material. (**a**) Chronic inflammatory infiltrate due to the presence of suture thread (blue arrows) in the oral mucosa (H&E; 100×). (**b**) Granulomatous inflammatory reaction due to graft material consistent with Bio-Oss® (green asterisks). Observe the basophilic amorphous material surrounded by histiocytic infiltrate (blue arrow) (H&E; 100×)

Table 14.1 Summary of the main immunohistochemical reactions and histological stains that can be used for characterizing the inflammatory infiltrate in granulomatous foreign body reactions

Antibody/stain	Most frequent results	Pattern	Objective
CD20	Positive	Membrane	To characterize B lymphocyte infiltrates
CD3	Positive	Membrane	To characterize T lymphocyte infiltrates
CD138	Positive	Membrane	To characterize plasma cell infiltrates
CD68	Positive	Cytoplasm	To demonstrate the presence of macrophages, multinucleated giant cells, and granulomas
PAS[a]	Negative	–	To exclude the presence of microorganisms
Grocott-Gomori[a]	Negative	–	To exclude the presence of microorganisms

[a]Histological stain

14.3 Immunohistochemistry and/or Genetics

The H&E microscopic analysis, together with clinical and laboratory data, is usually enough to establish the final diagnosis of granulomatous foreign body reaction. However, the immunohistochemical analysis using histiocytic markers like CD68 and CD163 can be useful to demonstrate the presence of the granulomatous nature of the infiltrate and the multinucleated giant cells when they are not prominent. The search for microorganisms may also be important in cases where foreign bodies are not easily observed under H&E stain, and the use of histochemical reactions like PAS and Grocott-Gomory stains can be useful to rule out possible infectious diseases (Table 14.1, Fig. 14.7).

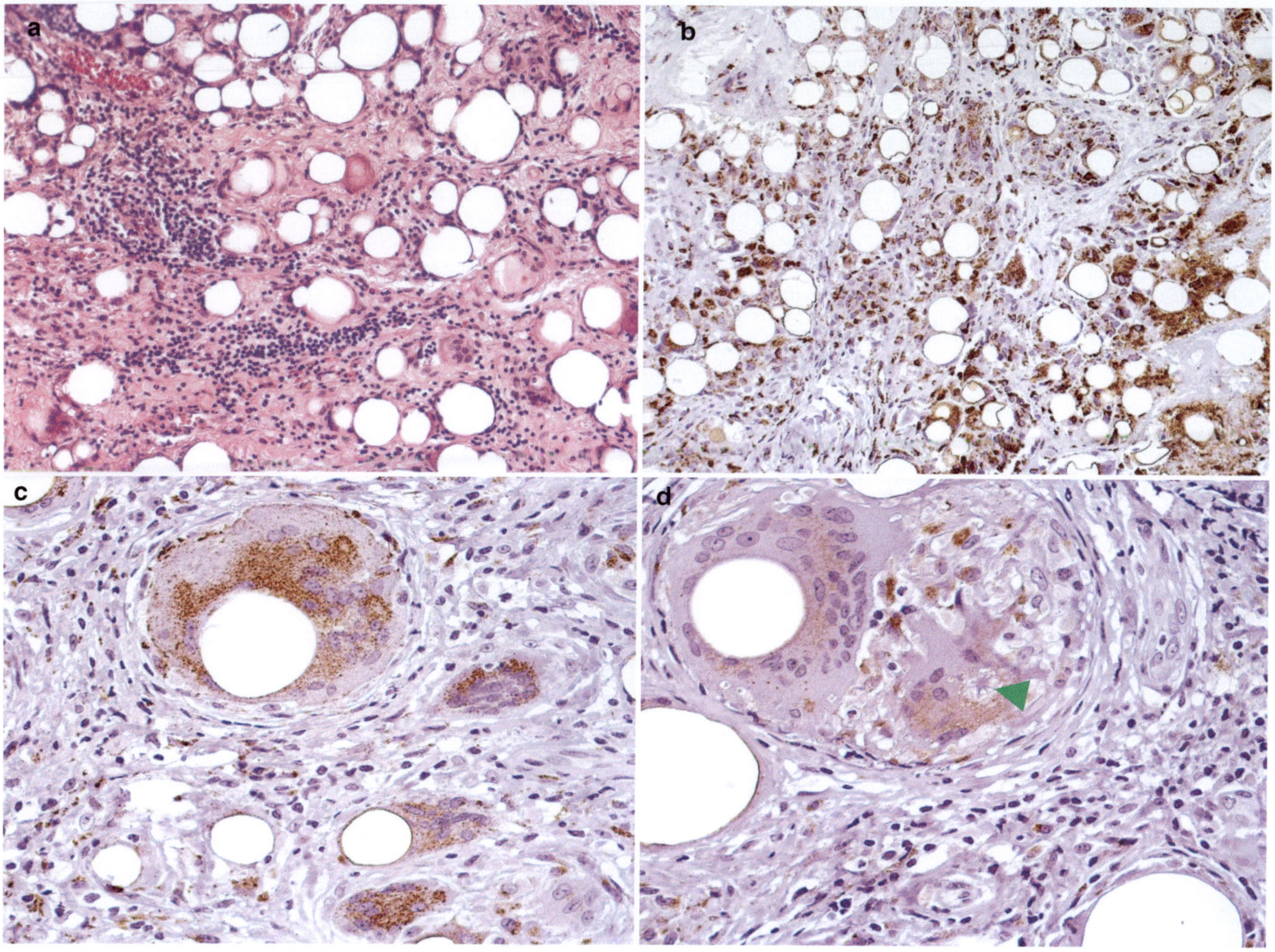

Fig. 14.7 Histologic and immunohistochemical features of oral granulomatous reaction due to cosmetic foreign body material. (**a**) The cosmetic filler presented as round whitish structures is surrounded by foreign body-type multinucleated giant cells. Lymphocytic infiltrate is also present (H&E; 100×). (**b**) The expression of CD68 better demonstrates the granulomatous nature of the inflammatory infiltrate (DAB; 100×). (**c**) Note the cytoplasmic expression of CD68 in the multinucleated giant cell surrounding a foreign body structure (DAB; 400×). (**d**) A steroid body (green arrow) can be seen in the cytoplasm of a multinucleated giant cell stained by CD68 protein (DAB; 400×)

Sources

1. Stewart CM, Watson RE. Experimental oral foreign body reactions. Commonly employed dental materials. Oral Surg Oral Med Oral Pathol. 1990;69:713–9. https://doi.org/10.1016/0030-4220(90)90354-u.
2. Jham BC, Nikitakis NG, Scheper MA, Papadimitriou JC, Levy BA, Rivera H. Granulomatous foreign-body reaction involving oral and perioral tissues after injection of biomaterials: a series of 7 cases and review of the literature. J Oral Maxillofac Surg. 2009;67:280–5. https://doi.org/10.1016/j.joms.2008.01.052.
3. Shahrabi Farahani S, Sexton J, Stone JD, Quinn K, Woo SB. Lip nodules caused by hyaluronic acid filler injection: report of three cases. Head Neck Pathol. 2012;6:16–20. https://doi.org/10.1007/s12105-011-0304-9.
4. Faria KM, Fonseca FP, Silva WG, Silva RN, Vargas PA, Almeida OP, et al. Fine needle aspiration cytology in the diagnosis of perioral adverse reactions to cosmetic dermal fillers. Oral Surg Oral Med Oral Pathol Oral Radiol. 2014;117:e393–5. https://doi.org/10.1016/j.oooo.2013.07.029.
5. Shahrabi-Farahani S, Lerman MA, Noonan V, Kabani S, Woo SB. Granulomatous foreign body reaction to dermal cosmetic fillers with intraoral migration. Oral Surg Oral Med Oral Pathol Oral Radiol. 2014;117:105–10. https://doi.org/10.1016/j.oooo.2013.10.008.
6. Müller S. Non-infectious granulomatous lesions of the orofacial region. Head Neck Pathol. 2019;13:449–56. https://doi.org/10.1007/s12105-018-00997-w.
7. Alawi F, Shields BE, Omolehinwa T, Rosenbach M. Oral granulomatous disease. Dermatol Clin. 2020;38:429–39. https://doi.org/10.1016/j.det.2020.05.004.
8. Rosen Y, Garcia PM, Navale P. Pulse/hyaline ring granuloma revisited: etiologic role of seed-derived storage cells. Virchows Arch. 2022;480:499–508. https://doi.org/10.1007/s00428-021-03222-2.
9. Rosendy G, Cavalcante IL, Barros CCDS, López-Labady J, González N, Pérez-Alfonzo R, et al. Adverse reactions associated with dermal fillers in the oral and maxillofacial region: a Venezuelan experience. Head Neck Pathol. 2023;17:631–7. https://doi.org/10.1007/s12105-023-01563-9.

10. Saoud C, Lossos C, Ali SZ. Polymethylmethacrylate-induced foreign body reaction presenting as bilateral parotid lesions: a case report of dermal filler adverse reaction diagnosed on fine needle aspiration. Cytopathology. 2023;34:385–7. https://doi.org/10.1111/cyt.13233.
11. Alamoudi WA, Abdelsayed RA, Sollecito TP, Alhassan GA, Kulkarni R, Bindakhil MA. Causes of oral granulomatous disorders: an update and narrative review of the literature. Head Neck Pathol. 2024;18:72. https://doi.org/10.1007/s12105-024-01678-7.
12. Pires FR, Said AMT, Netto JNS, da Cruz Perez DE, Bonan PRF, Martins HDD, et al. Oral/perioral reactions to injectable soft tissue fillers: a clinicopathological multicentric study. Oral Dis. 2024;31:899–910. https://doi.org/10.1111/odi.15143.
13. Santos LG, Jardim LC, Schuch LF, Silveira FM, Wagner VP, Pires FR, et al. Foreign body reactions related to orofacial esthetic fillers: a systematic review. Oral Dis. 2024;30:855–64. https://doi.org/10.1111/odi.14541.
14. Hisatomi M, Takeshita Y, Yanagi Y, Okada S, Fujikura M, Yoshida S, et al. Imaging characteristics of incidentally detected cosmetic surgery-derived foreign bodies on CT images in the maxillofacial region. Oral Radiol. 2024;40:277–84. https://doi.org/10.1007/s11282-023-00734-2.
15. Bezerra HKF, Faustino ISP, Santos-Silva AR, Vargas PA, Perez DEDC, Lopes MA. Submucosal nodule on the dorsal tongue. Oral Surg Oral Med Oral Pathol Oral Radiol. 2024;137:3–5. https://doi.org/10.1016/j.oooo.2023.08.015.

15 Granulomatosis with Polyangiitis

Ricardo Santiago Gomez, Wagner Henriques de Castro, Bruno Augusto Benevenuto de Andrade, and Felipe Paiva Fonseca

15.1 General Overview and Clinical Presentation

Systemic vasculitides are pathological processes characterized by inflammation and necrosis of blood vessel walls, leading to blood vessel destruction and impaired blood supply to affected tissues. They comprise a large number of disorders with very distinct clinicopathological manifestations that may vary from diseases limited to a single organ up to life-threatening conditions with unsatisfactory response to currently available therapies and a poor prognosis. The anti-neutrophil cytoplasmic antibodies (ANCA)-associated vasculitides represent a subgroup of systemic vasculitides that are typically associated with the presence of vasculitis in small- and medium-sized blood vessels and comprise three different entities with distinct clinical and microscopic manifestations: granulomatosis with polyangiitis, microscopic polyangiitis, and eosinophilic granulomatosis with polyangiitis.

Granulomatosis with polyangiitis was originally reported by the German pathologist Friedrick Wegener in 1937 and represents a systemic autoimmune disorder characterized by the occurrence of aseptic, necrotizing granulomatous vasculitis of small- and medium-sized vessels. Its etiology is largely unknown, and theories regarding the possible role played by yet unidentified infectious, environmental, chemical, toxic, or pharmacological agents are frequently reported in the literature. The pathogenesis of this condition is also not completely understood, but the importance of ANCA is well known since its first description in 1982, which is present in most of the granulomatosis with polyangiitis cases, more frequently, Proteinase 3 (PR3). Patients affected by granulomatosis with polyangiitis may demonstrate different clinical presentations, varying from limited to generalized manifestations that may also have a high risk of mortality if patients are not treated.

Patients are also frequently diagnosed with other rheumatologic conditions, especially rheumatoid arthritis, but the predisposing importance of these disorders for the development of granulomatosis with polyangiitis remains to be validated. It more commonly shows involvement of the upper and lower airways, lungs, and kidneys, although any other organ can also be involved, which leads to a wide variation in clinical manifestations that frequently include general malaise, myalgia, arthralgia, anorexia, fever, fatigue, weight loss, and pyrexia. Coexistence of intestinal bowel disease and granulomatosis with polyangiitis is uncommon but well described and may be explained by common underlying inflammatory responses and cytokine profiles polarized toward either Th1 or Th2, and in these cases, the possibility of oral manifestations of intestinal bowel disease should be ruled out by diagnosticians.

There is no significant sex predilection, and adults are the most commonly affected individuals with a wide age range and a mean age at diagnosis between 40 and 55 years-old, while cases affecting infants are only rarely reported. Current diagnostic criteria for ANCA-associated vasculitides, including granulomatosis with polyangiitis, is based on the American College of Rheumatology/European Alliance for Associations for Rheumatology (ACR/EULAR) guidelines that comprise a diagnostic algorithm that investigates the occurrence of 10 possible clinical, imaging, laboratorial, and microscopic features, demanding a final score of ≥5 to confirm the diagnosis of granulomatosis with polyangiitis. This algorithm includes the search for nasal lesions, cartilage manifestations, hearing loss,

R. S. Gomez (✉)
Department of Oral Surgery and Pathology, School of Dentistry, Universidade Federal de Minas Gerais, Belo Horizonte, Brazil

Medical School, Minas Gerais Medical Science, Belo Horizonte, Brazil

W. H. de Castro · F. P. Fonseca
Department of Oral Surgery and Pathology, School of Dentistry, Universidade Federal de Minas Gerais, Belo Horizonte, Brazil

B. A. B. de Andrade
Department of Oral Diagnosis and Pathology, School of Dentistry, Universidade Federal do Rio de Janeiro, Rio de Janeiro, Brazil

© The Author(s), under exclusive license to Springer Nature Switzerland AG 2025
F. P. Fonseca et al. (eds.), *Lymphoproliferative and Granulomatous Disorders of the Oral Cavity*,
https://doi.org/10.1007/978-3-031-98844-8_15

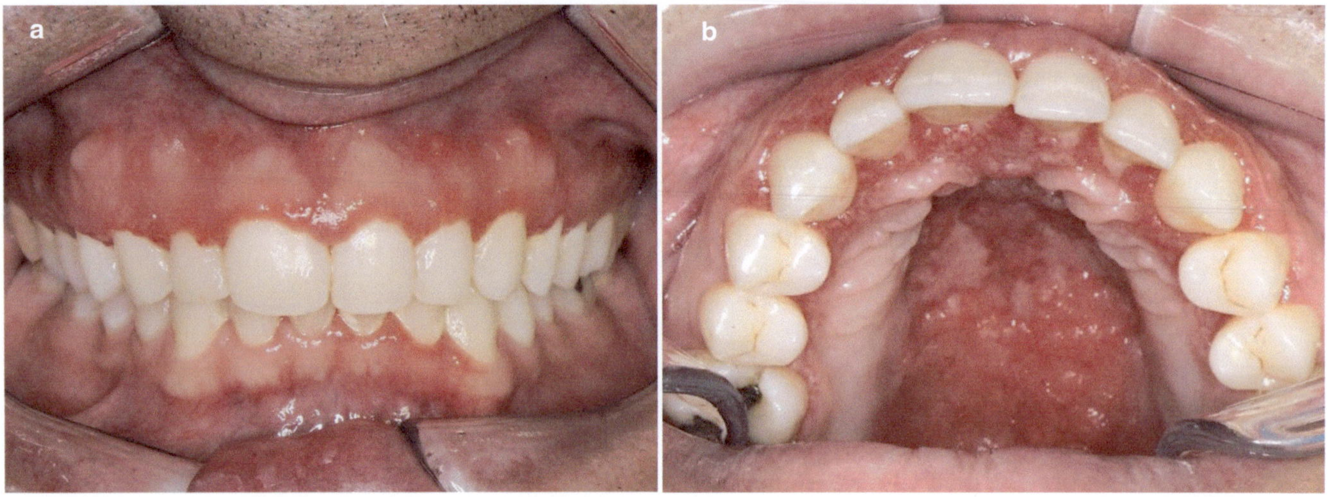

Fig. 15.1 Clinical presentation of granulomatosis with polyangiitis affecting the oral cavity. (**a**) Male patient diagnosed with granulomatosis with polyangiitis affecting the lungs and the kidneys, showing oral manifestations of the disease. There is a diffuse involvement of the gingival free margin that presented as painful, swollen, and erythematous. Observe the linear involvement of the gingiva. (**b**) The patient also had a diffuse involvement of the palatine mucosa that presented as strongly erythematous. Observe in this occlusal view the involvement of the palatine and vestibular gingiva

positivity for cytoplasmic (c)ANCA (Proteinase 3—PR3), chest imaging findings, the presence of granuloma on biopsy, sinus imaging alterations, pauci-immune glomerulonephritis on biopsy, positivity for perinuclear (p)ANCA (myeloperoxidase—MPO), and blood eosinophils ($\geq 1 \times 10^9$/L).

In the head and neck, manifestations include sinusitis, nasal obstruction, epistaxis, ocular inflammation, and otitis media. It is estimated that the oral cavity is affected in approximately 6–13% of all cases, representing the first manifestation of the disease in some instances. Oral manifestations more often occur in the gingival tissue, which usually present a diffuse involvement of either the lower or the upper gingivae or even the involvement of both simultaneously. The affected tissue manifests as enlarged, painful, erythematous interdental papillae, with red to purple gingival tissue containing petechiae and a granular surface interspersed with yellow or dark red punctate foci. This appearance, known as strawberry-like gingivitis, is typically associated with granulomatosis with polyangiitis but should be differentiated from other conditions with similar manifestations, such as paracoccidioidomycosis, oral squamous cell carcinoma, and leukemic infiltrates. The palate and other regions of the oral mucosa can also be affected less often. When the palate is affected, leishmaniasis should be included in the differential diagnosis, and in the presence of palatine perforation, the diagnosis of extranodal NK/T cell lymphoma should be carefully ruled out. Gingival bleeding is a common finding, mucosal ulceration may also occur, and different degrees of alveolar bone loss may be found, causing tooth mobility in some patients. Involvement of the oral cavity by other types of ANCA-associated vasculitides, such as eosinophilic granulomatosis with polyangiitis and microscopic polyangiitis, has also been reported but is very rare, more often presenting as unspecific oral ulcers.

A rapid therapeutic approach is necessary for these patients, and the use of oral or pulsed intravenous cyclophosphamide and corticosteroid combination is considered the gold standard therapy that comprises an initial induction phase, followed by a maintenance protocol that may include the use of azathioprine, methotrexate, and rituximab. Prognosis of the patients improved with the development of steroids and cytotoxic/immunosuppressives in the 1970s, but therapeutic toxicity represents a significant adverse effect, which, together with secondary infections, may still lead patients to death (Fig. 15.1).

15.2 Microscopic Findings

- Overlying epithelium hyperplasia with exocytosis and pseudoepitheliomatous growth.
- In the lamina propria, there is an intense chronic inflammatory infiltrate.
- Erythrocyte extravasation.
- Presence of well-formed granulomas in the connective tissue. In some cases, it is not possible to observe well-formed granulomas.
- Presence of lymphocytes, eosinophils, plasma cells, and histiocytes.
- Areas containing microabscesses can also be present in oral mucosa biopsies.
- Presence of multinucleated giant cells.
- Small vessel vasculitis is a typical finding, but in oral biopsies, it may be very difficult to identify this feature.
- The presence of fibrinotic necrosis in the vascular walls, as well as geographic necrosis, can be found in some cases, especially in lung biopsies (Figs. 15.2, 15.3, 15.4, 15.5, and 15.6).

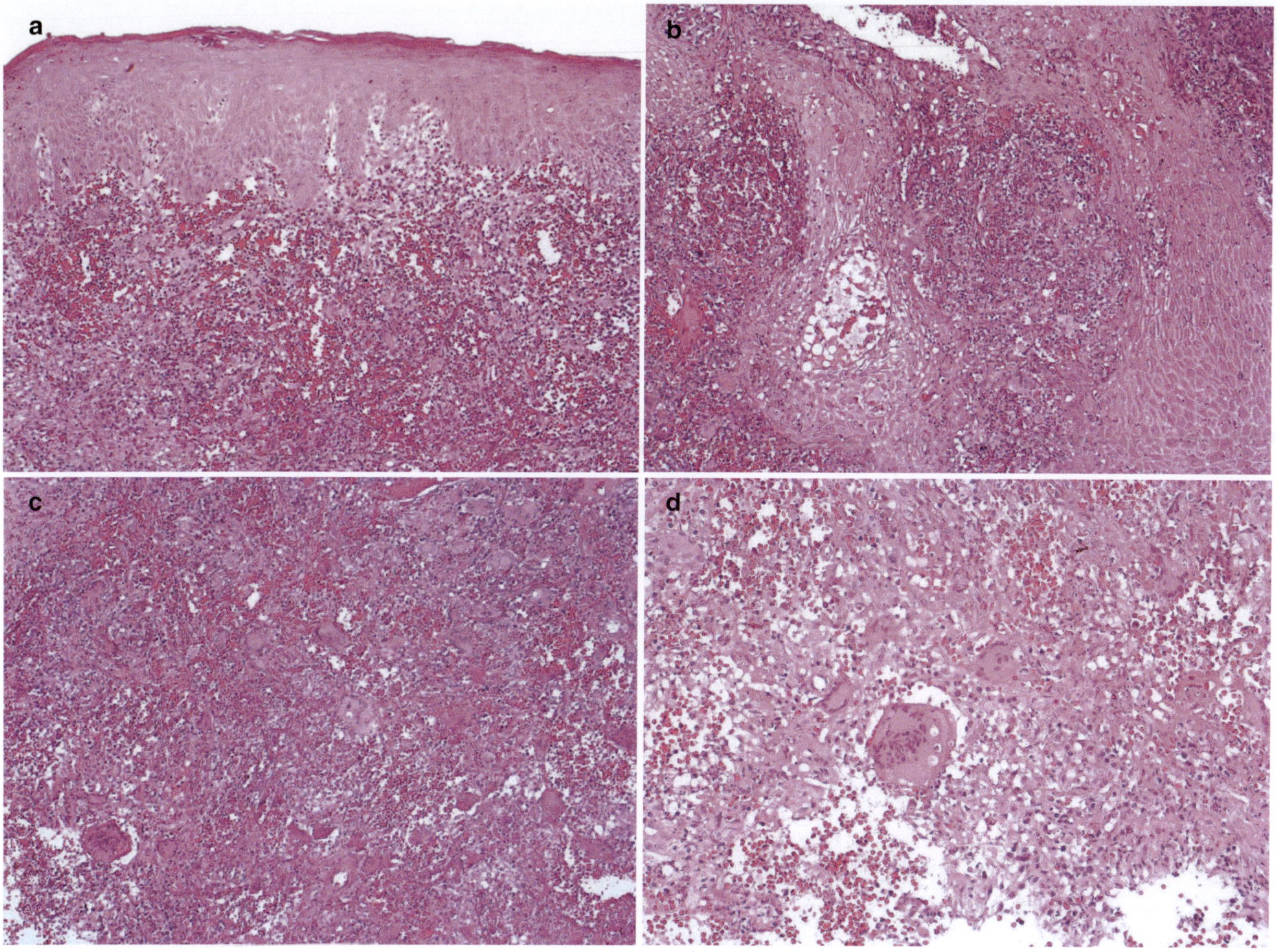

Fig. 15.2 Microscopic features of granulomatosis with polyangiitis affecting the oral cavity. (**a**) Observe the overlying squamous epithelium and the lamina propria showing a dense inflammatory infiltrate (H&E; 50X). (**b**) In some regions the epithelium is hyperplastic (H&E; 100X). (**c**) Dense inflammatory infiltrate in the lamina propria containing multinucleated giant cells (H&E; 100X). (**d**) Multinucleated giant cells, predominantly of the foreign body-type (H&E; 200X). There was no evidence of microorganisms in this sample

15.3 Immunohistochemistry and/or Genetics

The H&E microscopic analysis, together with clinical and laboratory data, is usually enough to establish the final diagnosis of granulomatosis with polyangiitis. However, the immunohistochemical analysis of this disease can be useful to demonstrate the polymorphic infiltrate when the granulomatous component of the disorder is not evident. The search for microorganisms or foreign bodies may also be important in challenging cases, and the use of histochemical reactions like PAS, Grocott-Gomory, and Ziehl-Neelsen stains can be useful to rule out possible infectious diseases (Table 15.1).

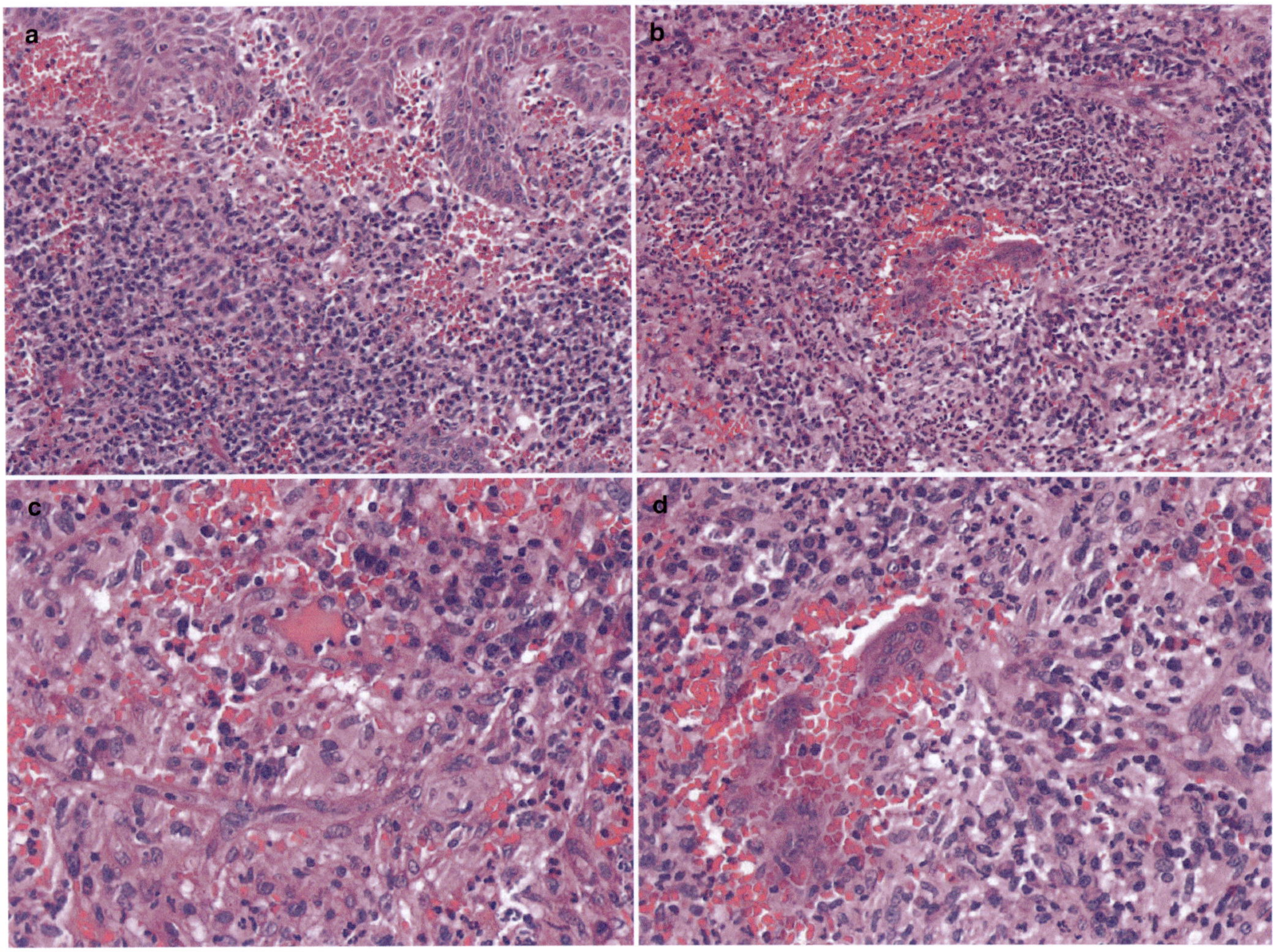

Fig. 15.3 Microscopic features of granulomatosis with polyangiitis affecting the oral cavity. (**a**) Note the dense inflammatory infiltrate located in the lamina propria, containing lymphocytes, plasma cells, macrophages and eosinophils (H&E; 100X). (**b**) The polymorphic inflammatory infiltrate of the disorder also contains multinucleated giant cells (H&E; 100X). (**c**) Extravasated erythrocytes and a perivascular distribution pattern of the inflammatory infiltrate (H&E; 200X). (**d**) Observe the multinucleated giant cells (H&E; 200X)

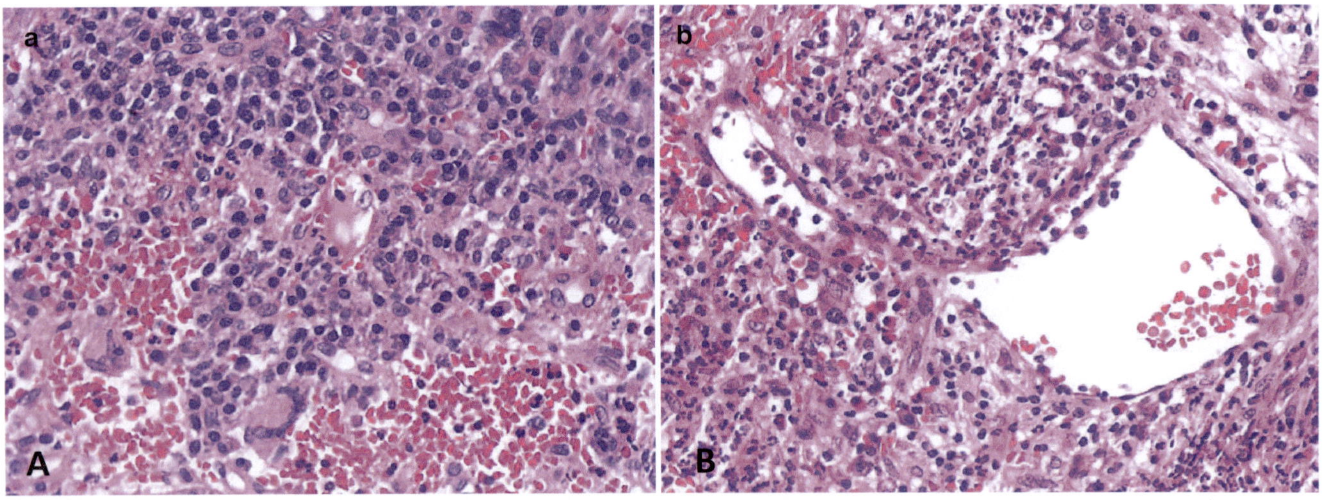

Fig. 15.4 Microscopic features granulomatosis with polyangiitis affecting the oral cavity. (**a**) Dense inflammatory infiltrate with the presence of many plasma cells and lymphocytes. Note the presence of multinucleated giant cells (H&E; 200X). (**b**) Although it is usually very difficult to observe the presence of vasculitis in oral biopsies, in this image we can appreciate the perivascular distribution of the inflammatory component (H&E; 200X)

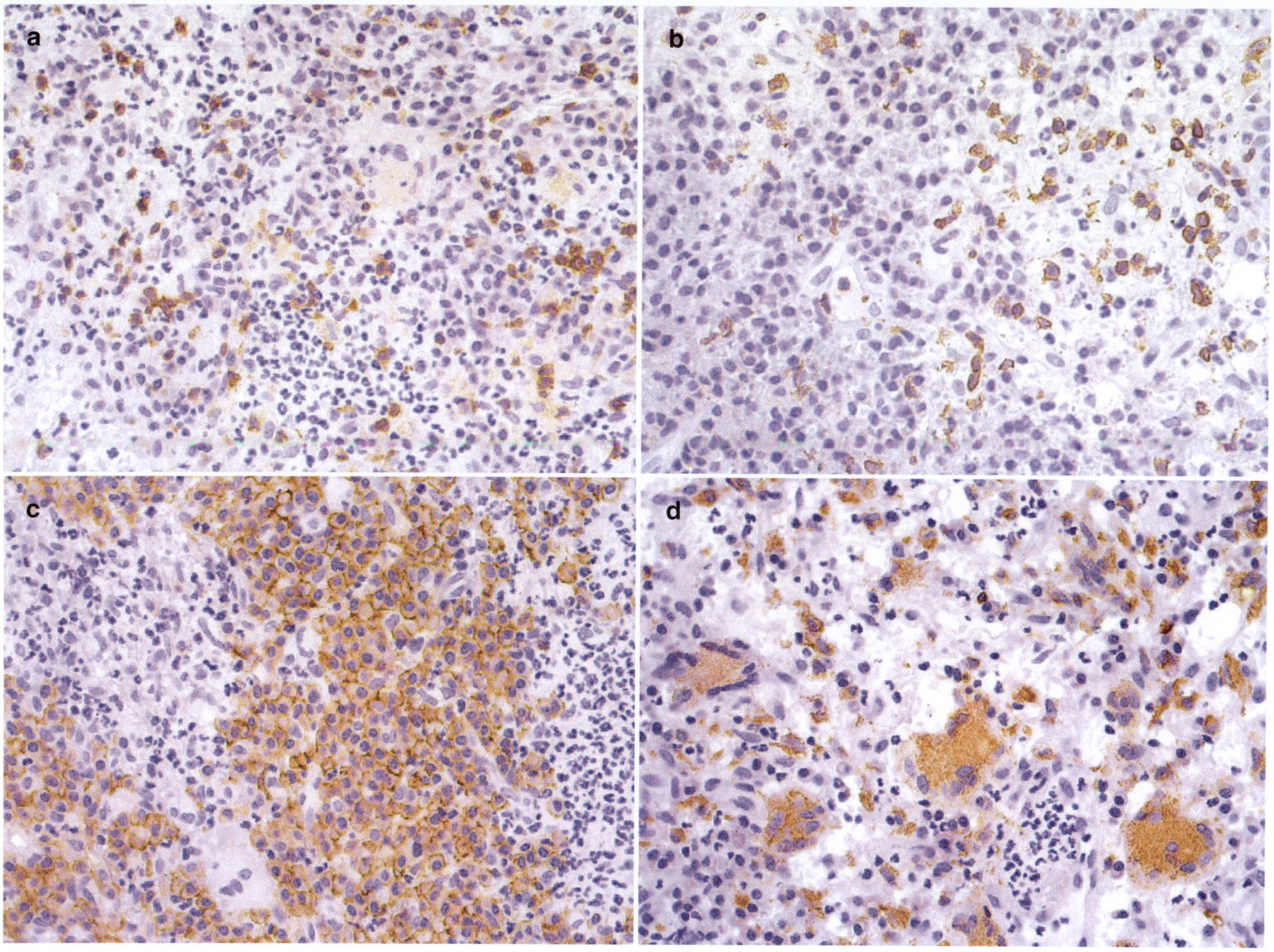

Fig. 15.5 Immunohistochemical features of granulomatosis with polyangiitis affecting the oral cavity. (**a**) Note the distribution of B lymphocytes demonstrated by CD20 expression (DAB; 100X). (**b**) The presence of T lymphocytes is demonstrated by CD3 expression (DAB; 100X). (**c**) The large number of plasma cells is demonstrated investigating CD138 protein expression (DAB; 100X). (**d**) Macrophages and multinucleated giant cells are illustrated by CD68 expression (DAB; 200X)

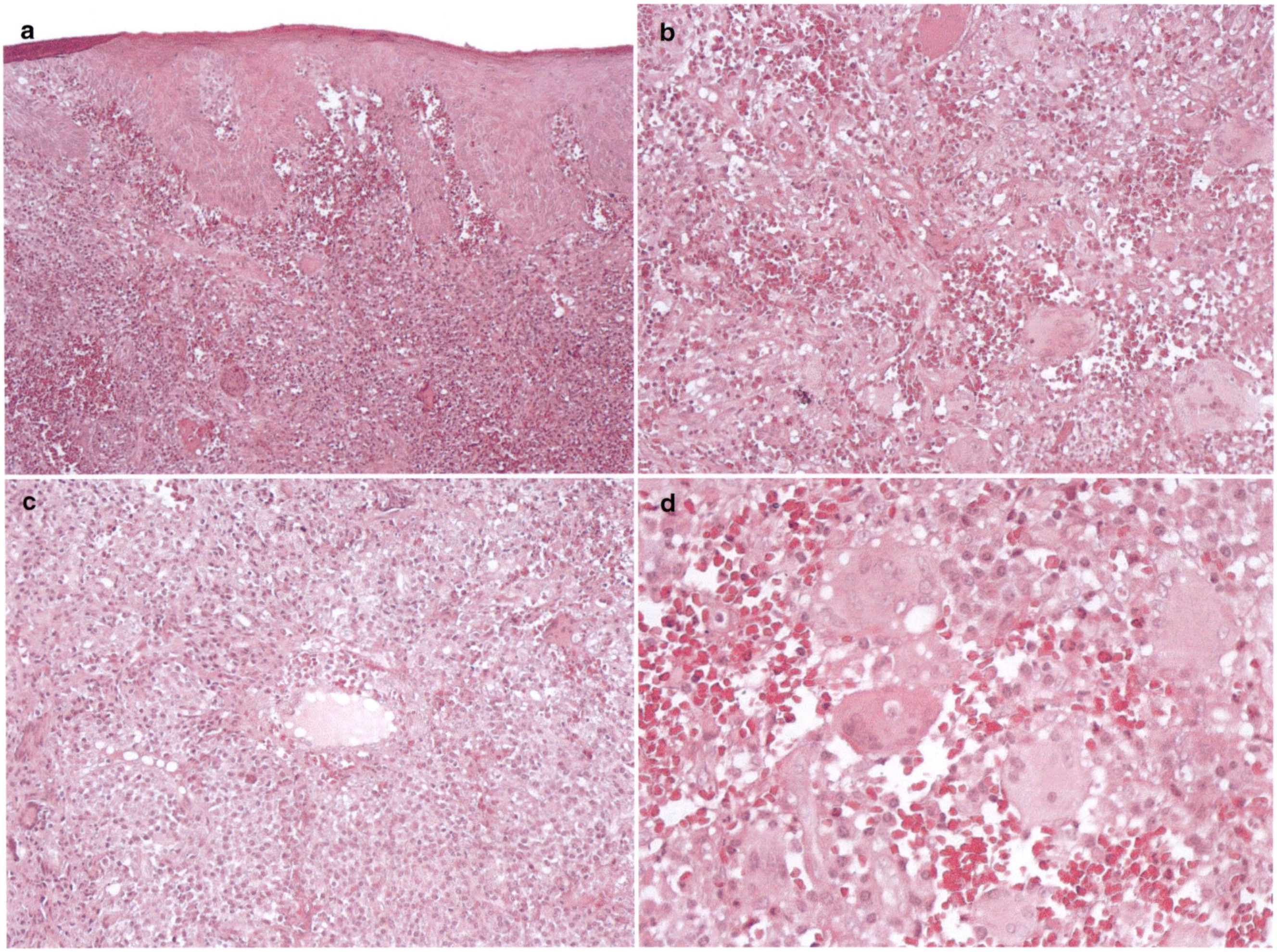

Fig. 15.6 Microscopic features of oral granulomatosis with polyangiitis affecting the gingiva of an adult female patient. (**a**) Overlying squamous epithelium and dense inflammatory infiltrate predominantly composed of mononuclear cells and scattered multinucleated giant cells (H&E; 100×). (**b**) Erythrocytes extravasation, lymphocytes, and multinucleated giant cells (H&E; 100×). (**c**) Predominance of plasma cells in some regions of the lesion, with the presence of multinucleated giant cells (H&E; 100×). (**d**) Under higher magnification, it is possible to observe that multinucleated giant cells have their nuclei randomly distributed in the cytoplasm of the cells, which is consistent with foreign-body type giant cells. PAS, Grocott-Gomori methenamine silver, Giemsa, and Ziehl-Neelsen histological reactions were negative (H&E; 200×)

Table 15.1 Summary of the main immunohistochemical reactions and histological stains used for granulomatosis with polyangiitis diagnosis

Antibody/stain	Most frequent results	Pattern	Objective
CD20	Positive	Membrane	To characterize the B lymphocyte infiltrate
CD3	Positive	Membrane	To characterize the T lymphocyte infiltrate
CD138	Positive	Membrane	To characterize the plasma cell infiltrate
CD68	Positive	Cytoplasm	To demonstrate the presence of histiocytes, multinucleated giant cells, and granulomas
Kappa/lambda	Polyclonal	Cytoplasm	To demonstrate the polyclonal nature of the infiltrate
PAS[a]	Negative	–	To exclude the presence of microorganisms
Grocott-Gomori[a]	Negative	–	To exclude the presence of microorganisms
Ziehl-Neelsen[a]	Negative	–	To exclude the presence of microorganisms

[a]Histological stain

Sources

1. Fonseca FP, Benites BM, Ferrari ALV, Sachetto Z, Campos GV, Almeida OP, et al. Gingival granulomatosis with polyangiitis (Wegener's granulomatosis) as a primary manifestation of the disease. Aust Dent J. 2017;62(1):102–6. https://doi.org/10.1111/adj.12441.
2. Ghiasi M. Strawberry gingivitis in granulomatosis with polyangiitis. N Engl J Med. 2017;377(21):2073. https://doi.org/10.1056/NEJMicm1706987.
3. Flores IL, Alves de Mesquita R, Uchoa Vasconcelos AC, Chaves Tarquinio SB, Neutzling Gomes AP. Destructive and painful ulcer in the posterior oral cavity and oropharynx. J Am Dent Assoc. 2017;148(9):678–83. https://doi.org/10.1016/j.adaj.2017.06.018.
4. Msallem B, Bassetti S, Matter MS, Thieringer FM. Strawberry gingivitis: challenges in the diagnosis of granulomatosis with polyangiitis on gingival specimens. Oral Surg Oral Med Oral Pathol Oral Radiol. 2019;128(6):e202–7.
5. Patrick A, Altman K. Granulomatosis with polyangiitis: potentially lethal gingival lesions presenting to the dentist. BMJ Case Rep. 2019;12(4):e229607. https://doi.org/10.1136/bcr-2019-229607.
6. Apoita-Sanz M, Blanco-Jauset P, Polis-Yanes C, Penin-Mosquera RM, Montserrat-Gomá G, Pozuelo-Arquimbau L, et al. Granulomatosis with Poliangeitis (Wegener's granulomatosis): orofacial manifestations. Systematic review and case report. Oral Health Prev Dent. 2020;18(4):929–43. https://doi.org/10.3290/j.ohpd.a45433.
7. Nico MMS, Pinto NT, Lourenço SV. From strawberry gingivitis to palatal perforation: the clinicopathological spectrum of oral mucosal lesions in granulomatosis with polyangiitis. J Oral Pathol Med. 2020;49(5):443–9. https://doi.org/10.1111/jop.13008.
8. Zhou Z, Yang C, Ye J. Perforation of palate in granulomatosis with polyangiitis. J Clin Rheumatol. 2020;26(3):e54. https://doi.org/10.1097/RHU.0000000000000842.
9. Kertesz T, Soowamber M, Bubola J, Psutka DJ, Bradley G. Gingival swelling as the initial manifestation of granulomatosis with polyangiitis. Head Neck Pathol. 2021;15(1):244–53. https://doi.org/10.1007/s12105-020-01144-0.
10. Ahmed A, Yein K, Ullah S. Strawberry gums as an initial presentation of severe granulomatosis with polyangiitis. Rheumatology (Oxford). 2021;60(3):1568. https://doi.org/10.1093/rheumatology/keaa601.
11. Noda S, Komiya Y, Soejima M. A case of eosinophilic granulomatosis with polyangiitis presented with blisters on the tongue. Clin Rheumatol. 2022;41(6):1925–6. https://doi.org/10.1007/s10067-022-06121-2.
12. Strouse J, Rajan A, Chang HB, Dimachkie MD, Halbur C, Bettendorf B. Clinical images: extranodal natural killer/T cell lymphoma as a rare mimicker of granulomatosis with polyangiitis. Arthritis Rheumatol. 2022;74(3):474. https://doi.org/10.1002/art.41956.
13. Fillingim SE, Artz C, Rambhatla P. Granulomatosis with polyangiitis presenting with strawberry gums. JAMA Dermatol. 2023;159(5):554. https://doi.org/10.1001/jamadermatol.2022.5839.
14. Labrador AJP, Valdez LHM, Marin NRG, Ibazetta KAR, Chacón JAL, Fernandez AJV, et al. Oral granulomatosis with polyangiitis a systematic review. Clin Exp Dent Res. 2023;9(1):100–11. https://doi.org/10.1002/cre2.706.
15. Rathmann J, Mohammad AJ. Classification criteria for ANCA associated vasculitis – ready for prime time? Curr Rheumatol Rep. 2024;26:332–42. https://doi.org/10.1007/s11926-024-01154-9.

Orofacial Granulomatosis

16

Adalberto A. Mosqueda-Taylor, Fabio Ramôa Pires, and Felipe Paiva Fonseca

16.1 General Overview and Clinical Presentation

Orofacial granulomatosis is an uncommon disorder characterized by the occurrence of persistent and/or recurrent enlargement of the oral and maxillofacial soft tissues with microscopic features showing the presence of chronic non-caseous granulomatosis. This term was originally proposed in 1985 to encompass the previously described diseases granulomatous cheilitis of Miescher and Melkersson–Rosenthal syndrome; therefore, orofacial granulomatosis shows multiple clinical phenotypes and its incidence is largely unknown, mostly because of the neglected nature of this disorder that is poorly recognized by clinicians, but also as a consequence of the wide variability of the diagnostic criteria applied to these entities, which very often have clinical and morphological overlapping, becoming unclear how to distinguish them in many instances.

Granulomatous cheilitis of Miescher is diagnosed when the tissue swelling is restricted to just one (more commonly) or to both (very rare) lips, more often painless, non-pruritic, and with an acute onset. It can be intermittent or persistent, and when pronounced, the swollen lip shows a fissure in the midline referred to as median cheilitis or at the buccal angles, potentially leading to aesthetic and functional impairments. Rarely, patients may complain of burning mouth sensation and of systemic symptoms like malaise, fever, and/or regional lymphadenopathy; there seems to be no race or sex predilection, and patients are usually young, between 20 and 40 years old. Oral ulceration and gingival enlargement may also occur in a subset of the patients. Granulomatous cheilitis of Miescher is sometimes considered an incomplete variant of Melkersson–Rosenthal syndrome, which may develop in many of these patients as the first manifestation or later during follow-up.

Melkersson–Rosenthal syndrome is defined as a neuromucocutaneous disorder, typically characterized by the triad of orofacial granulomatosis, cranial nerve involvement, and fissured tongue, although not all these features may be simultaneously present. The most affected sites are the upper lip, lower lip, gingivae, palate, cheeks, and nasolabial fold. The zygomatic, frontal, peri-orbital, or chin/submental region can also be affected. Patients are also young, usually starting in the second decade of life, and there is no sex predilection. Facial nerve paralysis occurs suddenly, before or after the orofacial swellings, it is usually unilateral, but it can be observed bilaterally, recurrently, or persistently, and the involvement of other cranial nerves has also been reported less commonly in approximately 30% of the cases, causing different symptoms like dysphagia, dysarthria, altered vision, and impaired eye motility.

Most cases of orofacial granulomatosis are considered idiopathic, not being associated with granulomatous cheilitis nor Melkersson–Rosenthal syndrome, and its pathogenesis

A. A. Mosqueda-Taylor (✉)
Department of Health Care, Universidad Autónoma Metropolitana Xochimilco, Mexico City, Mexico
e-mail: mosqueda@correo.xoc.uam.mx

F. R. Pires
Oral Pathology, School of Dentistry, Universidade do Estado do Rio de Janeiro, Rio de Janeiro, Brazil

F. P. Fonseca
Department of Oral Surgery and Pathology, School of Dentistry, Universidade Federal de Minas Gerais, Belo Horizonte, Brazil

© The Author(s), under exclusive license to Springer Nature Switzerland AG 2025
F. P. Fonseca et al. (eds.), *Lymphoproliferative and Granulomatous Disorders of the Oral Cavity*,
https://doi.org/10.1007/978-3-031-98844-8_16

is poorly understood, with several etiologic agents proposed as possible causes or triggering factors, including genetic predisposition, allergies to food or dental materials, and infectious or immunological agents. However, only a limited number of works have provided support for these hypotheses.

Orofacial granulomatosis is also frequently associated with Crohn's disease, and currently, it is not clear if these disorders represent the same condition or if they should be considered distinct entities, but in the presence of a diagnosis of orofacial granulomatosis, patients should undergo a detailed gastrointestinal and systemic evaluation to rule out a more specific etiology for the disorder, since about 40% of the infants and up to 50% of adults also demonstrate features of Crohn's disease, and these values may still be underestimated given that Crohn's disease is usually not systematically assessed in the absence of intestinal complains, the follow-up for the patients is usually very short, and because some treatment approaches for orofacial granulomatosis manifestations might have silenced the intestinal disease. On the other hand, some authors recommend that orofacial granulomatosis diagnosis should be reserved only for those idiopathic cases of the orofacial region, suggesting that the final diagnosis should be revised and modified if a systemic disorder is present.

Inflammatory bowel disease, including Crohn's disease and ulcerative colitis, is known to be associated with extraintestinal manifestations, most often affecting musculoskeletal, dermatologic, hepatobiliary, ocular, renal, and pulmonary systems. Crohn's disease is considered a relapsing/remitting systemic inflammatory disease, which predominantly affects the gut, especially the terminal ileum, and is usually associated with symptoms like abdominal pain, fever, and altered bowel habits. The oral manifestations of Crohn's disease include ulceration, diffuse swellings of the lips, cheeks and gingiva, "cobblestoning" mucosal lesions, mucosal tags, vertical lip fissures, angular cheilitis, and dysgeusia. Peri-oral erythema and cervical lymphadenopathy are also common findings.

Few cases of orofacial granulomatosis have been reported to be associated with a spontaneous resolution of the clinical manifestations, while many different therapeutic approaches have been described in the literature with widely different results and consensus among clinicians. The exposure to a restrictive diet by the patients and the use of low-level laser therapy have been investigated, but without a good and convincing response in most of the studies. The use of steroids represents the most widely used approach for these patients, associated or not with different types of immunosuppressants (e.g., azathioprine, methotrexate, thalidomide, and tacrolimus). Although systemic administration of steroids has shown partial to complete remission of the lesions in some studies, it is also frequently associated with side effects and recurrences after therapy. The intralesional administration of triamcinolone acetonide 10–40 mg/mL, in multiple affected sites for 2–3 weeks, has shown the best results, possibly because it releases higher concentrations of the drug in the affected site. Vitamin B and systemic steroids have also been used to manage the facial paralysis observed in cases of Melkerson–Rosenthal syndrome, while surgical cheiloplasty is recommended for unresponsive cases, although the follow-up behavior of these patients is unpredictable. For all those patients with oral manifestations of Crohn's disease, effective therapy depends on the correction of the gastrointestinal disorder (Figs. 16.1, 16.2, and 16.3).

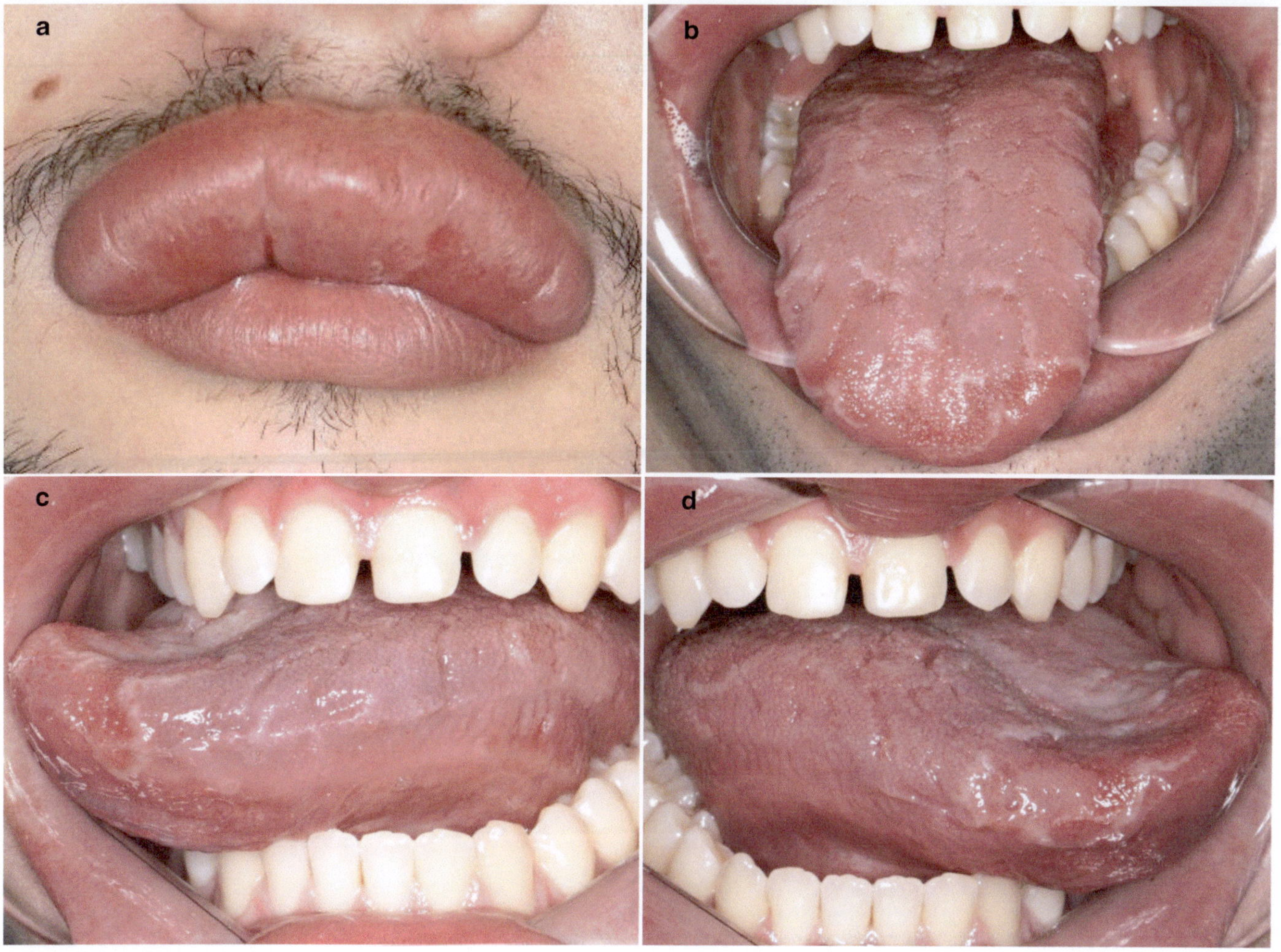

Fig. 16.1 Clinical presentation of orofacial granulomatosis in a 20-year-old male patient who also had facial paralysis of the left side and fissured tongue, consistent with Melkerson–Rosenthal syndrome. (**a**) Frontal view of the patient presenting an asymptomatic, large swelling of the upper lip. (**b**) Geographic tongue and fissured tongue were present on the dorsal surface of the tongue. (**c**) Geographic and fissured tongue on the left side and also (**d**) on the right side of the patient's tongue

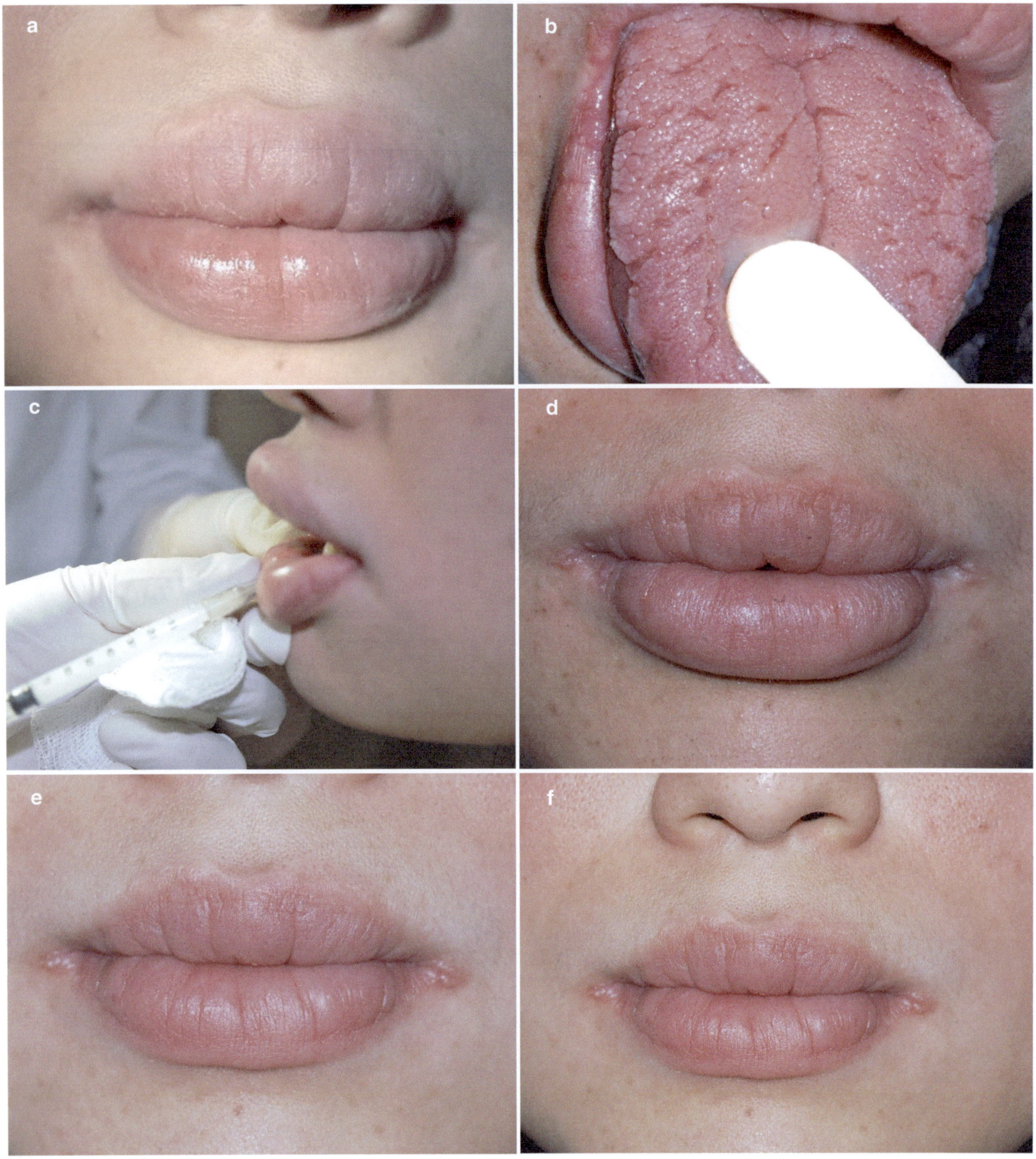

Fig. 16.2 Clinical presentation of orofacial granulomatosis in a 24-year-old female. (**a**) The patient had a 6-month history of asymptomatic recurrent upper and lower lip swellings. (**b**) Intra-oral exam depicted the presence of a fissured tongue. (**c**) Treatment comprised the use of intralesional injection of triamcinolone acetonide (10 mg/2 cm^3). (**d**) Observe the clinical presentation 1 week post-steroid infiltration. (**e**) Two weeks after treatment. Note residual commissural cheilitis, which resolved spontaneously after some days. (**f**) Final appearance of the patient after treatment

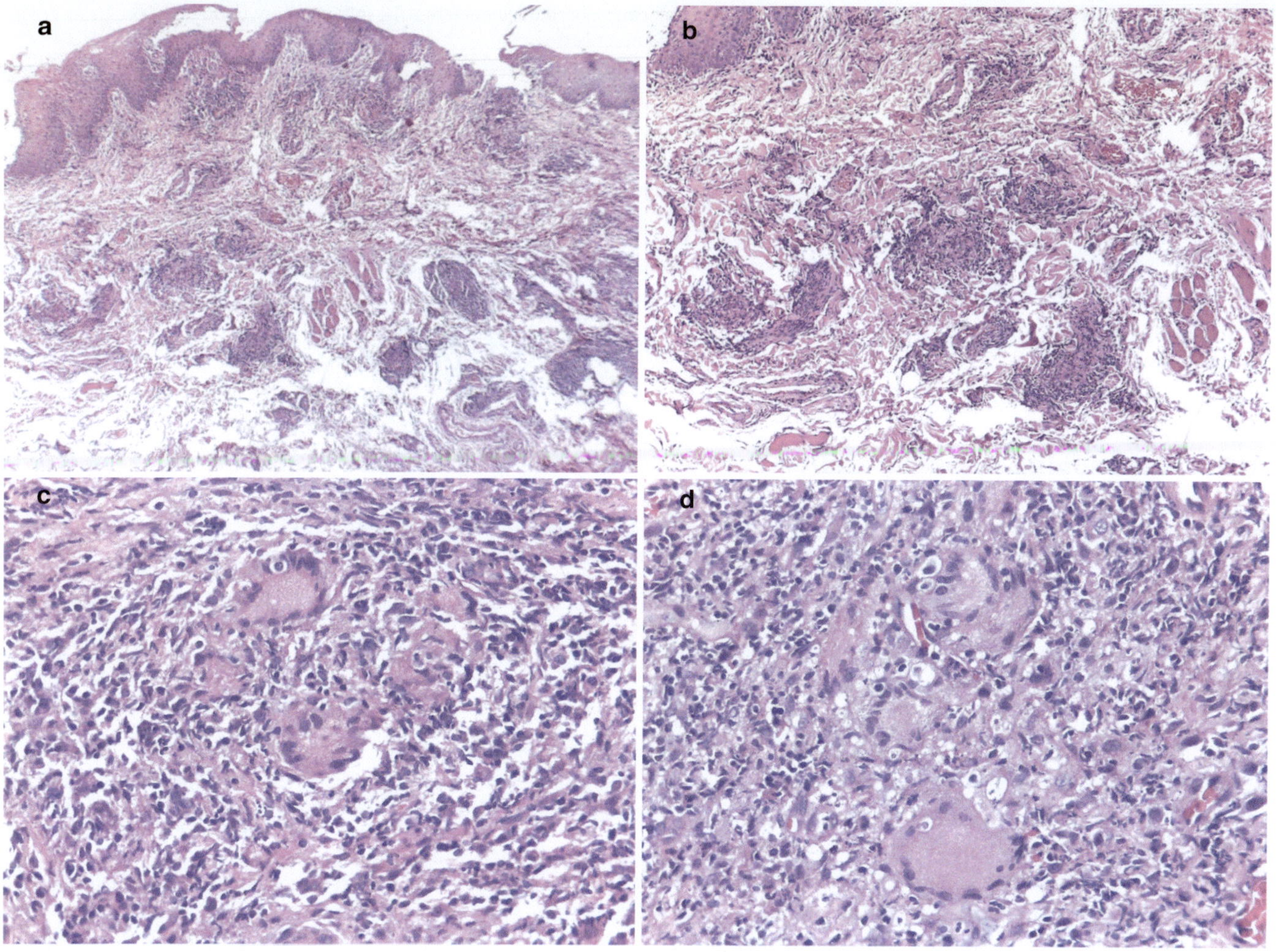

Fig. 16.3 Microscopic features identified in orofacial granulomatosis. (**a**) Oral mucosa biopsy showing the overlying epithelium and a chronic inflammatory infiltrate in the lamina propria (H&E; 25×). (**b**) The chronic inflammatory infiltrate consisted of lymphocytes and macrophages and in some regions demonstrated a perivascular distribution (H&E; 50×). (**c**) Presence of multinucleated giant cells and macrophages in a granulomatous inflammatory infiltrate (H&E; 100×). (**d**) Note the multinucleated giant cells, lymphocytes, and macrophages in the inflammatory infiltrate. Special histological stains did not reveal any microorganism in the lesion (H&E; 100×)

16.2 Microscopic Findings

- Histopathological features of orofacial granulomatosis and Crohn's disease are considered indistinguishable.
- The overlying epithelium may show different degrees of hyperkeratosis, acanthosis, spongiosis, mild to moderate lymphocyte exocytosis, and rete pegs hyperplasia.
- Sub-epithelial edema and an increased number of dilated lymphatic vessels are observed.
- Chronic inflammation with predominance of macrophages and lymphocytes.
- Perivascular lymphocytic infiltrate is frequently found.
- In many cases, there is a granulomatous infiltrate with non-necrotic, non-caseous granulomas, although not all cases demonstrate this feature, and its absence does not rule out these diagnoses.
- Epithelioid macrophages with large eosinophilic cytoplasm and round to oval nuclei are present in the granulomas.
- Multinucleated giant cells are usually present in the granulomas.
- Those cases without well-formed granulomas usually have nonspecific chronic inflammation with predominance of lymphocytes and macrophages.
- Microorganisms should not be present in the lesions.

Table 16.1 Summary of the main immunohistochemical reactions that can be used to characterize the inflammatory infiltrate of orofacial granulomatosis and Crohn's disease. The results of histological stains are also described

Antibody/stain	Most frequent results	Pattern	Objective
CD20	Positive	Membrane	To demonstrate the presence of B lymphocytes
CD3	Positive	Membrane	To demonstrate the presence of T lymphocytes
CD138	Positive	Membrane	To demonstrate the presence of plasma cells
CD68	Positive	Cytoplasm	To demonstrate the presence of histiocytes, macrophages, and multinucleated giant cells.
PAS[a]	Negative	–	To show the absence of microorganisms
Grocott-Gomori[a]	Negative	–	To show the absence of microorganisms
Ziehl-Neelsen[a]	Negative	–	To show the absence of microorganisms

PAS Periodic-Acid Schiff
[a]Histological stains

16.3 Immunohistochemistry and/or Genetics

The diagnosis of orofacial granulomatosis (including granulomatous cheilitis of Miescher or Melkersson–Rosenthal syndrome) and Crohn's disease is usually based on clinical data supported by morphological findings, while immunohistochemistry has a limited value for the diagnostic approach of these disorders. Immunoprofile of the inflammatory infiltrate depicts a granulomatous reaction with positivity for CD68, revealing the presence of histiocytes and a variable distribution of CD20-positive B lymphocytes and CD3-positive T lymphocytes, as well as a minor plasmacytic component demonstrated by CD138 or other plasma cell markers. These reactions may be more useful in those cases without well-organized granulomas, when the inflammatory infiltrate is nonspecific. Histologic stains like PAS, Grocott-Gomori methenamine silver, and Ziehl-Neelsen should be negative and are important to exclude possible infectious agents (Table 16.1).

Sources

1. Harty S, Fleming P, Rowland M, Crushell E, McDermott M, Drumm B, et al. A prospective study of the oral manifestations of Crohn's disease. Clin Gastroenterol Hepatol. 2005;3(9):886–91. https://doi.org/10.1016/s1542-3565(05)00424-6.
2. Zbar AP, Ben-Horin S, Beer-Gabel M, Eliakim R. Oral Crohn's disease: is it a separable disease from orofacial granulomatosis? A review. J Crohns Colitis. 2012;6(2):135–42. https://doi.org/10.1016/j.crohns.2011.07.001.
3. Al-Hamad A, Porter S, Fedele S. Orofacial granulomatosis. Dermatol Clin. 2015;33(3):433–46. https://doi.org/10.1016/j.det.2015.03.008.
4. Hullah EA, Escudier MP. The mouth in inflammatory bowel disease and aspects of orofacial granulomatosis. Periodontol 2000. 2019;80(1):61–76. https://doi.org/10.1111/prd.12264.
5. Galdiero MR, Maio F, Arcoleo F, Boni E, Bonzano L, Brussino L, et al. Orofacial granulomatosis: clinical and therapeutic features in an Italian cohort and review of the literature. Allergy. 2021;76(7):2189–200. https://doi.org/10.1111/all.14799.
6. Gavioli CF, Florezi GP, Lourenço SV, Nico MM. Clinical profile of Melkersson-Rosenthal syndrome/orofacial granulomatosis: a review of 51 patients. J Cutan Med Surg. 2021;25(4):390–6. https://doi.org/10.1177/1203475421995132.
7. Gavioli CFB, Nico MMS, Florezi GP, Lourenço SV. The histopathological spectrum of Melkersson-Rosenthal syndrome: analysis of 47 cases. J Cutan Pathol. 2020;47(11):1010–7. https://doi.org/10.1111/cup.13784.
8. Gavioli CFB, Nico MMS, Panajotopoulos N, Rodrigues H, Rosales CB, Valente NYS, et al. A case-control study of HLA alleles in Brazilian patients with Melkersson-Rosenthal syndrome. Eur J Med Genet. 2020;63(7):103879. https://doi.org/10.1016/j.ejmg.2020.103879.
9. Skaare AB, Hovden ES, Herlofson BB, Søland TM. Orofacial granulomatosis: a questionnaire study among Norwegian dental clinicians. Eur Arch Paediatr Dent. 2020;21(5):557–64. https://doi.org/10.1007/s40368-020-00511-3.
10. Wei M, Xie C, Liu Y, Wang Y, Wang Y, Wang X, et al. Characterizing disease manifestations and treatment outcomes among patients with orofacial granulomatosis in China. JAAD Int. 2020;1(2):126–34. https://doi.org/10.1016/j.jdin.2020.07.003.
11. Gavioli CFB, Florezi GP, Dabronzo MLD, Jiménez MR, Nico MMS, Lourenço SV. Orofacial granulomatosis and Crohn disease: coincidence or pattern? A systematic review. Dermatology. 2021;237(4):635–40. https://doi.org/10.1159/000513446.
12. Stoevesandt J, Keita DU, Goebeler M. Disease-related burden and long-term outcome in orofacial granulomatosis: observations from a large single-centre cohort. Clin Exp Dermatol. 2022;47(6):1169–73. https://doi.org/10.1111/ced.15124.
13. Phillips F, Verstockt B, Sladek M, de Boer N, Katsanos K, Karmiris K, et al. Orofacial granulomatosis associated with Crohn's disease: a multicentre case series. J Crohns Colitis. 2022;16(3):430–5. https://doi.org/10.1093/ecco-jcc/jjab158.
14. Joshi S, Mawdsley J, Hullah E, Ormond M, Carey B. Management of orofacial granulomatosis. Br J Hosp Med (Lond). 2023;29(3):1–16. https://doi.org/10.12968/hmed.2022.0416.
15. Wang Y, Xu H, Wei M, Wang Y, Wang W, Ju J, et al. Identification of putative bacterial pathogens for orofacial granulomatosis based on 16S rRNA metagenomic analysis. Microbiol Spectr. 2023;11(3):e02266–22. https://doi.org/10.1128/spectrum.02266-22.
16. Plemel DJA, Weis E, Punja KG, Ashenhurst ME, Mai DD, Kulaga A. Primary periocular orofacial granulomatosis: case series and systematic review. Ophthalmic Plast Reconstr Surg. 2024;40(1):11–7. https://doi.org/10.1097/IOP.0000000000002478.

Sarcoidosis

17

Madhu Shrestha, John M. Wright,
Cinthia Veronica Bardalez Lopez de Caceres,
and Felipe Paiva Fonseca

17.1 General Overview and Clinical Presentation

Sarcoidosis was first described in the nineteenth century and is currently recognized as an idiopathic multi-system granulomatous disease that more frequently affects the lungs and the lymph nodes of young adults between 25 and 35 years old. A second peak incidence occurs in individuals at 45–65 years, and females are slightly more affected. Its diagnosis is made by clinical and radiological findings, and the demonstration of non-caseating granulomas on biopsy tissue is mandatory, together with the exclusion of other diseases like tuberculosis, lymphomas, deep fungal infections, and other specific granulomatous disorders.

The disease may occur simultaneously with auto-immune disorders like lupus erythematosus, Sjögren disease, and rheumatoid arthritis, and the occurrence of sarcoidosis preceding or following the diagnosis of lymphoma is also known and has been termed as sarcoidosis-lymphoma syndrome. Sarcoidosis is believed to result from the exposure of genetically susceptible individuals to an unknown antigenic agent. A positive family history increases the risk of developing sarcoidosis twofold. Various human leukocyte antigen (HLA) variants are associated with the risk, type of organ, and severity of the disease. Various studies have highlighted the role of HLA-DRB1*07, *14, *15, *01, and *03 and DQB1*0602 to be associated with an increased risk of progressive pulmonary sarcoidosis. Different genetic, infectious, and environmental factors have been postulated as possible causes of the disease, including mycobacteria, dust containing silica, iron, or titanium, products of wood combustion, and insecticides, among others, whose etiological potential, however, still demands further validation. The affected tissues are characterized by the infiltration of activated Th1 lymphocytes and histiocytes that secrete biological mediators including IL-2, IL-12, IFN-c, and TNF-α, which will induce the formation of a non-caseating granulomatous reaction that may lead to fibrosis and organ dysfunction.

Involvement of the eyes, nervous system, and heart is observed. Patients usually demonstrate constitutional manifestations like fatigue, fever, cough, weight loss, and chest pains, while cutaneous complaints are found in approximately 37% of the cases, more often in the face and neck, ranging from erythema nodosum, hyper- or hypopigmentation, keloids, subcutaneous nodules, to maculopapular lesions. Head and neck sarcoidosis may occur primarily or in combination with CNS sarcoidosis and systemic diseases in 10–15% of cases, and salivary glands are the most affected structures, which may be associated with local swelling and xerostomia. When minor glands of patients affected by sarcoidosis are microscopically examined, non-caseating granulomatous reactions may be observed in up to 60% of the patients.

Sarcoidosis of the oral cavity is even rarer and mostly occult and often presents as solitary or multiple lesions. Oral lesions could be the first manifestation of systemic involvement in 35–58% cases without any obvious systemic presentation. The buccal mucosa, gingiva, lip, hard palate, and tongue are the most affected sites, and the lesions usually present as asymptomatic, normal-colored to reddish papules or nodules. Erythematous lesions containing a granular surface may also occur. Ulcerated lesions may be present and cause pain. Gingival hyperplasia, gingival redness/inflammation, and gingival ulcers, frequently associated with pain and bleeding, are possible oral manifestations of sarcoidosis. Gnathic bones can be affected, slightly more often in the maxilla, presenting an ill-defined radiolucency with erosions of the cortex, but usually without bone expansion. Tooth loosening and non-healing sockets may be found.

M. Shrestha (✉) · J. M. Wright
Department of Diagnostic Sciences, Texas A&M University, College Station (TAMU), School of Dentistry, Dallas, TX, USA
e-mail: madhushrestha@tamu.edu; john-m-wright@tamu.edu

C. V. B. L. de Caceres · F. P. Fonseca
Department of Oral Surgery and Pathology, School of Dentistry, Universidade Federal de Minas Gerais, Belo Horizonte, Brazil

© The Author(s), under exclusive license to Springer Nature Switzerland AG 2025

F. P. Fonseca et al. (eds.), *Lymphoproliferative and Granulomatous Disorders of the Oral Cavity*,
https://doi.org/10.1007/978-3-031-98844-8_17

Of note, clinicians and pathologists should be aware that the use of some types of drugs may lead to the development of a drug-induced sarcoidosis-like reaction. It is a granulomatous disorder that is indistinguishable from sarcoidosis and that occurs in a temporal relationship with the use of the etiologic drug, typically improving or resolving following the discontinuation of the offending drug. It more commonly affects the lungs, hilar lymph nodes, and skin, but several cases in the oral mucosa have been reported. Immune checkpoint inhibitors, highly active anti-retroviral therapy, interferons, and tumor necrosis factor-alpha antagonists are the most common drug categories associated with the drug-induced sarcoidosis-like reaction. Clinical and microscopic features are like sarcoidosis, and the exclusion of other more specific granulomatous conditions should also be made.

Treatment varies depending on the severity of the disease. Sarcoidosis cannot be cured, and treatment is more directed to control the symptoms, limit organ damage, or reduce a compromised quality of life. The overall arching goal of providing treatment is to prevent fibrosis development from the granulomatous inflammation in vital organs. Undoubtedly, corticosteroids remain the most efficient drug of choice. Other anti-inflammatory categories include anti-metabolites and biologic agents. A second line of treatment is often required for refractory or severe cases. These include but are not limited to Methotrexate, Hydroxychloroquine, Azathioprine, Leflunomide, Mycophenolate Mofetil, Infliximab, JAK-STAT inhibitors, etc. While sarcoidosis may occasionally be resolved on its own, more than 10% of patients progress to a severe form of the disease. Sarcoidosis has a mortality rate of approximately 7% within the first 5 years, but it may progress to more than 60% in cases with advanced pulmonary involvement.

17.2 Microscopic Findings

- For intraoral lesions, the overlying squamous epithelium may be atrophic, hyperplastic, or ulcerated.
- In the lamina propria, there is a typical dense granulomatous inflammatory infiltrate. However, a nonspecific mononuclear inflammatory infiltrate may precede granuloma formation and represent a diagnostic challenge for pathologists.
- The granulomas are typically compact, well-defined, and non-caseating and comprise epithelioid histiocytes and multinucleated giant cells, surrounded by lymphocytes, fibroblasts, and a varied degree of fibrosis.
- The granulomas show a predominance of CD4+ T lymphocytes in the central area and a rim of CD8+ T lymphocytes and B lymphocytes at the periphery.
- Although sarcoid granulomas can be angioinvasive, this finding is not usually found in oral biopsies.
- The occurrence of different inclusion bodies like asteroid bodies, Schaumann bodies, cockade-like structures, calcium oxalate crystals, and Hamazaki–Wesenberg bodies is frequently found in the multinucleated giant cells.
- Asteroid bodies are star-shaped, spiculated structures that can be found in the cytoplasm of the multinucleated giant cells in approximately 2–9% of the cases.
- Schaumann bodies (also known as conchoidal bodies) were first described in 1941 and present as round to oval shell-like concentric basophilic calcifications, possibly representing a residuum of lysosomal organelles activity. These inclusions are birefringent under polarized light and are present in approximately 48–88% of the cases.
- Birefringent calcium oxalate crystals are present in almost two-thirds of the cases, presenting as blocklike or irregular in configuration.
- Cockade-like structures are present in almost 12% of the cases, but their biological significance remains unknown.
- Hamazaki–Wesenberg bodies are present in approximately 16% of the cases. They are not birefringent structures. They present a round, oval, or spindle shape and stain yellow brown using the H&E technique. They possibly represent lysosome structures.
- Drug-induced sarcoidosis-like reaction is microscopically similar to sarcoidosis, exhibiting a non-caseating granulomatous reaction in the lamina propria, with the presence of Langhans-type multinucleated giant cells and a variable lymphoplasmacytic inflammatory infiltrate (Figs. 17.1, 17.2 and 17.3).

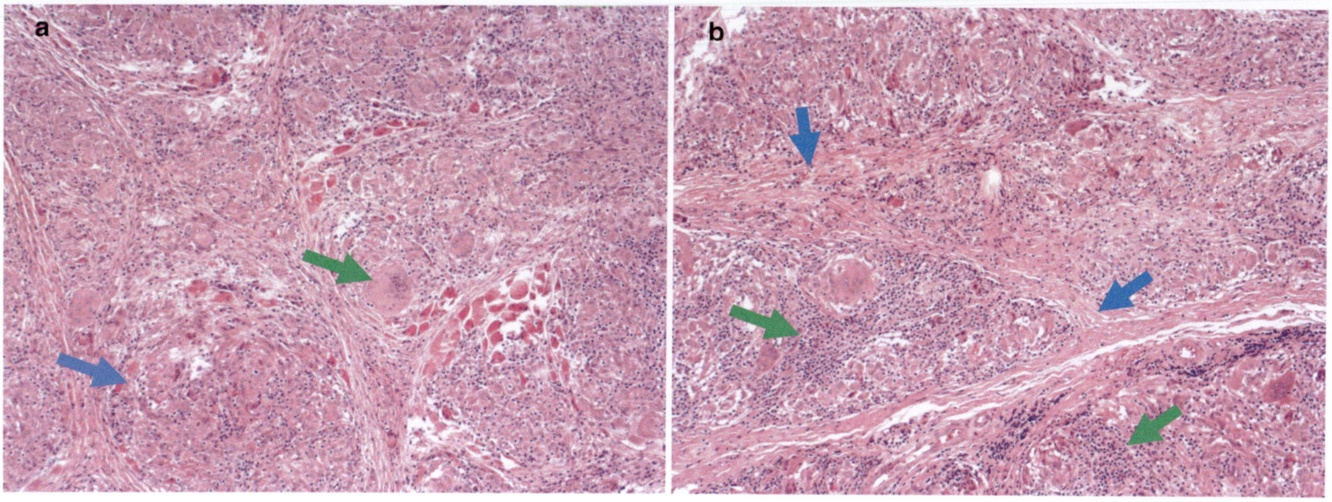

Fig. 17.1 Microscopic features of sarcoidosis affecting the oral cavity. (**a**) Diffuse granulomatous inflammatory infiltrate in the lamina propria. Note the presence of well-formed granulomas (blue arrow) and multinucleated giant cells (green arrows) (H&E; 100×). (**b**) A fibrous stroma is often observed (blue arrows). Note the presence of lymphocytes characterized by a more hyperchromatic appearance (green arrows) (H&E; 100×)

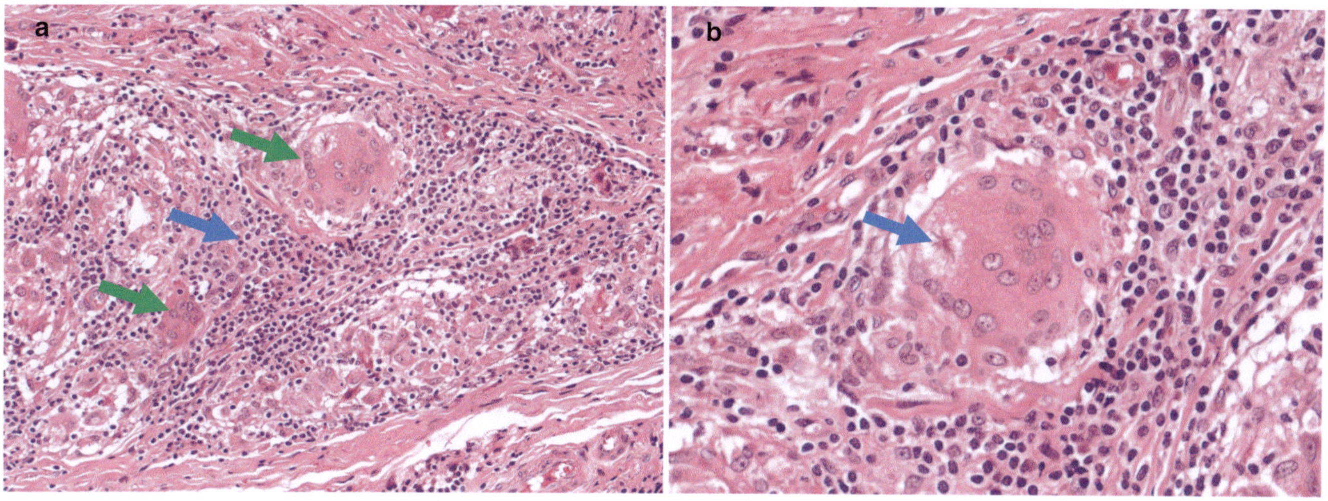

Fig. 17.2 Microscopic features of sarcoidosis affecting the oral cavity. (**a**) The presence of multinucleated giant cells (green arrows) is a typical microscopic finding in sarcoidosis, but in addition to the predominance of the histiocytic component, the inflammatory infiltrate is also composed of lymphocytes (blue arrow) (H&E; 200×). (**b**) Under high magnification, it is possible to observe the presence of an asteroid body (blue arrow) in the cytoplasm of a multinucleated giant cell (H&E; 400×)

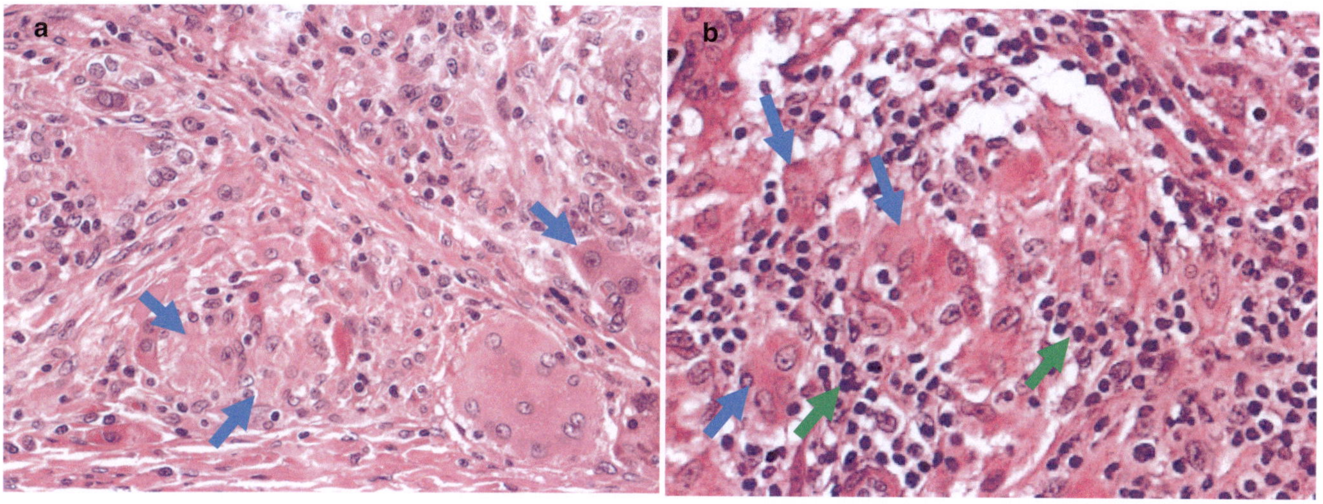

Fig. 17.3 Microscopic features of sarcoidosis affecting the oral cavity. (**a**) The granulomatous infiltrate is also characterized by the presence of epithelioid histiocytes that present a large eosinophilic cytoplasm (blue arrows) (H&E; 400×). (**b**) Note in this image the presence of aggregates of epithelioid histiocytes (blue arrows) surrounded by hyperchromatic lymphocytes (green arrows) (H&E; 400×)

17.3 Immunohistochemistry and/or Genetics

The diagnosis of the oral manifestations of sarcoidosis is based on clinical data supported by morphological findings, while immunohistochemistry has a limited value for diagnosis. Immunoprofile of the inflammatory infiltrate demonstrates a granulomatous reaction with positivity for CD68, revealing the presence of histiocytes and a variable distribution of CD20-positive B lymphocytes and CD3-positive T lymphocytes, as well as a plasmacytic component demonstrated by CD138 or other plasma cell markers. Histologic stains like PAS, Grocott-Gomori methenamine silver, and Ziehl-Neelsen should be negative and are important to exclude possible infectious agents (Figs. 17.4, 17.5, and 17.6, Table 17.1).

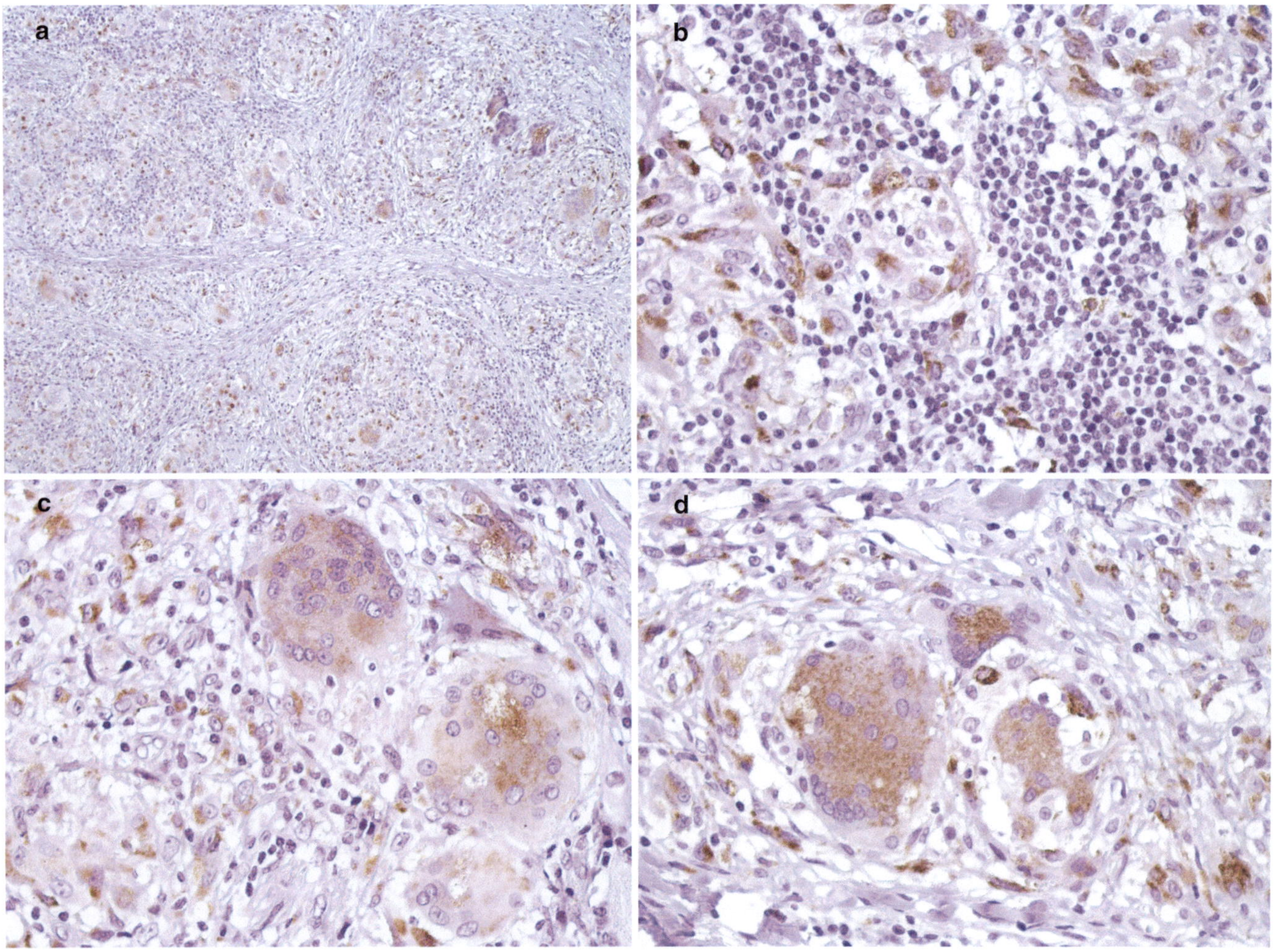

Fig. 17.4 Immunohistochemical features of sarcoidosis affecting the oral cavity. (**a**) The histiocytic component of the inflammatory infiltrate can be demonstrated by evaluating CD68 expression (DAB; 100×). (**b**) Note the expression of CD68 in the epithelioid histiocytes (DAB; 200×). (**c**) The multinucleated giant cells also express CD68 in the cytoplasm (DAB; 400×). (**d**) Observe the expression of CD68 in the multinucleated giant cells and in the epithelioid histiocytes (DAB; 400×)

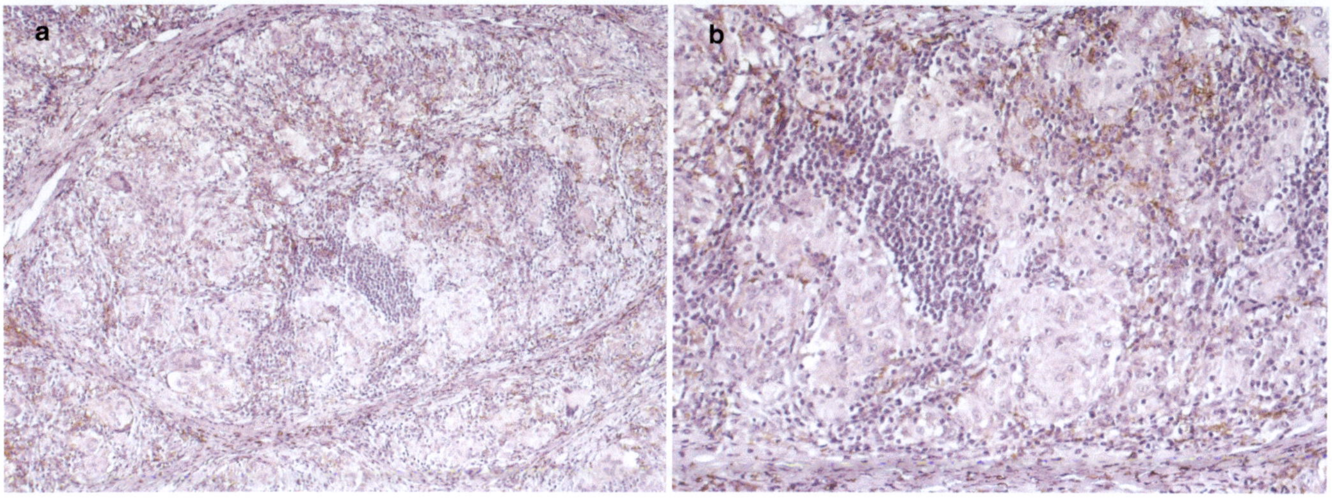

Fig. 17.5 Immunohistochemical features of sarcoidosis affecting the oral cavity. (**a**) The histiocytes are also positive for CD163 protein, considered a more specific marker for histiocytic differentiation than CD68 (DAB; 100×). (**b**) However, the multinucleated giant cells are negative or only faintly positive for CD163, as demonstrated in this image. Only the histiocytes resulted positive (DAB; 200×)

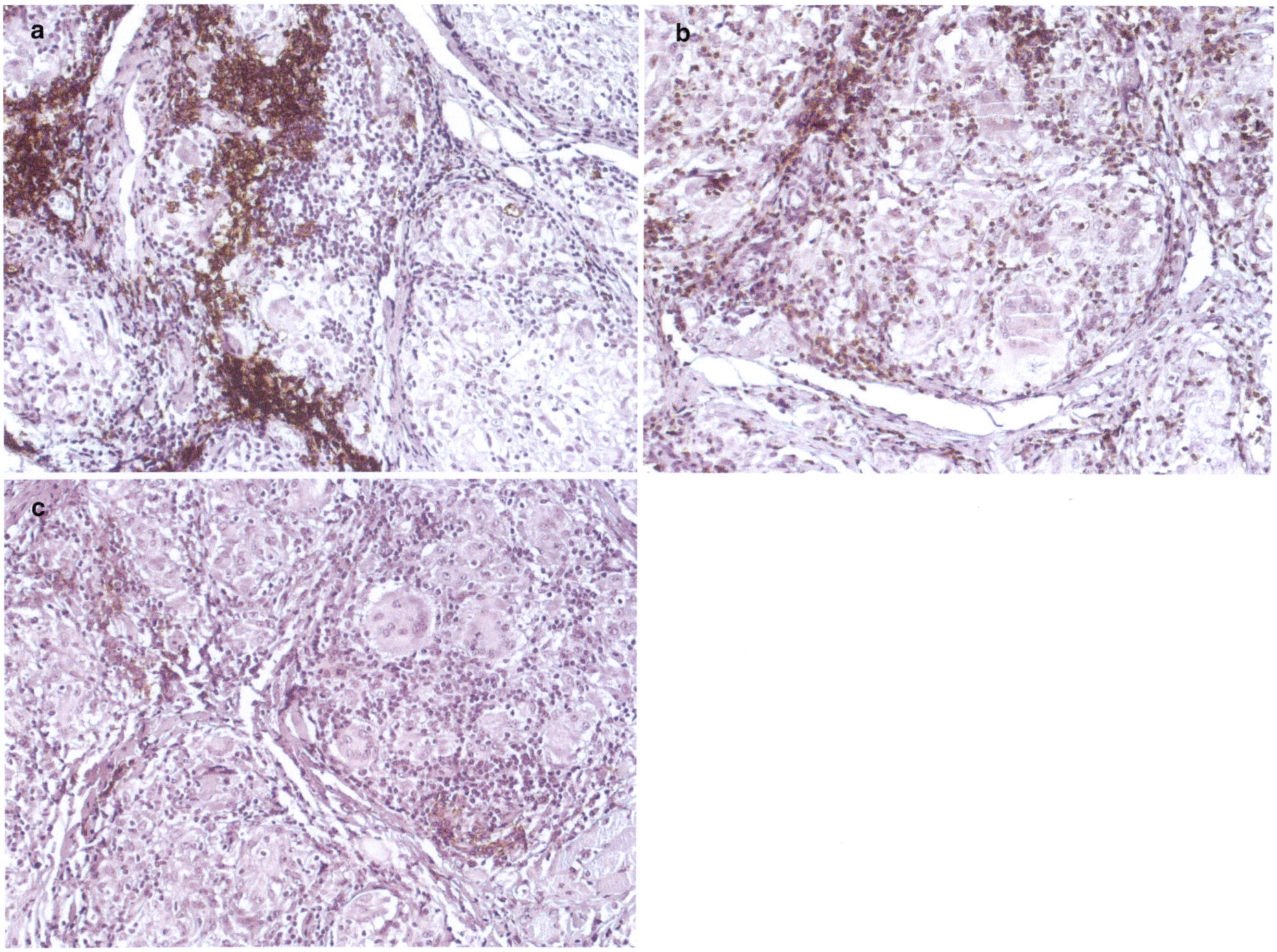

Fig. 17.6 Immunohistochemical features of sarcoidosis affecting the oral cavity. (**a**) Other cellular populations are also present in the granulomatous infiltrate of sarcoidosis. Observe the B lymphocytes expressing CD20 protein (DAB; 200×). (**b**) The CD3-positive T lymphocytes are also present (DAB; 200×). (**c**) Plasma cells express CD138 protein, but they represent a minor component of the inflammatory infiltrate (DAB; 200×)

Table 17.1 Summary of the main immunohistochemical reactions that can be used to characterize the inflammatory infiltrate of sarcoidosis. The results of histological stains are also described

Antibody/stain	Most frequent results	Pattern	Objective
CD20	Positive	Membrane	To demonstrate the presence of B lymphocytes
CD3	Positive	Membrane	To demonstrate the presence of T lymphocytes
CD138	Positive	Membrane	To demonstrate the presence of plasma cells
CD68	Positive	Cytoplasm	To demonstrate the presence of macrophages, multinucleated giant cells, and granulomas
PAS[a]	Negative	–	To show the absence of microorganisms
Grocott-Gomori[a]	Negative	–	To show the absence of microorganisms
Ziehl-Neelsen[a]	Negative	–	To show the absence of microorganisms

[a]Histological stains; *PAS* Periodic-Acid Schiff

Sources

1. Suresh L, Radfar L. Oral sarcoidosis: a review of literature. Oral Dis. 2005;11(3):138–45. https://doi.org/10.1111/j.1601-0825.2005.01014.x.
2. Kasamatsu A, Kanazawa H, Watanabe T, Matsuzaki O. Oral sarcoidosis: report of a case and review of literature. J Oral Maxillofac Surg. 2007;65(6):1256–9. https://doi.org/10.1016/j.joms.2005.09.028.
3. Antunes KB, Miranda AM, Carvalho SR, Azevedo AL, Tatakis DN, Pires FR. Sarcoidosis presenting as gingival erosion in a patient under long-term clinical control. J Periodontol. 2008;79(3):556–61. https://doi.org/10.1902/jop.2008.070139.
4. Bouaziz A, Le Scanf J, Chapelon-Abric C, Varron L, Khenifer S, et al. Oral involvement in sarcoidosis: report of 12 cases. Q J Med. 2012;105:755–67.
5. Motswaledi MH, Khammissa RA, Jadwat Y, Lemmer J, Feller L. Oral sarcoidosis: a case report and review of the literature. Aust Dent J. 2014;59(3):389–94. https://doi.org/10.1111/adj.12196.
6. London J, Grados A, Fermé C, Charmillon A, Maurier F, Deau B, et al. Sarcoidosis occurring after lymphoma: report of 14 patients and review of the literature. Medicine (Baltimore). 2014;93(21):e121. https://doi.org/10.1097/MD.0000000000000121.
7. Nico MM, Guimarães AL, Correa PY, Lourenço SV. Oral mucosal lesions in sarcoidosis: comparison with cutaneous lesions. Acta Derm Venereol. 2016;96(3):392–3. https://doi.org/10.2340/00015555-2262.
8. Ma Y, Gal A, Koss M. Reprint of: the pathology of pulmonary sarcoidosis: update. Semin Diagn Pathol. 2018;35(5):324–33. https://doi.org/10.1053/j.semdp.2018.09.001.
9. Ahmadzai H, Huang S, Steinfort C, Markos J, Allen RK, Wakefield D, et al. Sarcoidosis: a state-of-the-art review from the Thoracic Society of Australia and New Zealand. Med J Aust. 2018;208(11):499–504. https://doi.org/10.5694/mja17.00610.
10. Chopra A, Nautiyal A, Kalkanis A, Judson MA. Drug-induced sarcoidosis-like reactions. Chest. 2018;154(3):664–77. https://doi.org/10.1016/j.chest.2018.03.056.
11. Rodrigues-Fernandes CI, Migliorati CA, Gueiros LAM, de Lima Morais TM, Vargas PA, de Almeida OP, et al. Adalimumab-induced sarcoidosis-like reaction involving oral cavity in rheumatoid arthritis: a case-based review. Clin Rheumatol. 2021;40(9):3833–9. https://doi.org/10.1007/s10067-021-05654-2.
12. Belperio JA, Shaikh F, Abtin FG, et al. Diagnosis and treatment of pulmonary sarcoidosis: a review. JAMA. 2022;327(9):856–67. https://doi.org/10.1001/jama.2022.1570.
13. Grunewald J, Grutters JC, Arkema EV, et al. Sarcoidosis. Nat Rev Dis Primers. 2019;5:45. https://doi.org/10.1038/s41572-019-0096-x.
14. Papanikolaou IC, Antonakis E, Pandi A. State-of-the-art treatments for sarcoidosis. Methodist Debakey Cardiovasc J. 2022;18(2):94–105. https://doi.org/10.14797/mdcvj.1068. PMID: 35772032; PMCID: PMC9237819.

Drug-Induced Sarcoidosis-Like Reaction

18

Cesar Augusto Migliorati, Alan Roger Santos-Silva, Cinthia Veronica Bardalez Lopez de Caceres, Carla Isabelly Rodrigues-Fernandes, and Felipe Paiva Fonseca

18.1 General Overview and Clinical Presentation

Sarcoidosis is a rare disease of unknown cause. It is characterized by inflammation and the formation of granulomas. Although the most common areas of the human body affected are the lungs and the lymph nodes, it can occur in almost any organ. The cause of sarcoidosis is an active area of research. Experts believe that the disease can be of a genetic nature, but other factors such as microorganisms or chemicals may trigger the disease.

During the last decades, the occurrence of drug-induced sarcoidosis-like reaction (DISR) has been described to be associated with different classes of commonly used drugs. These medications are known to induce a systemic granulomatous inflammatory disorder considered to be clinically, biologically, radiologically, and microscopically indistinguishable from sarcoidosis. It occurs in a temporal relationship with the offending drug and can improve or resolve if the drug is discontinued. Because of the similarities between DISR and sarcoidosis, it is accepted that the only definite way to differentiate them is the resolution of the disorder after the drug discontinuation and its recurrence following rechallenge with the offending drug. The pathogenesis of DISR is complex and seems to vary depending on the drug category involved in the process. Cellular mechanisms involving the activation of T cell populations are usually described in most studies. A better understanding of the pathophysiology of DISR may contribute to a better understanding of the pathogenesis of sarcoidosis itself. Meanwhile, since the exact etiopathogenesis of sarcoidosis is still not completely understood, it is not clear if the drugs are truly causing sarcoidosis or if they are making the immune system more susceptible to the development of sarcoidosis. Nevertheless, it is unclear whether DISR is a distinct entity from sarcoidosis.

In an extensive search of the pharmacovigilance database from the World Health Organization, Cohen Hudson et al. were able to identify 2425 cases of DISR and 55 potential drugs between 1967 and 2019. Li et al. investigated the frequency of radiographically evident (CT chest, abdomen, and pelvis or whole body integrated 2-[18F]-fluoro-2-deoxy-D-glucose (FDG) positron-emission tomography (PET)/CT) DISR in 457 patients treated with anti-cytotoxic T-lymphocyte-associated antigen-4 (CTLA-4) therapy, anti-programmed cell death protein 1 (PD-1) therapy, or a combination of both. The authors identified radiological manifestations in 19 patients (4.1%), with a mean interval of 5.5 months from the initiation of immunotherapy to development of DISR. All patients exhibited pulmonary parenchymal findings like perifissural nodularity and ground-glass opacities. Moreover, Chorti et al. observed that 22% of their melanoma patients (10/45 cases) being treated with immune checkpoint inhibitors also developed DISR manifestations. These studies demonstrate the epidemiological importance of this condition.

Although the list of drugs associated with DISR is continuously expanding, which indicates that the granulomatous inflammation is not a drug-specific effect, the most frequently described drugs comprise combination antiretroviral therapy (cART), tumor necrosis factor alpha antagonists (Etanercept adalimumab, infliximab), interferons

C. A. Migliorati (✉)
Department of Oral and Maxillofacial Diagnostic Sciences, University of Florida College of Dentistry, Gainesville, FL, USA
e-mail: c.migliorati@dental.ufl.edu

A. R. Santos-Silva
Department of Oral Diagnosis (Semiology), Piracicaba Dental School, University of Campinas (UNICAMP), Piracicaba, Brazil
e-mail: madhushrestha@tamu.edu

C. V. B. L. de Caceres · F. P. Fonseca
Department of Oral Surgery and Pathology, School of Dentistry, Universidade Federal de Minas Gerais, Belo Horizonte, Brazil

C. I. Rodrigues-Fernandes
Department of Clinical and Preventive Dentistry, Oral Pathology Unit, Universidade Federal de Pernambuco, Recife, Pernambuco, Brazil

© The Author(s), under exclusive license to Springer Nature Switzerland AG 2025
F. P. Fonseca et al. (eds.), *Lymphoproliferative and Granulomatous Disorders of the Oral Cavity*,
https://doi.org/10.1007/978-3-031-98844-8_18

(interferon α is more frequently associated with DISR than interferon β), and immune checkpoint inhibitors (Nivolumab, Pembrolizumab, Atezolizumab, Avelumab, Durvalumab, Ipilimumab). It is important to highlight that some drugs can cause a single organ granulomatous reaction, most often of the skin, which may represent other entities like drug-induced accelerated rheumatoid nodulosis or granuloma annulare, in contrast to the occurrence of a multisystem involvement that is the most common presentation of DISR. The granulomatous response to BCG (Bacillus Calmette-Guérin) vaccine is also not defined as DISR.

Patients diagnosed with DISR more often demonstrate pulmonary and cutaneous manifestations, with the latter usually leading to the discovery of the lung disorder. The presence of intra-thoracic DISR-associated lymphadenopathy may be detected in approximately 5% of the individuals submitted to immune checkpoint inhibitors therapy. Patients may also develop other signs and symptoms like fever, extra-thoracic lymphadenopathy, uveitis, hypercalcemia, cough, dyspnea, headache, weakness, paresis, involvement of the nervous system, hepatosplenic system, muscles, and osteo-articular system. The presence of an elevated serum angiotensin-converting enzyme has also been described.

The oral manifestations of DISR are also known, but have been described in very few case reports. They are more commonly associated with the use of Adalimumab. Patients more often demonstrate painless diffuse swellings that may affect different regions of the oral mucosa, more frequently the gingival tissue, palate, cheek mucosa, and tongue. The lesions can be solitary or multiple; they are usually irregular and have a wide variation in size. There may be ulceration, usually covered by a fibrinous yellowish membrane.

Treatment approaches for DISR should take into consideration several factors, such as the prognosis of the underlying disease, the severity of DISR presentation, and treatment alternatives for the underlying disease. Specific therapeutic schemes include the use of topical corticosteroids, systemic corticosteroids, methotrexate, infliximab, and hydroxychloroquine. However, most cases are considered indolent and patients often demonstrate rapid resolution if the offending drug can be withdrawn. In general, patients have a good prognosis, with complications and poor response to steroid therapy occurring in less than 10% of the cases (Fig. 18.1).

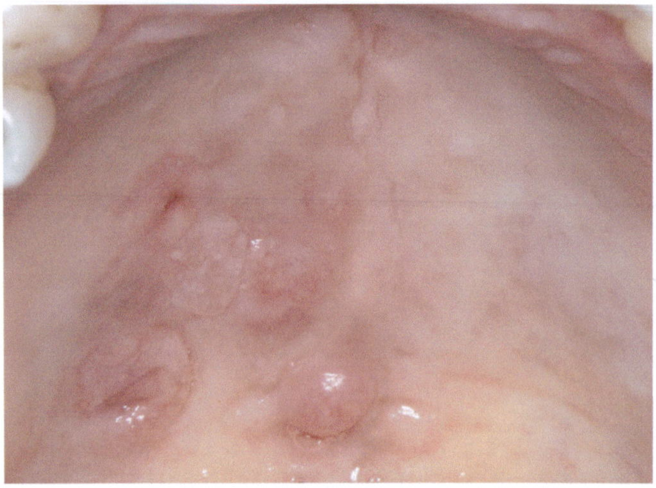

Fig. 18.1 Clinical presentation of DISR affecting the oral cavity

18.2 Microscopic Findings

- The overlying squamous epithelium is usually hyperplastic.
- Pseudo-epitheliomatous reaction of the epithelium may be present.
- The granulomatous reaction located in the lamina propria is similar to the inflammatory infiltrate described earlier for sarcoidosis.
- The occurrence of a granulomatous inflammation should also demand from pathologists a careful investigation for an infectious agent, which is even more important in HIV-positive patients with low levels of CD4+ T cell counts, when a (myco-)bacterial and fungal infection should be ruled out before a definitive diagnosis of DISR can be made.
- Although rare, sarcoid-like reaction to malignancies, especially lymphomas, should also be ruled out.
- There is a typical non-caseating granulomatous inflammatory infiltrate in the lamina propria.
- Multinucleated giant cells and epithelioid histiocytes are commonly observed, usually surrounded by a variable lymphoplasmacytic infiltrate.
- A fibrous stroma is typically observed (Figs. 18.2, 18.3, 18.4, and 18.5).

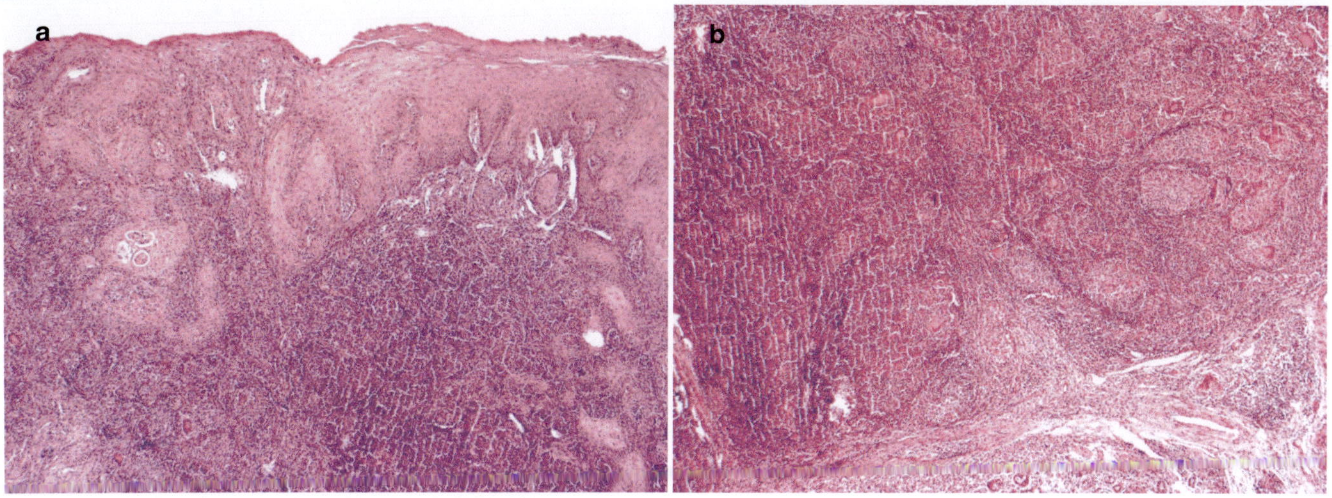

Fig. 18.2 Microscopic features of oral manifestations of DISR. (**a**) Reactive hyperplastic squamous epithelium with a severe inflammatory infiltrate in the lamina propria (H&E; 50×). (**b**) The inflammatory infiltrate in the lamina propria is dense and predominantly composed of lymphocytes (darker regions) and histiocytes (lighter regions) that give rise to granulomas (H&E; 50×)

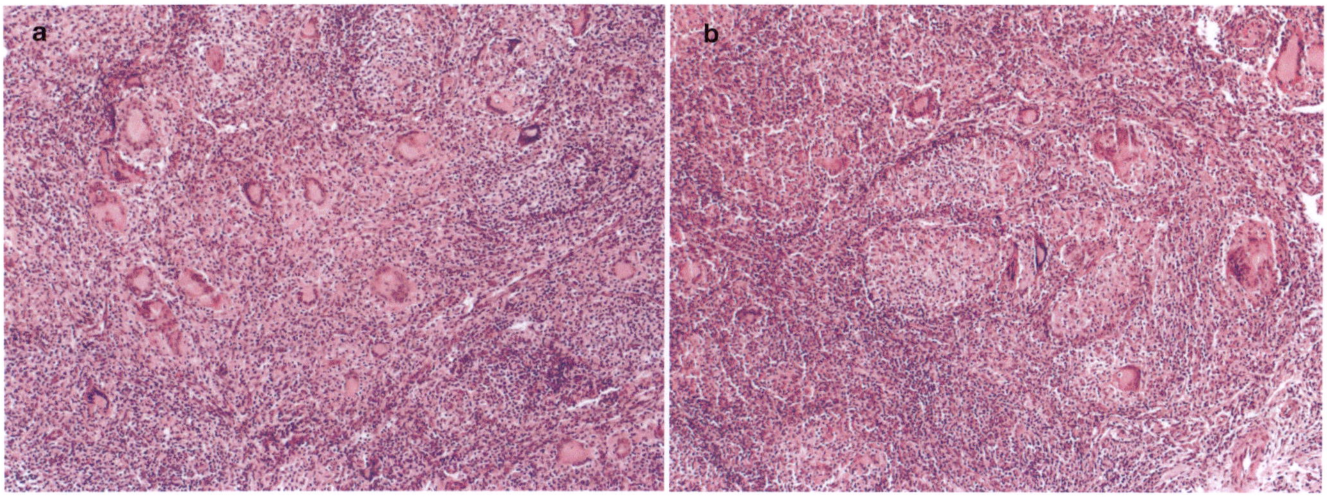

Fig. 18.3 Microscopic features of oral manifestations of DISR. (**a**) Inflammatory infiltrate in the lamina propria. Note the presence of granulomas and multinucleated giant cells. A strong lymphoplasmacytic infiltrate is also present (H&E; 100×). (**b**) Multiple granulomas are observed and surrounded by the lymphoplasmacytic infiltrate. The multinucleated giant cells are easily found (H&E; 100×)

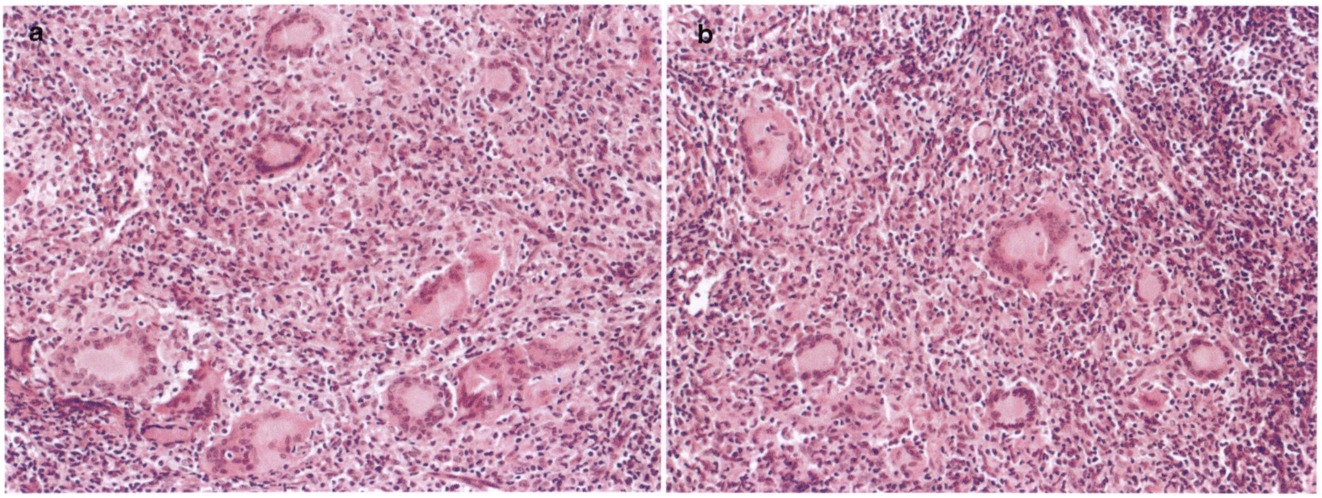

Fig. 18.4 Microscopic features of oral manifestations of DISR. (**a**) The epithelioid histiocytes have large eosinophilic cytoplasm and an oval to round nucleus (H&E; 200×). (**b**) Note the presence of several multinucleated giant cells (H&E; 200×)

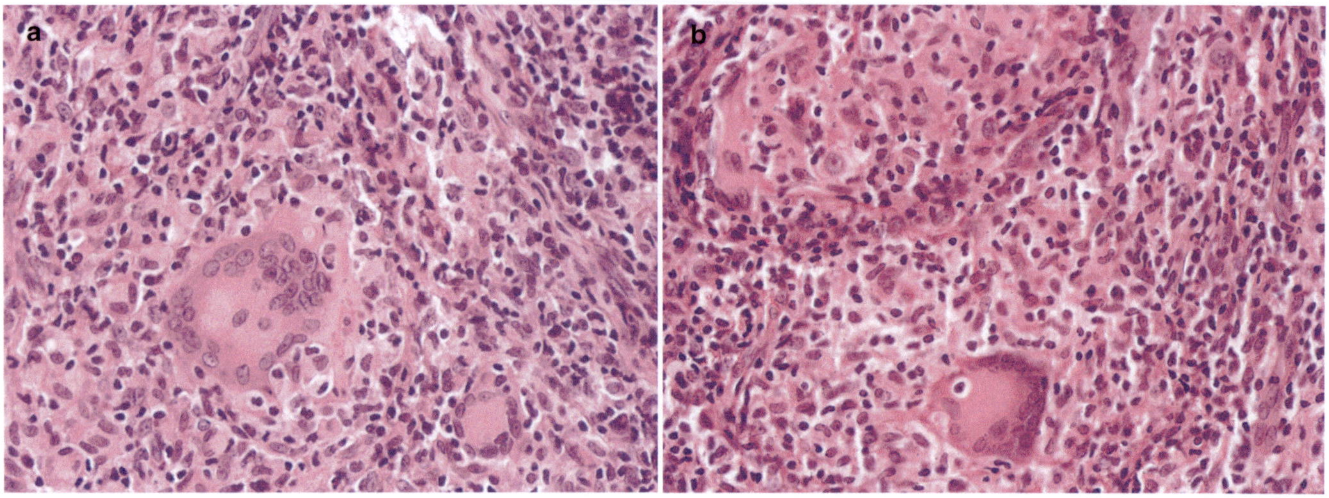

Fig. 18.5 Microscopic features of oral manifestations of DISR. (**a**) Under high magnification, the epithelioid histiocytes can be better appreciated. Note the large eosinophilic cytoplasm of these cells and the presence of multinucleated giant cells (H&E; 400×). (**b**) Well-formed granulomas containing the epithelioid histiocytes and multinucleated giant cells are a typical microscopic finding of DISR (H&E; 400×)

18.3 Immunohistochemistry and/or Genetics

The diagnosis of the oral manifestations of DISR is based on clinical findings that could support a direct association between the use of the drug and the development of the disease. Moreover, definitive diagnosis is further supported by morphological investigation that demonstrates the occurrence of a granulomatous inflammation with the absence of any detectable microorganism, and therefore, the use of special histological stains like PAS, Grocott-Gomori methenamine silver, and Ziehl-Neelsen is mandatory during microscopic examination. Immunohistochemistry has a limited value for the diagnostic approach of this disorder, but it can be useful to rule out sarcoid-like reaction to lymphomas and to characterize the inflammatory infiltrate that typically demonstrates positivity to CD68 protein, revealing histiocytes and multinucleated giant cells. The expression of the more specific histiocytic marker CD163 is better appreciated in the histiocytes, while multinucleated giant cells are usually negative. There is a variable distribution of CD20-positive B lymphocytes and a higher number of CD3-positive T lymphocytes. Plasma cells are demonstrated by CD138 or other plasma cell markers. These reactions may be more useful in those cases without well-formed granulomas (Table 18.1, Figs. 18.6 and 18.7).

Table 18.1 Summary of the main immunohistochemical reactions that can be used to characterize the inflammatory infiltrate of drug-induced sarcoidosis-like reaction. The results of histological stains are also described

Antibody/stain	Most frequent results	Pattern	Objective
CD20	Positive	Membrane	To demonstrate the presence of B lymphocytes
CD3	Positive	Membrane	To demonstrate the presence of T lymphocytes
CD138	Positive	Membrane	To demonstrate the presence of plasma cells
CD68	Positive	Cytoplasm	To demonstrate the presence of macrophages, multinucleated giant cells, and granulomas
CD163	Positive	Membrane	To demonstrate the presence of macrophages; the multinucleated giant cells are mostly negative
PAS[a]	Negative	–	To show the absence of microorganisms
Grocott-Gomori[a]	Negative	–	To show the absence of microorganisms
Ziehl-Neelsen[a]	Negative	–	To show the absence of microorganisms

PAS Periodic-Acid Schiff
[a]Histological stains

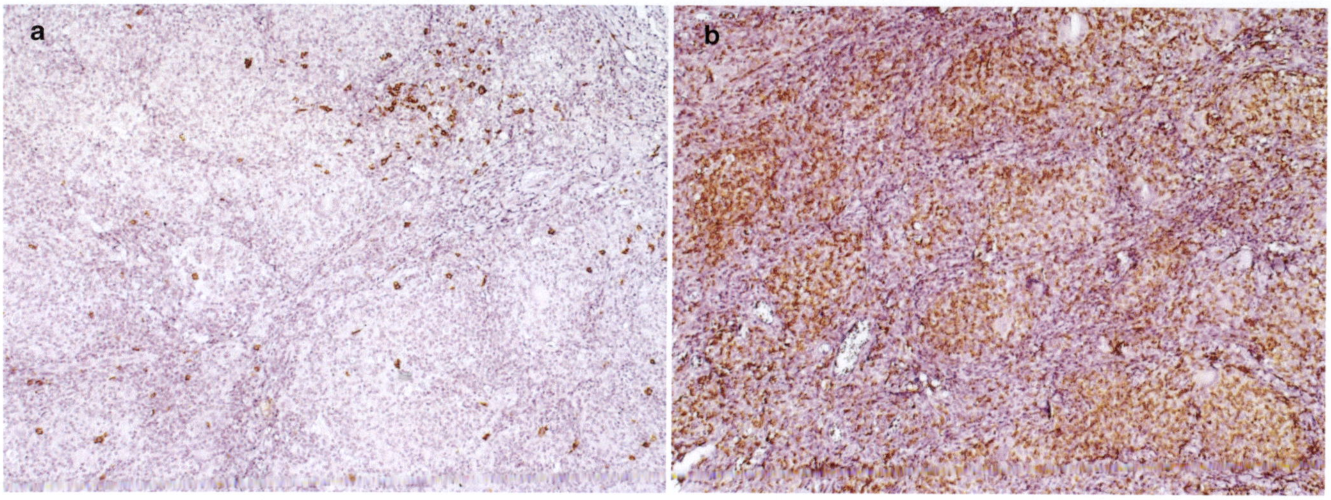

Fig. 18.6 Immunohistochemical features of oral manifestations of DISR. (**a**) Reactive B lymphocytes, demonstrated by CD20 expression, represent a minor component in the inflammatory infiltrate (DAB; 100×). (**b**) In contrast, the number of T lymphocytes is much higher, as demonstrated by CD3 expression (DAB; 100×)

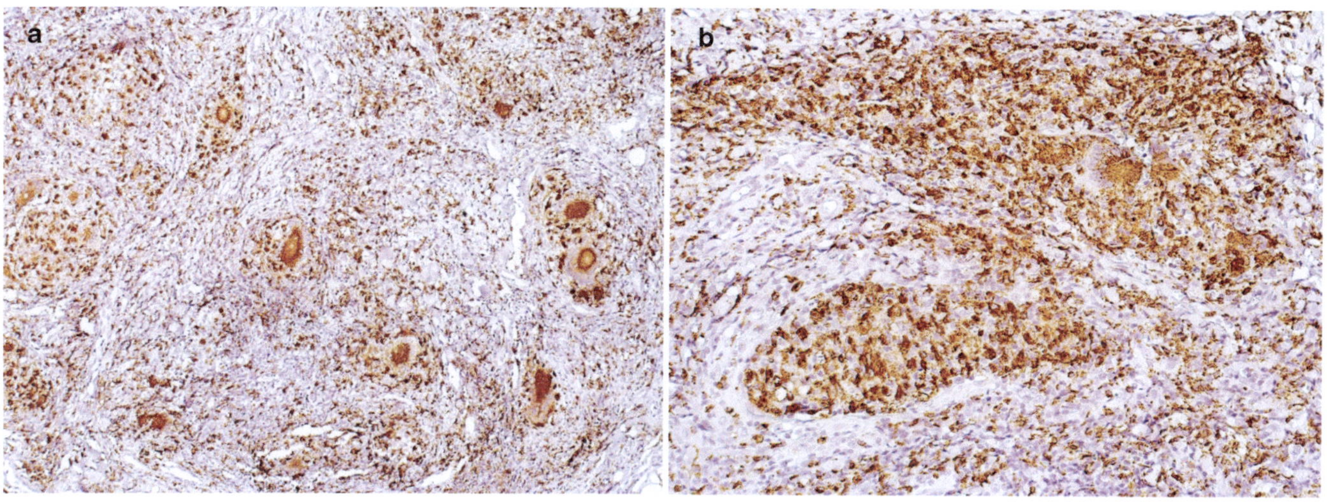

Fig. 18.7 Immunohistochemical features of oral manifestations of DISR. (**a**) The histiocytic component of the granulomatous infiltrate is demonstrated by CD68 immunoexpression. Note the diffuse staining pattern revealing the histiocytes with staining accentuation in multinucleated giant cells (DAB; 100×). (**b**) The expression of CD68 highlights the granulomas and the histiocytic component of the granulomatous infiltrate (DAB; 200×)

Sources

1. Christoforidou A, Goudakos J, Bobos M, Lefkaditis E, Vital V, Markou K. Sarcoidosis-like granulomatosis of the hypopharynx as a complication of anti-TNF therapy. Am J Otolaryngol. 2013;34(3):268–72. https://doi.org/10.1016/j.amjoto.2012.12.016.
2. Chopra A, Nautiyal A, Kalkanis A, Judson MA. Drug-induced sarcoidosis-like reactions. Chest. 2018;154:664–77. https://doi.org/10.1016/j.chest.2018.03.056.
3. Gkiozos I, Kopitopoulou A, Kalkanis A, Vamvakaris IN, Judson MA, Syrigos KN. Sarcoidosis-like reactions induced by checkpoint inhibitors. J Thorac Oncol. 2018;13(8):1076–82. https://doi.org/10.1016/j.jtho.2018.04.031.
4. Rambhia PH, Reichert B, Scott JF, Feneran AN, Kazakov JA, Honda K, et al. Immune checkpoint inhibitor-induced sarcoidosis-like granulomas. Int J Clin Oncol. 2019;24(10):1171–81. https://doi.org/10.1007/s10147-019-01490-2.
5. Cohen Aubart F, Lhote R, Amoura A, Valeyre D, Haroche J, Amoura Z, et al. Drug-induced sarcoidosis: an overview of the WHO pharmacovigilance database. J Intern Med. 2020;288(3):356–62. https://doi.org/10.1111/joim.12991.
6. Chorti E, Kanaki T, Zimmer L, Hadaschik E, Ugurel S, Gratsias E, et al. Drug-induced sarcoidosis-like reaction in adjuvant immunotherapy: increased rate and mimicker of metastasis. Eur J Cancer. 2020;131:18–26. https://doi.org/10.1016/j.ejca.2020.02.024.
7. Judson MA. The epidemic of drug-induced sarcoidosis-like reactions: a side effect that we can live with. J Intern Med. 2020;288(3):373–5. https://doi.org/10.1111/joim.13008.
8. Chanson N, Ramos-Casals M, Pundole X, Suijkerbuijk K, José de Barros E, Silva M, Lidar M, et al. Immune checkpoint inhibitor-associated sarcoidosis: a usually benign disease that does not require

immunotherapy discontinuation. Eur J Cancer. 2021;158:208–16. https://doi.org/10.1016/j.ejca.2021.05.041.
9. Miedema J, Nunes H. Drug-induced sarcoidosis-like reactions. Curr Opin Pulm Med. 2021;27(5):439–47. https://doi.org/10.1097/MCP.0000000000000800.
10. Rodrigues-Fernandes CI, Migliorati CA, Gueiros LAM, de Lima Morais TM, Vargas PA, de Almeida OP, et al. Adalimumab-induced sarcoidosis-like reaction involving oral cavity in rheumatoid arthritis: a case-based review. Clin Rheumatol. 2021;40(9):3833–9. https://doi.org/10.1007/s10067-021-05654-2.
11. Torres-Jiménez J, Esteban-Villarrubia J, García-Abellás P, Cortés-Salgado A, Soria-Rivas A, Gajate-Borau P, et al. Sarcoidosis-like reactions in cancer patients treated with immune checkpoint inhibitors: experience in a Spanish hospital. Clin Transl Oncol. 2021;23(7):1474–80. https://doi.org/10.1007/s12094-020-02546-w.
12. Li Y, Flavell RR, Juarez R, Chow M, Wu C, Tsai K, et al. Retrospective study of the incidence of sarcoidosis-like reaction in patients treated with immunotherapy. Clin Radiol. 2023;78(2):e131–6. https://doi.org/10.1016/j.crad.2022.09.127.
13. Simonato LE, de Arruda JAA, Louredo BVR, Vargas PA, Tomo S. Drug-induced sarcoidosis-like reaction to adalimumab in the oral mucosa of a patient with Crohn's disease. J Stomatol Oral Maxillofac Surg. 2024;125(5S2):101543. https://doi.org/10.1016/j.jormas.2023.101543.
14. Coelho RR, Pires Xavier S, Brandão JR, Furtado I. From fibrosis to granuloma: drug induced systemic sarcoidosis-like reaction after rituximab in a patient with primary Sjogren's syndrome. Eur J Case Rep Intern Med. 2024;11(12):005070. https://doi.org/10.12890/2024_005070.
15. Rizzo M, Pezzicoli G, Ganini C, Carone L, Caliò A, Brunelli M, et al. Sarcoidosis-like reactions in metastatic renal cell carcinoma patients treated with immune-based combinations. Immunotherapy. 2024;16(9):603–9. https://doi.org/10.1080/1750743X.2024.2342222.

Pyostomatitis Vegetans

19

Fabio Ramôa Pires, Roberta Rayra Martins-Chaves, and Felipe Paiva Fonseca

19.1 General Overview and Clinical Presentation

Pyostomatitis-pyodermatitis vegetans is a mucocutaneous disease first described in 1898 by François Hallopeau characterized by the occurrence of multiple pustules and considered a strong clinical marker for inflammatory bowel disease, which represents chronic inflammatory disorders of the digestive tract, more often comprising Crohn's disease and ulcerative colitis, and that are associated with several extraintestinal manifestations that also include erythema nodosum and Sweet syndrome. The etiology of pyostomatitis-pyodermatitis vegetans is still unknown, but immunological disturbances and microbial factors are usually speculated as possible causative factors. Similarly, the pathogenesis of the disease is also poorly understood; however, the importance of some interleukines like IL-6, IL-8, IL-36, and TNF-alpha, as well as the neutrophil extracellular traps (NETs) and the eosinophil extracellular traps (EETs), have recently been hypothesized to play some pathogenetic role in the innate immunity and autoinflammatory features of pyodermatitis-pyostomatitis vegetans.

The cutaneous manifestations of this condition are referred to as *pyodermatitis vegetans*, and more frequently present as erythematous, vesiculopustular, exudative, vegetating plaques more often affecting the inguinal and axillary folds. In the oral cavity, *pyostomatitis vegetans* more commonly manifests in the buccal and labial mucosa, followed by gingival tissues as edematous mucosa with multiple miliary sterile pustules that may rupture and result in confluent, painful, superficial yellowish pustules and erosions leading to the so-called "snail track" lesions. Male patients are slightly more affected than females, more often during the fourth to sixth decades of life. Simultaneous eosinophilia and cutaneous lesions are reported to be present in more than 50% of the cases affecting the oral mucosa.

In approximately 60% of patients, a diagnosis of intestinal bowel disease has already been established before pyostomatitis vegetans is identified. Nonetheless, clinicians should remain vigilant for patients without gastrointestinal symptoms, as the absence of such symptoms does not exclude the possibility of intestinal bowel disease. In these unusual cases, a diagnosis of oral pyostomatitis vegetans may prompt recognition of the underlying intestinal disorder.

The main differential diagnosis for pyostomatitis vegetans is represented by pemphigus vegetans, a rare variant of pemphigus vulgaris that may occur in the oral cavity and demonstrates intercellular deposition of immunoglobulin G by direct immunofluorescence, which may also occur in rare examples of pyoestomatitis vegetans, leading some authors to speculate whether these disorders could represent the spectrum of the same entity. Therefore, a strict clinical correlation of the oral manifestations with the gastrointestinal status of the patients is mandatory to aid in the differential diagnosis.

Although pyostomatitis vegetans can be effectively controlled by intestinal bowel disease treatment, there is currently no standard protocol established for managing these patients. Different therapeutic protocols are reported in the literature, ranging from topical and/or systemic steroids, monoclonal antibodies, immunosuppressive agents, antibiotics, or a combination of these different approaches. Although good clinical improvement is usually observed when therapy is done, relapses may occur during tapering or withdrawal of medication (Fig. 19.1).

F. R. Pires (✉)
Oral Pathology, School of Dentistry, Universidade do Estado do Rio de Janeiro, Rio de Janeiro, Brazil

R. R. Martins-Chaves
Medical School, Faculdade Ciências Médicas de Minas Gerais, Belo Horizonte, Brazil
e-mail: roberta.chaves@cienciasmedicasmg.edu.br

F. P. Fonseca
Department of Oral Surgery and Pathology, School of Dentistry, Universidade Federal de Minas Gerais, Belo Horizonte, Brazil

© The Author(s), under exclusive license to Springer Nature Switzerland AG 2025
F. P. Fonseca et al. (eds.), *Lymphoproliferative and Granulomatous Disorders of the Oral Cavity*,
https://doi.org/10.1007/978-3-031-98844-8_19

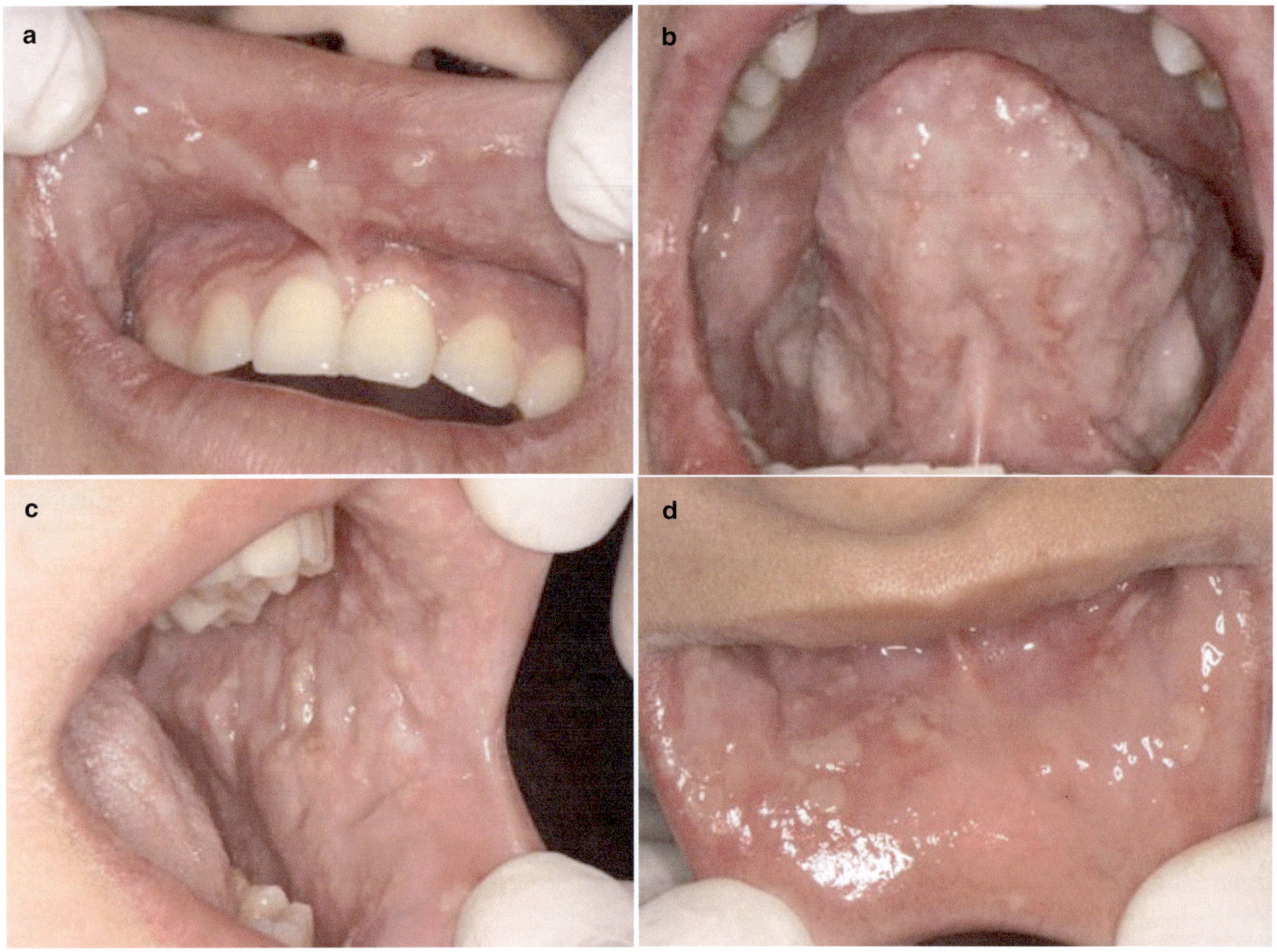

Fig. 19.1 Clinical presentation of pyostomatitis vegetans in the oral cavity. (**a**) The patient exhibited multiple ulcerations in the form of pustules with a typical yellowish aspect in the oral mucosa. Observe the involvement of the upper lip. (**b**) The tongue was also affected, especially the ventral surface. (**c**) The left buccal mucosa exhibited multiple pustules. (**d**) The lower lip mucosa was also affected by the disease

19.2 Microscopic Findings

- Epithelial acanthosis with neutrophilic and eosinophilic spongiosis is observed.
- Presence of intra-epithelial clefts.
- Acantholytic epithelial cells.
- Presence of a dense inflammatory infiltrate of neutrophils and eosinophils in the epithelial cleft and in the lamina propria below the epithelium.
- Chronic inflammatory cells like histiocytes, lymphocytes, and plasma cells can also be present, but in a lower number.
- Eosinophilic and neutrophilic microabscesses are frequent (Figs. 19.2 and 19.3).

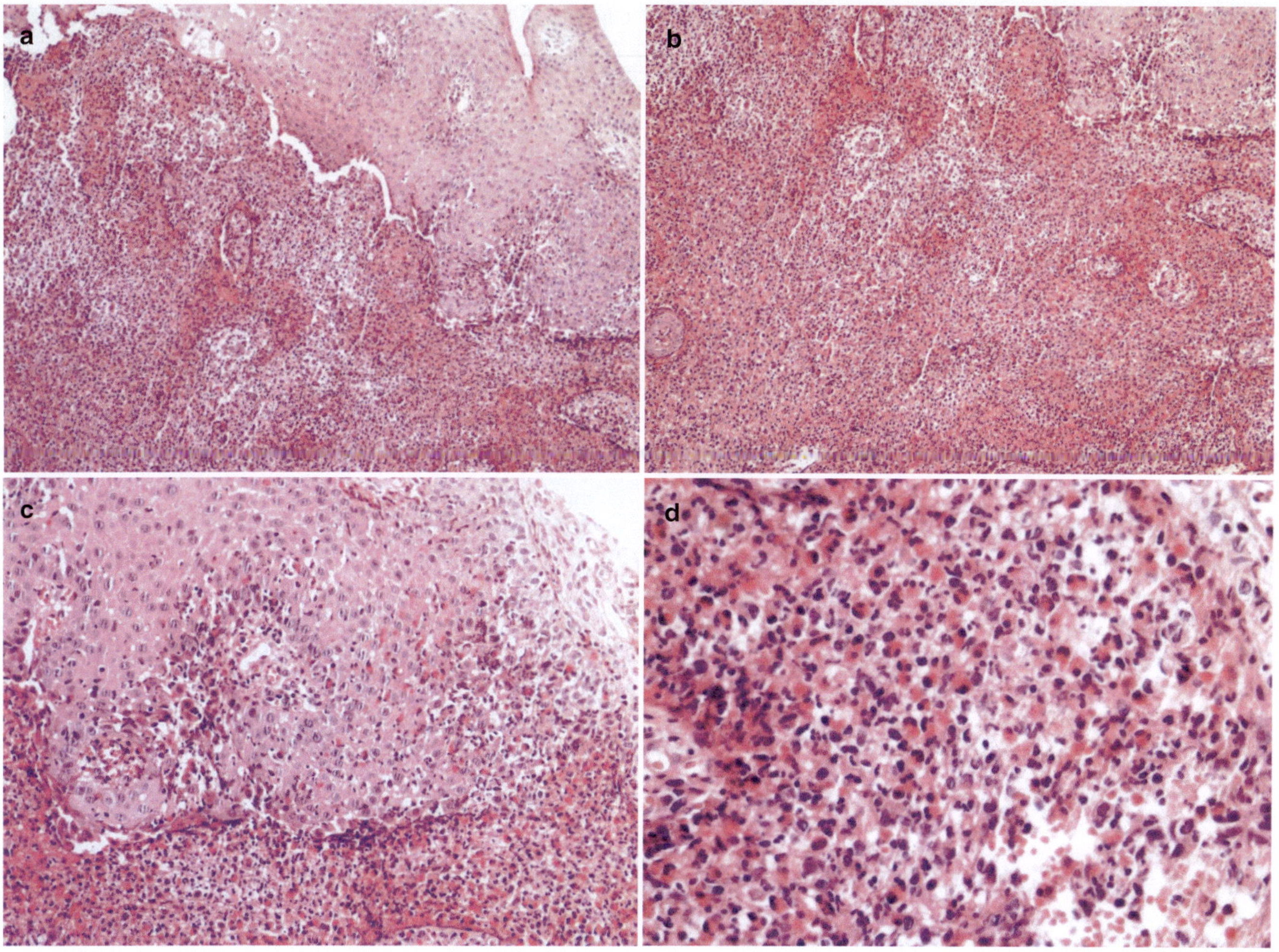

Fig. 19.2 Microscopic features of pyostomatitis vegetans in the oral cavity. (**a**) Overlying squamous epithelium with the presence of an epithelial cleft and a dense inflammatory infiltrate in the lamina propria (H&E; 50×). (**b**) Observe the connective tissue containing a very dense inflammatory infiltrate containing lymphocytes, macrophages, plasma cells, and, especially, eosinophils (H&E; 50×). (**c**) There is a large number of eosinophils in the inflammatory infiltrate. It is possible to observe an eosinophilic exocytosis, with the presence of these cells in the epithelium (H&E; 100×). (**d**) In the lamina propria, neutrophils and eosinophils are also present, together with other inflammatory cells (H&E; 200×)

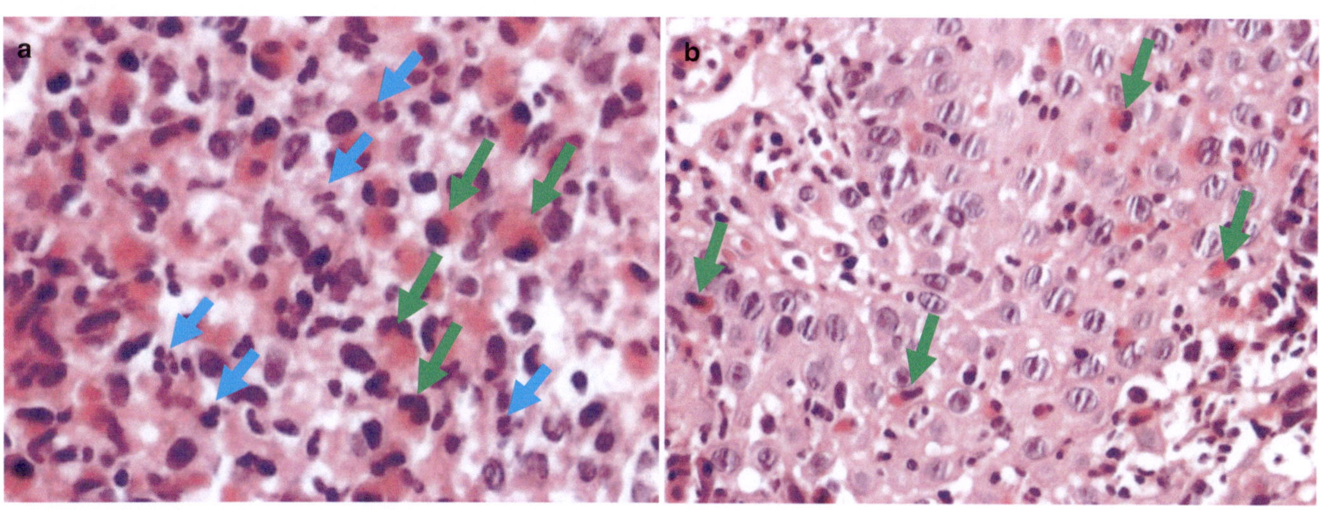

Fig. 19.3 Microscopic features of pyostomatitis vegetans in the oral cavity. (**a**) In the lamina propria, there is a dense inflammatory infiltrate with a large number of neutrophils (blue arrows) and eosinophils (green arrows) (H&E; 400×). (**b**) Note the presence of eosinophils in the overlying epithelium (green arrows) (H&E; 400×)

Table 19.1 Summary of the main immunohistochemical reactions that can be used in cases of pyostomatitis-pyodermatitis vegetans to better illustrate the inflammatory component of the disease

Antibody	Most frequent results	Pattern	Objective
CD15	Positive	Membrane	To demonstrate the presence of neutrophils and eosinophils
CD20	Positive	Membrane	To demonstrate the presence of B lymphocytes
CD3	Positive	Membrane	To demonstrate the presence of T lymphocytes
CD138	Positive	Membrane	To demonstrate the presence of plasma cells
CD68	Positive	Cytoplasm	To demonstrate the presence of macrophages
AE1/AE3	Positive	Cytoplasm	To better demonstrate the presence of the epithelial cleft

19.3 Immunohistochemistry and/or Genetics

The diagnosis of pyostomatitis-pyodermatitis vegetans is usually based on clinical data supported by morphological findings, while immunohistochemistry has a limited value for the diagnostic approach of this disorder. The use of AE1/AE3 may help to highlight the presence of the epithelial cleft, while the reactive inflammatory infiltrate will show the presence of histiocytes (CD68 positivity), a variable distribution of B lymphocytes (CD20 positivity) and T lymphocytes (CD3 positivity), plasma cells (CD138 positivity), and abundant eosinophils (CD15 positivity) (Table 19.1).

Sources

1. Hegarty AM, Barrett AW, Scully C. Pyostomatitis vegetans. Clin Exp Dermatol. 2004;29(1):1–7. https://doi.org/10.1111/j.1365-2230.2004.01438.x.
2. Femiano F, Lanza A, Buonaiuto C, Perillo L, Dell'Ermo A, Cirillo N. Pyostomatitis vegetans: a review of the literature. Med Oral Patol Oral Cir Bucal. 2009;14(3):E114–7.
3. Ficarra G, Baroni G, Massi D. Pyostomatitis vegetans: cellular immune profile and expression of IL-6, IL-8 and TNF-alpha. Head Neck Pathol. 2010;4(1):1–9. https://doi.org/10.1007/s12105-009-0149-7.
4. Nico MM, Hussein TP, Aoki V, Lourenço SV. Pyostomatitis vegetans and its relation to inflammatory bowel disease, pyoderma gangrenosum, pyodermatitis vegetans, and pemphigus. J Oral Pathol Med. 2012;41(8):584–8. https://doi.org/10.1111/j.1600-0714.2012.01152.x.
5. Clark LG, Tolkachjov SN, Bridges AG, Camilleri MJ. Pyostomatitis vegetans (PSV)-pyodermatitis vegetans (PDV): a clinicopathologic study of 7 cases at a tertiary referral center. J Am Acad Dermatol. 2016;75(3):578–84. https://doi.org/10.1016/j.jaad.2016.03.047.
6. Mizukami Y, Imanishi H, Tateishi C, Kaneshiro S, Sowa-Osako J, Ohsawa M, et al. Successful treatment of pyostomatitis vegetans with ulcerative colitis using dapsone without systemic steroids. J Dermatol. 2019;46(9):e316–7. https://doi.org/10.1111/1346-8138.14885.
7. Gara S, Souissi A, Mokni M. Pyodermatitis pyostomatitis vegetans. JAMA Dermatol. 2020;156(3):335. https://doi.org/10.1001/jamadermatol.2019.3515.
8. Nusbaum KB, Korman AM, Chung CG. Pyostomatitis vegetans with extensive tongue involvement. Int J Dermatol. 2020;59(7):e263–5. https://doi.org/10.1111/ijd.14932.
9. Petruzzi M, Della VF. Pyostomatitis vegetans. N Engl J Med. 2021;385(22):e77. https://doi.org/10.1056/NEJMicm2108327.
10. Stagg B, Simpson A, Sidhu S. Similar but different: distinguishing between pemphigus vegetans and pyostomatitis-pyodermatitis vegetans. BMJ Case Rep. 2021;14(4):e242162. https://doi.org/10.1136/bcr-2021-242162.
11. Zeng X, Hua H, Hu X. Rare mucocutaneous manifestations of ulcerative colitis: a case report of pyostomatitis vegetans and sweet syndrome. Oral Surg Oral Med Oral Pathol Oral Radiol. 2022;134(4):e256–60. https://doi.org/10.1016/j.oooo.2022.06.004.
12. Chrcanovic BR, Martins-Chaves RR, Pontes FSC, Fonseca FP, Pontes HAR, Gomez RS. Pyodermatitis-pyostomatitis vegetans: a case report and systematic review focusing on oral involvement. Oral Maxillofac Surg. 2024;28(3):1405–14. https://doi.org/10.1007/s10006-024-01234-1.
13. Kim TH, Kim SC. Pyodermatitis-pyostomatitis vegetans associated with Crohn's disease. Ann Dermatol. 2015 Oct;27(5):624–5. https://doi.org/10.5021/ad.2015.27.5.624.
14. O'Gorman C, Smyth S, Willis A. Unusual presentation of pyostomatitis vegetans and its management. BMJ Case Rep. 2023;16(9):e256318. https://doi.org/10.1136/bcr-2023-256318.
15. Yamamoto T. Local neutrophil and eosinophil extracellular traps formation in pyodermatitis pyostomatitis vegetans. Exp Dermatol. 2024;33(1):e14931. https://doi.org/10.1111/exd.14931.

Actinic Prurigo

20

María Elisa Vega-Memije,
Adalberto A. Mosqueda-Taylor, and Felipe Paiva Fonseca

20.1 General Overview and Clinical Presentation

Actinic prurigo is a chronic, idiopathic inflammatory photodermatosis that affects photo-exposed areas of the skin, lower lip, and conjunctiva, and it is considered an example of subtype A and B of type IV hypersensitivity reaction. The first report of actinic prurigo is unknown, but Robert Willan (1798) described a skin disease caused by the sun that he called "*eczema solaris*" and that could have represented the first description of this entity, but Jonathan Hutchinson's report about "summer prurigo" in 1878 is sometimes considered the first reference for this disease, while actinic prurigo is a term first used by Londoño in the Spanish literature. Many other terms have been used for this condition, including solar dermatitis, light-sensitive eruptions in American Indians, familial actinic prurigo, hereditary polymorphic light eruption, and solar prurigo of high plateaus, among others.

Actinic prurigo has a strong predilection for the Mestizo populations of the Latin American countries, especially from Mexico, Guatemala, Colombia, Honduras, Ecuador, Peru, and Bolivia, which represent the regions with the highest incidence of this disorder. Many of these patients live at high altitudes (>1000 m), improving the clinical symptoms when moving to lower altitudes closer to sea level. Although very uncommon, patients affected by actinic prurigo in many other parts of the world have already been reported, frequently as a consequence of migratory processes; therefore, clinicians and pathologists must be aware of this condition independently of their geographical location. A prompt diagnosis significantly benefits patients and improves their quality of life, while preventive measures can be implemented in susceptible populations.

The pathogenesis of actinic prurigo is not completely understood, although a strong etiological association with ultraviolet sun exposure is well recognized. This association is supported by the anatomical sites affected, seasonal differences in disease behavior, and the ability to reproduce lesions using artificial ultraviolet sources. Mast cells have been shown to be more numerous in actinic prurigo than in normal skin tissue, and elevated IgE levels were associated with moderate to severe clinical lesions. Some studies have demonstrated a potential genetic predisposition, possibly due to some ethnic heredity of the patients, although familial association has been found in only 4.3–25% of the cases in large series, suggesting different genetic susceptibility among individuals of the same family. A pathological link with human leukocyte antigen (HLA) gene, more specifically the HLA-DR4 allele, has been demonstrated, suggesting an autoimmune basis for this disorder. In Mexico, for instance, approximately 90–92.8% of the patients affected by the disease have this allele, and HLA-DRB1*0407 is the most frequent subtype. Similarly, the haplotype DRB1*0407/DQB1*0302/DPB1*0402 was found in 68.8% of Colombian patients and only in 12.5% of the controls. In addition to solar exposure, some other environmental risk factors have been proposed for the development of actinic prurigo, like cohabitation with domestic animals or farm animals, and exposure to wood smoke, but their role as predisposing or triggering factors has not been proved.

According to many epidemiological studies, females are more frequently affected by actinic prurigo, and in most of the cases, the disease manifests at a young age, usually ranging from 6 to 8 years old, although older individuals can also be affected, and in these cases, it tends to be more persistent.

M. E. Vega-Memije (✉)
Department of Dermatology, Hospital General "Dr. Manuel Gea González", Mexico City, Mexico

A. A. Mosqueda-Taylor
Department of Health Care, Universidad Autónoma Metropolitana Xochimilco, Mexico City, Mexico
e-mail: mosqueda@correo.xoc.uam.mx

F. P. Fonseca
Department of Oral Surgery and Pathology, School of Dentistry, Universidade Federal de Minas Gerais, Belo Horizonte, Brazil

© The Author(s), under exclusive license to Springer Nature Switzerland AG 2025
F. P. Fonseca et al. (eds.), *Lymphoproliferative and Granulomatous Disorders of the Oral Cavity*,
https://doi.org/10.1007/978-3-031-98844-8_20

The disease usually runs a chronic clinical course, often exacerbating after sun exposure. The prominent areas of the face, including the dorsum of the nose, malar regions, lower lip, and superciliary arches, are the most affected regions. In the skin, actinic prurigo more often manifests as macules, papules, plaques, excoriations, serohematic crusts, areas of lichenification, scars, and hypo- or residual hyperpigmentation. When it affects, the vermilion border of the lower lip produces edema, scaling, fissures, ulceration with serohematic crusts, and residual hyperpigmentation. Severe pruritus of the lower lip occurs in over 80% of cases, and patients may also complain of tingling and pain. The labial lesions are present in 84% of the cases and may be the only manifestation of the disease in approximately 27–56% of the patients. Actinic prurigo cheilitis should be differentiated from other affections of the lips, such as polymorphous light eruption, frictional (traumatic) cheilitis, actinic cheilitis, contact cheilitis, and nonspecific and granulomatous cheilitis, which carry different etiologies and clinicopathological features.

The eyes are affected in 45–62% of the cases, and conjunctiva involvement is considered the most serious manifestation of the disease, with patients usually demonstrating hyperemia, photophobia, increased lacrimation, progression to brown pigmentation, and pseudopterygium. Severe cases may interfere with normal vision. An uncommon intra-oral finding was reported in 2002 in patients who also manifested anterior gingival overgrowth, which was speculated to be a consequence of the result of mouth-breathing associated with the intense pruritus and lip sucking habits.

Treatment of actinic prurigo is considered challenging and begins with protection against sun exposure. This includes wearing protective clothing, wide-brimmed hats, and sunglasses, as well as applying photoprotective lip balms and broad-spectrum sunscreens with a high sun protection factor. In addition, many attempts with different approaches like the use of antihistamines, antimalarials, tetracycline, vitamin E, β-carotenes, Psoralen Ultraviolet A therapy, systemic corticosteroids, antibiotics, and sunscreens have been tried with only partial resolution of the symptoms. Treatment modalities may vary depending on the severity of the disease. In general, early lesions benefit from topical steroids and sun protection, whereas chronic and aggressive cases are better treated with thalidomide combined or not with steroids and protective measures. Phototherapy, narrow-band UVB, has been used successfully in some patients, but usually with limited remission of the lesions.

Thalidomide, a synthetic derivative of glutamic acid that holds an immunomodulatory and anti-inflammatory potential, very often leads to excellent response of the lesions, which has also been described as a diagnostic marker for actinic prurigo, but caution should be taken due to its possible important side effects. It was demonstrated that keratinocytes of the overlying squamous epithelium of actinic prurigo have a strong immunoreactivity for tumor necrosis factor-α (TNF-α), which may partially explain the clinical efficacy of thalidomide as a TNF-α inhibitor (Figs. 20.1 and 20.2).

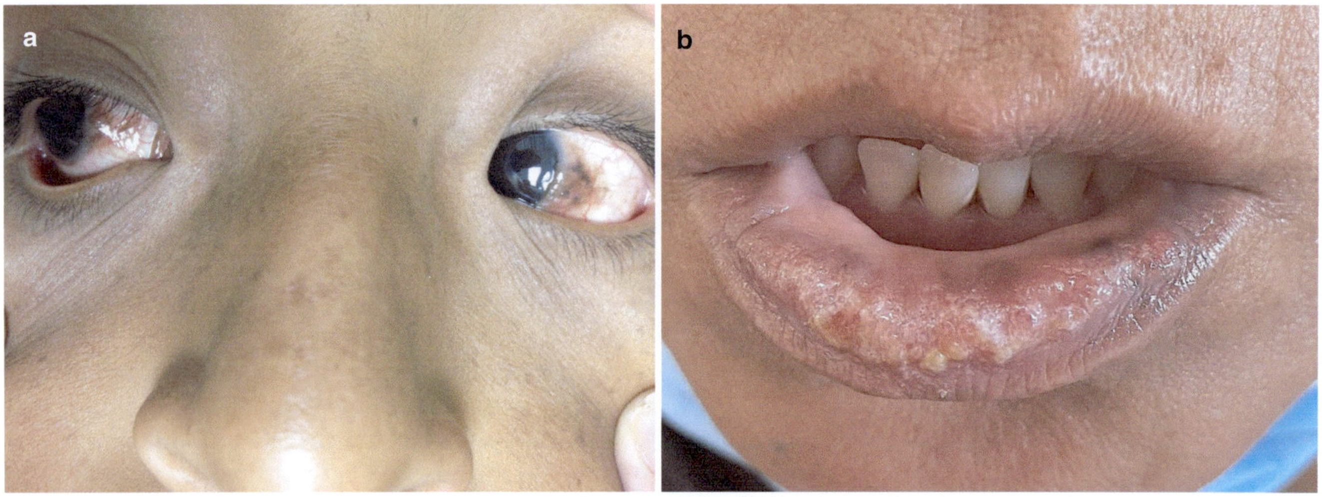

Fig. 20.1 Clinical manifestation of actinic prurigo. (**a**) Actinic prurigo conjunctivitis with hyperpigmentation and pseudopterygion. (**b**) Actinic prurigo cheilitis. Note swelling, erythema, scaling, hyperpigmentation, and serohematic crust formation on the lower lip

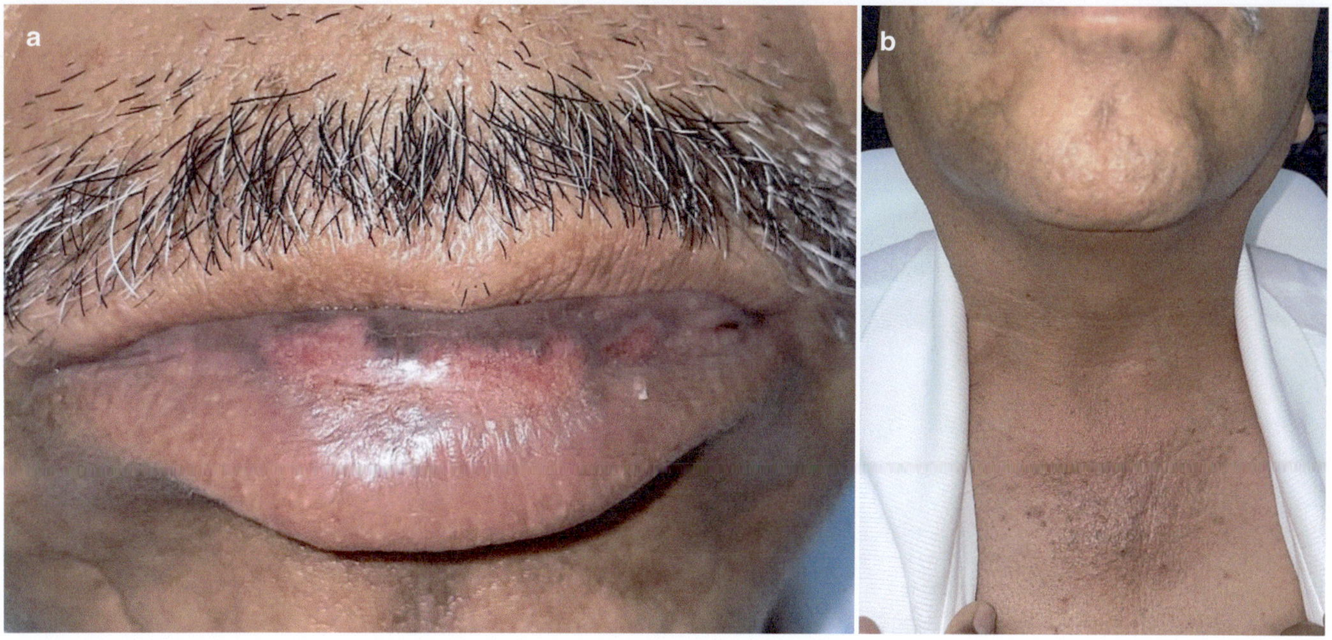

Fig. 20.2 Clinical manifestation of actinic prurigo. (**a**) Actinic prurigo cheilitis in a 58-year-old man. (**b**) Skin lesions in the sun-exposed areas of the chest in the same patient

20.2 Microscopic Findings

- The histopathological study of actinic prurigo cheilitis more frequently shows the characteristic features of this condition, while biopsies of skin lesions usually present a nonspecific lymphoid infiltrate.
- Ulceration of the labial epithelial surface.
- Presence of acanthosis, exocytosis, spongiosis, and basal cell vacuolation of the epithelium.
- In the lamina propria, there is a marked edema and a prominent vascularization.
- Dense and predominantly lymphocytic inflammatory infiltrate in the lamina propria.
- Presence of well-formed lymphoid follicles, many of them with germinal center formation.
- Some cases are devoid of lymphoid follicles, which may be partially explained by the location where the biopsy is done.
- Variable numbers of eosinophils and melanin-containing macrophages near the epithelium.
- Although actinic prurigo is strongly associated with sun exposure, significant solar elastosis is usually not detected, possibly because of the skin phototype and the fact that most patients have a short period of sun exposure, whereas actinic cheilitis is associated with chronic exposure in people with white skin (Figs. 20.3, 20.4, 20.5 and 20.6).

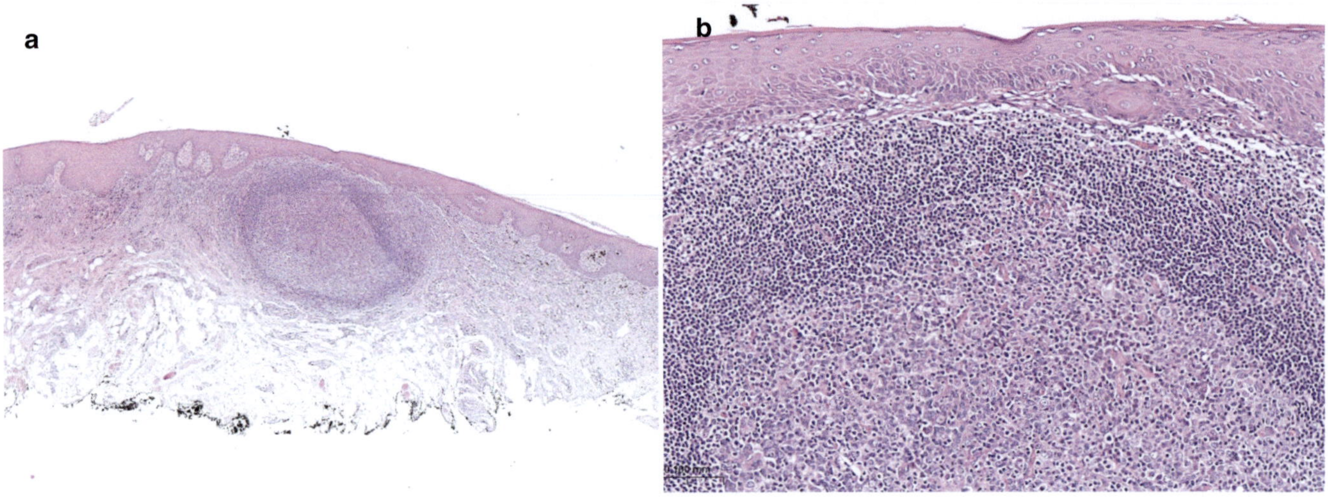

Fig. 20.3 Microscopic features of actinic prurigo. (**a**) Low power view of actinic prurigo cheilitis showing a well-formed lymphoid follicle in the lamina propria and abundant melanin located in the right part of the section (H&E; 20×). (**b**) Lymphoid follicle in actinic prurigo cheilitis demonstrating a mature, well-developed structure (H&E; 200×)

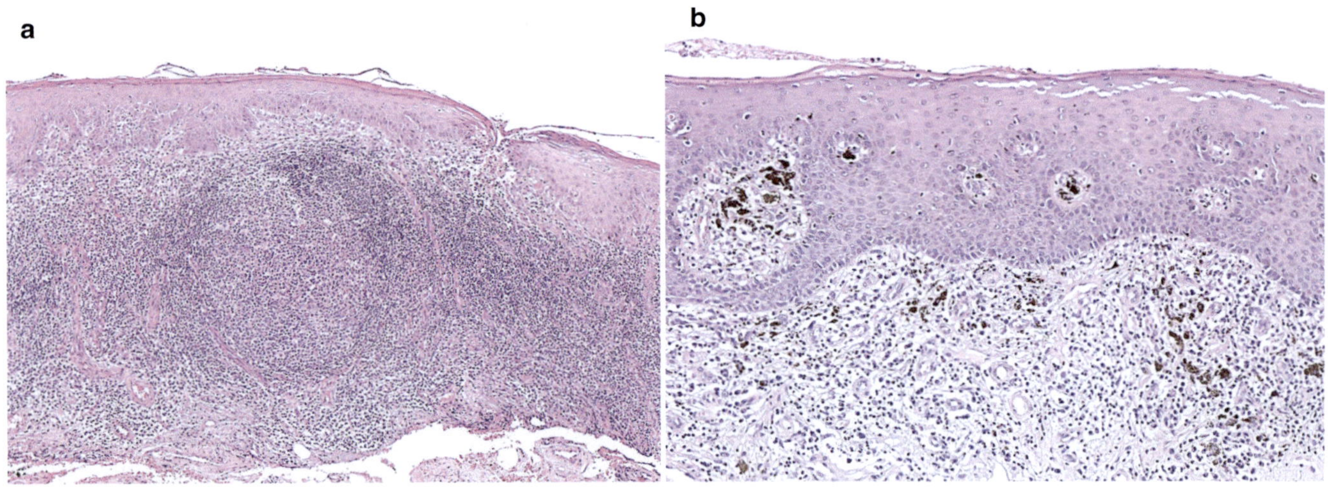

Fig. 20.4 Microscopic features of actinic prurigo. (**a**) Small area of ulceration with acanthosis, spongiosis, and basal cell vacuolation of the epithelium. The lamina propria presents a diffuse lymphocytic infiltrate overlying a lymphoid follicle (H&E; 50×). (**b**) Numerous melanin-containing macrophages located in the upper layer of the lamina propria (H&E; 100×)

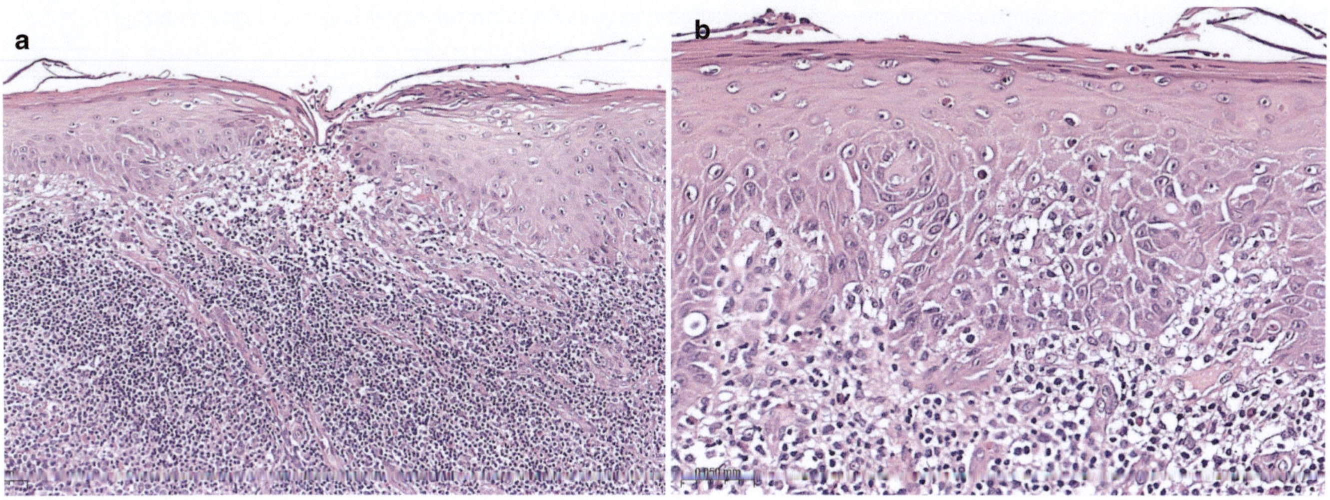

Fig. 20.5 Microscopic features of actinic prurigo. (**a**) Closer view of Fig. 4. Note the diffuse lymphocytic infiltrate overlying part of a lymphoid follicle on the lower left corner (H&E; 100×). (**b**) Edema of the lamina propria with a diffuse lymphocytic inflammatory infiltrate. Note the presence of some eosinophils. The epithelial surface exhibits spongiosis, exocytosis, and basal cell vacuolation (H&E; 200×)

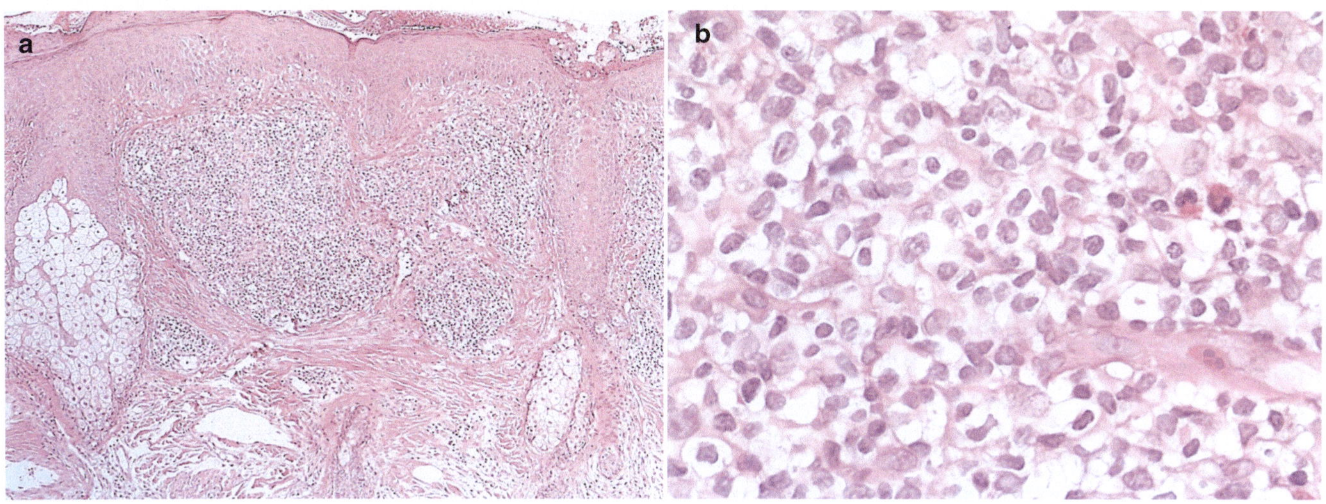

Fig. 20.6 Microscopic features of the cutaneous manifestation of actinic prurigo. (**a**) Skin biopsy of actinic prurigo showing a predominantly lymphocytic inflammatory infiltrate in the superficial dermis. The epithelium shows spongiosis and areas of vacuolar degeneration of the basal layer (H&E; 40×). (**b**) Higher power revealing some eosinophils scattered among the lymphohistiocytic inflammatory infiltrate (H&E 400×)

20.3 Immunohistochemistry and/or Genetics

Immunohistochemistry is useful to demonstrate the reactive nature of the dense inflammatory infiltrate usually present in cases of actinic prurigo and to rule out other reactive lesions that may develop lymphoid follicles, such as lymphocytoma cutis, drug-induced pseudolymphoma syndrome, and a possible marginal zone lymphoma or a follicular lymphoma/cutaneous follicle center lymphoma. The lymphoid follicles in actinic prurigo are benign in nature and show the normal distribution of the cellular populations, with the presence of B lymphocytes in the follicles and T lymphocytes in the interfollicular regions. BCL2 expression is observed predominantly in the interfollicular region, and a high Ki67 expression is observed in the germinal centers (Table 20.1).

Table 20.1 Summary of the main immunohistochemical reactions used to characterize the inflammatory infiltrate of actinic prurigo

Antibody	Most frequent results	Pattern	Objective
CD20	Positive	Membrane	To demonstrate B lymphocytes in the follicles
CD3	Positive	Membrane	To demonstrate T lymphocytes in the interfollicular regions
CD68	Positive	Cytoplasm	To demonstrate the presence of reactive histiocytes
BCL2	Positive in the interfollicular zone	Cytoplasm	To demonstrate the reactive nature of the lymphoid follicles
Ki67	High in the germinal centers	Nucleus	To characterize the proliferative rate of the germinal centers

Sources

1. Vega-Memije ME, Mosqueda-Taylor A, Irigoyen-Camacho ME, Hojyo-Tomoka MT, Domínguez-Soto L. Actinic prurigo cheilitis: clinicopathologic analysis and therapeutic results in 116 cases. Oral Surg Oral Med Oral Pathol Oral Radiol Endod. 2002;94(1):83–91. https://doi.org/10.1067/moe.2002.123539.
2. Vera Izaguirre DS, Zuloaga Salcedo S, González Sánchez PC, Sánchez Lara K, Chávez Tapia N, Hojyo Tomoka MT, et al. Actinic prurigo: a case-control study of risk factors. Int J Dermatol. 2014;53(9):1080–5. https://doi.org/10.1111/ijd.12168.
3. Valbuena MC, Muvdi S, Lim HW. Actinic prurigo. Dermatol Clin. 2014;32(3):335–44, viii. https://doi.org/10.1016/j.det.2014.03.010.
4. Martínez-Luna E, Bologna-Molina R, Mosqueda-Taylor A, Cuevas-González JC, Rodríguez-Lobato E, Martínez-Velasco MA, et al. Inmunohistochemical detection of mastocytes in tissue from patients with actinic prurigo. J Clin Exp Dent. 2015;7(5):e656–9. https://doi.org/10.4317/jced.52823.
5. Plaza JA, Toussaint S, Prieto VG, Mercadillo P, Diez de Medina JC, Lourenco S, et al. Actinic prurigo cheilitis: a clinicopathologic review of 75 cases. Am J Dermatopathol. 2016;38(6):418–22. https://doi.org/10.1097/DAD.0000000000000459.
6. Macfarlane L, Hawkey S, Naasan H, Ibbotson S. Characteristics of actinic prurigo in Scotland: 24 cases seen between 2001 and 2015. Br J Dermatol. 2016;174(6):1411–4. https://doi.org/10.1111/bjd.14444.
7. Chen YA, Yang CC, Ting SW, Lee JY, Chen W. Adult-onset actinic prurigo: report of 19 patients from Taiwan. J Eur Acad Dermatol Venereol. 2016;30(11):e140–2. https://doi.org/10.1111/jdv.13450.
8. Chen Q, Shen M, Heng YK, Theng TSC, Tey HL, Ren EC, et al. Actinic prurigo in Singaporean Chinese: a positive association with HLA-DRB1*03:01. Photochem Photobiol. 2016;92(2):355–9. https://doi.org/10.1111/php.12569.
9. Cuevas-Gonzalez JC, Lievanos-Estrada Z, Vega-Memije ME, Hojyo-Tomoka MT, Dominguez-Soto L. Correlation of serum IgE levels and clinical manifestations in patients with actinic prurigo. An Bras Dermatol. 2016;91(1):23–6. https://doi.org/10.1590/abd1806-4841.20163941.
10. Sitek JC. Actinic prurigo in Scandinavian adolescent successfully treated with cyclosporine A. Dermatol Reports. 2017;9(1):7050. https://doi.org/10.4081/dr.2017.7050.
11. Vega Memije ME, Cuevas Gonzalez JC, Hojyo-Tomoka MT, Rodríguez LE. Actinic prurigo as a hypersensitivity reaction type 4. Int J Dermatol. 2017;56(6):e135–6. https://doi.org/10.1111/ijd.13550.
12. Cuevas-González JC, Rodríguez-Lobato E, Hojyo-Tomoka MT, Vega-Memije ME. Actinic prurigo: a condition that affects the Latin American population. Int J Dermatol. 2019;58(11):e220–1. https://doi.org/10.1111/ijd.14600.
13. Valbuena MC, Rolon CM. Epidermal Langerhans cells resistance to solar-simulated radiation in actinic prurigo patients with low minimal erythema dose. Photodermatol Photoimmunol Photomed. 2020;36(2):105–10. https://doi.org/10.1111/phpp.12514.
14. Watts-Santos A, Martinez-Rico JC, Gomez-Flores M, Ocampo-Candiani J, Alba-Rojas E. Thalidomide: an option for the pediatric patient with actinic prurigo. Pediatr Dermatol. 2020;37(2):362–5. https://doi.org/10.1111/pde.14086.
15. Pardo-Zamudio AC, Valbuena MC, Jiménez-Torres HD, Colmenares-Mejía CC. Actinic prurigo in a dermatological reference center in Colombia: 108 cases. Biomedica. 2020;40(3):487–97. https://doi.org/10.7705/biomedica.5139.
16. Sangmala S, Wongpraparut C, Silpa-Archa N, Chaiyabutr C. Exploring adult-onset actinic prurigo in Thailand. Dermatol Reports. 2023;16(3):9810. https://doi.org/10.4081/dr.2023.9810.
17. Alamillo-Velazquez J, Ortiz-Morales G, Gonzalez-Gonzalez SE, Lopez-Altamirano DF, Rodríguez-Garcia A. Actinic conjunctivitis and its relationship with prurigo in an indigenous population from the highlands of Chiapas, Mexico. Int Ophthalmol. 2024;44(1):4. https://doi.org/10.1007/s10792-024-02925-0.

21 Systemic Lupus Erythematosus

Hercílio Martelli-Júnior, Bruno Augusto Benevenuto de Andrade, and Felipe Paiva Fonseca

21.1 General Overview and Clinical Presentation

Systemic lupus erythematosus is a multisystemic autoimmune disease, with the presence of autoantibodies towards nuclear antigens, immune complex deposition, and chronic inflammation that typically occurs in the skin, joints, and kidneys. Although epidemiologic data is difficult to be ascertained due to the complex diagnostic criteria for recognizing the disorder, it is estimated that systemic lupus erythematosus affects more than 3.4 million people in the world, with an incidence of 5.14 per 100,000 persons/year. There is a clear trend towards a higher incidence among females than males, and also among black people than white people, reaching up to 10 times higher in women and twice among black populations. Patients are usually between 15 and 44 years old, but younger patients can also be diagnosed with this disorder. The pathogenesis of the disease is very complex, but significant improvements in its understanding have been made during the last decades, especially regarding the molecular basis of the disease and the many genetic variants that can be identified, usually associated with alterations in specific immune pathways. Both innate and adaptive immune systems seem to be dysregulated in systemic lupus erythematosus, which ultimately induces a loss of immune self-tolerance.

Diagnosis of systemic lupus erythematosus may be a challenge, and the disease usually presents a wide range of clinical and laboratory manifestations that include constitutional (such as fatigue), musculoskeletal, or mucocutaneous symptoms, as well as organ-specific involvement. The American College of Rheumatology (ACR)/European League Against Rheumatism (EULAR) classification criteria published in 2019 are a very useful proposal to understand the spectrum of clinical and immunological manifestations of the disease. The presence of antinuclear antibodies (ANA) is a fundamental hallmark of systemic lupus erythematosus; some of them are considered more specific (anti-Sm and anti-double-stranded DNA [anti-ds] DNA), while others are less specific (anti-Ro/SSA and anti-La/SSB).

Regarding mucocutaneous manifestations, the butterfly-shaped rash over the cheeks and nose, called the malar rash, is considered a typical finding of these patients, which can also present other cutaneous lesions. Oral mucosa manifestation is estimated to occur in up to 40% of the patients, although the exact frequency varies depending on the methodologies used by each study to diagnose the disorder. Patients may reveal single or multiple oral mucosa sites affected and lesions can be asymptomatic or painful. The palate is the most affected site in the oral cavity, followed by the lips, buccal mucosa, gingiva and tongue. Oral lesions are more often reported as unspecific ulcers, but erythematous erosions, bullae, crust, macule and whitish striated lesions have also been reported. Desquamative gingivitis has also been described in systemic lupus erythematosus, and the differential diagnosis with oral lichen planus, pemphigus vulgaris, membrane pemphigoid, and other conditions may be very challenging and a multidisciplinary approach involving rheumatologists, dermatologists, oral medicine specialists, and oral pathologists is recommended to achieve correct diagnosis (Fig. 21.1).

Several studies have already demonstrated an increase in the risk for oral cancer development among patients affected by systemic lupus erythematosus, which has been further illustrated by recently published systematic reviews with meta-analysis that compiled available literature data and confirmed the elevated risk for oral cancer onset. Moreover,

H. Martelli-Júnior (✉)
Health Science/Primary Care Postgraduate Program, State University of Montes Claros (Unimontes), Montes Claros, Brazil

B. A. B. de Andrade
Department of Oral Diagnosis and Pathology, School of Dentistry, Universidade Federal do Rio de Janeiro, Rio de Janeiro, Brazil

F. P. Fonseca
Department of Oral Surgery and Pathology, School of Dentistry, Universidade Federal de Minas Gerais, Belo Horizonte, Brazil

© The Author(s), under exclusive license to Springer Nature Switzerland AG 2025

F. P. Fonseca et al. (eds.), *Lymphoproliferative and Granulomatous Disorders of the Oral Cavity*,
https://doi.org/10.1007/978-3-031-98844-8_21

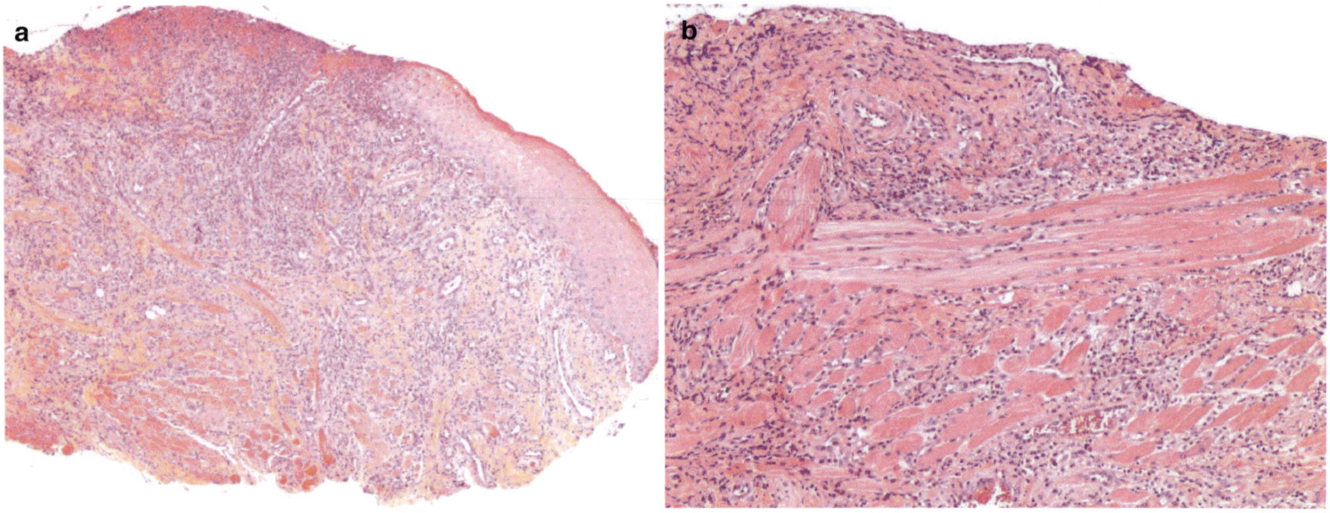

Fig. 21.1 Microscopic features of systemic lupus erythematosus affecting the oral cavity. (**a**) Oral mucosa with the overlying squamous epithelium and an ulcerated area. Note a diffuse inflammatory infiltrate in the lamina propria. (**b**) The inflammatory infiltrate is located near the epithelium and also deeper in the lamina propria surrounding muscular fibers and blood vessels

this group of patients also seems to carry an elevated risk for the occurrence of non-Hodgkin lymphomas, which may be 3- to four-fold higher than the general population. Therefore, a continuous and careful systemic and oral mucosa monitoring for early diagnosis of cancer has been recommended for individuals affected by systemic lupus erythematosus.

Most of the patients affected by systemic lupus erythematosus are treated by hydroxychloroquine, which has proven to be effective in controlling the disease; however, the combination with other immunosuppressive drugs like glucocorticoid and other more modern drugs like belimumab and anifrolumab, is also a common therapeutic approach. A well-known side effect that is related to the use of hydroxychloroquine is the dark to blue-grayish pigmentation of the oral mucosa. First described in the 1940s, the exact mechanisms that lead to mucosa pigmentation caused by the use of hydroxychloroquine are not yet fully established, although it is believed that the drug stimulates melanin production by melanocytes. These alterations are generally reversible when the medication is discontinued. The hard palate is typically involved, but there is still no clear explanation for the sparing of the soft palate, and the involvement of other sites like the lips, gingiva, and buccal mucosa is very rare. Cutaneous pigmentation and reversible graying of hair, beard, eyelashes and eyebrows have also been described in chronic therapy, while the occurrence of ocular complications is considered a special issue that may be associated with irreversible retinopathy, ultimately leading to blindness. The diagnosis of hydroxychloroquine-induced oral hyperpigmentation is usually based on medical history and clinical presentation, but a biopsy can be helpful to confirm the diagnosis in atypical cases, revealing the deposition of melanin and/or hemosiderin in the lamina propria. Although these pigments are easily observed under H&E staining, Fontana-Masson and Perls' histological reactions can be used to characterize their biological origin as either melanin (dark brown stain) or hemosiderin (bluish stain), respectively, and positive results are described for both reactions (Fig. 21.2).

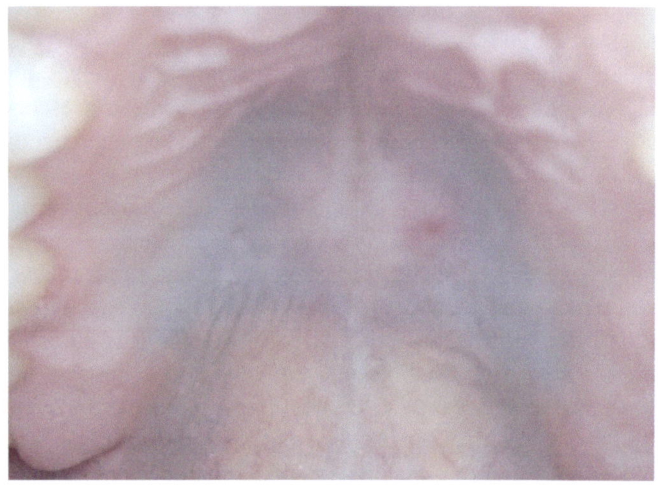

Fig. 21.2 Clinical presentation of oral pigmentation due to hydroxychloroquine use for treating systemic lupus erythematosus. Female patient exhibiting a dark pigmentation of the hard palate that spares the soft palate

Systemic lupus erythematosus is still considered an incurable disease despite the improvements in the treatment options, and currently available therapeutic approaches aim to control patients' symptoms and reduce the disease flare-ups. As a consequence of the disease activity and the side-effects of the immunomodulatory activity of the therapeutic schemes used, patients very often develop comorbidities that include a higher risk of infection, premature menopause affects fertility, bone density, diabetes risk, coronary heart disease and cerebrovascular disease, chronic renal disease, among others, which negatively impact patients' quality of life and mortality rates.

21.2 Microscopic Findings

- The overlying squamous epithelium may show pseudoepitheliomatous hyperplasia and hyperkeratosis with keratin plugging.
- Exocytosis and acanthosis of the overlying squamous epithelium may also occur.
- In the epithelium, there are apoptotic keratinocytes and hydropic degeneration of the basal layer.
- The characteristic PAS-positive stain in the basement membrane zone is usually observed.
- Presence of an intense chronic inflammatory infiltrate in the lamina propria below the epithelium.
- Predominance of lymphocytes, but also with scattered plasma cells and macrophages (Figs. 21.3, 21.4, 21.5, and 21.6).
- In the mucosal hyperpigmentation due to the use of hydroxychloroquine for systemic lupus erythematosus treatment, the presence of dark granules in the lamina propria is observed, which are more often located among collagen fibers, but may also be found phagocytized by macrophages (Fig. 21.7).

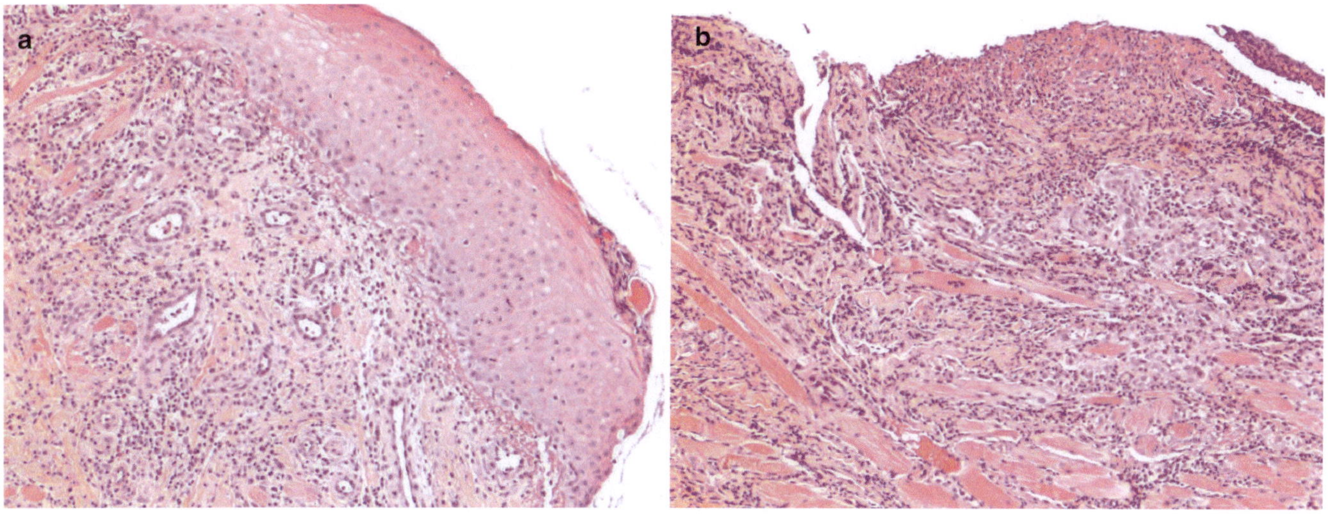

Fig. 21.3 Microscopic features of systemic lupus erythematosus affecting the oral cavity. (**a**) Below the overlying squamous epithelium there is a prominent eosinophilic layer representing the basal membrane (H&E; 100X). (**b**) Observe the ulcerated region containing a higher number of polymorphonuclear cells and the chronic inflammatory infiltrate deeper in the lamina propria (H&E; 100X)

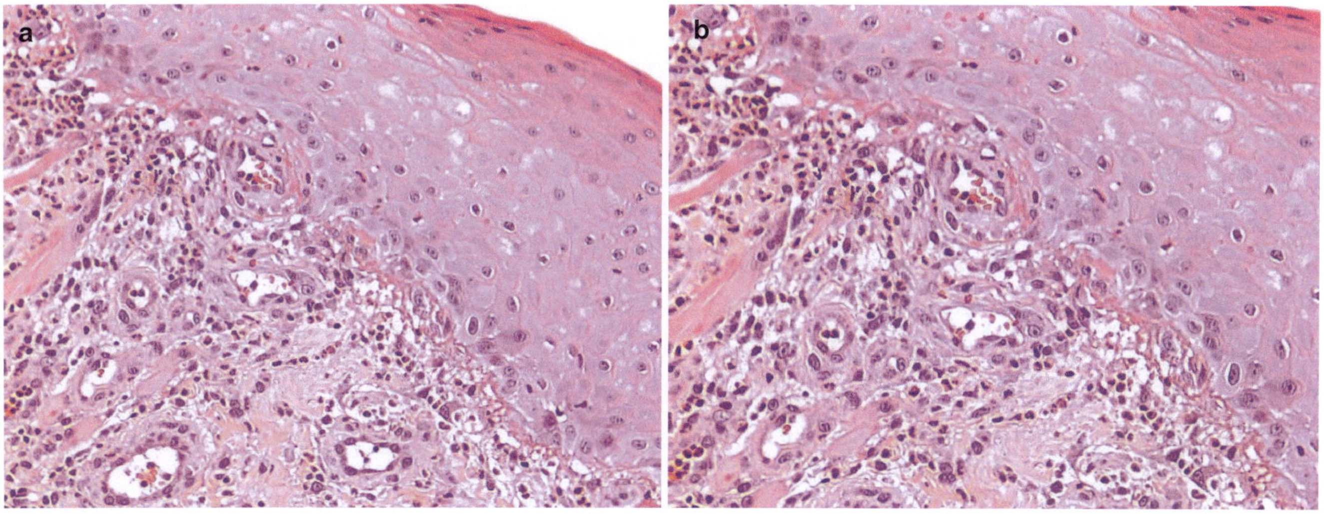

Fig. 21.4 Microscopic features of systemic lupus erythematosus affecting the oral cavity. (**a**) The presence of a thicker layer of basal membrane is observed in many cases consistent with lupus erythematosus (H&E; 100X). (**b**) Observe the amorphous eosinophilic layer beneath the squamous epithelium representing the basal membrane (H&E; 200X)

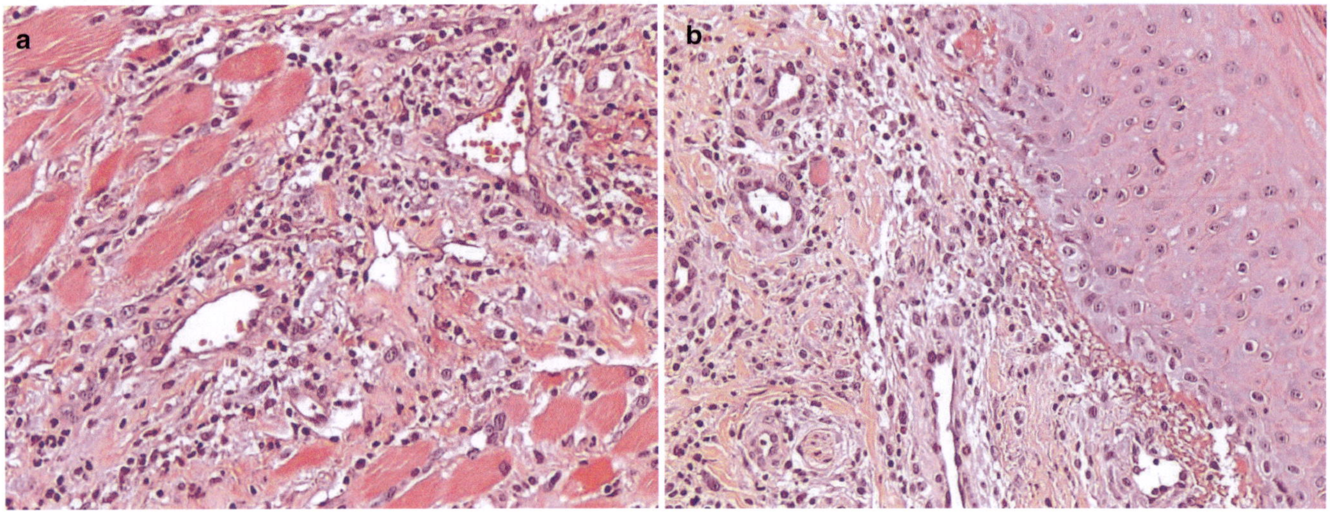

Fig. 21.5 Microscopic features of systemic lupus erythematosus affecting the oral mucosa. (**a**) An example of oral manifestation of systemic lupus erythematosus with chronic inflammatory infiltrate in the lamina propria (H&E; 200X). (**b**) Observe the prominent amorphous eosinophilic layer of basal membrane (H&E; 200X)

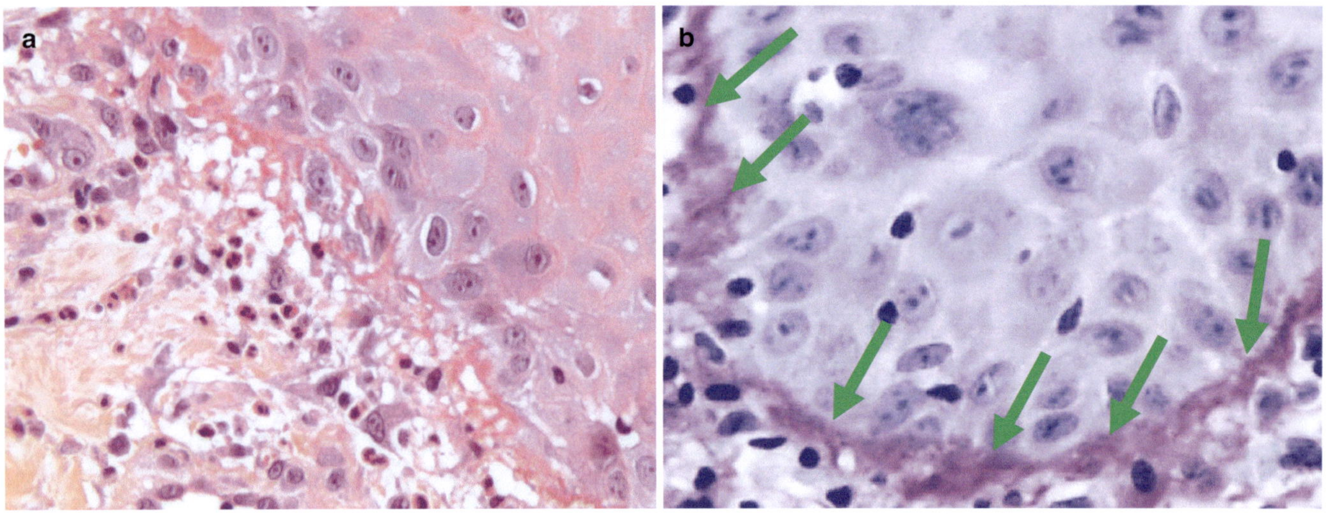

Fig. 21.6 Microscopic features of systemic lupus erythematosus affecting the oral mucosa. (**a**) Under higher magnification, note the eosinophilic basal membrane (H&E; 400X). (**b**) The basal membrane is highlighted using PAS staining (green arrows) (PAS; 400X)

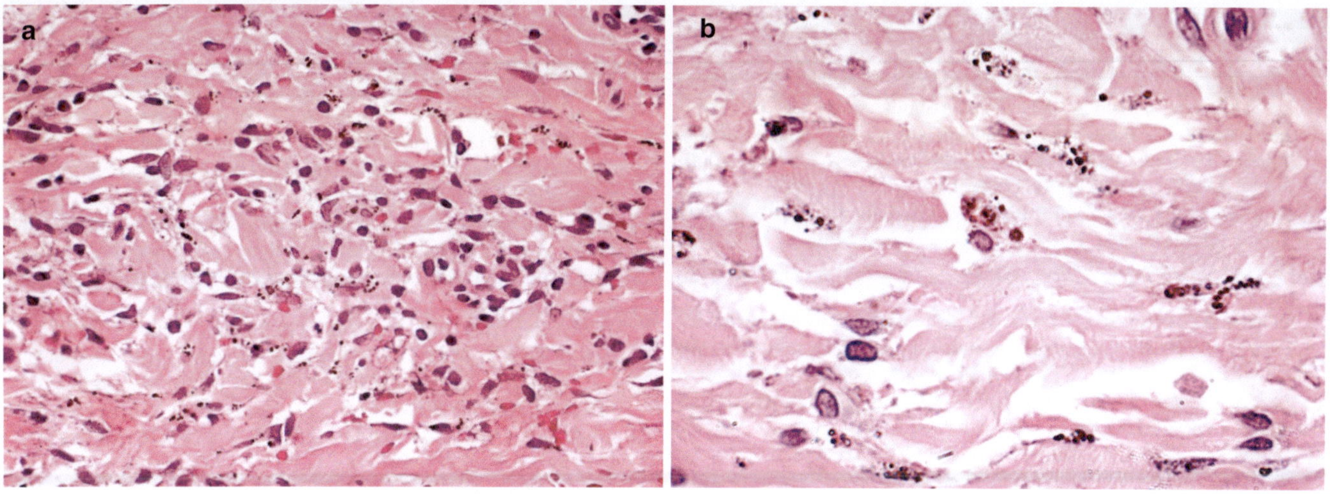

Fig. 21.7 Microscopic features of oral pigmentation due to hydroxychloroquine use for treating systemic lupus erythematosus. (**a**) Deposition of dark brown granules in the lamina propria of the oral mucosa. Few inflammatory cells are present (H&E; 100×). (**b**) The granules are located in the connective tissue (H&E; 200×)

21.3 Immunohistochemistry and/or Genetics

The diagnosis of systemic lupus erythematosus is based on clinical and laboratory data, while microscopic features obtained from cutaneous or mucosal biopsies have a more limited importance given their less specific characteristics. The use of immunohistochemistry for these cases is also limited and can only confirm the polymorphic and non-neoplastic nature of the lymphoid infiltrate. Regarding the oral hyperpigmentation associated with the use of hydroxychloroquine, Fontana-Masson and Perls' histological reactions are useful for better appreciating the granules and to define their origin. Most of the cases stain positively for Fontana-Masson as dark brown staining granules, and the speculated pathogenesis for the melanin production is based on the fact that antimalarial drugs would stimulate melanocytes to produce this pigment either directly and/or by elevating levels of androgens, while rare cases described positivity for Perls reaction, which presents as bluish staining. In these instances, it is hypothesized that iron chelation by the drug or its metabolite would lead to deposition of hemosiderin in the lamina propria (Table 21.1).

Table 21.1 Summary of the main immunohistochemical reactions and special histological stains that can be used to characterize the inflammatory infiltrate of systemic lupus erythematosus and the hydroxychloroquine-induced oral hyperpigmentation

Antibody/stain	Most frequent results	Pattern	Objective
CD20	Positive	Membrane	To characterize the B lymphocyte infiltrate
CD3	Positive	Membrane	To characterize the T lymphocyte infiltrate
CD138	Positive	Membrane	To characterize the plasma cell infiltrate
CD68	Positive	Cytoplasm	To demonstrate the presence of macrophages
Kappa/Lambda	Polyclonal	Cytoplasm	To demonstrate the polyclonal nature of the infiltrate
PAS[a]	Positive	Basal membrane	To demonstrate the presence of a thick basal membrane
Fontana-Masson[a]	Positive	Dark brown stain in the granules	To better appreciate the granules in the lamina propria and to demonstrate that they represent melanin deposition
Perls[a]	Positive	Bluish stain in the granules	To better appreciate the granules in the lamina propria and to demonstrate that they represent hemosiderin deposition

[a]Histological stain

Sources

1. López-Labady J, Villarroel-Dorrego M, González N, Pérez R, Mata de Henning M. Oral manifestations of systemic and cutaneous lupus erythematosus in a Venezuelan population. J Oral Pathol Med. 2007;36(9):524–7. https://doi.org/10.1111/j.1600-0714.2007.00569.x.
2. de Andrade BA, Fonseca FP, Pires FR, Mesquita AT, Falci SG, Dos Santos Silva AR, et al. Hard palate hyperpigmentation secondary to chronic chloroquine therapy: report of five cases. J Cutan Pathol. 2013;40(9):833–8. https://doi.org/10.1111/cup.12182.
3. Jallouli M, Francès C, Piette JC, Huong du LT, Moguelet P, Factor C, et al. Hydroxychloroquine-induced pigmentation in patients with systemic lupus erythematosus: a case-control study. JAMA Dermatol. 2013;149(8):935–40. https://doi.org/10.1001/jamadermatol.2013.709.
4. Bahloul E, Jallouli M, Garbaa S, Marzouk S, Masmoudi A, Turki H, et al. Hydroxychloroquine-induced hyperpigmentation in systemic diseases: prevalence, clinical features and risk factors: a cross-sectional study of 41 cases. Lupus. 2017;26(12):1304–8. https://doi.org/10.1177/0961203317700486.
5. Bae EH, Lim SY, Han KD, Jung JH, Choi HS, Kim CS, et al. Systemic lupus erythematosus is a risk factor for cancer: a nationwide population-based study in Korea. Lupus. 2019;28(3):317–23. https://doi.org/10.1177/0961203319826672.
6. Westermann R, Zobbe K, Cordtz R, Haugaard JH, Dreyer L. Increased cancer risk in patients with cutaneous lupus erythematosus and systemic lupus erythematosus compared with the general population: a Danish nationwide cohort study. Lupus. 2021;30(5):752–61. https://doi.org/10.1177/0961203321990106.
7. Silva PUJ, Oliveira MB, Vieira W, Cardoso SV, Blumenberg C, Franco A, et al. Oral pigmentation as an adverse effect of chloroquine and hydroxychloroquine use: a scoping review. Medicine (Baltimore). 2022;101(11):e29044. https://doi.org/10.1097/MD.0000000000029044.
8. Marques NP, Marques NCT, Lucena EHG, Martelli DRB, Oliveira EA, Martelli-Junior H. The continuous increase in the number of systemic lupus erythematosus cases in Brazil in the COVID-19 era. Braz Oral Res. 2023;37:e066. https://doi.org/10.1590/1807-3107bor-2023.vol37.0066.
9. Martelli Júnior H, Marques NP, Marques NCT, Gomes de Lucena E, Martelli DRB, Oliveira EA. Correspondence on 'clinical course of coronavirus disease 2019 (COVID-19) in a series of 17 patients with systemic lupus erythematosus under long-term treatment with hydroxychloroquine'. Ann Rheum Dis. 2023;82(11):e225. https://doi.org/10.1136/annrheumdis-2021-220410.
10. Rodrigues LRS, Ferraz DLF, de Oliveira CRG, Evangelista K, Silva MAG, Silva FPY, et al. Risk and prevalence of oral cancer in patients with different types of lupus erythematosus: a systematic review and meta-analysis. Oral Surg Oral Med Oral Pathol Oral Radiol. 2023;136(5):595–605. https://doi.org/10.1016/j.oooo.2023.07.007.
11. Hoi A, Igel T, Mok CC, Arnaud L. Systemic lupus erythematosus. Lancet. 2024;403(10441):2326–38. https://doi.org/10.1016/S0140-6736(24)00398-2.
12. de Arruda JAA, Villarroel-Dorrego M, Freire CH, Molina-Ávila I, Pimentel-Solá JM, Gilligan G, et al. Oral lesions of systemic lupus erythematosus: a collaborative Latin American study. Lupus. 2024;33(8):864–73. https://doi.org/10.1177/09612033241252042.
13. Siegel CH, Sammaritano LR. Systemic lupus erythematosus: a review. JAMA. 2024;331(17):1480–91.
14. Hartanto FK, Sufiawati I. Oral lesions in adult- and juvenile-onset systemic lupus erythematosus patients: a case series report. Dent Med Probl. 2024;61(1):145–52. https://doi.org/10.17219/dmp/132242.
15. Pettigrew B, Piragic N, Ouanounou A. Systemic lupus erythematosus: clinical manifestations, medical management, and dental treatment modifications. Compend Contin Educ Dent. 2024;45(8):403–8.
16. Amaral-Sobrinho LFD, Lima FS, Santos DBDN, Cavalcante IL, de Arruda JAA, Netto JNS, et al. Oral lesions of immune-mediated and autoimmune diseases: a 12-year experience at a single Brazilian referral center. Head Neck Pathol. 2024;18(1):49. https://doi.org/10.1007/s12105-024-01654-1.
17. Parodis I, Girard-Guyonvarc'h C, Arnaud L, Distler O, Domján A, Van den Ende CHM, et al. EULAR recommendations for the non-pharmacological management of systemic lupus erythematosus and systemic sclerosis. Ann Rheum Dis. 2024;83(6):720–9. https://doi.org/10.1136/ard-2023-224416.

Eosinophilic Ulcer

22

Márcio Ajudarte Lopes, Alan Roger Santos-Silva, Felipe Nör, and Felipe Paiva Fonseca

22.1 General Overview and Clinical Presentation

Eosinophilic ulcer, also called traumatic granuloma of the tongue, eosinophilic ulcer of the tongue, and traumatic granuloma with stromal eosinophilia, was first described by Popoff in 1956 and recognized as an independent entity in 1970. It represents a lesion that typically affects the tongue and that demonstrates a rapid onset, with some weeks of duration before spontaneous regression. It is accepted that eosinophilic ulcer had already been described among infants and neonates since the end of the nineteenth century, being labeled as Riga's disease, sublingual growth in infants, sublingual ulcer/granuloma, and reparative lesion of the tongue. The clinical description of this lesion in infants made by Riga in 1881 was followed by its histological characterization by Fede in 1890, and the term Riga-Fede disease represents a variant of eosinophilic ulcer found in the first 2 years of life. In these patients the lesion manifests as an isolated ulcer affecting the ventral surface of the tongue as a consequence of the chronic mucosal trauma caused by the anterior primary teeth.

The exact pathogenesis of eosinophilic ulcer is still poorly understood and different etiologies have been proposed including non-specific infections and local traumatic events like sharp tooth margins and ill-fitting dentures, although most of the cases are deficient of obvious clinical causes to confirm the traumatic origin of the lesion. It is characterized by the presence of a dense inflammatory infiltrate containing a variable number of eosinophils that more often surround muscular fibers. It has been demonstrated that the inflammatory component is mainly composed of cytotoxic T lymphocytes, mast cells, and macrophages.

The expression of the transmembrane protein CD30 is observed in many different lesions ranging from reactive conditions to T- or B-cell lymphomas, and the presence of a few large atypical cells positive for CD30 as either scattered or clustered infiltrates in eosinophilic ulcers led some authors to hypothesize the possibility of this lesion to represent a spectrum of the CD30+ lymphoproliferative disorders, like lymphomatoid papulosis, affecting the oral cavity; however, the true origin of these cells remains largely debatable, possibly representing histiocytic, dermal dendrocytic, or myofibroblastic cells; moreover, larger series demonstrated that this lesion commonly behaves as a benign, reactive disorder, with no tendency for recurrences and without a clear association with the presence of cutaneous lesions. However, in the presence of skin disorders, genetic analysis to investigate the clonality status of T-cell receptor (TCR) may aid in final diagnosis. Moreover, eosinophilic ulcers have microscopic features that may overlap with angiolymphoid hyperplasia with eosinophilia, which, however, typically manifests as a nodule rather than an ulcer, not being clear whether these entities represent different diseases or variants of the same condition.

Eosinophilic ulcer usually shows an equal sex distribution, more often affecting those patients in the fifth and seventh decades of life. Although the tongue is the most affected site, especially the dorsum and the tip of the tongue, any mucosal location can be affected, including the buccal mucosa, retromolar area, floor of the mouth, vestibular mucosa, gingiva, and palatal mucosa. An asymptomatic, solitary, persistent ulcer in the oral mucosa is the main clinical presentation of this entity, but painful and multiple ulcerations may also be reported, often leading to significant

M. A. Lopes (✉) · A. R. Santos-Silva
Department of Oral Diagnosis (Semiology), Piracicaba Dental School, University of Campinas (UNICAMP), Piracicaba, Brazil
e-mail: malopes@fop.unicamp.br; malopes@unicamp.br; alan@unicamp.br

F. Nör
Department of Periodontics and Oral Medicine, University of Michigan School of Dentistry, Ann Arbor, MI, USA
e-mail: fenor@umich.edu

F. P. Fonseca
Department of Oral Surgery and Pathology, School of Dentistry, Universidade Federal de Minas Gerais, Belo Horizonte, Brazil

© The Author(s), under exclusive license to Springer Nature Switzerland AG 2025

F. P. Fonseca et al. (eds.), *Lymphoproliferative and Granulomatous Disorders of the Oral Cavity*,
https://doi.org/10.1007/978-3-031-98844-8_22

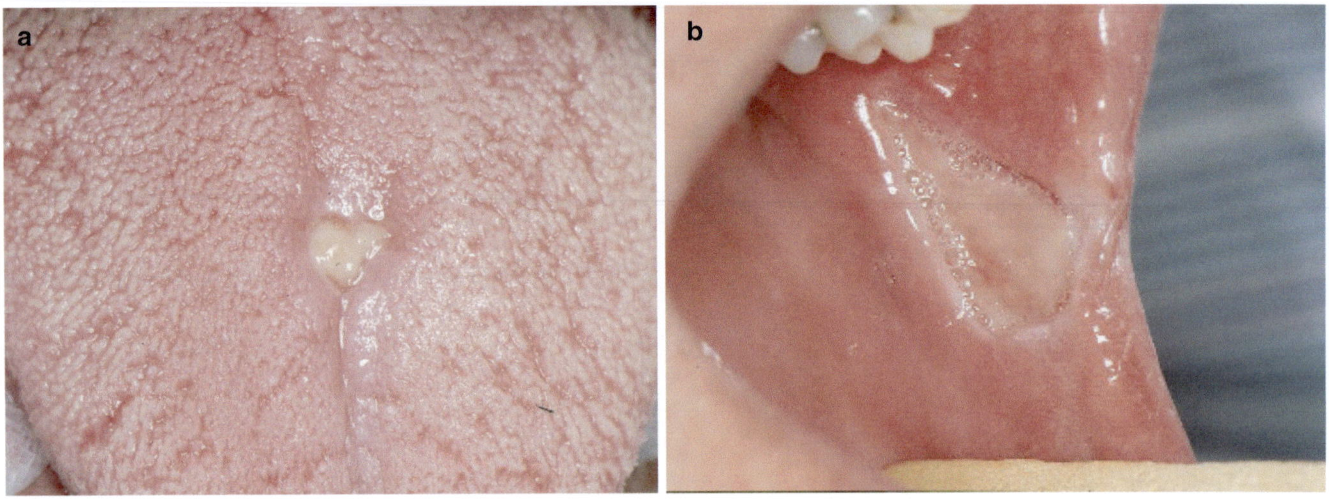

Fig. 22.1 Clinical presentation of eosinophilic ulcers. (**a**) Round ulceration in the central area of the dorsum of the tongue covered by a yellowish fibrinous membrane. (**b**) A male patient showing a painful ulceration in the cheek mucosa

impairment of food intake, and many differential diagnoses can be considered, ranging from neoplastic to infectious processes. The lesion exhibits variable size and shape, with large ulcers with central areas covered by a yellowish fibrinopurulent pseudomembrane being reported in the literature. Because of its elevated and indurated borders, eosinophilic ulcers particularly affecting the lateral border and the venter of the tongue, or the floor of the mouth, may strongly resemble squamous cell carcinoma, and misdiagnoses are frequent among clinicians not familiarized with this entity. Other differential diagnoses usually include deep fungal infections, necrotizing bacterial infections, syphilis, and granulomatous disorders due to the slow-healing process.

A careful clinical and histopathological correlation is very important to achieve the correct diagnosis of this disorder and to avoid unnecessary aggressive surgical approaches, since eosinophilic ulcers commonly demonstrate a benign, self-limited behavior. Its clinical resemblance to other conditions almost always demands that an incisional biopsy be done, but the lesions usually heal after biopsy in 1–2 weeks of follow-up and recurrences are very uncommon. This healing process, however, may take some months, and it has been speculated that the delayed healing of eosinophilic ulcers would be associated with the lack of secretion of transforming growth factor (TGF)-a and TGF-b by the eosinophils that typically infiltrate these lesions (Fig. 22.1).

22.2 Microscopic Findings

- Depending on the site of the biopsy, there may or may not be an ulcerated surface.
- In the connective tissue, there is an intense, reactive chronic inflammatory infiltrate (granulation tissue).
- The inflammatory infiltrate is distributed throughout the lamina propria and usually surrounds and damages deep muscular fibers.
- Presence of reactive lymphocytes, plasma cells and histiocytes.
- In the regions near the ulcers, the presence of neutrophils predominates.
- The presence of eosinophils is typically observed, but the number of these cells varies and can be very high in some cases.
- Eosinophils are more commonly located around striated muscle fibers.
- The occurrence of angiocentric distribution of the inflammatory cells has rarely been described in eosinophilic ulcers and should not be misinterpreted as evidence of a malignant neoplasm.
- Larger CD30-positive atypical cells are occasionally seen, some featuring multiple or lobulated nuclei, with large eosinophilic cytoplasm (Figs. 22.2, 22.3 and 22.4).

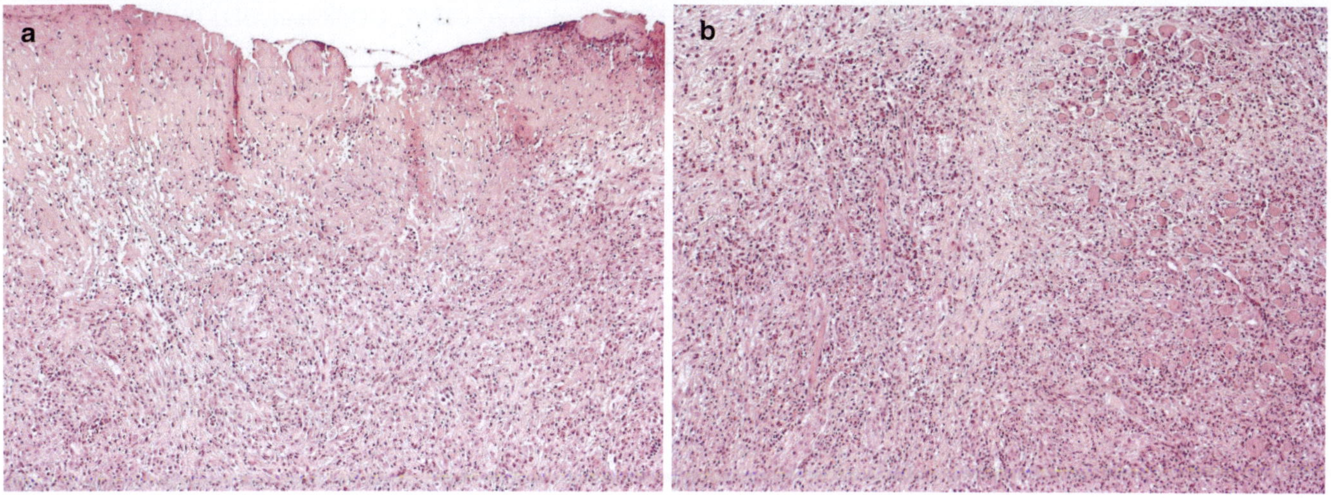

Fig. 22.2 Microscopic features of eosinophilic ulcer. (**a**) Ulcerated surface covered by a fibrinous pseudomembrane and the presence of a mixed inflammatory infiltrate just beneath the pseudomembrane containing a large number of neutrophils and lymphocytes (H&E; 50×). (**b**) The inflammatory infiltrate extends deeper toward the lamina propria surrounding muscle bundles (H&E; 50×)

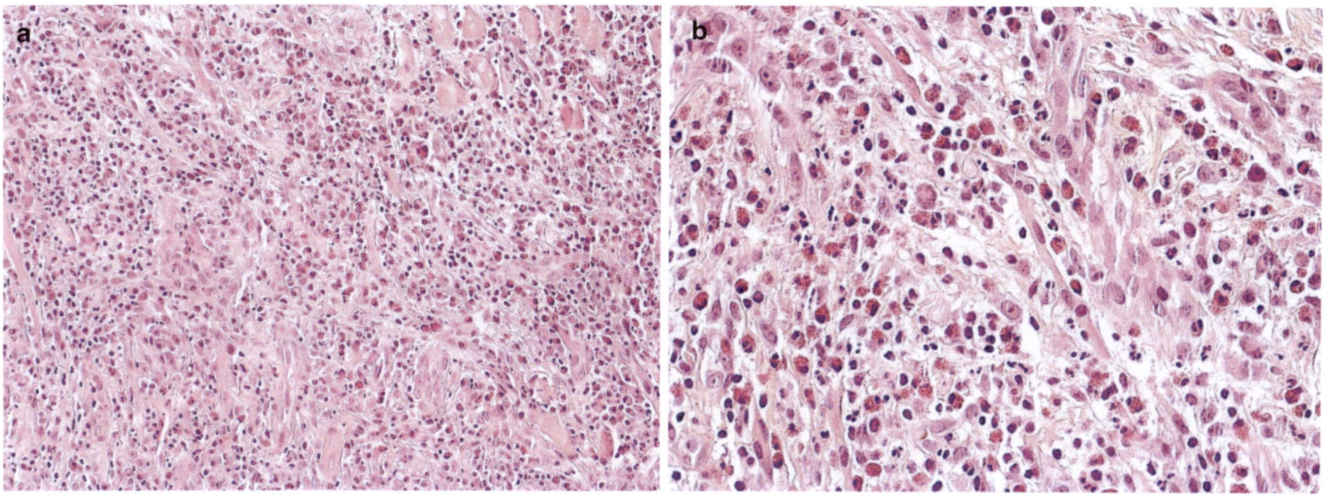

Fig. 22.3 Microscopic features of eosinophilic ulcer. (**a**) In the deeper region of the specimen, the presence of lymphocytes and eosinophils predominates in the inflammatory infiltrate (H&E; 100×). (**b**) Observed under higher-magnification the presence of innumerable eosinophils (H&E; 200×)

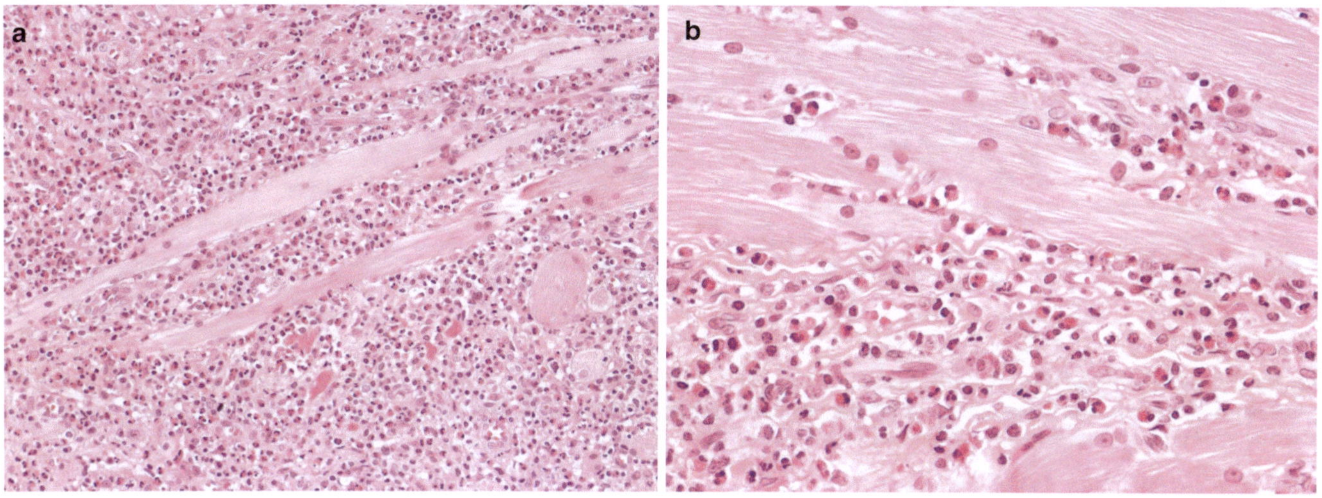

Fig. 22.4 Microscopic features of eosinophilic ulcer. (**a**) The muscular fibers are frequently surrounded by the inflammatory cells (H&E; 100×). (**b**) The presence of eosinophils is even higher near the muscular bundles (H&E; 200×)

22.3 Immunohistochemistry and/or Genetics

The diagnosis of eosinophilic ulcers is usually established through H&E-based histological analysis combined with clinical data. Immunohistochemistry is useful in demonstrating that the inflammatory component of this lesion is polymorphous in nature and in ruling out possible mimickers in challenging cases. The presence of CD20 expression reveals B lymphocytes, while CD3 demonstrates that T lymphocytes usually predominate in the lesion, which are more often cytotoxic, as shown by Granzyme B, TIA-1 or Perforin expression. Other inflammatory components like neutrophils/eosinophils, histiocytes, and plasma cells can be easily identified using CD15, CD68 and CD138/MUM1 expressions, respectively, among other possible markers. Scattered or clustered cells may express CD30; these are more often small cells, but larger atypical cells containing a round nucleus, fine chromatin and abundant cytoplasm are also frequently identified. This staining pattern is different from the more diffuse expression pattern observed in anaplastic large cell lymphoma, and eosinophilic ulcers lack ALK-1 protein expression. Proliferative index is variable, and EBV is not expected to be present (Table 22.1, Figs. 22.5, 22.6, 22.7 and 22.8). Available studies that used PCR assay to investigate the clonality of the T-cell receptor (TCR) in eosinophilic ulcers demonstrated a predominance of polyclonal status for TCR.

Table 22.1 Summary of the main immunohistochemical reactions used to characterize the inflammatory infiltrate of eosinophilic ulcers

Antibody/probe	Most frequent results	Pattern	Objective
CD20	Positive	Membrane	To demonstrate B lymphocytes
CD3	Positive	Membrane	To demonstrate T lymphocytes
CD4/CD8	Positive	Membrane	To demonstrate the predominance of cytotoxic CD8+ T cells
Granzyme B	Positive	Cytoplasm	To demonstrate cytotoxic T lymphocytes
Perforin	Positive	Cytoplasm	To demonstrate cytotoxic T lymphocytes
TIA-1	Positive	Cytoplasm	To demonstrate cytotoxic T lymphocytes
CD138	Positive	Membrane	To demonstrate plasma cell lymphocytes
CD15	Positive	Membrane	To demonstrate neutrophils/eosinophils lymphocytes
CD68	Positive	Cytoplasm	To demonstrate the presence of histiocytes
CD30	Positive	Membrane	Present in scattered small and larger atypical cells
ALK	Negative	Variable	To differentiate the lesion from ALCL
Ki67	~20–30%	Nucleus	To illustrate the proliferative index of the lesion
EBER[a]	Negative	Nucleus	To exclude an EBV+ lymphoproliferative disorder

The EBV status is also described
ALCL Anaplastic large cell lymphoma
[a]Investigated by in situ hybridization

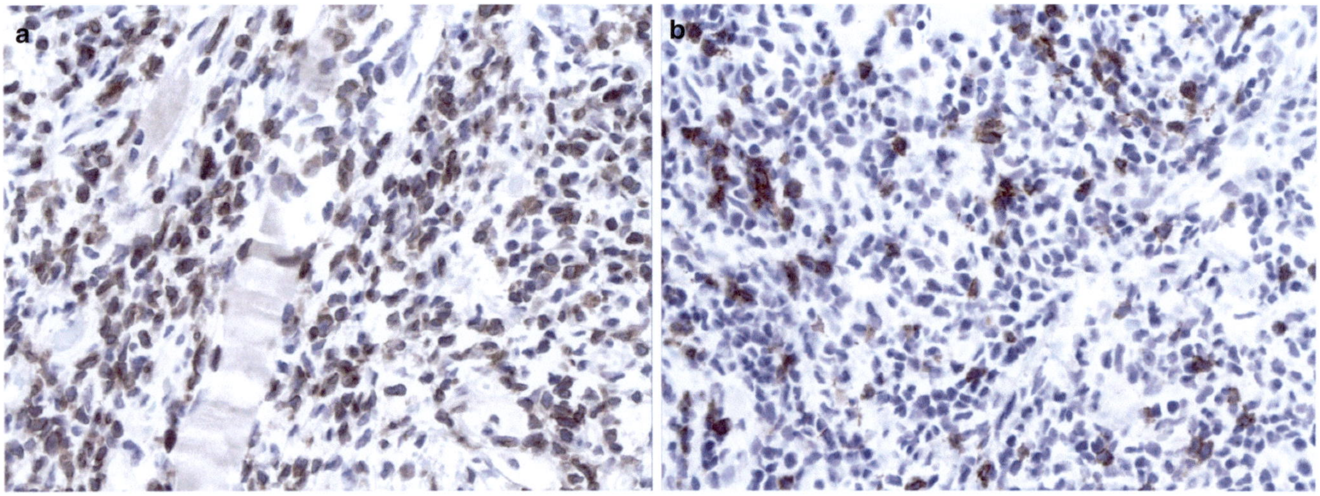

Fig. 22.5 Immunohistochemical findings of eosinophilic ulcer. (**a**) T lymphocytes predominate in the inflammatory infiltrate of eosinophilic ulcers as shown in this image using CD3 staining (DAB; 200×). (**b**) A smaller subset of lymphocytes are B cells and stain positively for CD20 protein (DAB; 200×)

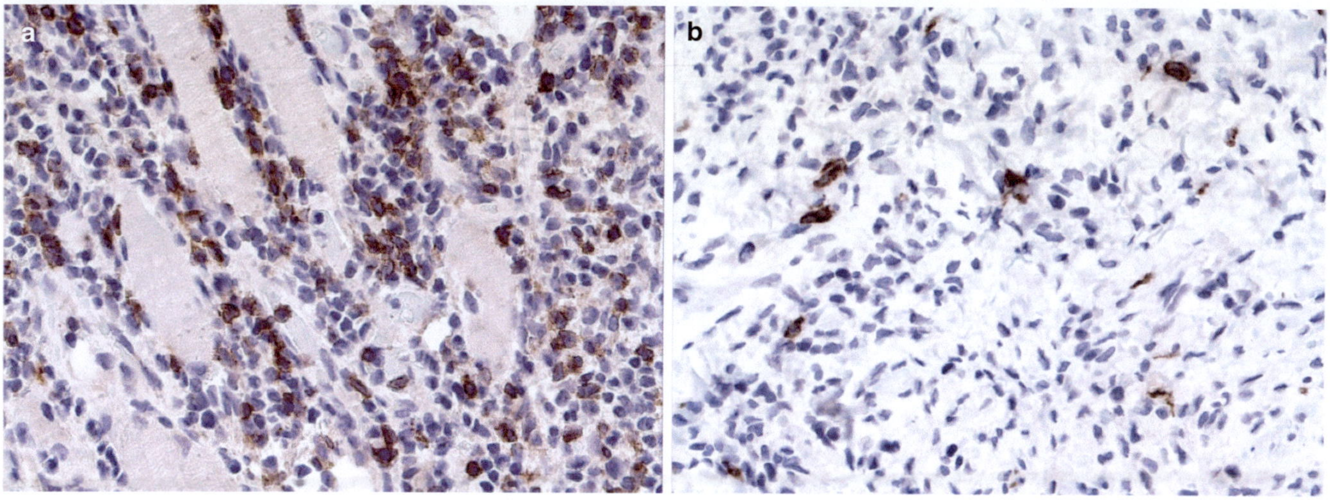

Fig. 22.6 Immunohistochemical findings of eosinophilic ulcer. (**a**) The T lymphocytes are predominantly cytotoxic and are positive for CD8 (DAB; 200×). (**b**) Mast cells are also found (DAB; 200×)

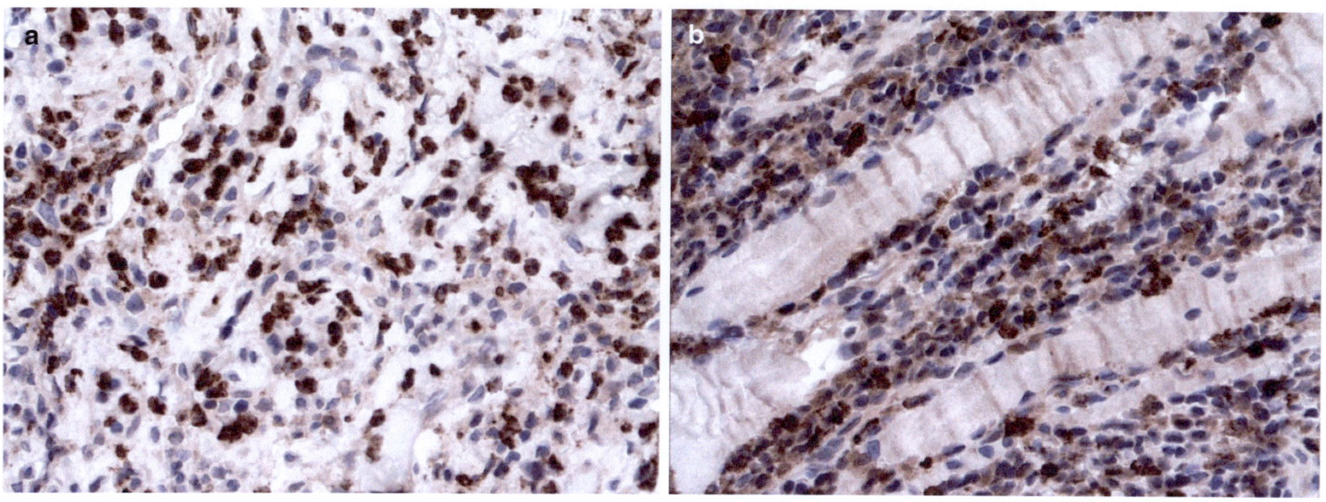

Fig. 22.7 Immunohistochemical findings of eosinophilic ulcer. (**a**) Myeloperoxidase expression, although not specific for eosinophils, highlights the presence of these cells in the lesion (DAB; 200×). (**b**) It can be seen in this image a high expression of Myeloperoxidase around the muscular fibers (DAB; 200×)

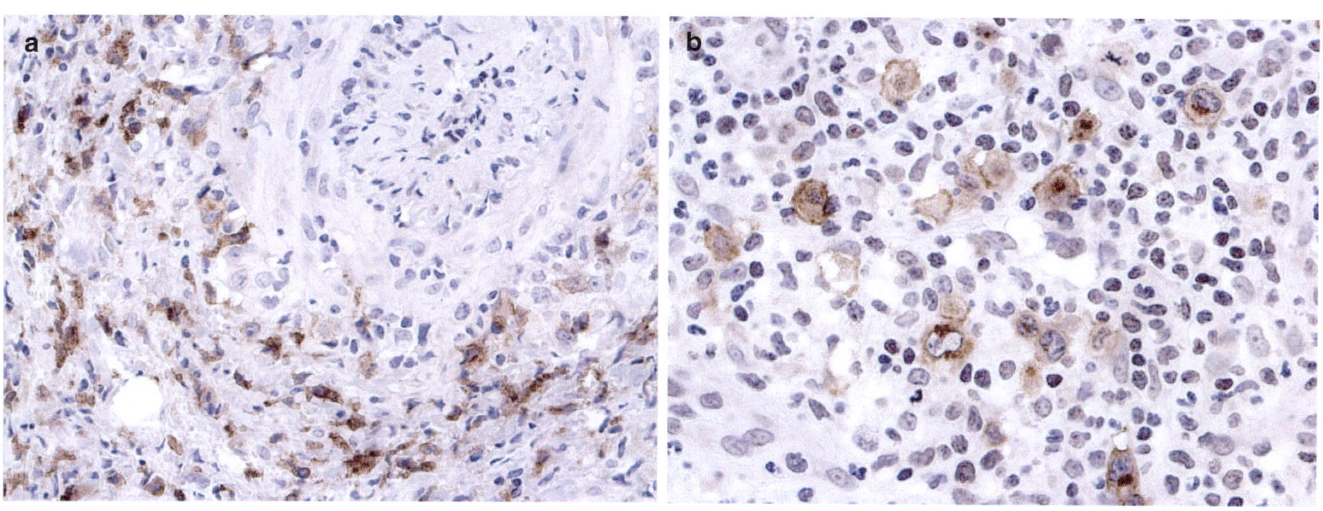

Fig. 22.8 Immunohistochemical findings of eosinophilic ulcer. (**a**) Scattered large and atypical cells are often present in eosinophilic ulcers. Most of them and also some smaller cells are positive for CD30 expression (DAB; 200×). (**b**) It is possible to observe CD30 membrane and dot-like staining pattern in atypical cells (DAB; 200×)

Sources

1. Salisbury CL, Budnick SD, Li S. T-cell receptor gene rearrangement and CD30 immunoreactivity in traumatic ulcerative granuloma with stromal eosinophilia of the oral cavity. Am J Clin Pathol. 2009;132(5):722–7. https://doi.org/10.1309/AJCPX3S5MSOVVLOP.
2. Fonseca FP, Andrade BAB, Coletta RD, Vargas PA, Lopes MA, Almeida OP, et al. Clinicopathological and immunohistochemical analysis of 19 cases of oral eosinophilic ulcers. Oral Surg Oral Med Oral Pathol Oral Radiol. 2013;115:532–40.
3. Aizic A, Raiser V, Solar I, Aharon Z, Shlomi B, Kaplan I. Traumatic ulcerative granuloma with stromal eosinophilia: CD30 analysis and clonality for T cell receptor gene rearrangement. Acta Histochem. 2019;121(8):151450. https://doi.org/10.1016/j.acthis.2019.151450.
4. Hamie L, Hamie M, Kurban M, Abbas O. Eosinophilic ulcer of the oral mucosa: an update on clinicopathologic features, pathogenesis, and management. Int J Dermatol. 2022;61(11):1359–63. https://doi.org/10.1111/ijd.15986.
5. el-Mofty SK, Swanson PE, Wick MR, Miller AS. Eosinophilic ulcer of the oral mucosa. Report of 38 new cases with immunohistochemical observations. Oral Surg Oral Med Oral Pathol. 1993;75(6):716–22. https://doi.org/10.1016/0030-4220(93)90429-8.
6. Segura S, Romero D, Mascaró JM Jr, Colomo L, Ferrando J, Estrach T. Eosinophilic ulcer of the oral mucosa: another histological simulator of CD30+ lymphoproliferative disorders. Br J Dermatol. 2006;155(2):460–3. https://doi.org/10.1111/j.1365-2133.2006.07331.x.
7. Ficarra G, Prigmano F, Romagnoli P. Traumatic eosinophilic granuloma of the oral mucosa: a CD-30+ (Ki-1) lymphoproliferative disorder? Oral Oncol. 1997;33:375–9.
8. Segura S, Pujol RM. Eosinophilic ulcer of the oral mucosa: a distinct entity or a non-specific reactive pattern? Oral Dis. 2008;14(4):287–95. https://doi.org/10.1111/j.1601-0825.2008.01444.x.
9. Brasileiro BF, Alves DB, Andrade BA, Vargas PA, León JE, Almeida OP. Traumatic ulcerative granuloma with stromal eosinophilia of the palate showing an angiocentric/angiodestructive growth pattern. Contemp Clin Dent. 2012;3(Suppl 1):S109–11. https://doi.org/10.4103/0976-237X.95118.
10. Benitez B, Mülli J, Tzankov A, Kunz C. Traumatic ulcerative granuloma with stromal eosinophilia – clinical case report, literature review, and differential diagnosis. World J Surg Oncol. 2019;17(1):184. https://doi.org/10.1186/s12957-019-1736-z.
11. Shen WR, Chang JY, Wu YC, Cheng SJ, Chen HM, Wang YP. Oral traumatic ulcerative granuloma with stromal eosinophilia: a clinicopathological study of 34 cases. J Formos Med Assoc. 2015;114(9):881–5. https://doi.org/10.1016/j.jfma.2013.09.012.
12. Shah A, Kurago Z, Bindakhil M. Clinical considerations associated with traumatic ulcerative granuloma with stromal eosinophilia. Int J Dermatol. 2022;61:e272–4. https://doi.org/10.1111/ijd.15732.
13. Mohamad AF, Abdul Rahman NR, Ch'ng ES. A case report of traumatic ulcerative granuloma with stromal eosinophilia (TUGSE): clinical and histopathological diagnostic challenges. Cureus. 2023;15(11):e48481. https://doi.org/10.7759/cureus.48481.
14. Axelrod B, Reddy R, Steinberg M. An unusual clinical presentation of traumatic ulcerative granuloma with stromal eosinophilia. J Oral Maxillofac Surg. 2024;31:S0278-2391(24)00337-9. https://doi.org/10.1016/j.joms.2024.05.012.
15. Bordignon NC, Correia-Neto IJ, Gondak R, de Albuquerque-Júnior RL. Traumatic ulcerative granuloma with stromal eosinophilia mimicking a squamous cell carcinoma. J Clin Exp Dent. 2024;16(3):e377–82. https://doi.org/10.4317/jced.61322.
16. Lee YP, Hwang MJ, Jin YT, Chiang CP. Traumatic ulcerative granuloma with stromal eosinophilia at the lateral border of the tongue. J Dent Sci. 2024;19(1):701–3. https://doi.org/10.1016/j.jds.2023.09.001.

Immunodeficiency-Associated Lymphoproliferative Disorder

23

André Caroli Rocha, Guilherme Rossi Assis de Mendonça, Pablo Agustin Vargas, and Felipe Paiva Fonseca

23.1 General Overview and Clinical Presentation

Immune deficiency and dysregulation-associated lymphoproliferative disorders encompass a heterogeneous group of conditions that may develop in the context of different immunodeficiencies. Current nomenclature proposed by the fifth edition of the World Health Organization classification guidelines recommends a three-part standardization for these entities: (1) the name of the histological lesion; (2) the presence or absence of oncogenic virus(es); and (3) the clinical setting/immunodeficiency background. Most of the immunodeficiency-associated lymphoproliferative disorders in the oral cavity arise in the setting of the human immunodeficiency virus (HIV) infection, which clinical scenario was discussed with more details in Chap. 2, or develop as a post-transplant complication (Table 23.1).

The *EBV-positive mucocutaneous ulcer* represents an important entity that may arise in the oral mucosa of immunosuppressed patients and will be discussed in Chap. 24. Different *lymphoma subtypes can also develop in an immunosuppression setting*, more frequently diffuse large B-cell lymphoma and classic Hodgkin lymphoma, but the discussion of the clinicopathological features of each lymphoma subtype manifesting in the oral cavity will be provided in their respective Chapters. *Lymphoproliferative disorders arising in the context of an inborn error of immunity* manifesting in the oral cavity are very rare and, therefore, will not be addressed in this textbook.

Table 23.1 Classification of lymphoid proliferations and lymphomas arising in the setting of immunodeficiency

Lymphoid hyperplasias arising in immunodeficiency
Polymorphic lymphoproliferative disorder arising in immunodeficiency
EBV-positive mucocutaneous ulcer
Lymphomas arising in the setting of immunodeficiency
Inborn errors of immunity-associated lymphoid proliferations and lymphomas

Hyperplasias arising in the context of immunodeficiency are predominantly composed of small lymphocytes and polytypic plasma cells (example of current nomenclature: plasmacytic hyperplasia, EBV+, presumed immune senescence), a lymphoplasmacytic proliferation with more prominent immunoblasts resembling infectious mononucleosis (example of current nomenclature: infectious mononucleosis-like hyperplasia, EBV+, post-transplant setting); or marked follicular hyperplasia (example of current nomenclature: follicular hyperplasia, EBV+, autoimmune setting), among other presentations. These non-clonal diseases are variably associated with EBV or HHV8 infections, do not cause normal tissue architecture destruction and are more commonly diagnosed in the lymph nodes. In the oral cavity, these conditions are rare and are more frequently found in the Waldeyer's ring region, especially in the tonsils. In contrast, *polymorphic lymphoproliferative disorders arising in the setting of immunodeficiency* are characterized by effacement of normal architecture of the affected tissues, with the presence of polymorphic lymphoid cells, plasma cells, immunoblasts and Hodgkin/Reed-Sternberg-like cells, as well as angioinvasion and tissue necrosis, but not fulfilling the criteria for an overt lymphoma. It occurs following a depletion of T-cell

A. C. Rocha (✉)
Oral and Maxillofacial Surgery and Traumatology Service, Hospital das Clínicas of the University of São Paulo Medical School, São Paulo, Brazil

G. R. A. de Mendonça
Department of Pathology, School of Medical Sciences, University of Campinas, Campinas, Brazil

P. A. Vargas
Oral and Maxillofacial Division, Piracicaba Dental School, State University of Campinas (UNICAMP), Piracicaba, Brazil
e-mail: pavargas@fop.unicamp.br

F. P. Fonseca
Department of Oral Surgery and Pathology, School of Dentistry, Belo Horizonte, Brazil

© The Author(s), under exclusive license to Springer Nature Switzerland AG 2025
F. P. Fonseca et al. (eds.), *Lymphoproliferative and Granulomatous Disorders of the Oral Cavity*,
https://doi.org/10.1007/978-3-031-98844-8_23

immunosurveillance, and it may regress if the immunological status of the patient is reestablished. Infection by EBV is very common, more often demonstrating a Latency type III, but this virus can be absent in up to 40% of the cases.

For post-transplant patients, different factors impact the risk of developing a lymphoproliferative disorder, including the type of organ transplanted. Once this complication predominates among patients submitted to bowel recipients (20% of patients), followed by heart, lung, liver, kidney, and, less often, bone marrow transplants. Younger patients also have a higher risk of developing a post-transplant lymphoproliferative disorder than adults, which may also vary depending on the patient's previous exposure to EBV infection. Most of the cases manifest in the gastrointestinal tract, followed by the chest, and the head and neck. In the oral and maxillofacial region, post-transplant lymphoproliferative disorder is uncommon, but several cases have already been described in different locations, including the tonsils, tongue, gingiva, palate and other less common sites. A strict clinical and pathological correlation is necessary for correct diagnosis, and in the absence of clinical information, a high level of diagnostic suspicion is necessary from pathologists to consider the possibility of an immunodeficiency-associated lymphoproliferative disorder.

Clinical presentation of oral lesions may range from mucosal hyperplasia to painful mucosal ulcerations covered by yellowish necrosis or fibrinopurulent membrane, usually with a short period of duration. Therefore, it is recommended that all oral lesions in transplanted patients be biopsied and microscopically evaluated to rule out a possible lymphoma or other malignancy.

In mild lymphoproliferative disorders the immunosuppressant dose is lowered and that is usually enough for the patient to go into remission. In severe lymphoproliferative disorders, surgery, radiotherapy, and chemotherapy may be necessary and will depend on the subtype diagnosed. Similarly, prognosis varies significantly, ranging from a remissive lesion after immunosuppression therapy is stopped to an aggressive neoplasm associated with a poor survival when high-grade monomorphic lymphomas develop. The use of antiviral agents (acyclovir or ganciclovir), either as lymphoproliferative disorders chemoprophylaxis or treatment, is still controversial (Figs. 23.1 and 23.2).

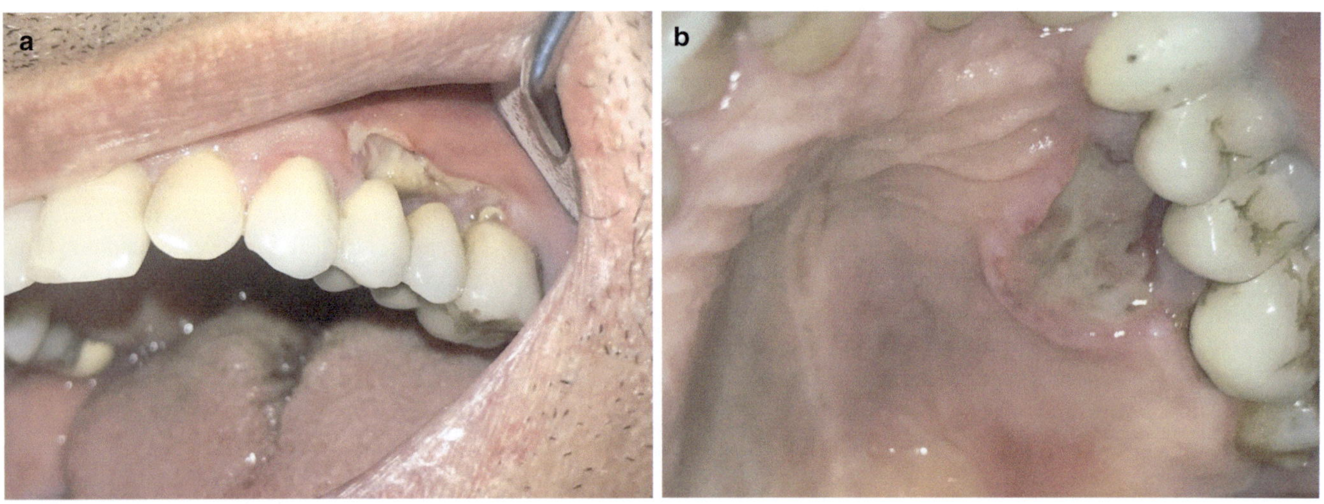

Fig. 23.1 Clinical manifestation of a post-transplant polymorphic lymphoproliferative disorder affecting the oral cavity of a patient submitted to renal transplant. (**a**) Large ulcerated lesion affecting the upper left gingiva. (**b**) The lesion extended towards the palate, where an ulcerated region with well-demarcated borders could also be observed

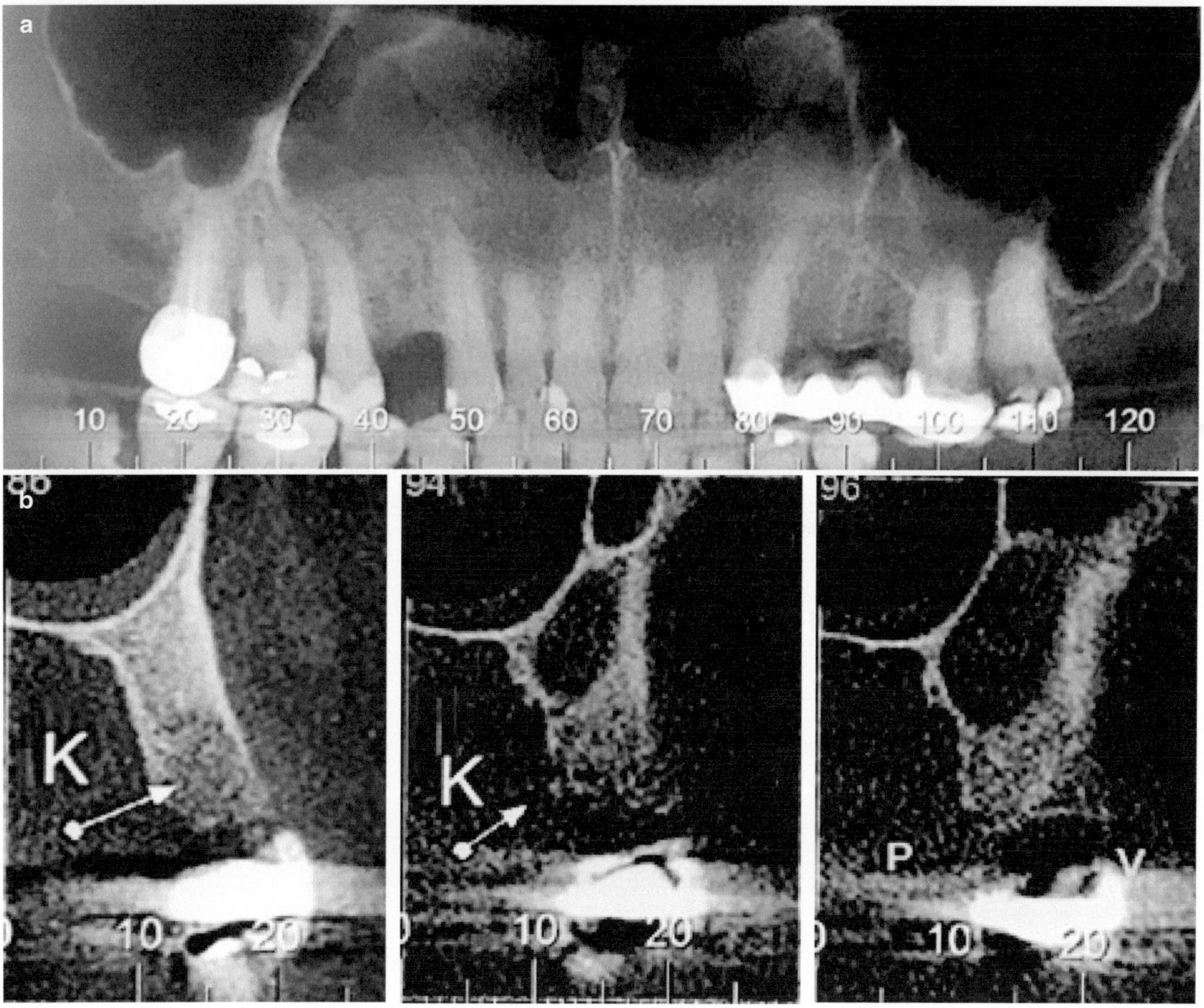

Fig. 23.2 Computed tomography evaluation of the same case as Fig. 23.1. (**a**) Panoramic image does not show any important bone involvement. (**b**) Coronal sections of the alveolar bone adjacent to the ulcerated lesions depicted slight superficial resorptions

23.2 Microscopic Findings

- Microscopic features are highly variable and depend on the subtype diagnosed.
- The main *Hyperplasias* are characterized by:
  - Plasmacytic hyperplasia associated with immunodeficiency: Diffuse proliferation of plasma cells.
  - Infectious mononucleosis-like hyperplasia associated with immunodeficiency: Diffuse proliferation of lymphocytes and plasma cells.
  - Follicular hyperplasia associated with immunodeficiency: Nodular proliferations of lymphocytes.
- Polymorphic lymphoproliferative disorder is characterized by: Diffuse proliferation of lymphoid cells, with infiltration and destruction of the surrounding normal tissues.
- Lymphomas arising in the setting of immunodeficiency will have the same microscopic findings as those described for immunocompetent patients, and they will be described in detail in their respective chapters.
- In the oral cavity most cases are polymorphic lymphoproliferative disorders.
- Presence of large lymphocytes (centroblasts, immunoblasts) mixed with small lymphocytes (centrocytes), predominantly from the B-cell lineage.
- Presence of other inflammatory cells like T lymphocytes, epithelioid macrophages, neutrophils, plasma cells and scattered eosinophils.
- Hodgkin-like cells can be found, presenting as a large cell with a round nucleus and a centrally located prominent nucleolus.
- Reed-Sternberg-like cells may also be found, presenting as a large cell with two nuclei containing prominent nucleoli surrounded by a clear perinuclear halo.
- Necrosis can be present in some cases, as well as a variable degree of cellular pleomorphism and a variable number of mitotic figures (Figs. 23.3 and 23.4).

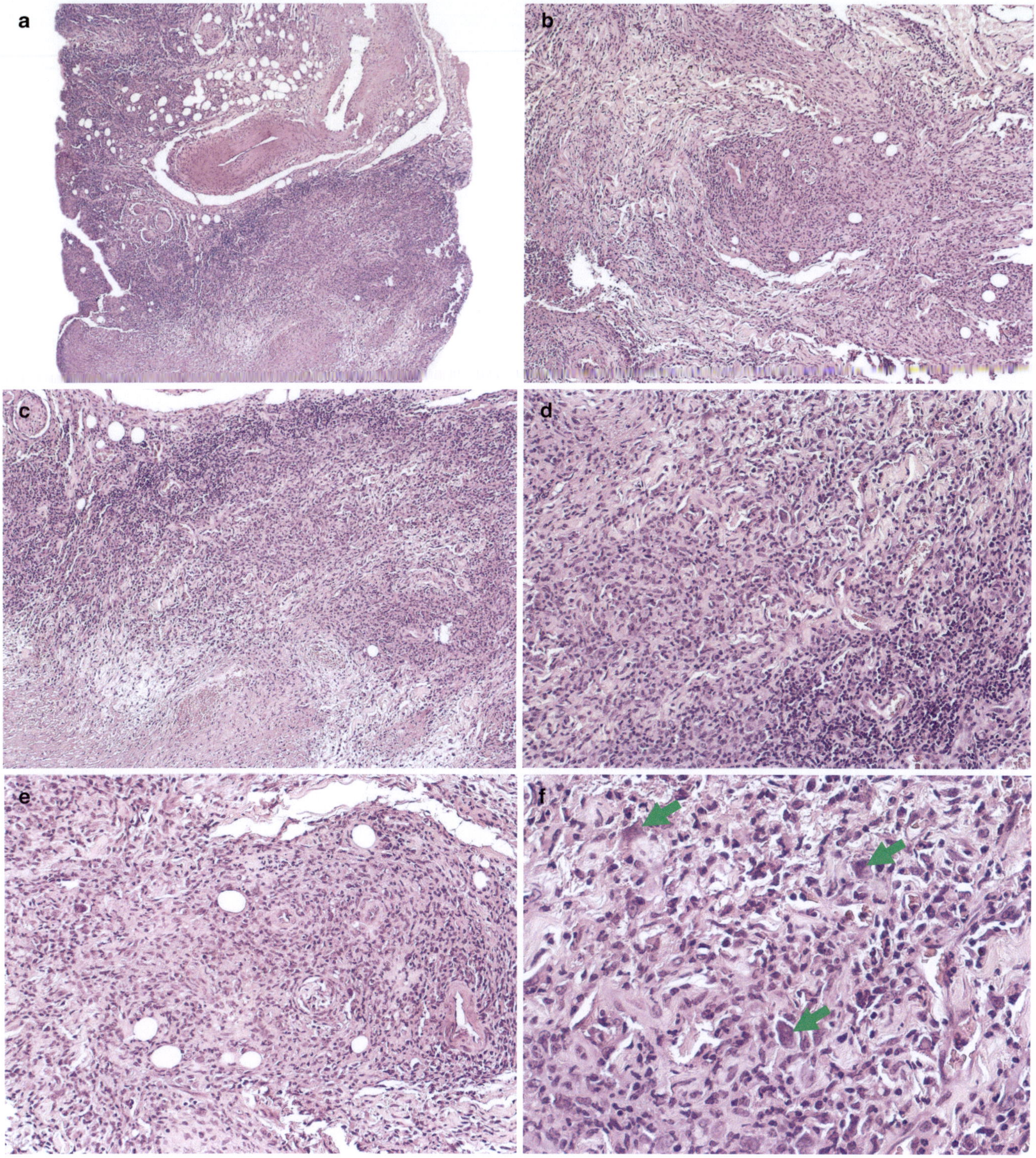

Fig. 23.3 Microscopic features of post-transplant polymorphic lymphoproliferative disorder affecting the oral cavity. (**a**) The lesion is characterized by a diffuse proliferation of lymphoid cells in a fibrotic stroma (H&E; 25×). (**b**) The lymphoid cells surround normal structures like blood vessels, muscular fibers and mature adipocytes (H&E; 50×). (**c**) Diffuse polymorphic proliferation of lymphoid cells (H&E; 50×). (**d**) It is possible to observe scattered large atypical cells (H&E; 100×). (**e**) The lymphoid infiltrate is characterized by small to large cells, few of them present pleomorphism (H&E; 100×). (**f**) Under higher magnification it is possible to observe the presence of several pleomorphic cells that are large, atypical and hyperchromatic (green arrow) (H&E; 200×)

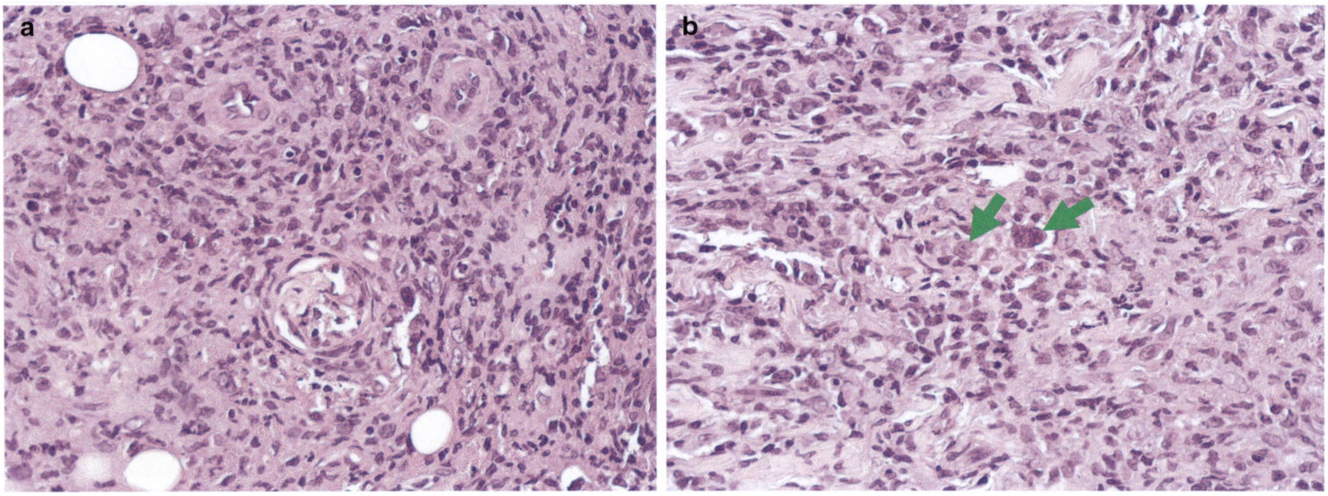

Fig. 23.4 Microscopic features of post-transplant polymorphic lymphoproliferative disorder affecting the oral cavity. (**a**) The lymphoid cells surround blood vessels and small nerve bundles (H&E; 200×). (**b**) Observe the variability in the morphological features of the lymphoid cells that vary from small to large size, containing scattered pleomorphic cells (green arrow) (H&E; 200×)

23.3 Immunohistochemistry and/or Genetics

Immunohistochemical reactions are mandatory for the diagnosis of lymphoproliferative disorders associated with immunodeficiency; however, the results are highly variable depending on the subtype diagnosed. In the hyperplasias there will be a predominance of CD20, CD3 or plasma cell markers expression depending on the subtype, while the lymphoma subtypes will present mostly the same immunophenotype as observed in immunocompetent individuals.

Polymorphic lymphoproliferative disorders associated with immunosuppression will have a highly variable and non-specific immunohistochemical profile, most often characterized by CD20 diffuse staining (B lymphocytes), CD3 (T lymphocytes) positivity in a lower proportion, as well as CD68 (macrophages) and plasma cell markers (CD138/MUM1/VS38c). These lesions are frequently CD30 positive. Proliferative index is variable and usually high, achieving approximately 50% in some cases. EBER is frequently positive and is very useful in confirming the diagnosis. A strict and careful clinical correlation is necessary to confirm this diagnosis.

Polymorphic lymphoproliferative disorders demonstrate either a monoclonal or an oligoclonal immunoglobulin rearrangement (Table 23.2, Figs. 23.5, 23.6, 23.7 and 23.8).

Table 23.2 Summary of the main immunohistochemical reactions used for the diagnosis of polymorphic lymphoproliferative disorders associated with immunosuppression

Antibody/probe	Most frequent results	Pattern	Objective
CD20	Positive	Membrane	To demonstrate the predominance of B lymphocytes
CD3	Positive	Membrane	To demonstrate the presence of T lymphocytes
Granzyme B	Positive	Cytoplasm	To demonstrate the presence of cytotoxic T lymphocytes
TIA-1	Positive	Cytoplasm	To demonstrate the presence of cytotoxic T lymphocytes
Perforin	Positive	Cytoplasm	To demonstrate the presence of cytotoxic T lymphocytes
CD30	Positive	Membrane	Characteristically present in polymorphic lymphoproliferative disorders
CD68	Positive	Cytoplasm	To demonstrate the presence of macrophages
CD138	Positive	Membrane	To demonstrate the presence of plasma cells
Ki67	~40–50%	Nucleus	To demonstrate the proliferative index of the lesion
EBER[a]	Positive (~60% of the cases)	Nucleus	To demonstrate the presence of EBV

The result of EBV investigation is also described
[a]Investigated by in situ hybridization

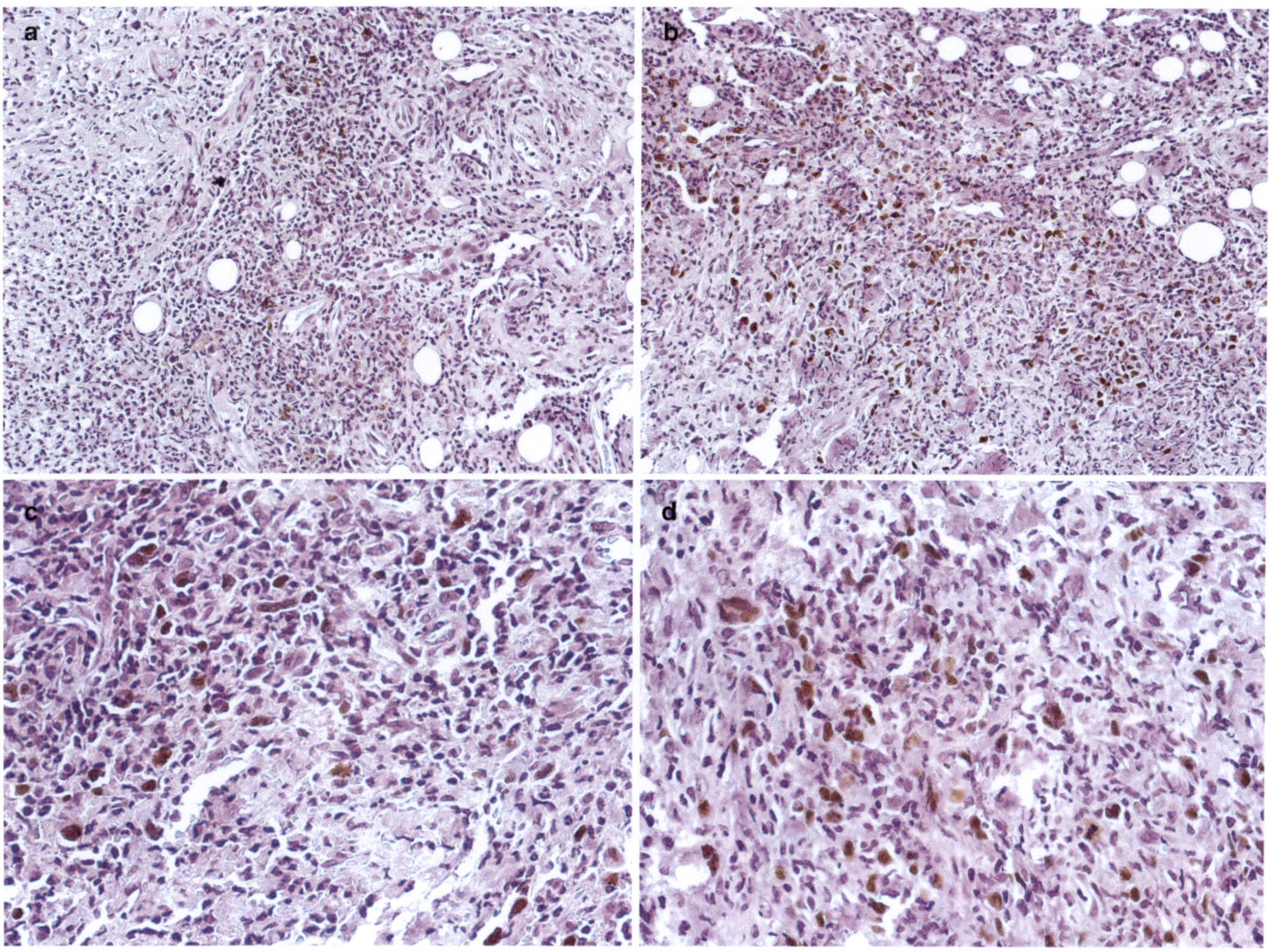

Fig. 23.5 Immunohistochemical features of post-transplant polymorphic lymphoproliferative disorder affecting the oral cavity. (**a**) Some lymphoid cells express mature B-cell markers like CD20 (DAB; 100×), (**b**) and PAX5 (DAB; 100×). (**c**) PAX5 expression is observed both in the small cells and in the scattered large atypical cells (DAB; 200×). (**d**) Therefore, these more pleomorphic component is considered to be of Bcell lineage. Observe the nuclear expression of PAX5 in the atypical cells (DAB; 200×)

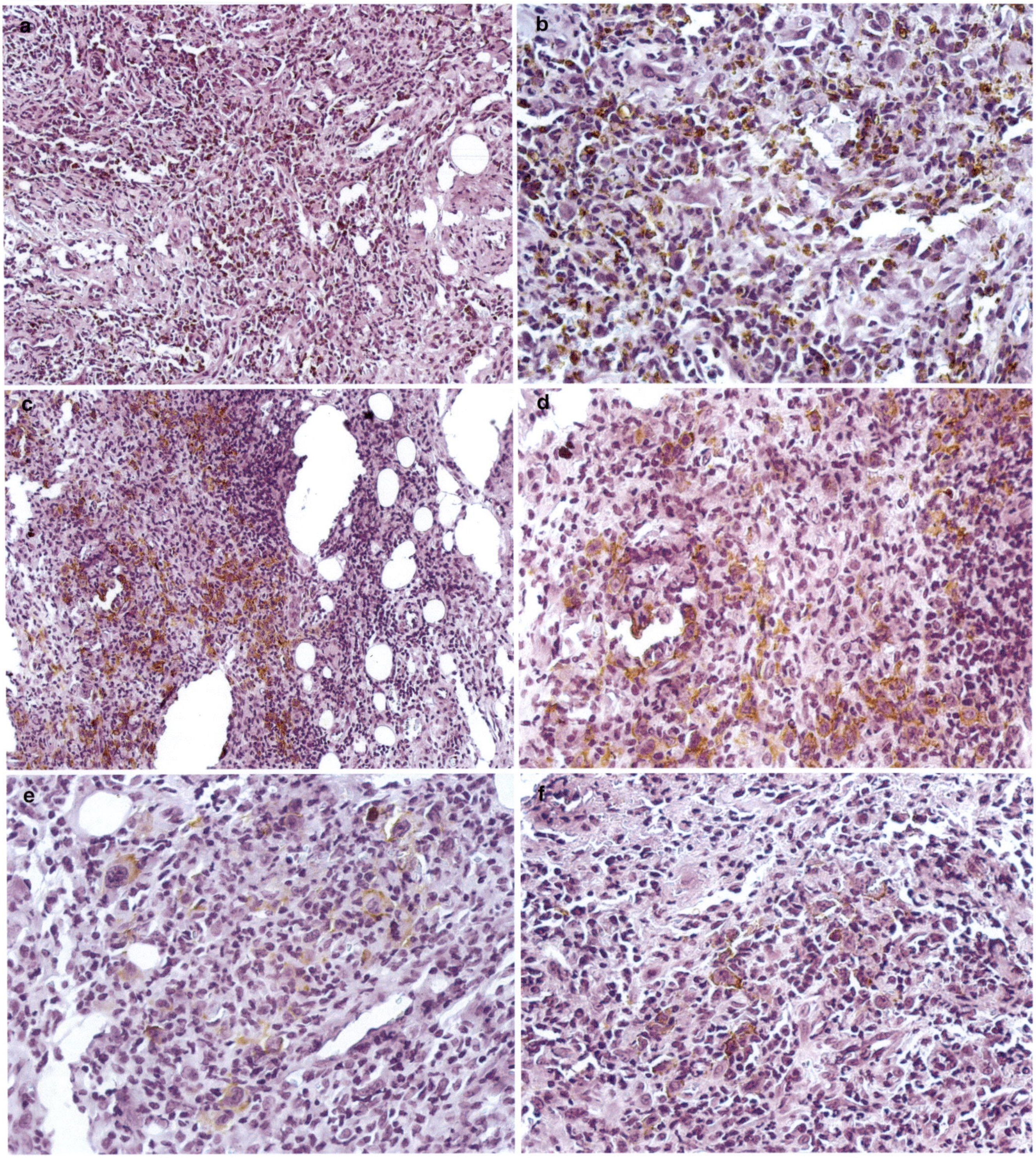

Fig. 23.6 Immunohistochemical features of post-transplant polymorphic lymphoproliferative disorder affecting the oral cavity. (**a**) Many lymphoid cells present in the lesion express the mature T-cell marker CD3 (DAB; 100×), (**b**) while a large number of cells express CD68 and prove to be of macrophage lineage. This expression pattern of B lymphocytes, T lymphocytes and macrophages, as well as the presence of plasma cells, demonstrates the polymorphic nature of the lymphoproliferative disorder (DAB; 200×). (**c**) CD30 expression is frequently observed in PTLD. Observe the membrane staining pattern of CD30 in this case (DAB; 100×). (**d**) CD30 expression is observed in some small cells and in the large atypical cells (DAB; 200×). (**e**) CD30 expression is typically observed in the large atypical cells (DAB; 200×). (**f**) In some areas the expression of CD30 is more focal and predominates in the large atypical cells, with few small cells also expressing this protein (DAB; 200×)

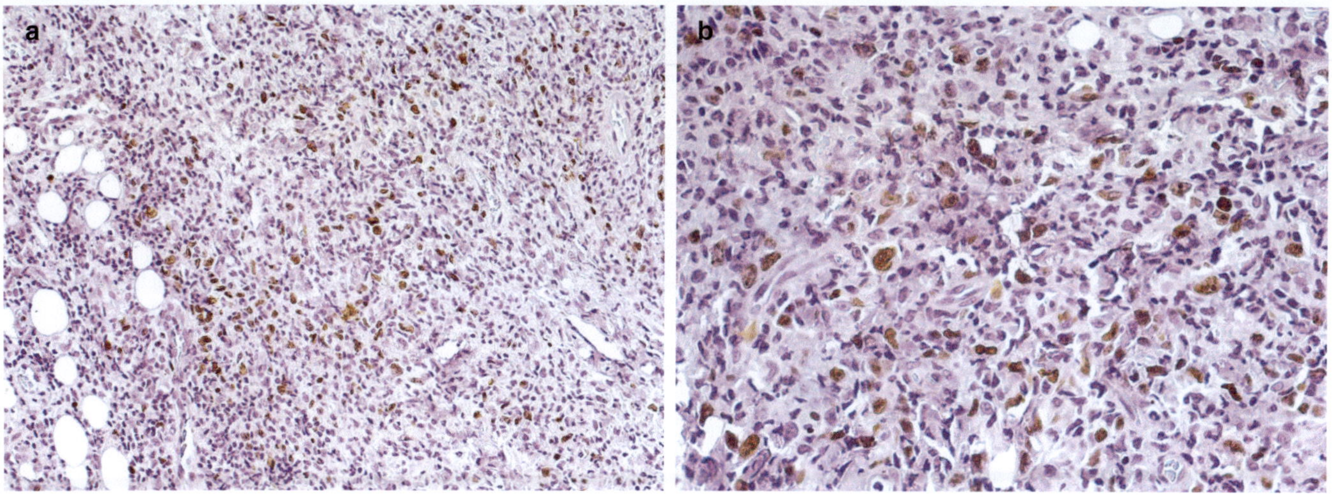

Fig. 23.7 Immunohistochemical features of post-transplant polymorphic lymphoproliferative disorder affecting the oral cavity. (**a**) The proliferative index measured by Ki67 varies significantly from case to case, and also in the same case, it is higher in some regions but lower in others (DAB; 100×). (**b**) Observe the nuclear expression of Ki67 in the small and large cells of this PTLD (DAB; 200×)

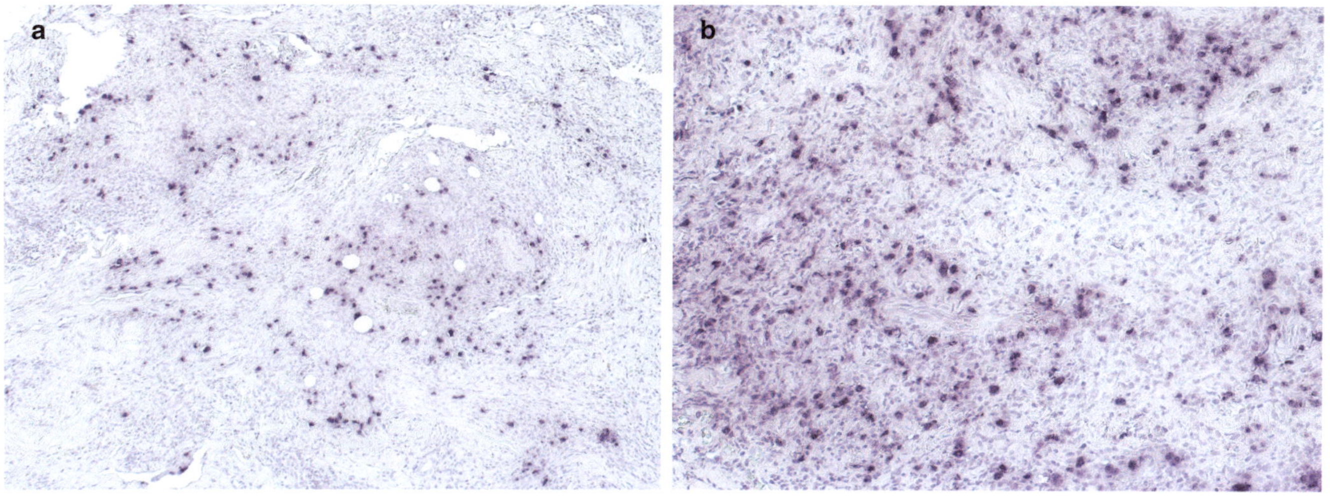

Fig. 23.8 In situ hybridization for EBV detection (EBER) in the post-transplant polymorphic lymphoproliferative disorder affecting the oral cavity. (**a**) The presence of EBV is demonstrated in the dark blue nuclei of this PTLD affecting the gingival tissue of a previously renal transplanted patient (EBER; 50×). (**b**) Observe the nuclear presence of EBV in this polymorphic PTLD (EBER; 100×)

Sources

1. Ojha J, Islam N. Post-transplant lymphoproliferative disorders of oral cavity. Oral Surg Oral Med Oral Pathol Oral Radiol Endod. 2008;105(5):589–96.
2. León JE, Takahama Júnior A, Vassallo J, Soares FA, de Almeida OP, Lopes MA. EBV-associated polymorphic posttransplant lymphoproliferative disorder presenting as gingival ulcers. Int J Surg Pathol. 2011;19(2):241–6. https://doi.org/10.1177/1066896909353599.
3. Akbas A, Tiede C, Lemound J, Maecker-Kolhoff B, Kreipe H, Hussein K. Post-transplant lymphoproliferative disorders with naso- and oropharyngeal manifestation. Transpl Int. 2015;28:1299–307. https://doi.org/10.1111/tri.12632.
4. Krasuska-Sławińska E, Minko-Chojnowska I, Pawłowska J, Dembowska-Bagińska B, Pronicki M, Olczak-Kowalczyk D. Post-transplant lymphoproliferative disorder (PTLD) manifesting in the oral cavity of a 13-year-old liver transplant recipient (LTx). Ann Transplant. 2015;20:478–82. https://doi.org/10.12659/AOT.893497.
5. Amorim Pellicioli AC, Luciano AA, Rangel AL, de Oliveira GR, Santos Silva AR, de Almeida OP, et al. Epstein-Barr virus (EBV)--associated posttransplant lymphoproliferative disorder appearing as mandibular gingival ulcers. Oral Surg Oral Med Oral Pathol Oral Radiol. 2016;121(4):e80–6. https://doi.org/10.1016/j.oooo.2015.07.029.
6. Natkunam Y, Gratzinger D, Chadburn A, Goodlad JR, Chan JKC, Said J, et al. Immunodeficiency-associated lymphoproliferative disorders: time for reappraisal? Blood. 2018;132(18):1871–8. https://doi.org/10.1182/blood-2018-04-842559.
7. Kawaharada M, Maruyama S, Abé T, Yamazaki M, Kurokawa A, Katagiri W, et al. Other iatrogenic immunodeficiency-associated lymphoproliferative disorders in the oral cavity: a clinicopathologic study of 4 cases and literature review. Oral Surg Oral Med Oral Pathol Oral Radiol. 2021;132(6):687–97. https://doi.org/10.1016/j.oooo.2021.05.015.

8. Quintanilla-Martinez L, Swerdlow SH, Tousseyn T, Barrionuevo C, Nakamura S, Jaffe ES. New concepts in EBV-associated B, T, and NK cell lymphoproliferative disorders. Virchows Arch. 2023;482:227–44.
9. Atallah-Yunes SA, Salman O, Robertson MJ. Post-transplant lymphoproliferative disorder: update on treatment and novel therapies. Br J Haematol. 2023;201(3):383–95. https://doi.org/10.1111/bjh.18763.
10. Gross TG, Rubinstein JD. Post-transplant lymphoproliferative disease in children, adolescents, and young adults. Hematol Oncol. 2023;41(Suppl 1):48–56. https://doi.org/10.1002/hon.3139.
11. Mah JK, Tam PCK, Chang YC, Saullo JH, Baker AW, Maziarz EK, et al. Limited utility of Epstein-Barr virus (EBV) surveillance for predicting post-transplant lymphoproliferative disorders in adult EBV seropositive lung transplant recipients. J Clin Virol. 2024;176:105758. https://doi.org/10.1016/j.jcv.2024.105758.
12. Toh J, Reitsma AJ, Tajima T, Younes SF, Ezeiruaku C, Jenkins KC, et al. Multi-modal analysis reveals tumor and immune features distinguishing EBV-positive and EBV-negative post-transplant lymphoproliferative disorders. Cell Rep Med. 2024;5(12):101851. https://doi.org/10.1016/j.xcrm.2024.101851.
13. El-Mallawany NK, Rouce RH. EBV and post-transplant lymphoproliferative disorder: a complex relationship. Hematology Am Soc Hematol Educ Program. 2024;2024(1):728–35. https://doi.org/10.1182/hematology.2024000583.
14. Volaric AK, Fedoriw Y. Epstein-Barr virus-associated B-cell lymphoproliferative disorders and lymphomas: diagnostic overlaps and defining features. Hum Pathol. 2025;156:105697. https://doi.org/10.1016/j.humpath.2024.105697.

EBV-Positive Mucocutaneous Ulcer

24

Irene Lafuente Ibáñez de Mendoza,
Pablo Aguirre-Echevarría, José Manuel Aguirre Urizar,
Bruno Augusto Benevenuto de Andrade,
and Felipe Paiva Fonseca

24.1 General Overview and Clinical Presentation

The Epstein-Barr virus (EBV)-positive mucocutaneous ulcer is a benign lymphoproliferative disorder first reported by Dojcinov et al. in 2010 who described 26 patients with ulcerative lesions limited to the oropharynx, skin, and gastrointestinal tract. This condition was then accepted as a distinct clinicopathological entity and recognized by the World Health Organization classification of lymphoid tumors and lesions in its revised fourth edition published in 2017. It is defined as a mucosal or cutaneous ulcer that is histologically characterized by a polymorphous lymphoid infiltrate containing proliferating EBV-positive atypical large B cells and/or Hodgkin/Reed-Sternberg-like cells, more often affecting immunosuppressed patients.

Although it may histologically resemble diffuse large B-cell lymphoma, this entity presents an indolent clinical course and, therefore, should be differentiated from a neoplastic disease. Clonality studies have demonstrated heterogeneous results, with approximately one-third of the cases being associated with clonal immunoglobulin rearrangement. Some reports have claimed local traumatic events in immunosuppressed patients as a possible adjuvant etiologic factor for EBV-positive mucocutaneous ulcers development, although this hypothesis remains to be fully validated. Patients usually do not demonstrate elevated EBV DNA counts in peripheral blood despite the positivity observed by immunohistochemistry and in situ hybridization in the biopsies, suggesting that this condition may rather represent an isolated mucosal EBV-driven lymphoproliferation than a response to a generalized, systemic infection as occurs in other post-transplant lymphoproliferative disorders.

The patients are usually immunosuppressed due to different causes including organ transplantation, age-related immunosenescence, human immunodeficiency virus/acquired immune deficiency syndrome (HIV/AIDS) and other iatrogenic immunosuppressions. Many cases have been reported associated with the use of immunosuppressive drugs such as azathioprine, cyclosporine, micophenolate and more specifically methotrexate (MTX) therapy for different rheumatological conditions, especially patients being treated for rheumatoid arthritis. Patients developing oral ulcerations in the setting of MTX use have been described before the recognition of EBV-positive mucocutaneous ulcer, but most of these lesions were usually not biopsied and microscopically evaluated. Females are usually more affected, and most of the individuals are elderly patients, with a median age of 77 years. The lesion usually manifests as a well-circumscribed, shallow, isolated ulcer in the oral and oropharyngeal mucosa, skin, and gastrointestinal tract, although deep ulcerations and sometimes lesions presenting as through-and-through defects from mucosa to skin have been reported. Cases manifesting as multiple simultaneous mucocutaneous lesions have also been reported. Any region of the oral cavity can be affected, but the tongue and the gingiva are the most common. Affected patients do not have systemic symptoms, lymphadenopathy, hepatosplenomegaly, or bone marrow involvement.

A study developed by Ohata et al. (2017) reported the clinicopathological features of 14 EBV-positive mucocutaneous ulcers in the oral cavity, and the authors stated that oral

I. Lafuente Ibáñez de Mendoza (✉) · J. M. Aguirre Urizar
Department of Stomatology, University of the Basque Country (UPV/EHU), Leioa, Spain
e-mail: irene.lafuente@ehu.eus; josemanuel.aguirre@ehu.eus

P. Aguirre-Echevarría
Pathological Anatomy Service, Donostia University Hospital Osakidetza, University of the Basque Country (UPV/EHU), Donostia, Spain
e-mail: pablo.aguirreechevarria@osakidetza.eus

B. A. B. de Andrade
Department of Oral Diagnosis and Pathology, School of Dentistry, Universidade Federal do Rio de Janeiro, Rio de Janeiro, Brazil

F. P. Fonseca
Department of Oral Surgery and Pathology, School of Dentistry, Universidade Federal de Minas Gerais, Belo Horizonte, Brazil

© The Author(s), under exclusive license to Springer Nature Switzerland AG 2025

F. P. Fonseca et al. (eds.), *Lymphoproliferative and Granulomatous Disorders of the Oral Cavity*,
https://doi.org/10.1007/978-3-031-98844-8_24

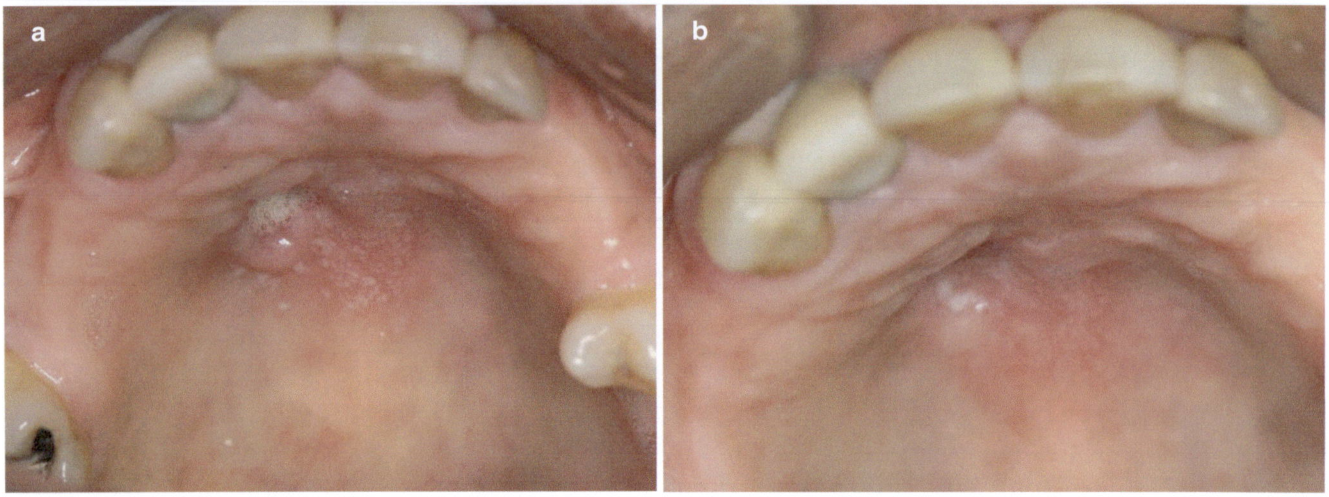

Fig. 24.1 Clinical presentation of EBV-positive mucocutaneous ulcer affecting the oral cavity. (**a**) Female patient on treatment with Methotrexate for rheumatoid arthritis complained of a painful ulcer in the palate with a duration of 2 months. Observe that the ulcer is well defined and superficial, partially covered by a yellowish membrane. (**b**) After 3 weeks of follow-up, the ulcer had already decreased in size without any treatment

EBV-positive B-cell lymphoid proliferation with polymorphous features would often fulfill the criteria for EBV-positive mucocutaneous ulcers, differentiating from diffuse large B-cell lymphomas by not presenting mutations in a specific group of oncogenes and behaving in a more indolent way. Therefore, clinical follow-up is very important for diagnostic confirmation of EBV-positive mucocutaneous ulcers, since the lesion may spontaneously regress and heal after some weeks upon reduction of immunosuppression.

Since EBV-positive mucocutaneous ulcer exhibits an indolent clinical course, conservative treatment strategies are initially recommended, and with the reduction of immunosuppression, remission of the lesion can be seen in most cases. Some authors, however, advocate the use of radiotherapy and chemotherapy for those more aggressive cases. Relapses occur in approximately 15% of the cases, more frequently associated with repeated immunosuppression, and evolution to an overt lymphoma has also been reported (Fig. 24.1).

24.2 Microscopic Findings

- Well-circumscribed ulceration covered by a fibrinopurulent membrane.
- Pseudoepitheliomatous proliferation of the overlying squamous epithelium may be present in some cases.
- Diffuse growth pattern of the lymphoid infiltrate in the lamina propria.
- Extensive to scant fibrous stroma.
- Areas of tissue necrosis and vascular thrombosis.
- The lymphoid infiltrate present in the connective tissue is polymorphous.
- Variable number of small cells, immunoblasts, large atypical B-cells, and Hodgkin or Reed-Sternberg-like cells.
- Variable number of inflammatory cells such as plasma cells, histiocytes, eosinophils and neutrophils.
- Apoptotic cells, necrosis and angioinvasion can be seen in some cases, and these cases should be differentiated from extranodal NK/T-cell lymphoma.
- The periphery and the base of the ulcer is usually well demarcated and well circumscribed, with the presence of many small lymphocytes, predominantly representing T lymphocytes.
- Ikeda et al. (2020) divided EBV-positive mucocutaneous ulcers in four different microscopic subtypes: (1) *Polymorphous type*, presents small to large atypical EBER-positive lymphoid cells, densely or scattered distributed, and with necrosis and angioinvasion; (2) *Large cell-rich type*, presents atypical lymphoid cells as large and monomorphic cells with dense proliferations, resembling diffuse large B-cell lymphoma; (3) *Classic Hodgkin lymphoma-like type*, presents many Hodgkin or Reed-Sternberg-like cells and various sized atypical lymphoid cells, and (4) *Mucosa-associated lymphoid tissue (MALT) lymphoma-like type*, presents small to medium sized atypical lymphoid cells, with centrocytic-like features, and/or plasmacytic features.
- EBV-positive mucocutaneous ulcers, comprised of small lymphocytic infiltration without cellular atypia, have also been reported (Figs. 24.2 and 24.3).

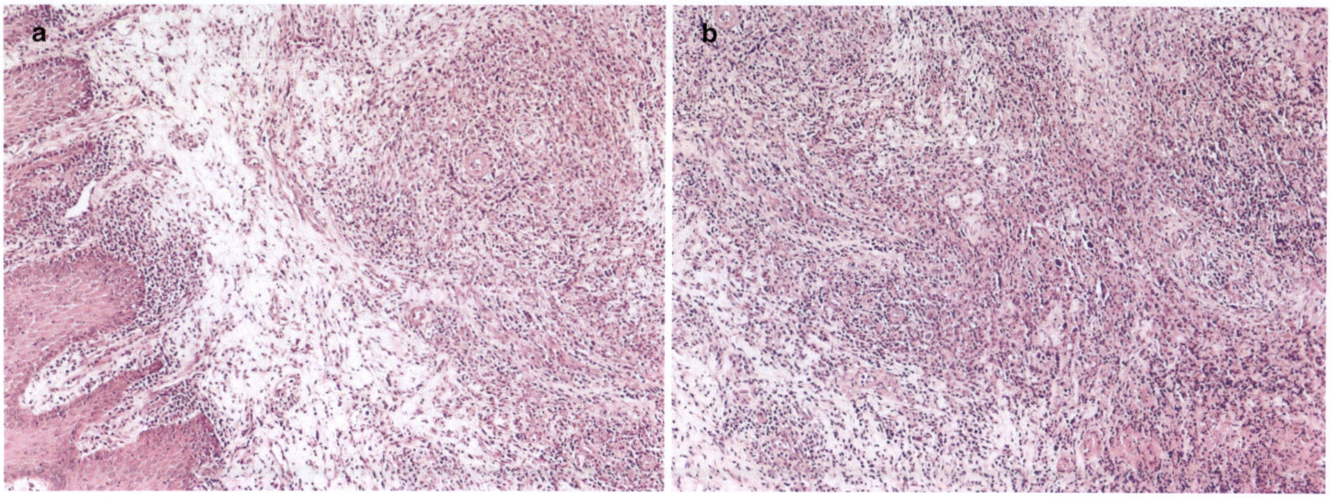

Fig. 24.2 Microscopic features of EBV-positive mucocutaneous ulcer affecting the oral cavity. (**a**) Squamous epithelium of the oral mucosa is seen in the left side of the image, while the lamina propria exhibits an intense lymphoid infiltrate that proliferates near to the epithelium d also deeper (H&E; 50×). (**b**) Diffuse proliferation of lymphoid cells in the lamina propria. There were scattered cells exhibiting pleomorphism. The stroma is fibrotic and there was no necrotic focus (H&E; 50×)

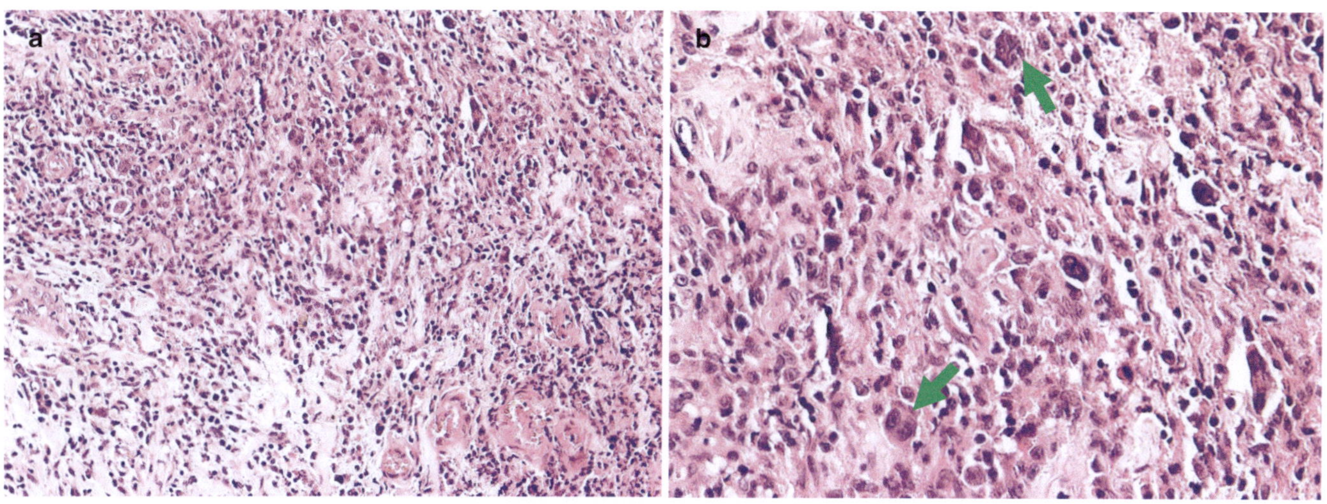

Fig. 24.3 Microscopic features of EBV-positive mucocutaneous ulcer affecting the oral cavity. (**a**) Lymphoid proliferation with the presence of scattered larger cells showing nuclear pleomorphism (H&E; 100×). (**b**) Reed-Sternberg-like cells with binucleated nucleus and prominent nucleoli (green arrow) is a frequent finding in EBV-positive mucocutaneous ulcers (H&E; 200×)

24.3 Immunohistochemistry and/or Genetics

The EBV-positive mucocutaneous ulcer reveals positivity to CD20 in both small B lymphocytes and in the large atypical cells resembling Hodgkin or Reed-Sternberg-like cells, which also demonstrate positivity to other mature Bcell markers like PAX5 and CD79a. The expression of CD3 is often observed in a varied number of small cells representing T lymphocytes. More often these T lymphocytes express CD8 protein and cytotoxic markers. The atypical cells are also frequently positive for CD30 protein, but they only unusually show CD15 expression. EBV is demonstrated by immunohistochemistry targeting LMP1 protein or by in situ hybridization (EBER), suggesting a predominance of Type II latency for the virus. The presence of other reactive cellular populations can be demonstrated by CD68 (histiocytes) and CD138/MUM1 (plasma cells). Proliferative index is variable and Ki67 expression can achieve up to 50% in some cases.

It is accepted that immunoglobulin gene rearrangements can be observed in a proportion of the cases, achieving up to 50% of the reports, which is speculated to be a consequence of possible clonal expansions of EBV-infected B cells; therefore, immunoglobulin rearrangement is not useful to differentiate EBV-positive mucocutaneous ulcer from diffuse large B-cell lymphoma. The occurrence of T-cell receptor rearrangements is reported to be present in up to 31% of the cases. Volaric et al. (2024) used Next Generation Sequency to investigate the molecular basis of 10 EBV-positive mucocutaneous ulcers, demonstrating the loss of function of *TET2* variants in up to 30% of their sample, in addition to loss of function in *DNMT3A* and missense variants in the *IRF8* gene; however, the authors stated that their findings were not specific, demanding further studies to elucidate any possible clinical significance (Table 24.1, Figs. 24.4, 24.5, 24.6, 24.7 and 24.8).

Table 24.1 Summary of the main immunohistochemical reactions used for EBV-positive mucocutaneous ulcer diagnosis

Antibody/probe	Most frequent results	Pattern	Objective
CD20	Positive	Membrane	To demonstrate the large atypical B cells in the lesion
CD3	Positive	Membrane	To demonstrate the T cells in the lesion
MUM1	Positive	Nucleus	To demonstrate the plasma cells in the lesion
CD68	Positive	Cytoplasm	To demonstrate the presence of histiocytes in the lesion
CD30	Positive	Membrane	Characteristically positive in the large B cells
CD15	Variably positive	Membrane	It is rarely positive in the large B cells
Ki67	Variable	Nucleus	To demonstrate the proliferative index of the lesion
LMP1	Positive	Membrane	To demonstrate the presence of EBV
EBER[a]	Positive	Nucleus	To demonstrate the presence of EBV

The EBV status is also described
[a]Investigated by in situ hybridization

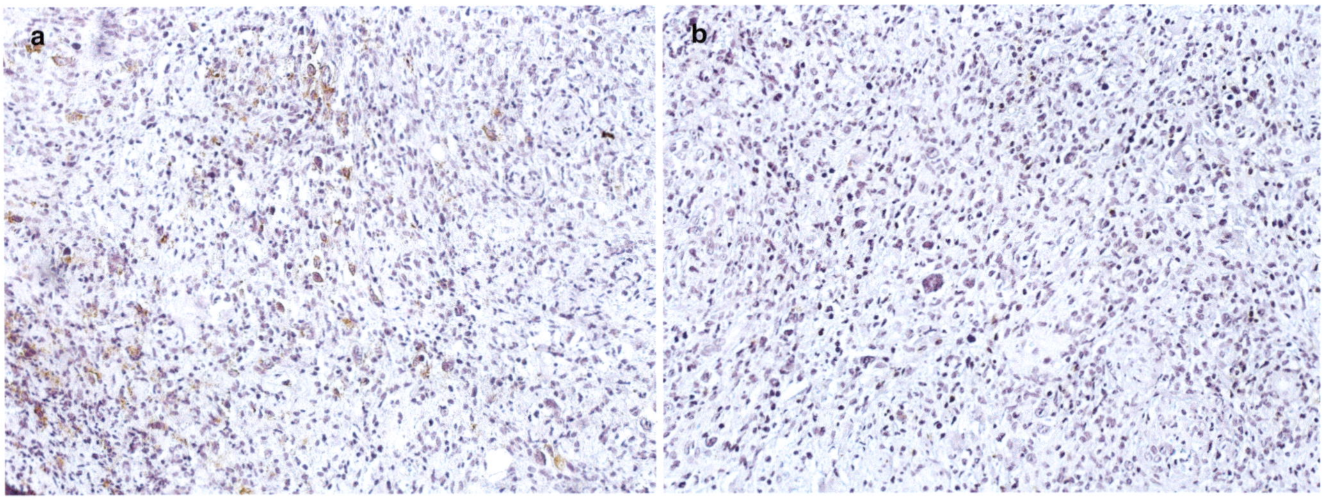

Fig. 24.4 Immunohistochemical features of EBV-positive mucocutaneous ulcer affecting the oral cavity. (**a**) The presence of B lymphocytes is demonstrated by CD20, which also stains positively the larger, pleomorphic cells (DAB; 100×). (**b**) The T-cell population is demonstrated by CD3 staining (DAB; 100×)

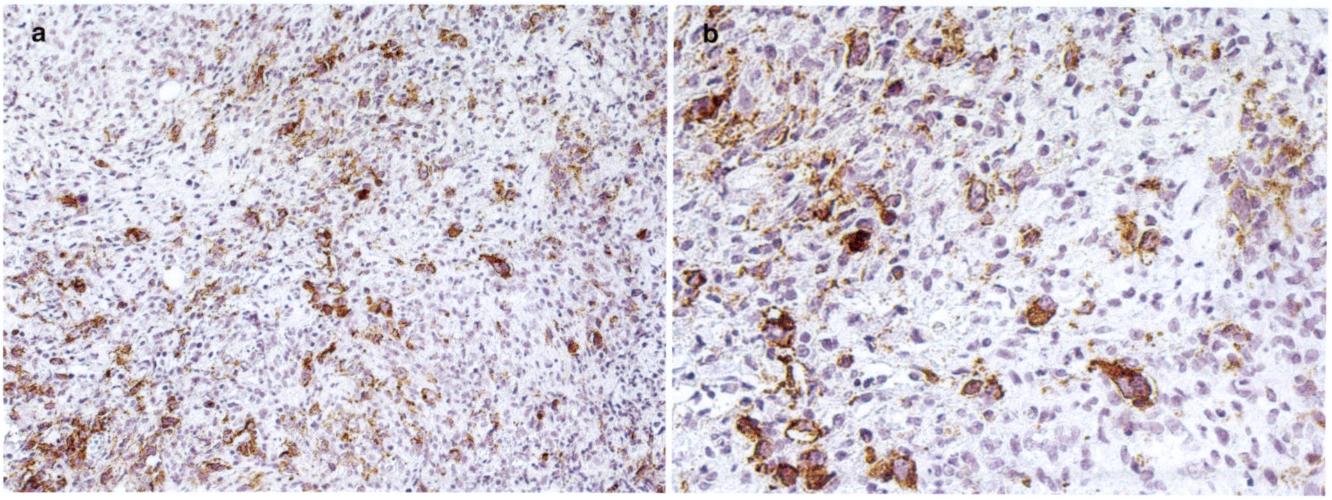

Fig. 24.5 Immunohistochemical features of EBV-positive mucocutaneous ulcer affecting the oral cavity. (**a**) The expression of CD30 in a variable number of cells is a common finding in EBV-positive mucocutaneous ulcers (DAB; 100×). (**b**) Observe that the larger, pleomorphic cells are also positive for CD30 expression (DAB; 200×)

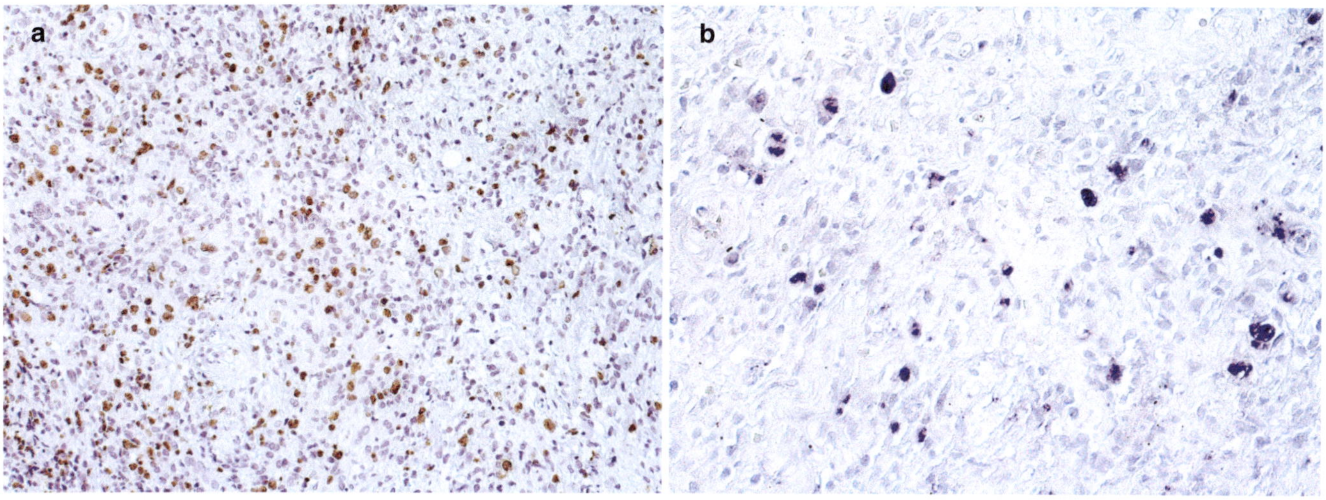

Fig. 24.6 Immunohistochemical features and EBV detection of EBV-positive mucocutaneous ulcer affecting the oral cavity. (**a**) The proliferative rate of EBV-positive mucocutaneous ulcers measured by Ki67 expression varies, but it can be high in some regions, resembling a malignant process (DAB; 100X). (**b**) The presence of EBV is demonstrated predominantly in the pleomorphic cells using in situ hybridization (EBER) (EBER; 200×)

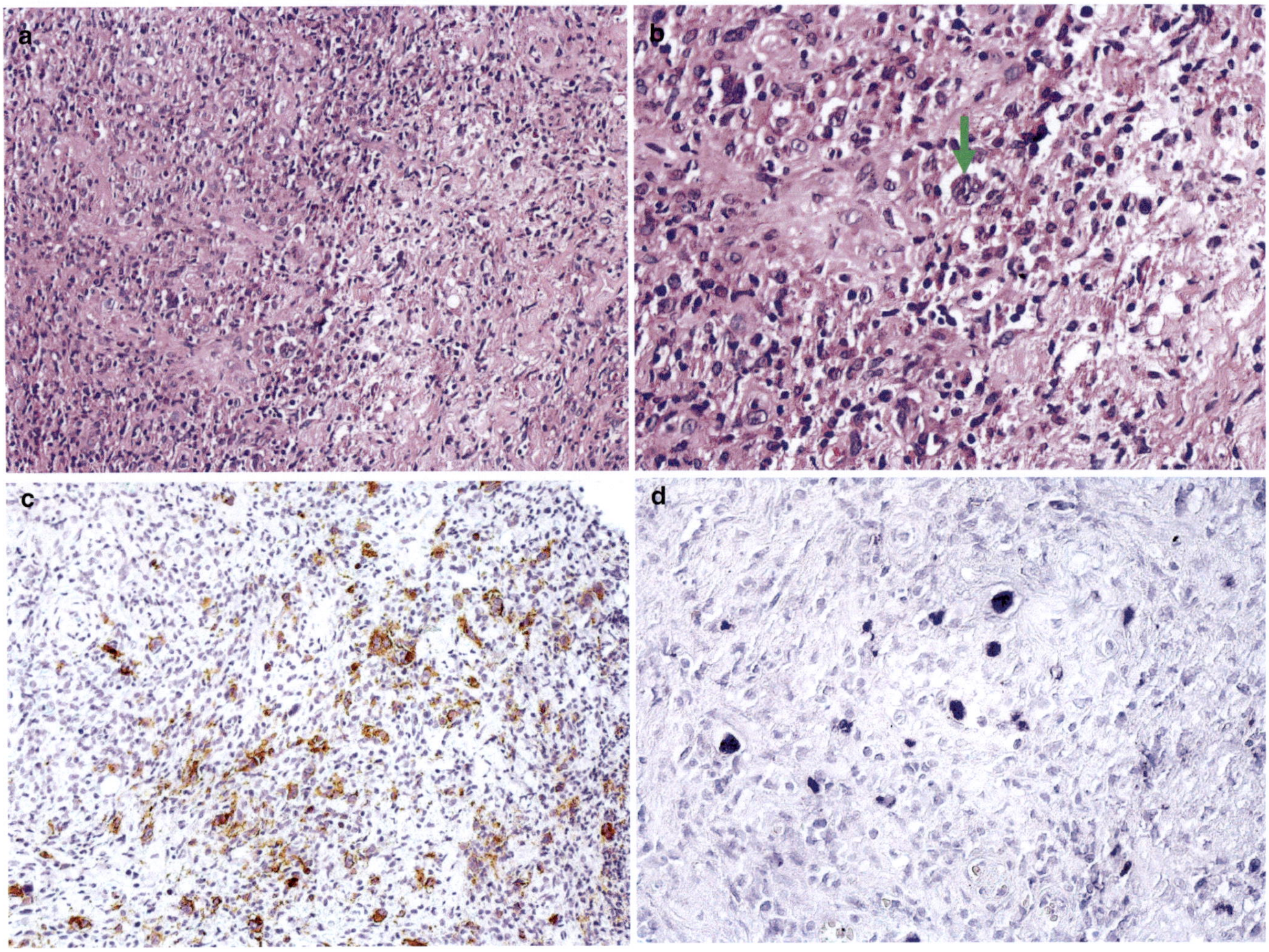

Fig. 24.7 Microscopic features of EBV-positive mucocutaneous ulcer affecting the oral cavity of a female patient. (**a**) Diffuse proliferation of lymphoid infiltrate (H&E; 50X). (**b**) Some of the lymphoid cells are larger with pleomorphism. Hodgkin-like and Reed-Sternberg-like cells can be found (green arrow) (H&E; 200X). (**c**) CD30 expression is observed in both small and large cells (DAB; 200X). (**d**) EBV is demonstrated by in-situ hybridization (EBER; 400X)

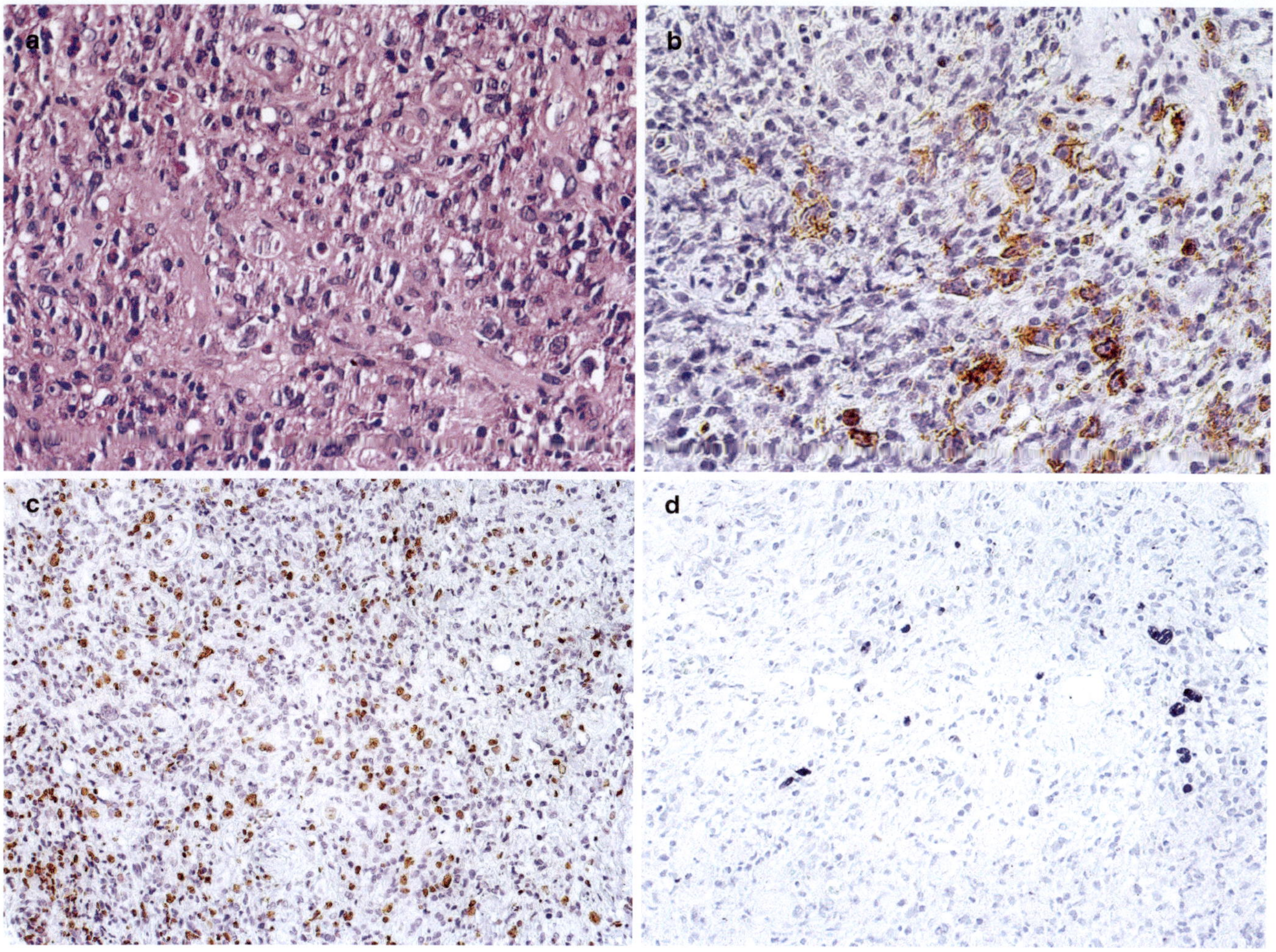

Fig. 24.8 Microscopic and Microscopic features of EBV-positive mucocutaneous ulcer affecting the oral cavity. (**a**) Diffuse proliferation of lymphoid cells. Some cells are large with a prominent centrally located nucleolus and abundant eosinophilic cytoplasm (H&E; 400X). (**b**) Observe the expression of CD30 protein (H&E; 400X). (**c**) This disorder may show a high proliferative rate, as demonstrated by the expression of Ki67 (DAB; 200X). (**d**) Scattered EBV-positive cells shown by in-situ hybridization (EBER; 200X)

Sources

1. Dojcinov SD, Venkataraman G, Raffeld M, Pittaluga S, Jaffe ES. EBV positive mucocutaneous ulcer—a study of 26 cases associated with various sources of immunosuppression. Am J Surg Pathol. 2010;34:405–17.
2. Hart M, Thakral B, Yohe S, Balfour HH Jr, Singh C, Spears M, et al. EBV-positive mucocutaneous ulcer in organ transplant recipients: a localized indolent posttransplant lymphoproliferative disorder. Am J Surg Pathol. 2014;38(11):1522–9. https://doi.org/10.1097/PAS.0000000000000282.
3. Bunn B, van Heerden W. EBV-positive mucocutaneous ulcer of the oral cavity associated with HIV/AIDS. Oral Surg Oral Med Oral Pathol Oral Radiol. 2015;120(6):725–32. https://doi.org/10.1016/j.oooo.2015.06.028.
4. Roberts TK, Chen X, Liao JJ. Diagnostic and therapeutic challenges of EBV-positive mucocutaneous ulcer: a case report and systematic review of the literature. Exp Hematol Oncol. 2016;5:13. https://doi.org/10.1186/s40164-016-0042-5.
5. Ohata Y, Tatsuzawa A, Ohyama Y, Ichikawa A, Mochizuki Y, Ishibashi S, et al. A distinctive subgroup of oral EBV+ B-cell neoplasm with polymorphous features is potentially identical to EBV+ mucocutaneous ulcer. Hum Pathol. 2017;69:129–39. https://doi.org/10.1016/j.humpath.2017.09.013.
6. Prieto-Torres L, Eraña I, Gil-Redondo R, Gómez de la Riva I, Manso R, Pajares R, et al. The Spectrum of EBV-positive mucocutaneous ulcer: a study of 9 cases. Am J Surg Pathol. 2019;43(2):201–10. https://doi.org/10.1097/PAS.0000000000001186.
7. Satou A, Banno S, Hanamura I, Takahashi E, Takahara T, Nobata H, et al. EBV-positive mucocutaneous ulcer arising in rheumatoid arthritis patients treated with methotrexate: single center series of nine cases. Pathol Int. 2019;69(1):21–8. https://doi.org/10.1111/pin.12745.
8. Ikeda T, Gion Y, Sakamoto M, Tachibana T, Nishikori A, Nishimura MF, et al. Clinicopathological analysis of 34 Japanese patients with EBV-positive mucocutaneous ulcer. Mod Pathol. 2020;33:2437–48. https://doi.org/10.1038/s41379-020-0599-8.
9. Li DTS, Lo AWI, Su YX. Oral Epstein-Barr virus-positive mucocutaneous ulcer: gingival presentation of a benign lymphoproliferative lesion. Int J Oral Maxillofac Surg. 2020;49(10):1351–4. https://doi.org/10.1016/j.ijom.2020.01.008.
10. Hyrcza MD, Lindenmuth TR, Auerbach A. Top ten lymphoproliferative lesions not to miss when evaluating oral ulcer biopsies. Head Neck Pathol. 2023;17(1):99–118. https://doi.org/10.1007/s12105-023-01532-2.
11. Sawada K, Momose S, Iijima Y, Takahashi T, Kaneko T, Yamamoto W, et al. EBV-positive mucocutaneous ulcer arising in methotrexate-treated rheumatoid arthritis patients: a clinicopathological study of 12 cases with analysis of PD-L1 expression. J Clin Exp Hematop. 2023;63(2):90–8. https://doi.org/10.3960/jslrt.22048.
12. Macklin PS, Fisher R, Stonard C, Matin RN, Ieremia E. Skin-limited, methotrexate-associated Epstein-Barr virus-positive mucocutaneous ulcer-a mimicker of high-grade lymphoma. A report of 4 cases and review of the literature. Am J Dermatopathol. 2023;45(8):519–31. https://doi.org/10.1097/DAD.0000000000002419.
13. Hong YR, Kwon JS, Ahn HJ, Han SY, Cho E, Kim BE. Importance of differential diagnosis of EBV mucocutaneous ulcer and EBV-positive diffuse large B-cell lymphoma: a case report. Medicine (Baltimore). 2024;103(8):e37243. https://doi.org/10.1097/MD.0000000000037243.
14. Volaric AK, Kumar J, Nicholas V, Saleem A, Fernandez-Pol S, Suarez CJ, et al. Targeted mutational profiling of Epstein Barr virus-positive mucocutaneous ulcer: implications for differential diagnosis with EBV-positive diffuse large B-cell lymphoma. Ann Diagn Pathol. 2024;73:152344. https://doi.org/10.1016/j.anndiagpath.2024.152344.
15. Alphonsus L, Zhang Q, Jairath V. Multifocal Epstein-Barr virus-positive mucocutaneous ulcers in a patient with Crohn's disease. ACG Case Rep J. 2024;11(9):e01468. https://doi.org/10.14309/crj.0000000000001468.
16. Lafuente-Ibáñez de Mendoza I, Aguirre-Echevarria P, Silva-Soria TM, Aisa FJV, de Larrinoa AF, Aguirre-Urizar JM. Peri-implant Epstein-Barr virus (+) mucocutaneous ulcer in an immunocompetent patient: case report and review of the literature. Clin Implant Dent Relat Res. 2025;27(1):e13440. https://doi.org/10.1111/cid.13440.

IgG4-Related Disease

25

Syed Ali Khurram, Luiz Alcino Monteiro Gueiros, Ciro Dantas Soares, and Felipe Paiva Fonseca

25.1 General Overview and Clinical Presentation

IgG4-related disease (IgG4-RD) is a fibroinflammatory, immune-mediated condition characterized by the formation of tumor-like sclerosing lesions. It is often misdiagnosed as aggressive neoplasms, infection or other immunological conditions due to its overlapping clinical features. First recognized as a distinct clinicopathological entity by a Japanese group in 2001, it was initially described in patients with sclerosing pancreatitis demonstrating elevated IgG4 levels. However, the pathogenesis of IgG4-RD remains poorly understood. Although the elevated IgG4 levels are commonly observed in this disorder, the precise role of IgG4 in its pathogenesis has not been definitively established. Current evidence suggests that elevated IgG4 is more accurately viewed as a marker of the disease rather than a causative factor, but further research is needed to clarify IgG4's role in the underlying mechanisms of the disorder. The exact incidence of IgG4-RD is unknown, and numerous cases have been reported in Asia, but it is still unclear if there is a true increased incidence of the disease in this region or if this high number of reports is a consequence of a higher awareness of the condition by clinicians and pathologists.

S. A. Khurram (✉)
School of Clinical Dentistry, Faculty of Health, University of Sheffield, Sheffield, UK
e-mail: s.a.khurram@sheffield.ac.uk

L. A. M. Gueiros
Department of Clinic and Preventive Dentistry, Federal University of Pernambuco, Recife, Pernambuco, Brazil
e-mail: luiz.mgueiros@ufpe.br

C. D. Soares
Laboratório de Patologia Getúlio Sales, Natal, Brazil

F. P. Fonseca
Department of Oral Surgery and Pathology, School of Dentistry, Universidade Federal de Minas Gerais, Belo Horizonte, Brazil

As understanding of IgG4-RD has evolved, several conditions previously considered distinct—such as Mikulicz's disease, Kuttner's tumor, autoimmune pancreatitis, interstitial nephritis, prostatitis, inflammatory aortic aneurysm, retroperitoneal fibrosis—are now recognized as part of the spectrum of IgG4-RD. These conditions are thought to represent various organ-specific manifestations of the same fibroinflammatory process. To standardize research and ensure consistent terminology in the literature, it is recommended to use the term "IgG4-related" followed by the appropriate organ inflammation designation (e.g., sialadenitis, pancreatitis, cholangitis, dacryoadenitis, thyroiditis, etc.) to describe specific clinical presentations. This approach improves clarity in diagnosis and communication within the medical community.

Initially, the diagnosis of IgG4-RD was primarily based on its histological features, which included a dense lymphoplasmacytic infiltrate with a high number of IgG4-positive plasma cells, abundant storiform fibrosis, and obliterative phlebitis, all of which can gradually lead to impaired organ function. However, microscopic evaluations were not always accessible, and these characteristics were not consistently present in all cases. As a result, in 2019, the American College of Rheumatology (ACR) and European League Against Rheumatism (EULAR) proposed a new set of classification criteria that incorporates a broader range of clinical and laboratorial features while ensuring the exclusion of other plausible diagnoses.

Additionally, the Ministry of Health, Labor and Welfare of Japan introduced a significant guideline in 2011, updated in 2021, which recommends a diagnostic approach based on three critical domains: (1) clinical and radiological features, (2) serological diagnosis, and (3) pathological findings. These guidelines highlight the complexity of diagnosing IgG4-RD and emphasize a multidimensional approach to accurately identify cases.

The disease presents with highly variable clinical and laboratorial manifestations, as it can affect nearly any organ.

© The Author(s), under exclusive license to Springer Nature Switzerland AG 2025

F. P. Fonseca et al. (eds.), *Lymphoproliferative and Granulomatous Disorders of the Oral Cavity*,
https://doi.org/10.1007/978-3-031-98844-8_25

The pancreas is the most commonly involved, while brain parenchyma, bone, and synovial tissue are rarely affected. Lymph nodes are also frequently implicated, and the head and neck region is the second most common site, particularly the major salivary glands. While serum IgG4 levels are often used for diagnosis, they have low specificity, as they can also be elevated in other conditions like rheumatoid arthritis, Castleman's disease and systemic sclerosis. Additionally, 30–50% IgG4-RD patients have normal IgG4 serum levels. It primarily affects middle-aged to elderly individuals, with a mean age of 53 years, being more common in females.

Oral lesions are typically asymptomatic and may appear as normal, reddish or red-purple rubbery swellings, usually on the palate, which can be unilateral or bilateral. Other common sites include the jaw bones and tongue, particularly the lateral borders and the ventral surfaces. Gingival involvement manifests as diffuse, erythematous swelling that may cause a burning sensation, while gnathic bone involvement leads to nonspecific bone destruction, demonstrating an ill-defined radiolucency. Up to 70% of patients with oral manifestations also exhibit other systemic signs of IgG4-RD, with nearly 80% having elevated serum IgG4 levels (>135 mg/dL).

The diagnostic utility of lower lip minor salivary gland biopsy for IgG4-RD has shown promising specificity and sensibility in some studies, but further validation is demanded. In major salivary glands, asymptomatic enlargement is the primary clinical feature, more often affecting the submandibular glands, whereas parotid involvement is less frequent. Formerly known as Kurtner's tumors or chronic sclerosing sialadenitis, these submandibular gland swellings are now considered part of the IgG4-RD spectrum, characterized by firm, persistent glandular enlargement.

Core needle biopsy provides a smaller pathology specimen to be microscopically evaluated compared to salivary gland surgical specimens, which may potentially limit the use of this scarless technique; however, a recent study demonstrated that when a navigation system was employed during submandibular gland core needle biopsy of suspected IgG4-RD cases, it was possible to obtain well representative samples for pathological analysis, claiming that this less-invasive diagnostic approach could be sufficient for the histological diagnosis of IgG4-RD in the submandibular glands.

IgG4-RD can present either as an indolent condition or with significant morbidity, potentially leading to organ failure due to the fibroinflammatory process. While spontaneous improvement has been reported, corticosteroids remain the standard treatment, often resulting in rapid lesion improvement, though recurrences are common. Alternative therapies include azathioprine, methotrexate, cyclophosphamide, mycophenolate mofetil, and also Rituximab, a monoclonal anti-CD20 antibody. In oral cavity lesions, surgery is frequently used due to initial misdiagnoses as other neoplastic and non-neoplastic conditions, with the final diagnosis based on surgical specimens.

25.2 Microscopic Findings

- Moderate to dense lymphoplasmacytic infiltrate.
- In the lamina propria there are many reactive lymphocytes, but the predominance of plasma cells is reported in most cases.
- Germinal centers and secondary follicles are also frequently observed.
- Fibrosis is commonly observed, but only a subset of these cases shows a storiform pattern of fibrosis.
- Obliterative phlebitis can be found. However, this feature is very difficult to be observed in oral biopsies.
- Pleomorphism or atypical mitoses are not found.
- A variable number of eosinophils is common (Figs. 25.1, 25.2 and 25.3).

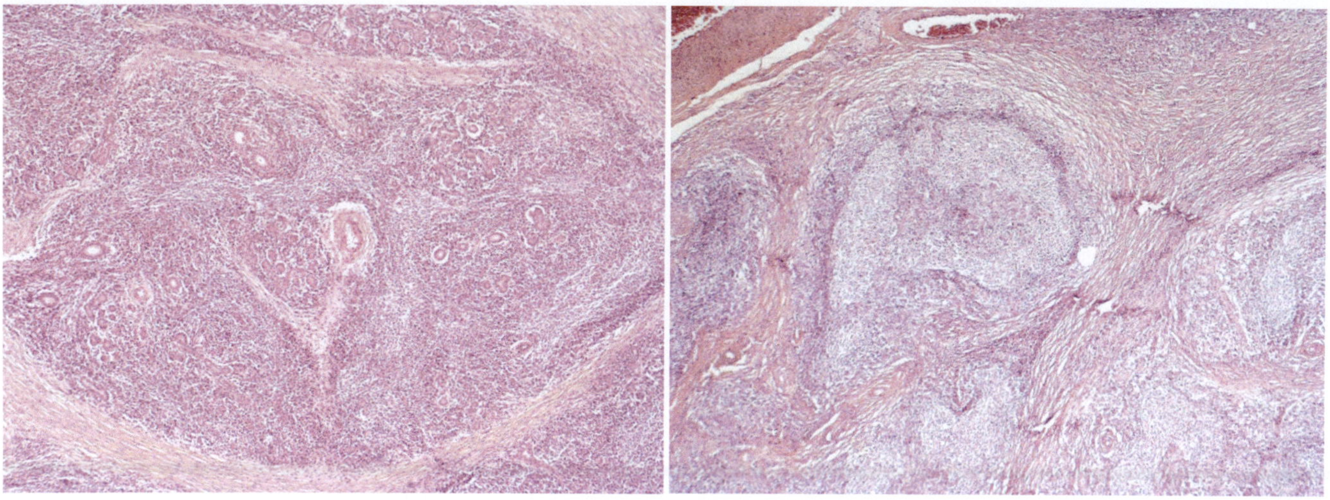

Fig. 25.1 Microscopic features of IgG4-related disease affecting minor salivary glands of the palate. (**a**) The disorder is characterized by a dense lymphoplasmacytic infiltration and extensive areas of stromal fibrosis. (**b**) The occurrence of secondary follicles with the presence of reactive germinal centers is a common finding in IgG4-related disease and, together with the presence of stromal fibrosis and a large amount of plasma cells, demands from pathologists a careful analysis to rule out a possible IgG4-related disease diagnosis

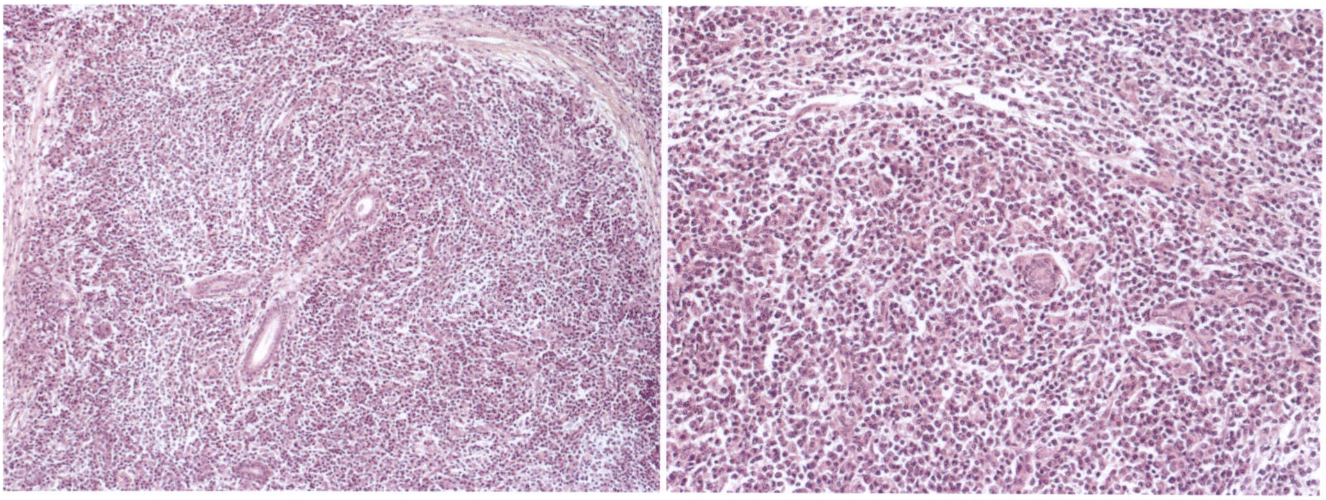

Fig. 25.2 Microscopic features of IgG4-related disease affecting minor salivary glands of the palate. (**a**) Presence of a dense lymphoplasmacytic infiltration surrounding residual atrophic salivary gland ducts. (**b**) There is a predominance of plasma cells in the lymphoplasmacytic infiltrate

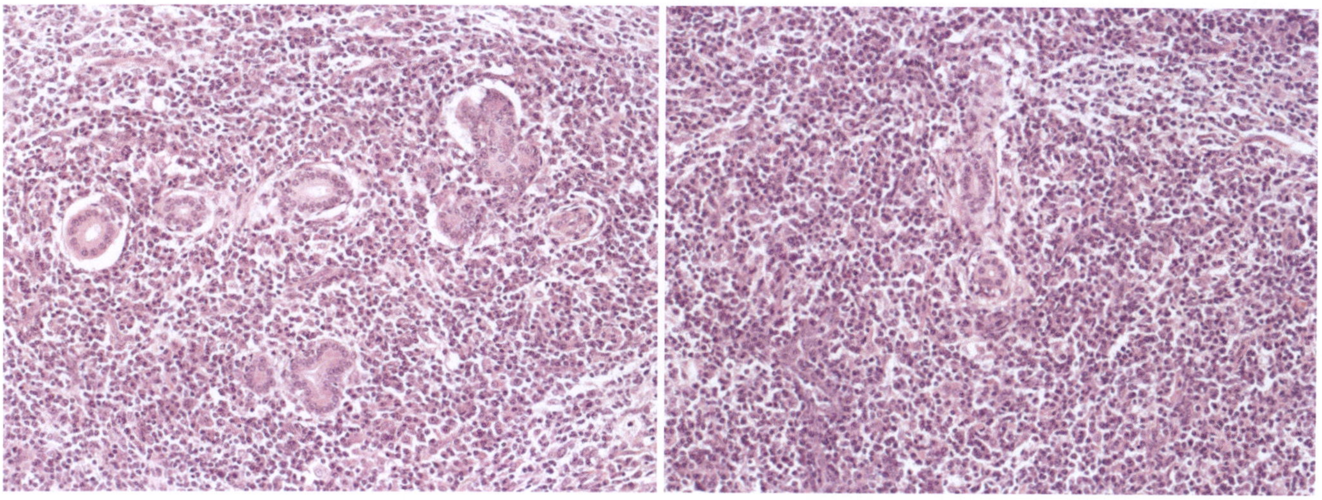

Fig. 25.3 Microscopic features of IgG4-related disease affecting minor salivary glands of the palate. (**a**) Observe the presence of residual atrophic salivary gland ducts surrounded by the lymphoplasmacytic infiltrate. (**b**) Large number of plasma cells in the IgG4-related disease

25.3 Immunohistochemistry

Immunohistochemistry is useful for detecting increased IgG4-positive plasma cells, but not all cases exhibit a high IgG4-positive/IgG-positive plasma cell ratio and the occurrence of IgG4-positive cells is not exclusively found in IgG4-RD specimens; for instance, an elevated number of IgG4-positive plasma cells has also been described in a few samples obtained from sialadenitis associated with sialolithiasis and from nonspecific forms of sialadenitis that do not comply with full diagnostic criteria for IgG4-RD.

It is accepted that a value exceeding 40% is more diagnostic valuable than the absolute count of IgG4-positive cells in a high-power field. Lower lip biopsies have shown potential diagnostic value for IgG4-RD, though their reproducibility and reliability require further validation. The immune infiltrate typically includes CD20-positive (B lymphocytes) and CD3-positive (T lymphocytes) cells, and many plasma cells that can be better appreciated by CD138/MUM1/EMA expression, supporting a reactive process, which is further demonstrated by the absence of Kappa and Lambda monoclonality. Additionally, BCL2-negative germinal centers and a variable proliferative index (Ki67 expression) further indicate a reactive process (Table 25.1, Figs. 25.4, 25.5, 25.6, 25.7 and 25.8).

Table 25.1 Summary of the main immunohistochemical reactions used for IgG4-RD microscopic characterization

Antibody	Main result	Pattern	Objective
CD20	Positive	Membrane	To investigate a possible B-cell lymphoma
CD3	Positive	Membrane	To investigate a possible T-cell lymphoma
MUM1	Positive	Nucleus	To demonstrate the plasm cell component
CD138	Positive	Membrane	To demonstrate the plasm cell component
EMA	Positive	Membrane	To demonstrate the plasm cell component
BCL2	Negative in the germinal center	Cytoplasm	To demonstrate the reactive nature of the secondary follicles
IgG	Positive	Cytoplasm	To investigate the proportion of IgG4 plasma cells
IgG4	Positive	Cytoplasm	To investigate the proportion of IgG4 plasma cells
Kappa	Polyclonal	Cytoplasm	To demonstrate the polyclonal nature of the lymphoplasmacytic infiltrate
Lambda	Polyclonal	Cytoplasm	To demonstrate the polyclonal nature of the lymphoplasmacytic infiltrate
Ki67	Variable	Nucleus	To demonstrate the proliferative potential of the disease

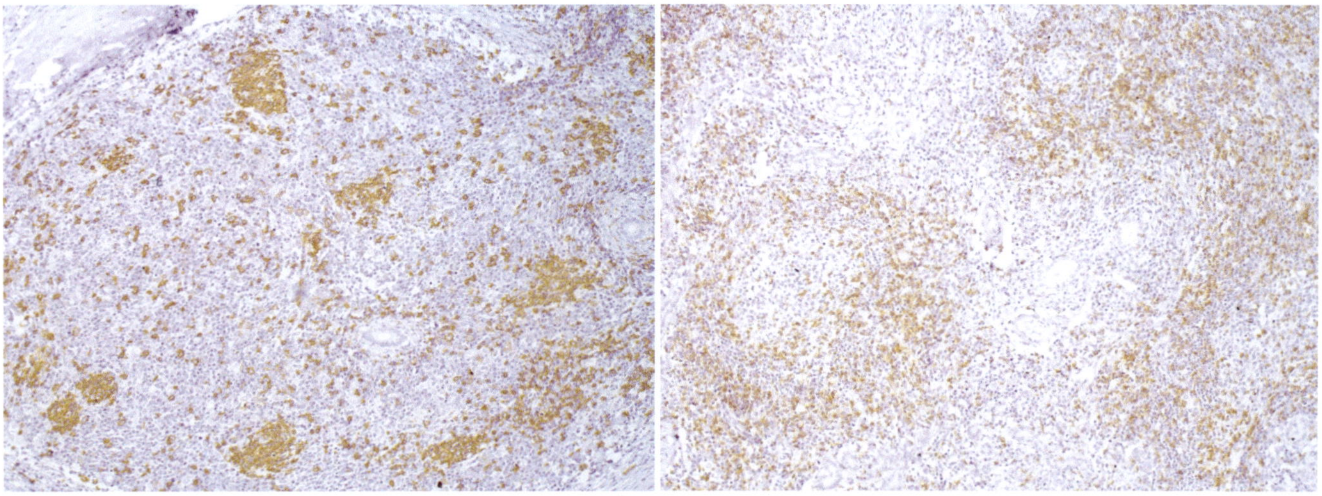

Fig. 25.4 Immunohistochemical features of IgG4-related disease. (**a**) The presence of reactive lymphoid follicles is demonstrated by CD20 expression, which is also expressed by other B lymphocytes distributed in the lymphoplasmacytic infiltrate. (**b**) The presence of T lymphocytes is mainly observed in the interfollicular regions, demonstrated using CD3 staining

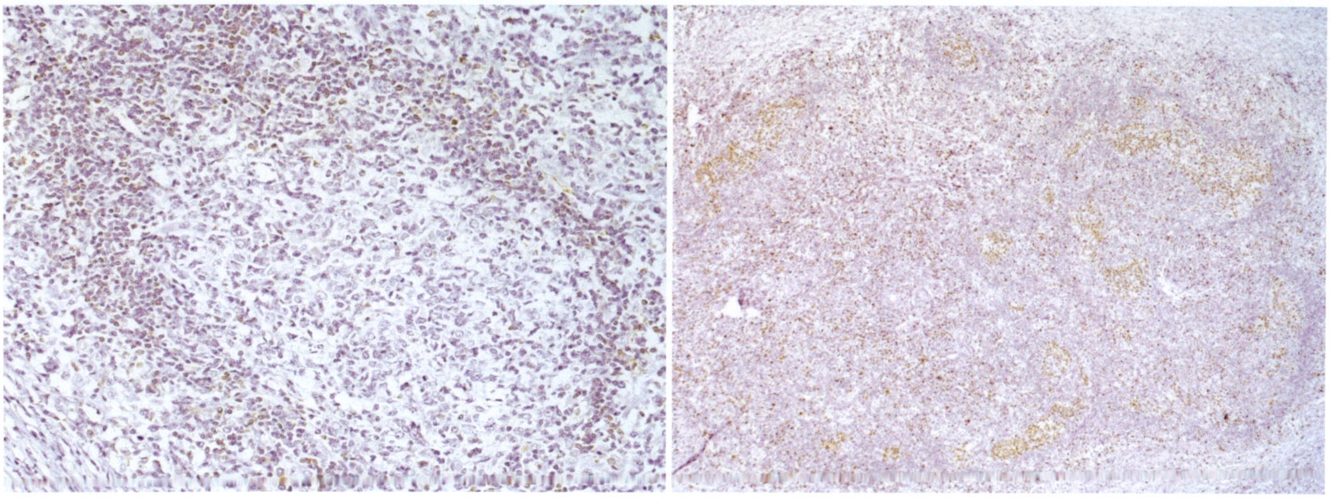

Fig. 25.5 Immunohistochemical features of IgG4-related disease. (**a**) The reactive nature of the lymphoid follicles present in the IgG4-related disease infiltrate is demonstrated by BCL2 expression located in the outer region of the follicles. (**b**) There is an increased proliferative index of cells located in the germinal centers, although many cells distributed through the lymphoplasmacytic infiltrate are also positive for Ki67

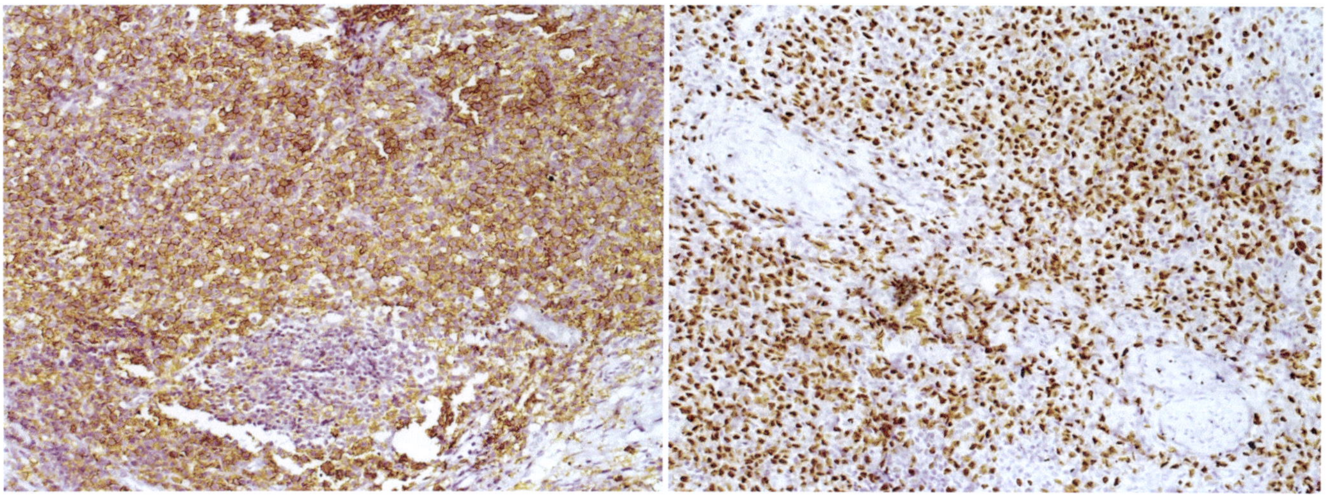

Fig. 25.6 Immunohistochemical features of IgG4-related disease. (**a**) The presence of a large number of plasma cells in the infiltrate can be determined using CD138 expression. (**b**) This finding is further supported by the nuclear expression of MUM1 by the plasma cells

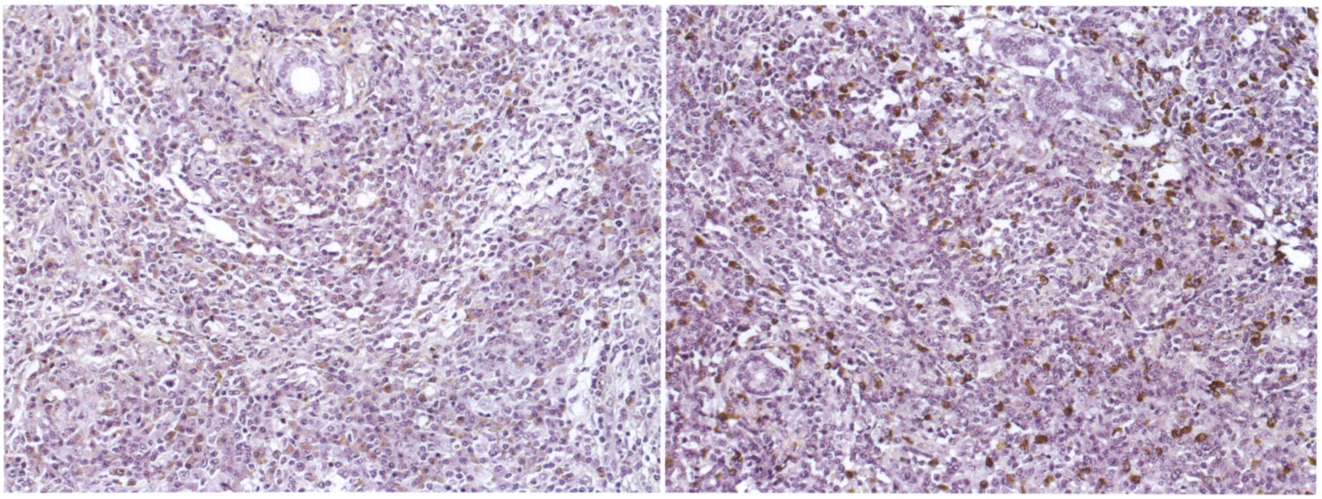

Fig. 25.7 Immunohistochemical features of IgG4-related disease. (**a**) The reactive nature of the plasma cell component present in the infiltrate is supported by the lack of monoclonality investigated using immunoglobulin light chains expression. Observe the expression of kappa light chain, (**b**) and lambda light chain in this case of IgG4-related disease

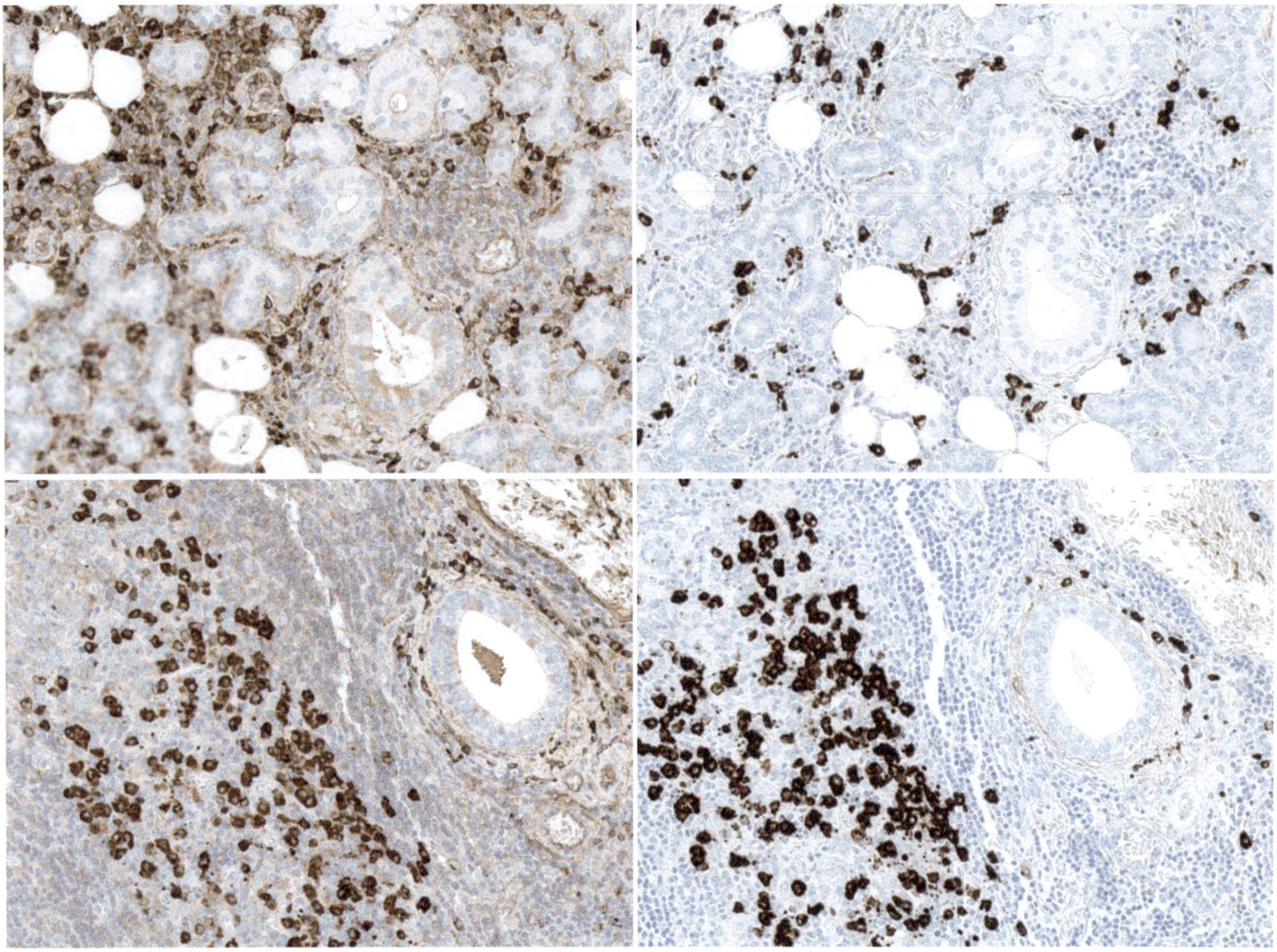

Fig. 25.8 Immunohistochemical features of IgG4-related disease. (**a**) Observe a large number of plasma cells expressing IgG protein. (**b**) Observe now that more than 40% of these cells are expressing IgG4 protein. (**c**) Another example of IgG4-related disease affecting the salivary glands with the expression of IgG. (**d**) In this case there was approximately 60% of IgG4 expression by plasma cells

Sources

1. Abe T, Sato T, Tomaru Y, Sakata Y, Kokabu S, Hori N, et al. Immunoglobulin G4-related sclerosing sialadenitis: report of two cases and review of the literature. Oral Surg Oral Med Oral Pathol Oral Radiol Endod. 2009;108(4):544–50. https://doi.org/10.1016/j.tripleo.2009.06.001.
2. Geyer JT, Ferry JA, Harris NL, Stone JH, Zukerberg LR, Lauwers GY, et al. Chronic sclerosing sialadenitis (Küttner tumor) is an IgG4-associated disease. Am J Surg Pathol. 2010;34(2):202–10. https://doi.org/10.1097/PAS.0b013e3181c811ad.
3. Khurram SA, Fernando M, Smith AT, Hunter KD. IgG4-related sclerosing disease clinically mimicking oral squamous cell carcinoma. Oral Surg Oral Med Oral Pathol Oral Radiol. 2013;115(2):e48–51. https://doi.org/10.1016/j.oooo.2012.04.011.
4. Khosroshahi A, Wallace ZS, Crowe JL, Akamizu T, Azumi A, Carruthers MN, et al. International consensus guidance statement on the management and treatment of IgG4-related disease. Arthritis Rheumatol. 2015;67(7):1688–99. https://doi.org/10.1002/art.39132.
5. Yang WT, Tsai KY. A rare case of oral tumor presenting as first sign of immunoglobulin G4-related disease. Oral Surg Oral Med Oral Pathol Oral Radiol. 2019;128(5):e187–90. https://doi.org/10.1016/j.oooo.2019.03.004.
6. Peuraharju E, Saarinen R, Aro K, Mäkinen LK, Tarkkanen J, Mäkitie A, et al. Sclerosing sialadenitis of the submandibular gland is rarely an immunoglobulin G4-related disease in the Finnish population. Mod Pathol. 2020;33(4):551–9. https://doi.org/10.1038/s41379-019-0395-5.
7. Wallace ZS, Naden RP, Chari S, Choi H, Della-Torre E, Dicaire JF, et al. The 2019 American College of Rheumatology/European League Against Rheumatism classification criteria for IgG4-related disease. Arthritis Rheumatol. 2020;72(1):7–19. https://doi.org/10.1002/art.41120.
8. Rampi A, Lanzillotta M, Mancuso G, Vinciguerra A, Dagna L. IgG4-related disease of the oral cavity. Case series from a large single-center cohort of Italian patients. Int J Environ Res Public Health. 2020;17(21):8179. https://doi.org/10.3390/ijerph17218179.
9. Umehara H, Okazaki K, Kawa S, Takahashi H, Goto H, Matsui S, et al. The 2020 revised comprehensive diagnostic (RCD) criteria for IgG4-RD. Mod Rheumatol. 2021;31(3):529–33. https://doi.org/10.1080/14397595.2020.1859710.
10. Pereira GG, Pontes FSC, Soares CD, de Carvalho MGF, da Silva TA, Calderaro DC, et al. Oral and maxillofacial manifestations of

IgG4-related disease: a clinicopathological study. J Oral Pathol Med. 2022;51(5):493–500. https://doi.org/10.1111/jop.13296.

11. Peuraharju E, Hagström J, Tarkkanen J, Haglund C, Atula T. IgG4-positive plasma cells in nonspecific sialadenitis and sialolithiasis. Mod Pathol. 2022;35(10):1423–30. https://doi.org/10.1038/s41379-022-01089-5.
12. Liu Z, Nie Y, Peng Y, Lu H, Zhang P, Li J, et al. The external validation of the 2019 ACR/EULAR classification criteria for IgG4-related disease in a large cohort from China. Semin Arthritis Rheum. 2023;61:152202. https://doi.org/10.1016/j.semarthrit.2023.152202.
13. Kogami M, Abe Y, Ando T, Makiyama A, Yamaji K, Tamura N. Performance of classification and diagnostic criteria for IgG4-related disease and comparison of patients with and without IgG4-related disease. Sci Rep. 2023;13(1):2509. https://doi.org/10.1038/s41598-023-29645-2.
14. Yamamoto H, Taniguchi Y. Clinical images: hard palate mass as an IgG4-related disease. Arthritis Rheumatol. 2023;75(9):1685. https://doi.org/10.1002/art.42517.
15. Li ZZ, Zhu H, Li W, Gao Y, Su JZ, Yu GY. Utility of navigation system-guided submandibular gland core needle biopsy in the diagnosis of immunoglobulin G4-related sialadenitis. Int J Oral Maxillofac Surg. 2023;52(9):1005–12. https://doi.org/10.1016/j.ijom.2023.01.007.
16. Azzi L, Magnoli F, Krepysheva D, Fontana F, Coppola A, Cappelli A, et al. The "great imitator": IgG4-related disease of the oral cavity. Two case reports and scoping review. Head Neck. 2024;46(6):1510–25. https://doi.org/10.1002/hed.27763.
17. Czarnywojtek A, Agaimy A, Pietrończyk K, Nixon IJ, Vander Poorten V, Mäkitie AA, et al. IgG4-related disease: an update on pathology and diagnostic criteria with a focus on salivary gland manifestations. Virchows Arch. 2024;484(3):381–99. https://doi.org/10.1007/s00428-024-03757-0.
18. Muniz VRVM, Altemani A, Freitas VS, Pires BC, de Santana DA, Couto LA, et al. Chronic sclerosing sialadenitis of the submandibular gland and its histopathological spectrum in the IgG4-related disease: a series of 17 cases. Head Neck Pathol. 2024;18(1):42. https://doi.org/10.1007/s12105-024-01651-4.

Sjögren Disease

26

Luiz Alcino Monteiro Gueiros,
Silvia Ferreira de Sousa,
and Felipe Paiva Fonseca

26.1 General Overview and Clinical Presentation

Sjögren disease, previously termed Sjögren syndrome, is a chronic multisystem autoimmune disorder characterized by the infiltration of lymphoid cells into exocrine gland parenchyma, in particular the salivary and lacrimal glands, leading to a sensation of dry eyes (keratoconjunctivitis sicca) and dry mouth (xerostomia), among other extraglandular manifestations. It is one of the most common rheumatological conditions with a prevalence of 60.8 (95% CI: 43.7–77.9) cases per 100,000 inhabitants, and its diagnosis is often delayed because of its initial presentation as common and isolated symptoms.

The etiology and the pathogenesis of Sjögren's disease have been better investigated during the last decades, but they remain to be fully understood. The development of this complex disease is currently recognized as a multistep disorder triggered by the interplay of environmental, hormonal, and genetic factors, which causes the innate and adaptive immune systems to initiate and perpetuate the pathological inflammatory process that characterizes this condition.

Sjögren disease more often occurs in the fourth to fifth decades of life, with a stronger female predilection (female-to-male ratio of 9:1). Apart from the usual sicca symptoms, Sjögren disease is frequently followed by fatigue and arthralgia. Also, patients may have local complaints such as asymptomatic glandular swellings, as well as several systemic clinical manifestations, including lymphadenopathy, peripheral neuropathy, hematologic disturbances, pulmonary involvement and pain. In addition, it seems to represent a cluster of autoimmunity, commonly overlapping with other autoimmune diseases like systemic lupus erythematosus, rheumatoid arthritis, systemic sclerosis and autoimmune thyroiditis.

Diagnosing Sjögren disease can often be challenging. Over the past few decades, several sets of clinical classification criteria have been proposed, reflecting the lack of a consensual understanding of the disease presentation. In 2016, the American College of Rheumatology and the European League Against Rheumatism (ACR/EULAR) introduced a new set of criteria aimed at standardizing the classification of individuals with suspected Sjögren disease. These criteria are based on five key tests: antinuclear autoantibody [anti-SSA(Ro)] serology, Schirmer's test, ocular staining score, unstimulated salivary flow rate, and minor salivary gland biopsy.

Although the parotid gland biopsy can be used as an auxiliary method for the diagnosis of Sjögren disease, a minor salivary gland biopsy of the lower lip is the standard method for allowing microscopic evaluation. Individuals with Sjögren disease exhibit focal lymphocytic inflammatory infiltration adjacent to the glandular parenchyma. Currently, the methods for morphologic evaluation of the salivary glands were meticulously described as part of the SICCA Alliance (a major research consortium) set of publications. Both parotid and minor salivary gland biopsies offer similar sensitivity and specificity for classifying Sjögren disease, ranging from 63.5% to 93.7% and from 61.2% to 100%, respectively. The use of imaging, particularly ultrasonography, has been increasing, and is now recommended alongside lip biopsy to improve diagnostic accuracy.

Patients with Sjögren disease have a significantly higher risk of developing non-Hodgkin lymphomas, as well as other hematological and non-hematological neoplasms. The pathogenetic pathways that lead to lymphoma development

L. A. M. Gueiros (✉)
Department of Clinic and Preventive Dentistry, Federal University of Pernambuco, Recife, Pernambuco, Brazil
e-mail: luiz.mgueiros@ufpe.br

S. F. de Sousa · F. P. Fonseca
Department of Oral Surgery and Pathology, School of Dentistry, Universidade Federal de Minas Gerais, Belo Horizonte, Brazil
e-mail: silviafsousa@ufmg.br

© The Author(s), under exclusive license to Springer Nature Switzerland AG 2025
F. P. Fonseca et al. (eds.), *Lymphoproliferative and Granulomatous Disorders of the Oral Cavity*,
https://doi.org/10.1007/978-3-031-98844-8_26

in Sjögren disease patients are also still elusive, although much effort has been made to identify risk factors that would allow a more reliable and precise risk stratification for malignancy onset in these patients. The reported prevalence of lymphoma among Sjögren disease patients ranges from 4% to 11%, representing an 8–16 times higher risk of lymphoma development compared to the general population. This risk seems to be significantly higher among women aged 40–49, and reduced after this interval. Non-Hodgkin lymphomas predominate and represent approximately 90% of all cases, while Hodgkin lymphoma accounts for 10% of the total number of lymphomas diagnosed in this group of patients. Among non-Hodgkin lymphomas, marginal zone lymphoma of the mucosa-associated lymphoid tissue (MALT) lymphoma and diffuse large B-cell lymphoma are the most frequently diagnosed subtypes. In addition, multiple myeloma, leukemia and solid tumors also present an increased risk of onset in Sjögren disease patients.

Since patients with Sjögren disease often present multiorgan involvement, multidisciplinary care is typically recommended and involves at least a rheumatologist, an ophthalmologist and an oral medicine specialist. Treatment protocols include the use of antimalarials, steroids and immunosuppressive agents, while various symptomatic treatments, such as artificial saliva, are commonly used to mitigate the effects of xerostomia. Long-term follow-up is essential, with particular attention to the increased risk of dental caries and lymphoma (Figs. 26.1 and 26.2).

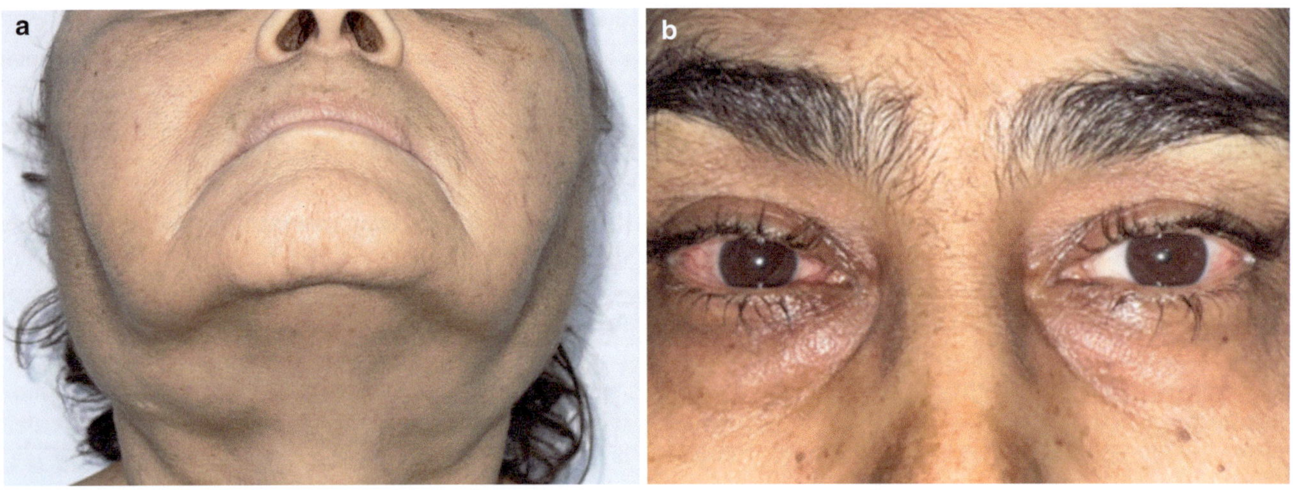

Fig. 26.1 Clinical manifestation of a female patient diagnosed with Sjögren disease. (**a**) Bilateral inflammatory parotitis. (**b**) Scleritis secondary to intense xerophthalmia

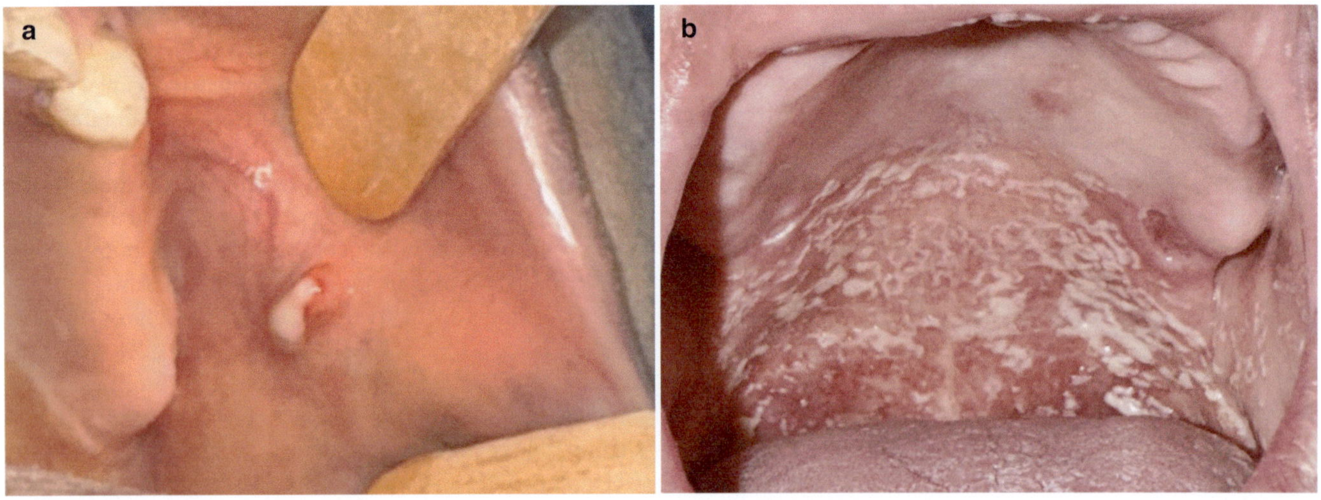

Fig. 26.2 Oral manifestation of patients diagnosed with Sjögren disease. (**a**) Purulent drainage through Stensen's duct in a patient with bacterial sialadenitis. (**b**) Oral candidiasis secondary to intense hyposalivation

26.2 Microscopic Findings

- Aggregates of mononuclear cells (mostly lymphocytes) with ≥50 cells.
- These aggregates predominate around ductal structures.
- Periductal lymphoid foci can be seen in both minor and major salivary glands.
- Degenerative findings like fibrosis or acinar necrosis are acceptable if alongside areas of focal lymphocytic sialadenitis.
- The foci are mainly composed of T- and B-lymphocytes with few other mononuclear cells, including histiocytes and follicular dendritic cells.
- A minority of plasma cells can also be found.
- Secondary lymphoid follicles may develop, with the presence of well-organized germinal centers.
- Lymphocytes exhibit normal morphological features.
- Lymphoepithelial lesions may occur.
- Lymphoepithelial lesions exhibit infiltration of lymphocytes in epithelial cells of ducts, which often show some degree of hyperplasia that may result in complete occlusion of the striated duct (present in approximately 33% of labial and 93% of parotid biopsies of Sjögren disease patients).
- Lymphoid aggregates are predominantly located adjacent to normal-appearing mucous acini, although some foci adjacent to areas with atrophy, duct dilation or interstitial fibrosis may occur.
- There seems to be a relative decrease in the concentration of IgA+ plasma cells and a relative increase of IgG+ and IgM+ plasma cells in Sjögren disease patients compared to normal individuals.
- The biological significance and interpretation of the microscopic presence of lymphocyte aggregates in lower lip biopsied tissue should be strictly correlated with clinical and laboratorial findings, since from 6.2% to 13.1% of the labial biopsies may also show focal lymphocytic sialadenitis in non-Sjögren disease patients.

26.2.1 Evaluating the Focus Score

The presence of focal lymphocytic sialadenitis in lower lip biopsies is a key indicator of Sjögren disease. To ensure accurate focus score quantification, it is recommended to examine at least four minor salivary glands, or six if they are small, with a minimum of 8 mm^2 of glandular tissue available for analysis. This area should exclude epithelium, adipose tissue, and other non-glandular structures. The focus score is determined by counting the lymphocytic sialadenitis foci per 4 mm^2 of glandular area, with a score of ≥1 in labial or parotid biopsies considered indicative of Sjögren disease. In cases where the focus score is between 10 and 12, the foci may merge, and an arbitrary maximum score of 12 is typically used. The diagnostic accuracy of biopsies can be improved by examining multiple tissue sections. If biopsies show varying patterns of lymphoid aggregates or degenerative changes, the diagnosis may be more accurately classified as non-specific chronic sialadenitis or sclerosing chronic sialadenitis, depending on the predominant features observed (Figs. 26.3, 26.4, 26.5, 26.6 and 26.7).

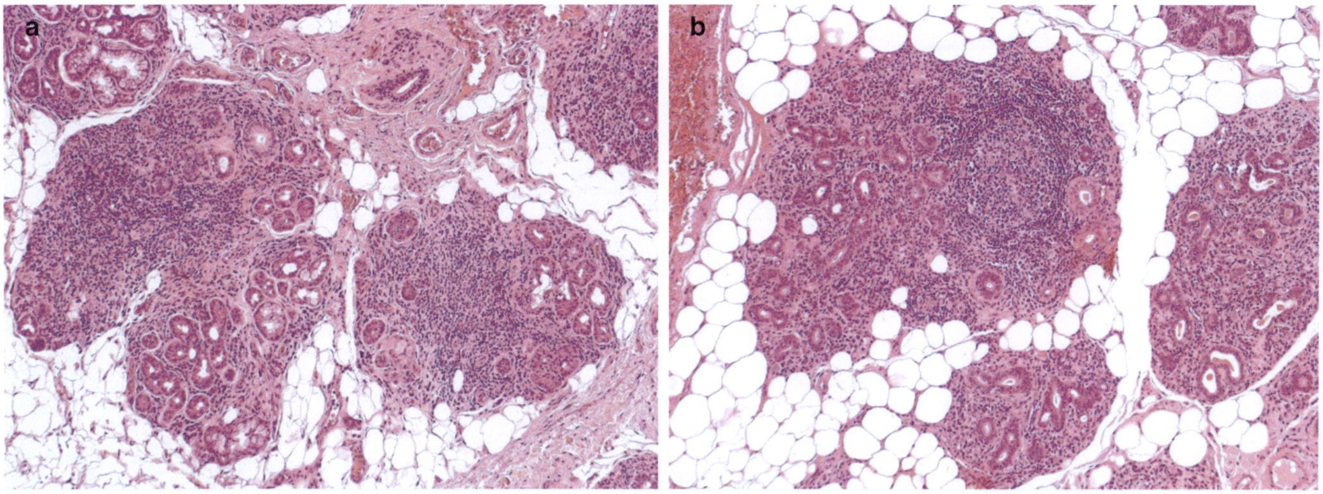

Fig. 26.3 Microscopic features observed after a lower lip biopsy obtained from a patient diagnosed with Sjögren disease. (**a**) Presence of several lymphoplasmacytic foci surrounding the glandular structures, especially the ductal component (H&E; 50×). (**b**) In one of these foci, it is possible to observe the development of a secondary follicle containing the germinal center in the central region (H&E; 50×)

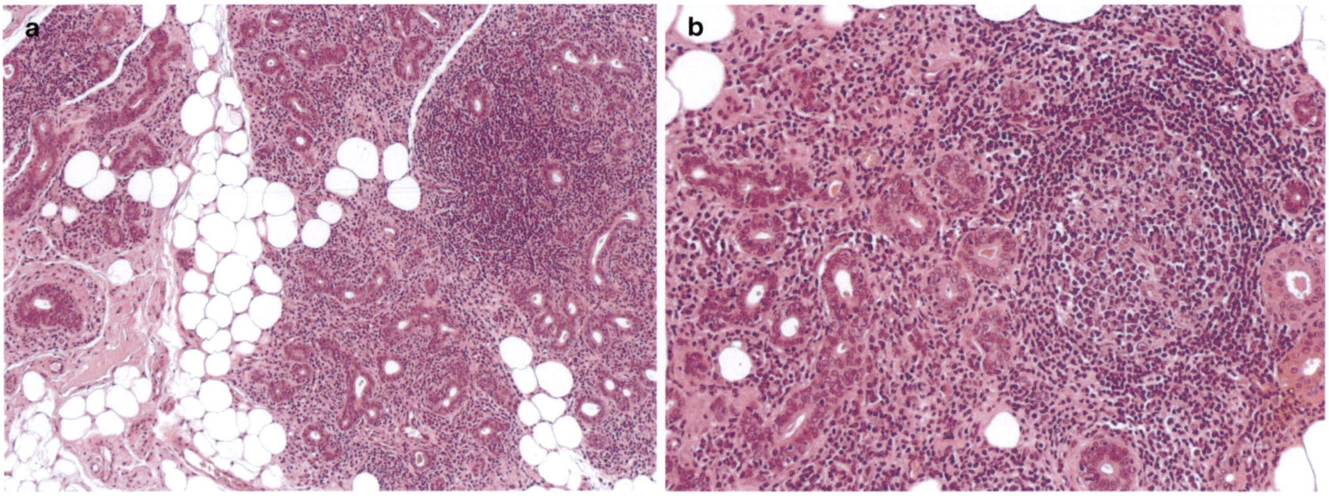

Fig. 26.4 Microscopic features observed after a lower lip biopsy obtained from a patient diagnosed with Sjögren disease. (**a**) The lymphoplasmacytic foci had more than 50 lymphocytes and could be easily observed in this patient surrounding the ductal structures of the salivary gland (H&E; 50×). (**b**) Observe the presence of a secondary follicle containing the germinal center (H&E; 100×)

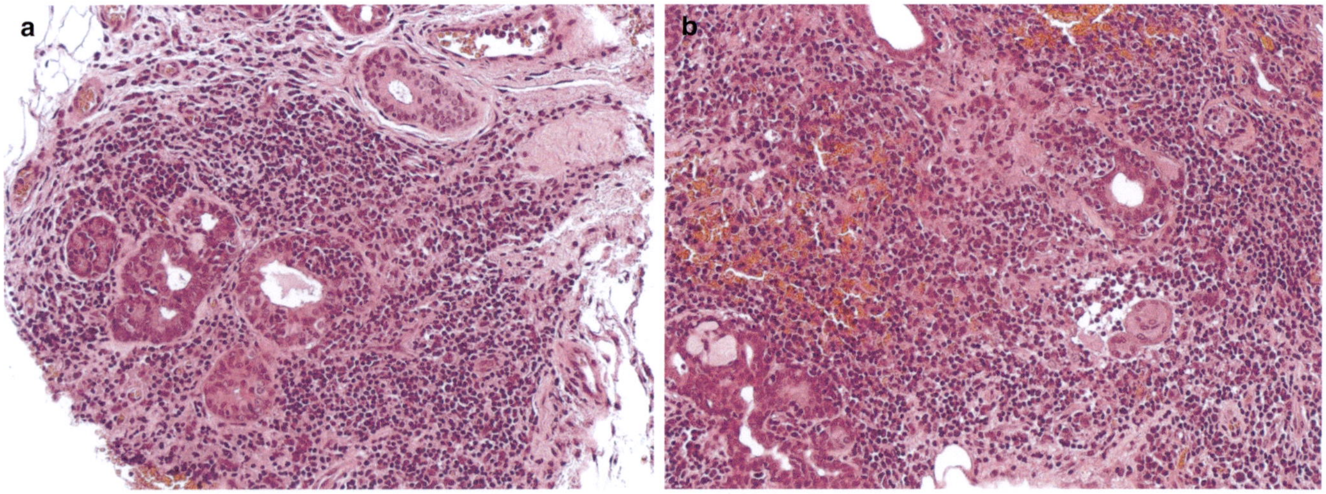

Fig. 26.5 Microscopic features observed after a lower lip biopsy obtained from a patient diagnosed with Sjögren disease. (**a**) The infiltration of lymphocytes towards the epithelial cells of the ductal structures led to the development of lymphoepithelial lesions, a common finding in these patients (H&E; 100×). (**b**) Observe in this focus the presence of lymphocytes and plasma cells surrounding the glandular ducts (H&E; 100×)

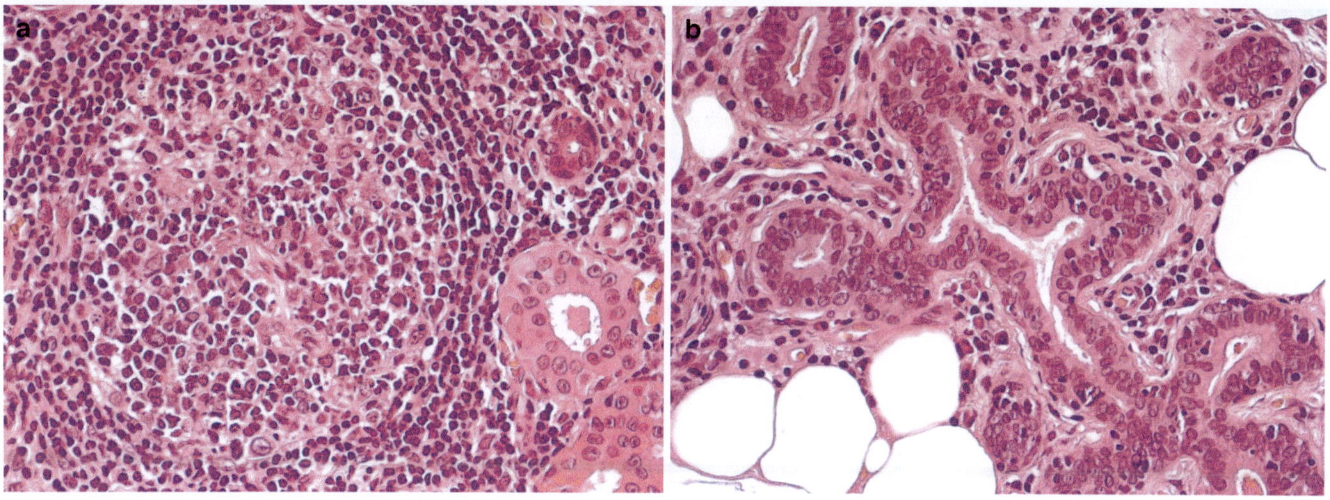

Fig. 26.6 Microscopic features observed after a lower lip biopsy obtained from a patient diagnosed with Sjögren disease. (**a**) The presence of a secondary follicle containing a germinal center with large and small cells. Observe the zonation pattern in the germinal center and the outer mantle zone. These features are consistent with a reactive process (H&E; 200×). (**b**) Presence of lymphocytes and plasma cells around the salivary gland ducts (H&E; 200×)

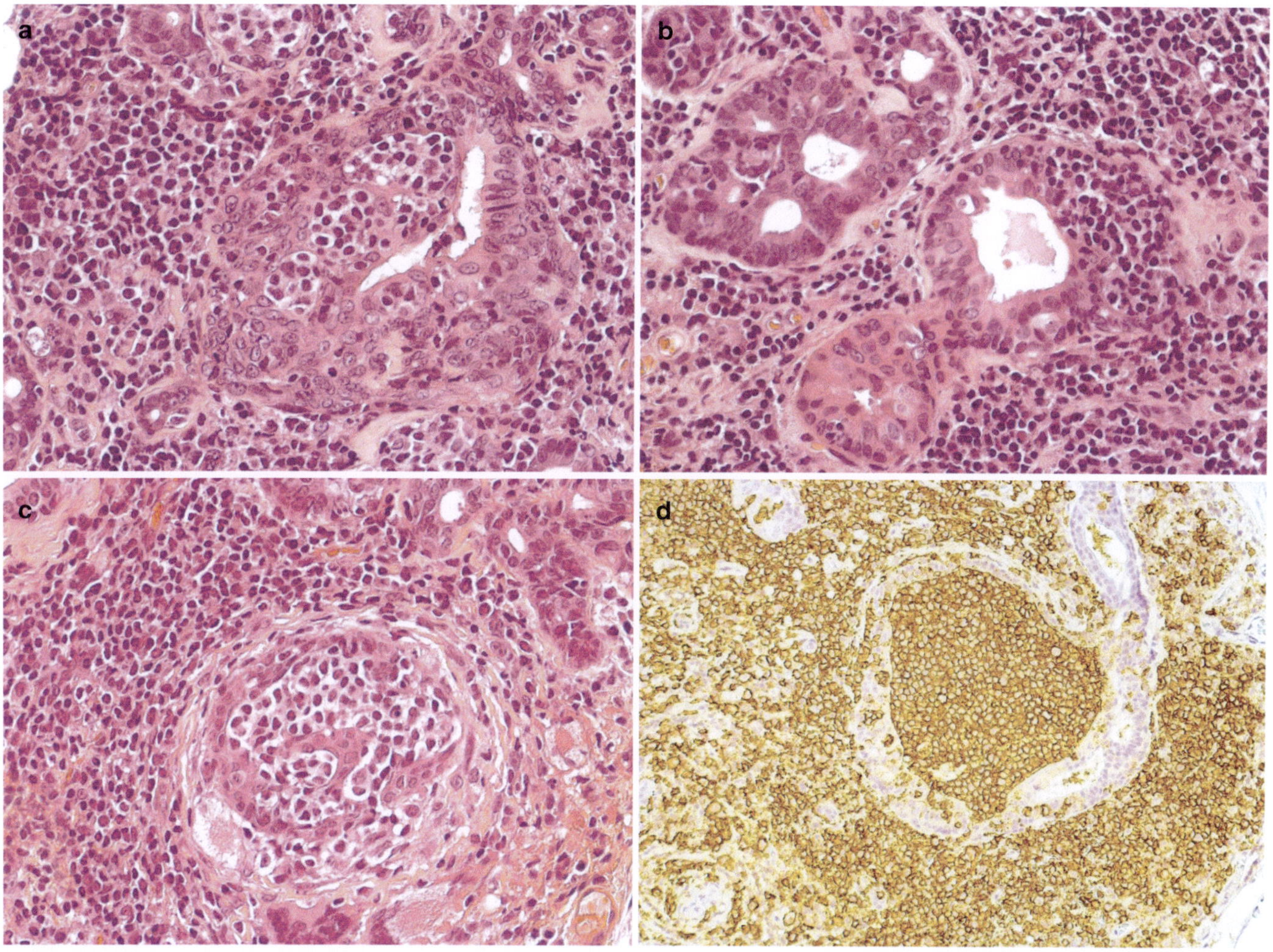

Fig. 26.7 Microscopic and immunohistochemical features observed after lower lip biopsy obtained from a patient diagnosed with Sjögren disease, highlighting the presence of lymphoepithelial lesions. (**a**) The lymphoid cells are closely associated with the salivary gland duct epithelium, frequently invading the epithelium and stimulating its proliferation (H&E; 200×). (**b**) Observe the close association between the lymphoid cells and the salivary duct epithelium in this image (H&E; 200×). (**c**) Lymphoid cells are located in the residual salivary gland duct epithelium (H&E; 200×). (**d**) Using Immunohistochemistry to detect CD20 expression, it is possible to observe the B lymphocytes inside the salivary gland duct epithelium in this lymphoepithelial lesion (DAB; 100×)

26.3 Immunohistochemistry and/or Genetics

Immunohistochemistry is useful for characterizing the presence and distribution of different cell populations in the lymphoid aggregates and investigating a possible diagnosis of lymphoma. Lymphoid follicles, when present, exhibit a comparable cellular distribution to normal follicles. There usually is a predominance of B lymphocytes, which are shown using CD20 staining, while the presence of the T lymphocytes is demonstrated by the expression of CD3 protein. A variable, usually a lower number of plasma cells, is usually found and can be shown by plasma cell, CD138 and/or EMA immunostaining. These cells are polyclonal and positivity to both immunoglobulin light chains is seen (kappa and lambda). The presence of germinal centers can be highlighted using follicular dendritic cell markers like CD21, CD23 and/or CD35 (Table 26.1, Figs. 26.8, 26.9 and 26.10). The reactive nature of the germinal centers is also demonstrated by the expression of BCL2 in the interfollicular region.

Table 26.1 Summary of immunohistochemical reactions that can be used for Sjögren disease microscopic evaluation

Antibody	Most frequent results	Pattern	Objective
CD20	Positive	Membrane	To demonstrate the B lymphocyte population
CD3	Positive	Membrane	To demonstrate the T lymphocyte population
CD138/EMA	Positive	Membrane	To demonstrate the plasma cell population
CD21/CD23	Positive	Membrane	To demonstrate the follicular dendritic cell population in germinal centers
CD68	Positive	Cytoplasm	To demonstrate the presence of histiocytes
BCL2	Positive in the interfollicular zone	Cytoplasm	To demonstrate the reactive nature of the germinal centers
Kappa/lambda	Polyclonal	Cytoplasm	To demonstrate the polyclonal nature of the plasma cells
Ki67	Positive	Nucleus	To demonstrate the proliferative patterns of the lymphoid aggregates

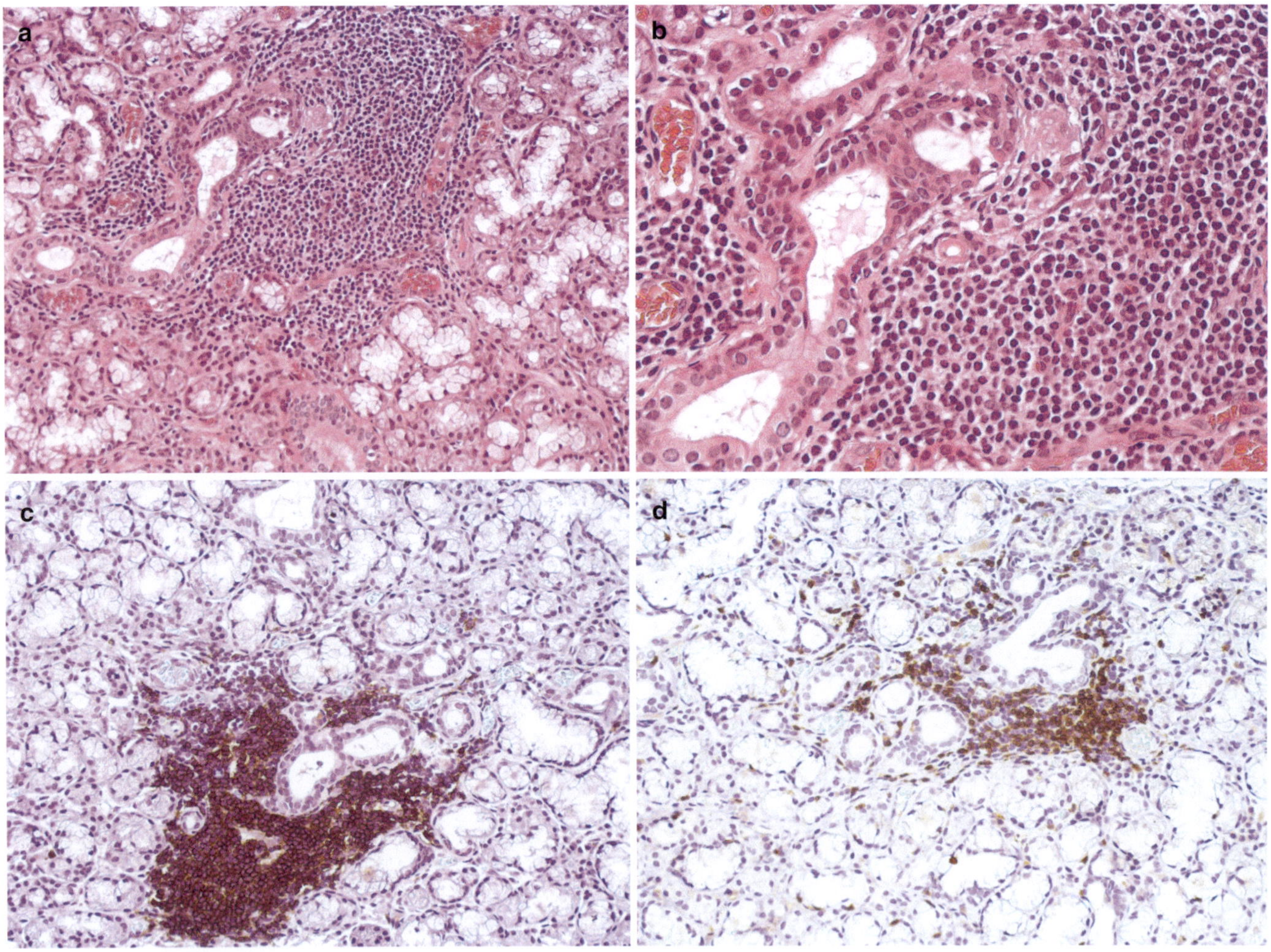

Fig. 26.8 Microscopic and immunohistochemical features observed in the lower lip biopsy of a patient diagnosed with Sjögren disease. (**a**) Focal lymphoid aggregates around ductal structures (H&E; 200×). (**b**) Predominance of lymphocytes in the aggregates (H&E; 400×). (**c**) Note the predominance of B lymphocytes demonstrated by CD20 expression (DAB; 200×); (**d**) but also with a large component of CD3-positive T lymphocytes (DAB; 200×)

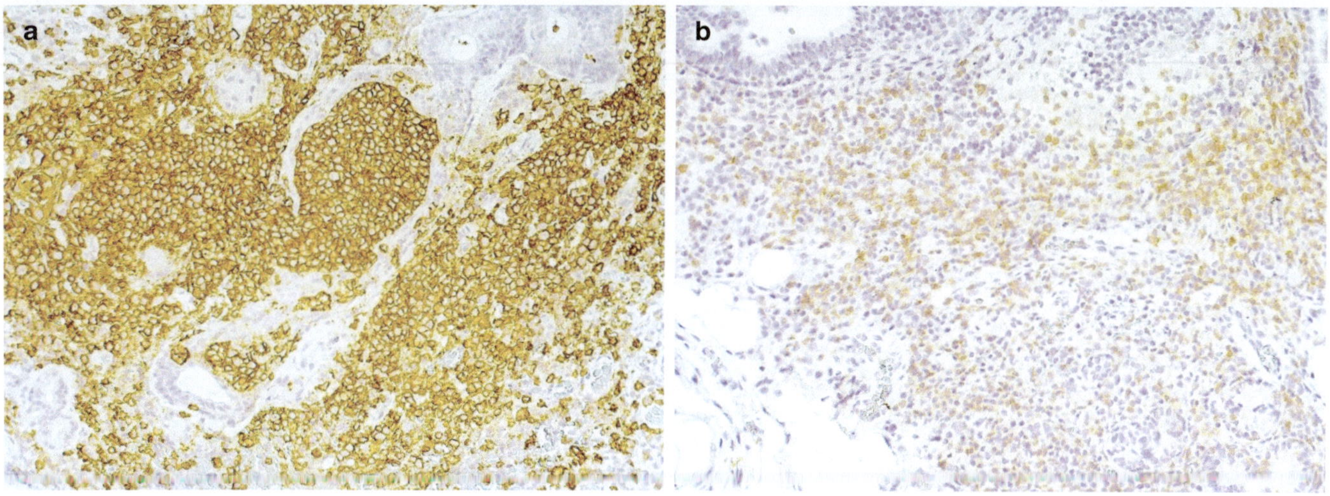

Fig. 26.9 Immunohistochemical features observed after lower lip biopsy obtained from a patient diagnosed with Sjögren disease. (**a**) The majority of the lymphocytes represent B cells, which are strongly and diffusely positive for CD20 (DAB; 100×). (**b**) The presence of T lymphocytes can also be demonstrated, especially in the interfollicular regions. Observe the expression of CD3 (DAB; 100×)

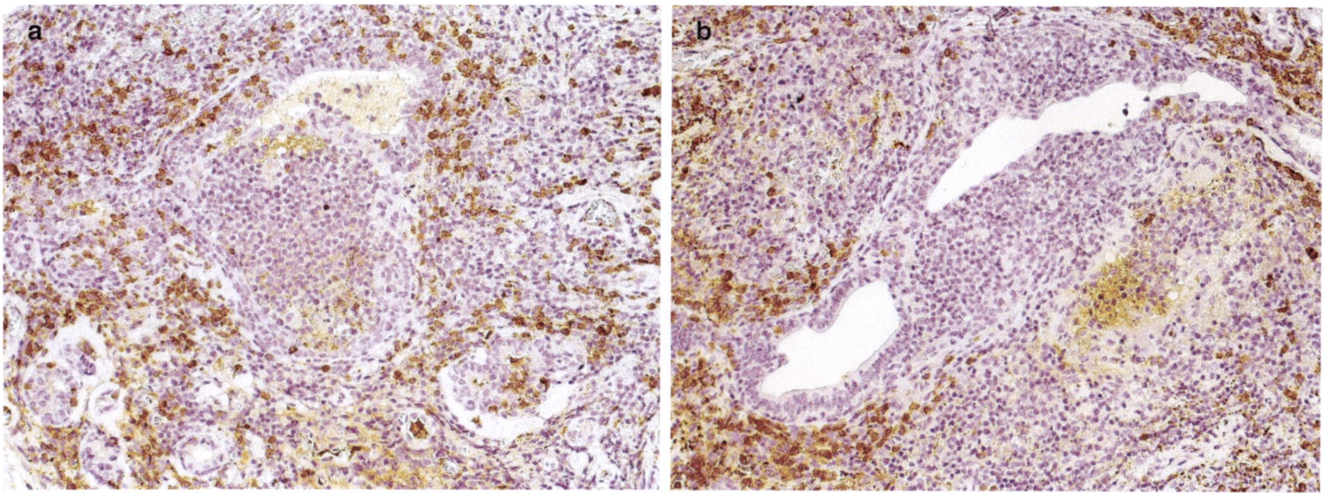

Fig. 26.10 Immunohistochemical features observed after lower lip biopsy obtained from a patient diagnosed with Sjögren disease. (**a**) The polyclonal nature of the lymphoid infiltrate can be demonstrated by investigating the expression of the immunoglobulin light chains. Observe the expression of kappa light chain (DAB; 100×). (**b**) The lambda light chain was also shown to be expressed in the reactive infiltrate (DAB; 100×)

Sources

1. Christodoulou MI, Kapsogeorgou EK, Moutsopoulos HM. Characteristics of the minor salivary gland infiltrates in Sjögren's syndrome. J Autoimmun. 2010;34:400–7.
2. Daniels TE, Cox D, Shiboski CH, Schiodt M, Wu A, Lanfranchi H, et al. Associations between salivary gland histopathologic diagnoses and phenotypic features of Sjögren's syndrome among 1,726 registry participants. Arthritis Rheum. 2011;63:2021–30.
3. Shiboski CH, Shiboski SC, Seror R, Criswell LA, Labetoulle M, Lietman TM, et al. 2016 American College of Rheumatology/European league against rheumatism classification criteria for primary Sjögren's syndrome: a consensus and data-driven methodology involving three international patient cohorts. Arthritis Rheumatol. 2017;69(1):35–45. https://doi.org/10.1002/art.39859.
4. Fisher BA, Jonsson R, Daniels T, Bombardieri M, Brown RM, Morgan P, et al. Standardisation of labial salivary gland histopathology in clinical trials in primary Sjögren's syndrome. Ann Rheum Dis. 2017;76(7):1161–8. https://doi.org/10.1136/annrheumdis-2016-210448.
5. Kroese FGM, Haacke EA, Bombardieri M. The role of salivary gland histopathology in primary Sjögren's syndrome: promises and pitfalls. Clin Exp Rheumatol. 2018;36 Suppl 112(3):222–33.
6. Takagi Y, Nakamura H, Sumi M, Shimizu T, Hirai Y, Horai Y, et al. Combined classification system based on ACR/EULAR and ultrasonographic scores for improving the diagnosis of Sjögren's syndrome. PLoS One. 2018;13(4):e0195113. https://doi.org/10.1371/journal.pone.0195113.
7. Retamozo S, Brito-Zerón P, Ramos-Casals M. Prognostic markers of lymphoma development in primary Sjögren syndrome. Lupus. 2019;28(8):923–36. https://doi.org/10.1177/0961203319857132.
8. Stergiou IE, Poulaki A, Voulgarelis M. Pathogenetic mechanisms implicated in Sjögren's syndrome lymphomagenesis: a review of the literature. J Clin Med. 2020;9(12):3794. https://doi.org/10.3390/jcm9123794.

9. Delli K, van Ginkel MS, Vissink A, Stel AJ, van der Vegt B, Spijkervet FKL, et al. Can salivary gland ultrasonography replace salivary gland biopsy in the diagnosis of Sjögren's syndrome? Clin Exp Rheumatol. 2022;40(12):2443–9. https://doi.org/10.55563/clinexprheumatol/xbcu8d.
10. Zhong H, Liu S, Wang Y, Xu D, Li M, Zhao Y, Zeng X. Primary Sjögren's syndrome is associated with increased risk of malignancies besides lymphoma: a systematic review and meta-analysis. Autoimmun Rev. 2022;21(5):103084. https://doi.org/10.1016/j.autrev.2022.103084.
11. Saleh W, Elashry MM, Winn N, Mona M, Katz J, Cha S. A lower prevalence of malignant lymphoma in Sjögren's syndrome patients: a cross-sectional study. Oral Dis. 2023;29:3313–24. https://doi.org/10.1111/odi.14435.
12. Zhan Q, Zhang J, Lin Y, Chen W, Fan X, Zhang D. Pathogenesis and treatment of Sjogren's syndrome: review and update. Front Immunol. 2023;14:1127417. https://doi.org/10.3389/fimmu.2023.1127417.
13. Baldini C, Chatzis LG, Fulvio G, La Rocca G, Pontarini E, Bombardieri M. Pathogenesis of Sjogren's disease: one year in review 2024. Clin Exp Rheumatol. 2024;42(12):2336–43. https://doi.org/10.55563/clinexprheumatol/i8iszc.
14. Tromby F, Manfrè V, Chatzis LG, Arends S, Tzioufas AG, Bootsma H, et al. Clinical manifestations, imaging and treatment of Sjogren's disease: one year in review 2024. Clin Exp Rheumatol. 2024;42(12):2322–35. https://doi.org/10.55563/clinexprheumatol/5xq3fb.
15. Liu S, Chen C, Zheng Q, Sun H, Yang C, Wang B, et al. Non-negligible prevalence of focal lymphocytic sialadenitis in minor salivary glands of non-Sjogren's disease individuals. Clin Exp Rheumatol. 2024;42(12):2499–506. https://doi.org/10.55563/clinexprheumatol/ou4fx6.
16. Al-Shahrestani F, Al-Khafaf AE, Asheer Z, Jelicic J, Chanchiri I, Blocher CE, et al. Lymphomas of the parotid gland in Denmark: a nationwide cohort study. Laryngoscope. 2024;135:1391–400. https://doi.org/10.1002/lary.31929.
17. Nayar S, Turner JD, Asam S, Fennell E, Pugh M, Colafrancesco S, et al. Molecular and spatial analysis of tertiary lymphoid structures in Sjogren's syndrome. Nat Commun. 2025;16(1):5. https://doi.org/10.1038/s41467-024-54686-0.

Part IV

Histiocytic and Dendritic Cell Lesions

Extranodal Rosai-Dorfman Disease

27

Lucas Lacerda de Souza, Javier Rendon Henao, and Felipe Paiva Fonseca

27.1 General Overview and Clinical Presentation

Rosai-Dorfman disease (RDD), sometimes referred to as Rosai-Dorfman-Destombes disease, is a non-Langerhans cell histiocytosis first recognized by Pierre-Paul Destombes, who reported four cases in 1965 and described it as *adenitis with lipid excess*. Rosai and Dorfman later reported 34 cases in 1969 and coined the name *sinus histiocytosis with massive lymphadenopathy*, which was later modified to RDD. With an estimated prevalence of approximately one case in 200,000 individuals, this condition has a broad spectrum of clinical manifestations, but it typically affects the lymph nodes. It may occur as a de novo disease in an otherwise healthy individual or it may be present in patients diagnosed with other disorders, including autoimmune, hereditary, or malignant conditions.

The etiology of RDD is poorly understood, although recent studies demonstrated that approximately one third of these patients harbor gene mutations involving the *MAPK/ERK* pathway, including *NRAS*, *KRAS*, *MAP2K1*, *MEK* and, more rarely, the *BRAF* mutation, suggesting that this family of genes are implicated in the pathogenesis of the condition and recent studies have investigated the possible efficacy of targeted therapies for affected patients. Although this is a reactive self-limited benign process in the majority of cases, a small subpopulation of patients may be refractory to conventional therapy and eventually die due to complications associated with the disease. Affected patients usually demonstrate massive, bilateral, painless cervical lymphadenopathy, occasionally showing fever, weight loss, leukocytosis, elevated erythrocyte sedimentation rate, anemia and hypergammaglobulinemia. The bone marrow infiltration is considered rare, and approximately 5% of the cases are known to involve the central nervous system, 75% as intracranial lesions and 25% the spine.

Adolescents and young adults are the most commonly affected individuals, with a mean age of 20 years old, although children and older patients can also be affected. Males are slightly more affected than females. The radiological findings of RDD are usually nonspecific and may potentially simulate malignant neoplasms. It usually demonstrates a homogeneous enhancement on computed tomography (CT) and magnetic resonance imaging (MRI), while ultrasonography reveals large and multiple lymphadenopathies, which shows hypermetabolic activity on FDG18-PET/CT. Therefore, radiologists should always include RDD in the list of potential diagnoses for massive painless bilateral cervical lymphadenopathy in young patients. Moreover, intraosseous involvement of RDD represents a well-known manifestation of the disorder, which more often occurs in the bones of the extremities, followed by the vertebra and the craniofacial bones, radiographically showing lytic well- or ill-defined images.

Although uncommon, extranodal presentation of the disease is well known, and it is present in approximately 43% of the cases. Patients usually have a mean age of 44 years at the moment of diagnosis, and most of the affected extranodal sites include the eyes, soft tissues of the head and neck, skin, and bone. In the head and neck regions the nasal cavity and paranasal sinuses are the most affected locations, leading to nasal obstruction and epistaxis. Oral manifestations have also been well documented, including cases affecting the mandible and maxilla. These lesions are almost always identified in association with nodal or other extranodal diseases. Jaw lesions present as well or ill-defined single or multiple radiolucent images that may be associated with loose teeth, and the

L. L. de Souza (✉)
Department of Oral Diagnosis, Piracicaba Dental School, University of Campinas, Piracicaba, Brazil

J. R. Henao
Department of Hematopathology and Flow Cytometry, Ayudas Diagnósticas Sura Center, Cartagena, Colombia

F. P. Fonseca
Department of Oral Surgery and Pathology, School of Dentistry, Universidade Federal de Minas Gerais, Belo Horizonte, Brazil

© The Author(s), under exclusive license to Springer Nature Switzerland AG 2025

F. P. Fonseca et al. (eds.), *Lymphoproliferative and Granulomatous Disorders of the Oral Cavity*,
https://doi.org/10.1007/978-3-031-98844-8_27

condition can easily be misinterpreted as dental-related inflammation. Gnathic RDD is frequently a locally destructive disease with cortical bone destruction, and in some cases, it may also be associated with extension to soft tissue, but it usually demonstrates a benign and self-limited clinical course. Association with a delayed healing of the alveolar bone in dental extraction sites has been reported, as well as the occurrence of the so-called 'floating tooth" appearance due to an extensive loss of alveolar bone around teeth.

In the oral mucosa, RDD is considered very rare and few case reports have described the disease as asymptomatic or painful swelling, or as an unspecific, non-healing, ulcer in the tongue. Patients with isolated oral RDD usually do not show any fever, malaise, weight loss, or nasal complaints. This unspecific clinical presentation associated with the complex microscopic features of the condition and the unawareness of pathologists to its oral manifestations makes the diagnosis of oral RDD a scenario likely underrecognized.

There is currently no standardized treatment for RDD; a watch-and-wait approach is considered for asymptomatic or mildly symptomatic patients since approximately 40% of these cases regress. Surgical resection is used for patients with unifocal diseases, while steroids use, external-beam radiation therapy, and different schemes of chemotherapy and immunotherapy have also been described in the literature. The use of the *MEK* inhibitor Cobimetinib has recently been described, but the use of target therapy for these patients remains to be validated and approved. Prognosis is usually favorable for cutaneous, nodal, and bone RDD; however, central nervous system (CNS) involvement with RDD has variable outcomes and bone marrow infiltration is associated with a worse prognosis. In most cases, patients have a good prognosis; however, some patients may have a progressive disease and rare cases may reveal a fatal course.

27.2 Microscopic Findings

- Mixed population of cells, including histiocytes, lymphocytes and plasma cells.
- The most distinctive cells are the histiocytes that are usually large with round-to-oval nuclei, dispersed chromatin, prominent nucleoli, and abundant clear-to-foamy or vacuolated cytoplasm.
- The distribution of the histiocytes may vary significantly in a single case, with areas containing histiocytic clustering and regions showing a more mixed cellularity, which may result in alternating dark and light regions when observed under low magnification.
- Cases affecting the mandible and maxilla should be carefully differentiated from dental inflammatory processes like periapical radicular granuloma that may contain numerous foamy histiocytes. A careful clinical and radiographic correlation, with evaluation of the dental pulp vitality, is strongly recommended.
- The presence of plasma cells may make it difficult to differentiate it from IgG4-related disease.
- Occurrence of emperipolesis is a typical histopathological finding of RDD that more often represents the presence of lymphocytes engulfed in the cytoplasm of the histiocytes; however, the engulfment of neutrophils and plasma cells may also be less commonly observed.
- In the emperipolesis process the engulfed cells remain viable and can exit histiocytes, in contrast to the process of phagocytosis.
- These findings are observed in both nodal and extranodal sites, but there is a greater degree of fibrosis and less emperipolesis in the extranodal manifestations.
- The strong expression of S100 by the histiocytes creates a clear "halo" aspect around the engulfed lymphocytes.
- The presence of stromal deposition of acellular eosinophilic material that stains positively for Congo red and exhibits apple-green birefringence under polarized microscopy consistent with amyloid deposition may also occur in a few cases.
- Eosinophils are rare.
- There is only rare or no mitosis or necrosis (Figs. 27.1, 27.2 and 27.3).

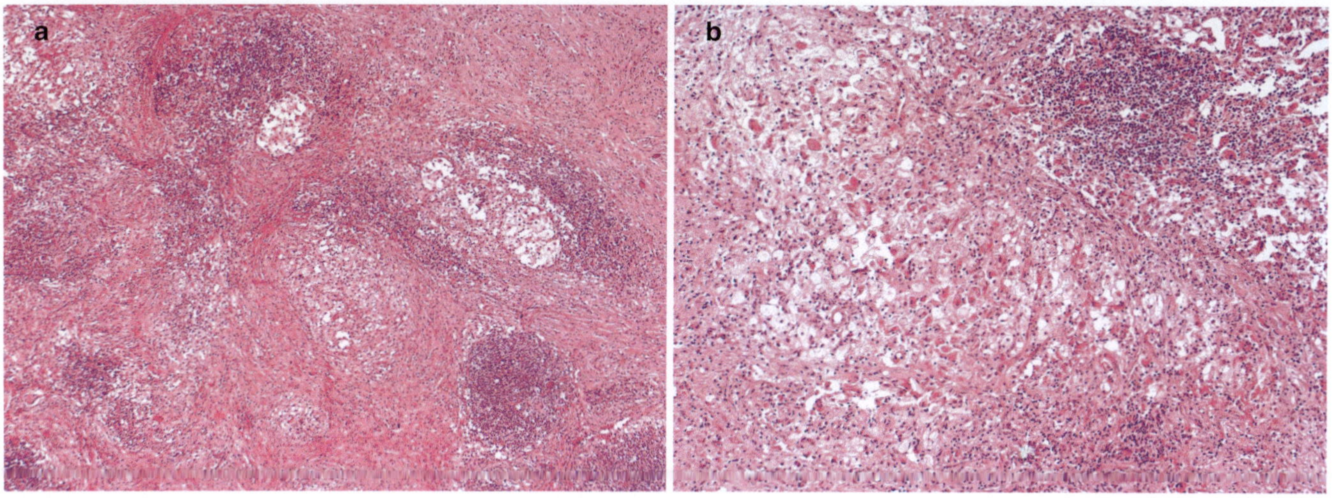

Fig. 27.1 Microscopic features of extranodal Rosai-Dorfman disease affecting the buccal space. (**a**) It is possible to observe the presence of various lymphoid aggregates and lighter areas consisting of foamy macrophages in a fibrous stroma (H&E; 50×). (**b**) Foamy macrophages proliferate in the specimen (H&E; 50×)

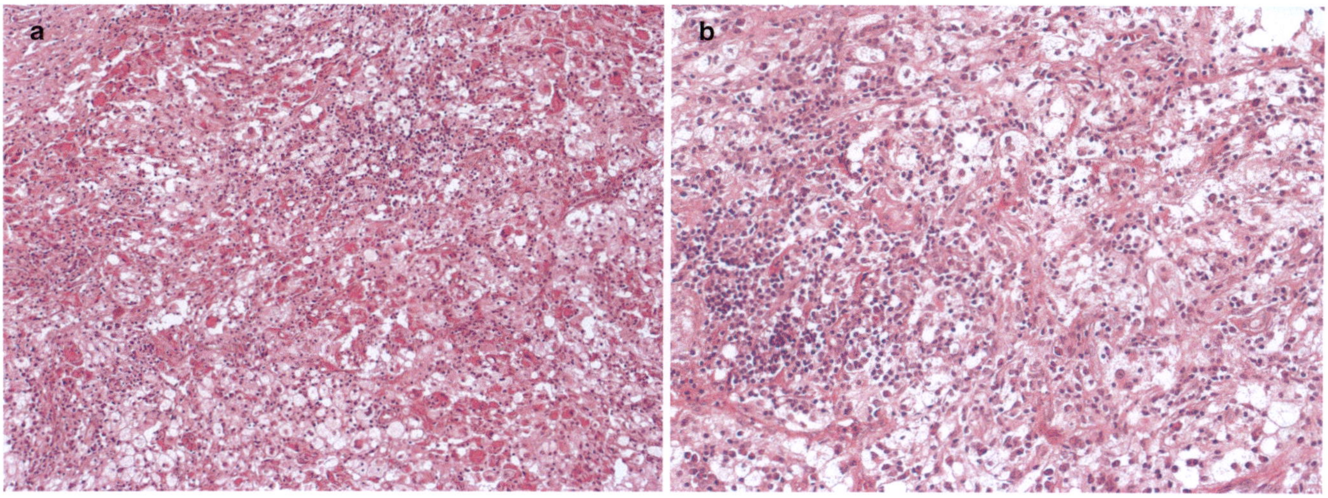

Fig. 27.2 Microscopic features of extranodal Rosai-Dorfman disease affecting the buccal space. (**a**) Diffuse proliferation of foamy histiocytes with reactive lymphoid cells (H&E; 100×). (**b**) Several histiocytes contain small mature lymphocytes engulfed in the cytoplasm (H&E; 100×)

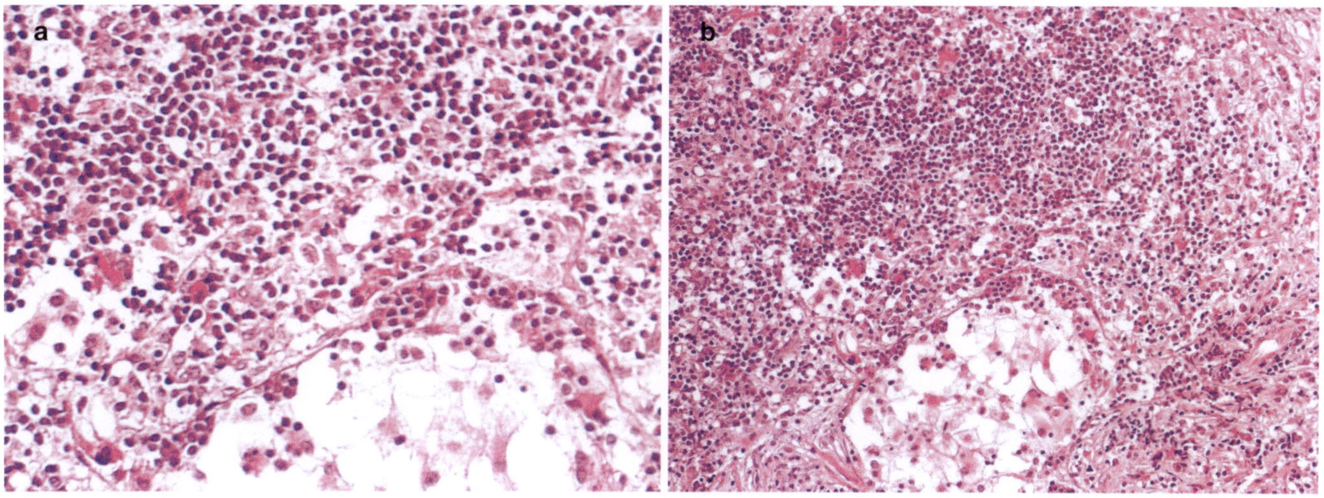

Fig. 27.3 Microscopic features of extranodal Rosai-Dorfman disease affecting the buccal space. (**a**) The presence of reactive plasma cells is a frequent finding in this lesion and should prompt pathologists to differentiate Rosai-Dorfman disease from IgG4-related disease and other lymphoproliferative disorders rich in this cell population (H&E; 200×). (**b**) The occurrence of emperipolesis can be seen in the lower part of this image (H&E; 100×)

27.3 Immunohistochemistry and/or Genetics

In the presence of a typical histological presentation, diagnosis is suggestive, but immunohistochemistry can aid in the identification of the process. Different markers may contribute to characterizing the process, although not all of them need to be investigated in one single case. The macrophages in the lesion show positivity for typical histiocytic markers like CD68 and CD163, but they lack the Langerhans' cells markers CD1a and CD207, as well as follicular dendritic cell markers CD21, CD23 and CD35. Positivity for S100 in the histiocytes is a typical finding. The occurrence of mutations in different *MAPK* components leads to activation of this pathway and expression of pErk protein. Cyclin D1 is also overexpressed in most cases. Plasma cells are present and are polyclonal, while the proliferative index is low (Table 27.1, Figs. 27.4, 27.5, 27.6 and 27.7).

Table 27.1 Summary of the main immunohistochemical reactions and histological stains that can be used for RDD diagnosis, and the main molecular events

Antibody/probe	Most frequent results	Pattern	Objective
CD20	Negative	Membrane	To demonstrate B lymphocytes and to exclude B-cell lymphomas
CD3	Negative	Membrane	To demonstrate T lymphocytes and to exclude T-cell lymphomas
S100	Positive	Cytoplasm/nucleus	To demonstrate the presence of histiocytes
CD68	Positive	Cytoplasm	To demonstrate the presence of histiocytes
CD163	Positive	Membrane	To demonstrate the presence of histiocytes
Cyclin D1	Positive	Nucleus	It is positive due to the mutational landscape of the disease
pERK	Positive	Nucleus	It is positive due to the mutational landscape of the disease
OCT2	Positive	Nucleus	Positive in RDD histiocytes
CD1a	Negative	Membrane	To exclude a Langerhans cell type histiocytosis
CD207	Negative	Cytoplasm	To exclude a Langerhans cell type histiocytosis
CD138	Negative	Membrane	To highlight the presence of plasma cells
IgG/IgG4	Variably positive	Cytoplasm	To exclude an IgG4-related disease
Kappa/lambda	Polyclonal	Cytoplasm	To demonstrate the polyclonal nature of plasma cells
Ki67	Low	Nucleus	To demonstrate the proliferative feature of the lesion
NRAS[a]	Variably positive	–	To characterize the molecular landscape of the lesion
KRAS[a]	Variably positive	–	To characterize the molecular landscape of the lesion
MAP2K1[a]	Variably positive	–	To characterize the molecular landscape of the lesion
BRAF[a]	Rarely positive	–	To characterize the molecular landscape of the lesion
PAS[b]	Negative	–	To exclude the presence of microorganisms
Grocott-Gomori[b]	Negative	–	To exclude the presence of microorganisms

RDD Rosai-Dorfman disease
[a]Investigated by PCR
[b]Histological stain

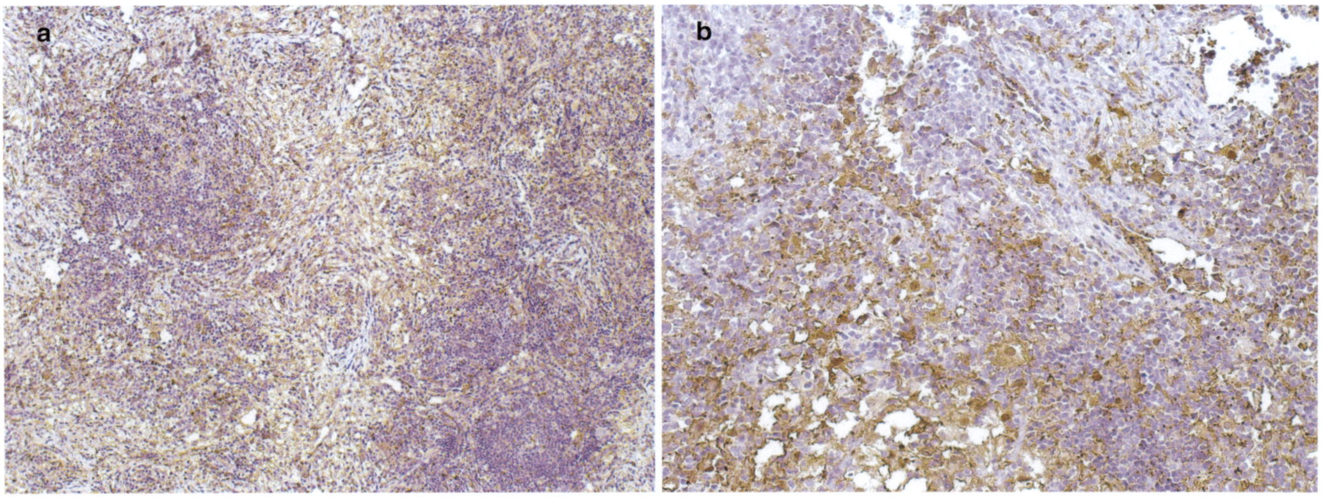

Fig. 27.4 Immunohistochemical features of extranodal Rosai-Dorfman disease affecting the buccal space. (**a**) CD68 is diffusely positive in RDD (DAB; 50×), (**b**) the histiocytes are also strongly positive for S100 protein (DAB; 100×)

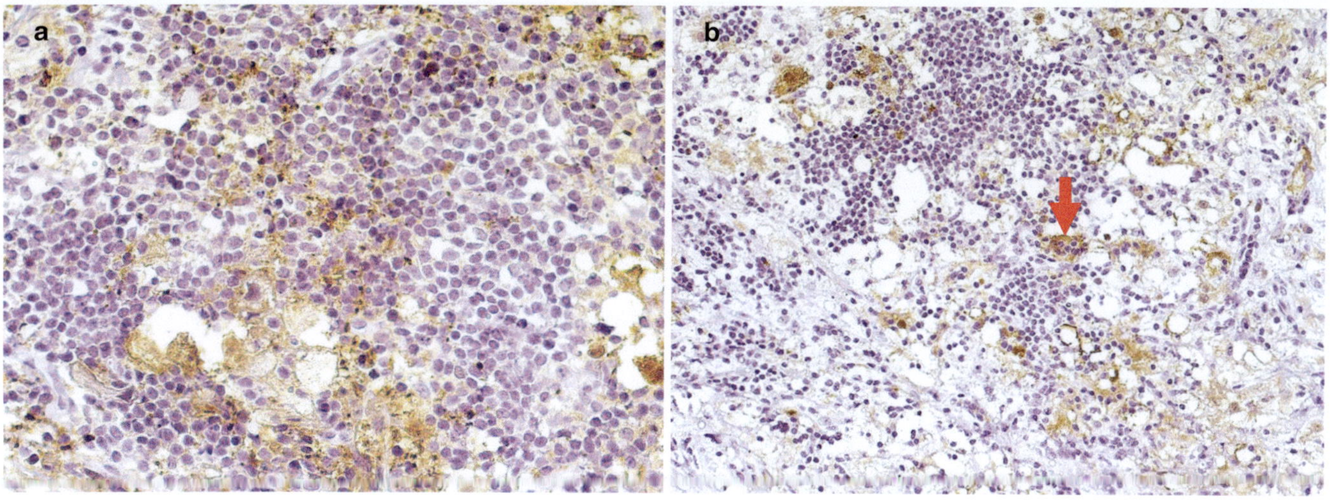

Fig. 27.5 Immunohistochemical features of extranodal Rosai-Dorfman disease affecting the buccal space. (**a**) S100 expression is observed in the histiocytes present in the disease, which are surrounded by a dense lymphoid infiltrate (DAB; 200×). (**b**) The S100 expression helps to demonstrate the occurrence of emperipolesis, with the presence of lymphocytes inside the histiocytic cells (red arrow) (DAB; 100×)

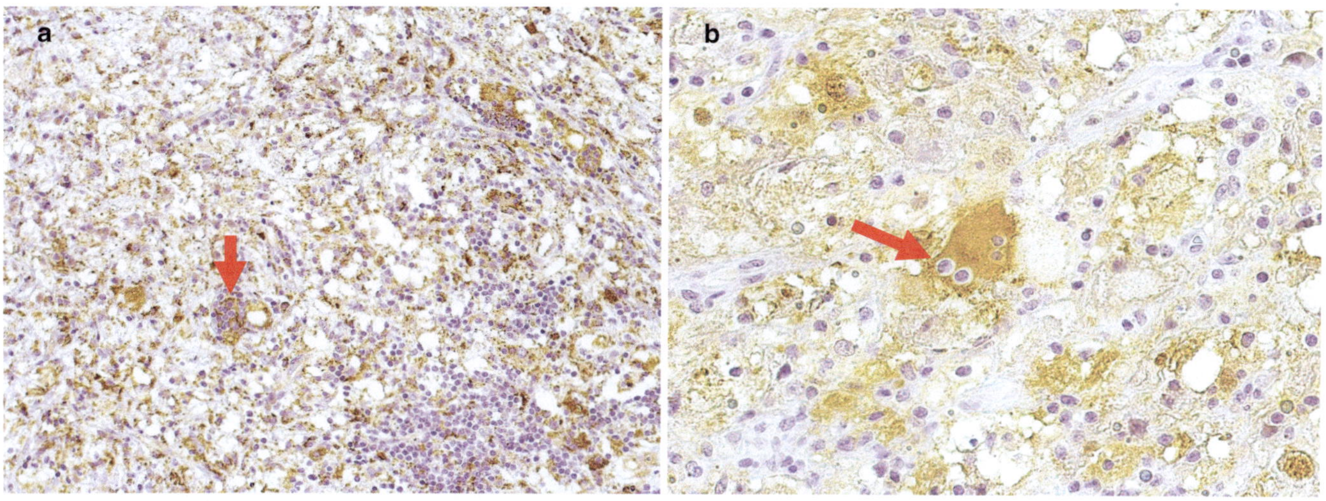

Fig. 27.6 Immunohistochemical features of extranodal Rosai-Dorfman disease affecting the buccal space. (**a**) S100 used to demonstrate the occurrence of emperipolesis in RDD, a phenomenon characteristically present in this disorder and that helps to confirm the diagnosis (red arrow) (DAB; 100×). (**b**) Under higher magnification, it is possible to observe an example of emperipolesis. Observe the presence of lymphocytes inside the histiocytic cell. There is a clear halo around the lymphocytes (red arrow) (DAB; 200×)

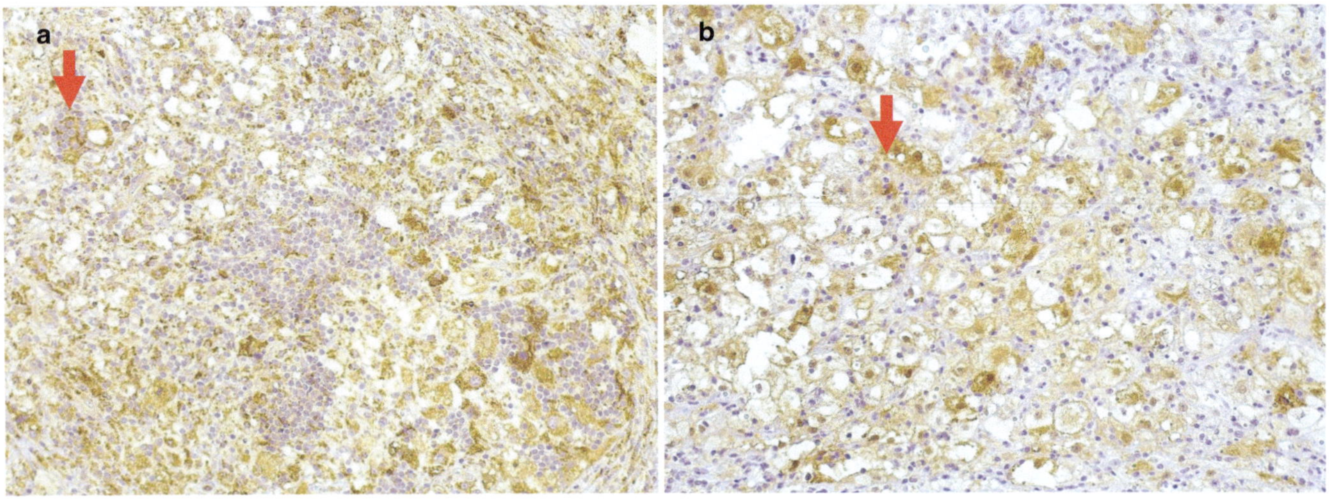

Fig. 27.7 Immunohistochemical features of extranodal Rosai-Dorfman disease affecting the buccal space. (**a**) CD68 expression can also be used to illustrate the histiocytic origin of the disease. There is a diffuse expression of this protein in the histiocytes and it is possible to observe an example of emperipolesis (red arrow) (DAB; 100×). (**b**) Diffuse expression of CD68 in a case of extranodal RDD and the presence of emperipolesis (red arrow) (DAB; 100×)

Sources

1. Röcken C, Wieker K, Grote HJ, Müller G, Franke A, Roessner A. Rosai-Dorfman disease and generalized AA amyloidosis: a case report. Hum Pathol. 2000;31(5):621–4. https://doi.org/10.1053/hp.2000.6705.
2. Alawi F, Robinson BT, Carrasco L. Rosai-Dorfman disease of the mandible. Oral Surg Oral Med Oral Pathol Oral Radiol Endod. 2006;102(4):506–12. https://doi.org/10.1016/j.tripleo.2005.
3. Güven G, Ilgan S, Altun C, Gerek M, Gunhan O. Rosai Dorfman disease of the parotid and submandibular glands: salivary gland scintigraphy and oral findings in two siblings. Dentomaxillofac Radiol. 2007;36(7):428–33. https://doi.org/10.1259/dmfr/39858276.
4. Demicco EG, Rosenberg AE, Björnsson J, Rybak LD, Unni KK, Nielsen GP. Primary Rosai-Dorfman disease of bone: a clinicopathologic study of 15 cases. Am J Surg Pathol. 2010;34(9):1324–33. https://doi.org/10.1097/PAS.0b013e3181ea50b2.
5. Kaltman JM, Best SP, McClure SA. Sinus histiocytosis with massive lymphadenopathy Rosai-Dorfman disease: a unique case presentation. Oral Surg Oral Med Oral Pathol Oral Radiol Endod. 2011;112(6):e124–6. https://doi.org/10.1016/j.tripleo.2011.06.018.
6. Miniello TG, Araujo JP, Sugaya NN, Elias FM, de Almeida OP, Alves FA. Rosai-Dorfman disease affecting the maxilla. Autops Case Rep. 2016;6(4):49–55. https://doi.org/10.4322/acr.2016.057.
7. Garces S, Medeiros LJ, Patel KP, Li S, Pina-Oviedo S, Li J, et al. Mutually exclusive recurrent KRAS and MAP2K1 mutations in Rosai-Dorfman disease. Mod Pathol. 2017;30(10):1367–77. https://doi.org/10.1038/modpathol.2017.55.
8. Cracolici V, Gurbuxani S, Ginat DT. Head and neck sinus histiocytosis with massive lymphadenopathy radiology-pathology correlation. Head Neck Pathol. 2019;13(4):656–60. https://doi.org/10.1007/s12105-018-0941-3.
9. Baraban E, Sadigh S, Rosenbaum J, Van Arnam J, Bogusz AM, Mehr C, et al. Cyclin D1 expression and novel mutational findings in Rosai-Dorfman disease. Br J Haematol. 2019;186(6):837–44. https://doi.org/10.1111/bjh.16006.
10. Ojha J, Rawal YB, Hornick JL, Magliocca K, Montgomery DR, Foss RD, et al. Extra nodal Rosai-Dorfman disease originating in the nasal and paranasal complex and gnathic bones: a systematic analysis of seven cases and review of literature. Head Neck Pathol. 2020;14(2):442–53. https://doi.org/10.1007/s12105-019-01056-8.
11. Azari-Yaam A, Abdolsalehi MR, Vasei M, Safavi M, Mehdizadeh M. Rosai-Dorfman disease: a rare clinicopathological presentation and review of the literature. Head Neck Pathol. 2021;15(1):352–60. https://doi.org/10.1007/s12105-020-01183-7.
12. Abeykoon JP, Rech KL, Young JR, Ravindran A, Ruan GJ, Dasari S, et al. Outcomes after treatment with Cobimetinib in patients with rosai-dorfman disease based on KRAS and MEK alteration status. JAMA Oncol. 2022;8(12):1816–20. https://doi.org/10.1001/jamaoncol.2022.4432.
13. Elbaz Younes I, Sokol L, Zhang L. Rosai-Dorfman disease between proliferation and neoplasia. Cancers (Basel). 2022;14(21):5271. https://doi.org/10.3390/cancers14215271.
14. Weng X, Yang Y, Zhang M, Cai C, Sun Y, Wu X, et al. Primary intraosseous Rosai-Dorfman disease: an analysis of clinicopathologic characteristics, molecular genetics, and prognostic features. Front Oncol. 2022;12:950114. https://doi.org/10.3389/fonc.2022.950114.
15. Zhang X, Yin W, Guo Y, He Y, Jiang Z, Li Y, Xie B, Zhang S, Jiang X, Liu Q, Yuan J. Rosai-Dorfman disease of the central nervous system: a clinical, radiological, and prognostic study of 12 cases. Front Oncol. 2022;12:1013419. https://doi.org/10.3389/fonc.2022.1013419.
16. Hyrcza MD, Lindenmuth TR, Auerbach A. Top ten lymphoproliferative lesions not to miss when evaluating oral ulcer biopsies. Head Neck Pathol. 2023;17(1):99–118. https://doi.org/10.1007/s12105-023-01532-2.
17. Charfeddine A, Omami M, Garma M, Bellalah A, Sioud S, Selmi J. Rosai-Dorfman disease of the oral cavity. Autops Case Rep. 2023;13:e2023463. https://doi.org/10.4322/acr.2023.463.
18. Moen FM, Youssef MM, Shukla M, Nierodzik ML, Mayerhoefer ME, Park C. BRAF V600E mutation and high expression of PD-L1 in Rosai-Dorfman disease: case report and review of the literature. J Hematop. 2024;17(4):183–9. https://doi.org/10.1007/s12308-024-00611-9.
19. Tran PTC, Din NU, Xu Z, Ahsan BU. Clinicopathological characteristics of extranodal Rosai-Dorfman disease: a retrospective case series of 25 patients. Ann Diagn Pathol. 2024;73:152377. https://doi.org/10.1016/j.anndiagpath.2024.152377.

Xanthoma

28

Danyel Elias da Cruz Perez,
Carla Isabelly Rodrigues-Fernandes,
Bruno Augusto Benevenuto de Andrade,
Mohammed N. Islam, and Felipe Paiva Fonseca

28.1 General Overview and Clinical Presentation

The term "xanthoma," from the Greek word *xanthos* or yellow, was coined in the nineteenth century to characterize yellow nodules of the skin. This designation describes the collection of yellowish and cholesterol-rich material in different parts of the body, more frequently soft tissues, but also in the bone.

Verruciform xanthoma of the oral cavity is a rare, benign mucocutaneous lesion first described in 1971 by Shafer that accounts for less than 0.05% of all oral lesions. Rare cases affecting extra-oral sites have been reported, especially in the skin and genital regions. The etiology of oral verruciform xanthoma remains unclear, and some hypotheses have been speculated in the literature, including inflammation, trauma, and an altered immunological response that releases lipid material or epithelial degeneration followed by lipid accumulation. Several cases have been reported in patients affected by different systemic inflammatory conditions.

Contrary to other dermal xanthomas (such as xanthelasma palpebrarum) that may indicate dyslipidemia, atherothrombotic disease or type II diabetes, there is no such association with verruciform xanthoma. However, verruciform xanthoma is part of the CHILD syndrome, a condition caused by mutations in the *3β-hydroxysteroid dehydrogenase (NSDHL)* gene located at chromosome Xq28 and involved in the cholesterol biosynthetic pathway. The occurrence of mutations in this gene has also been reported in a small subset of sporadic verruciform xanthomas. The search for HPV infection in verruciform xanthomas has been carried out, but the virus has not been consistently detected, therefore, not demonstrating any definitive viral etiology for this disorder.

The clinical diagnosis of oral verruciform xanthoma is usually not considered by clinicians, and the microscopic analysis is required for a definitive diagnosis. There is a similar distribution between males and females, with a slight female predominance described in some series and a male preponderance in others. Most of the patients are adults or elderly, with a mean age of 61 years, but with a wide age distribution ranging from 9 to 94 years old. The masticatory mucosa is the most affected location, especially the gingiva and hard palate, followed by the buccal mucosa. However, other locations can also be affected. The lesions are most frequently normal-colored, although red, white, or yellow lesions have been described. They usually manifest as asymptomatic, slow-growing, well-demarcated plaques or nodules that rarely exceed 2 cm in diameter and reveal a papillary or verrucous surface, often described as bumpy, rough, verrucoid and/or papillary lesions.

Intraosseous xanthoma is a rare benign entity characterized by bone destruction of variable severity that may also cause bone expansion or cortical perforation. The biological nature of this lesion is debatable, and intraosseous xanthoma may be associated with neoplasms or inflammatory processes in response to surgery or trauma, and can also be present in the context of metabolic diseases. It is hypothesized that a lipid leakage from blood vessels following a local trauma or hemorrhage would lead to macrophage phagocytosis of the deposited fat that would accumulate in the local

D. E. da Cruz Perez (✉) · C. I. Rodrigues-Fernandes
Department of Clinical and Preventive Dentistry, Oral Pathology Unit, Universidade Federal de Pernambuco, Recife, Pernambuco, Brazil
e-mail: danyel.perez@ufpe.br

B. A. B. de Andrade
Department of Oral Diagnosis and Pathology, School of Dentistry, Universidade Federal do Rio de Janeiro, Rio de Janeiro, Brazil

M. N. Islam
Department of Oral and Maxillofacial Pathology, University of Florida College of Dentistry, Gainesville, FL, USA
e-mail: mnislam@ufl.edu

F. P. Fonseca
Department of Oral Surgery and Pathology, School of Dentistry, Universidade Federal de Minas Gerais, Belo Horizonte, Brazil

© The Author(s), under exclusive license to Springer Nature Switzerland AG 2025
F. P. Fonseca et al. (eds.), *Lymphoproliferative and Granulomatous Disorders of the Oral Cavity*,
https://doi.org/10.1007/978-3-031-98844-8_28

tissue. Therefore, intraosseous xanthoma possibly represents a reactive or degenerative process rather than a true neoplastic entity. Moreover, intraosseous xanthoma should be differentiated from fibrohistiocytic conditions like the rare central benign fibrous histiocytoma, which may show some microscopic similarities, and the non-ossifying fibroma, whose terminology should be confined to metaphyseal lesions of the long bones.

Other non-gnathic bones can also be affected by intraosseous xanthoma, including the pelvis, rib, skull, ilium, and tibia. Cases affecting the jaws are available in the literature, with a predominance of lesions among young adults in their second to third decades of life, with no evidence of sex predilection. Most of the cases have been described in the posterior region of the mandible as an asymptomatic swelling, although these lesions can also be identified as incidental findings on panoramic radiographs. Radiographically, the lesions vary from well-defined radiolucent lesions with sclerotic margins to ill-defined radiolucent lesions. Multiple xanthomatous bone lesions may occur and have been associated with hyperlipidemic states, but such association with gnathic lesions is very uncommon and remains to be validated.

Verruciform xanthoma is treated with simple surgical removal and prognosis is considered excellent. However, very rare examples of recurrences have been reported. Intraosseous xanthoma is more often treated conservatively with curettage, and recurrences are very rare. Malignant transformation from xanthoma has not been reported (Figs. 28.1 and 28.2).

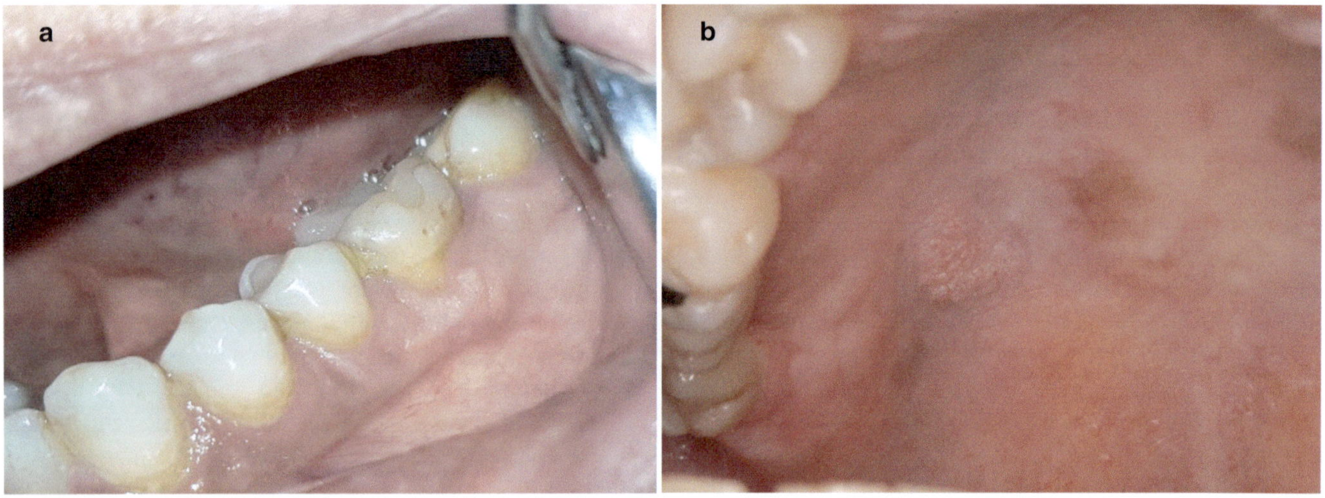

Fig. 28.1 Clinical presentation of verruciform xanthoma in the oral cavity. (**a**) Female patient with a whitish to yellowish plaque with rough surface affecting the lower left gingiva. (Image courtesy: Dr. Ellen Cortezzi). (**b**) A plaque-like lesion affecting the palate of a 42-year-old female patient exhibiting the verruciform surface

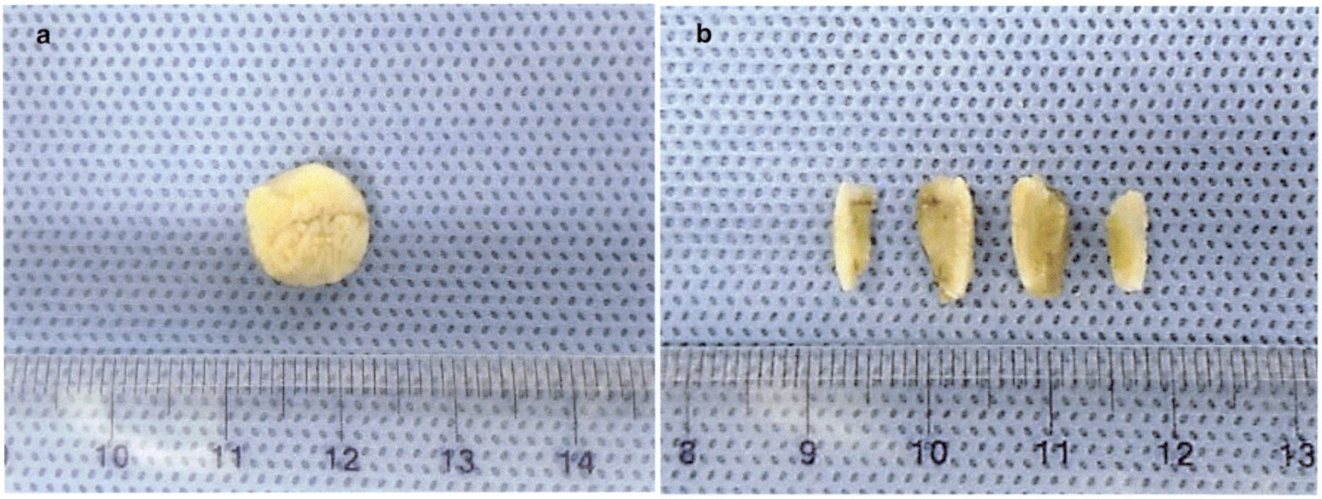

Fig. 28.2 Surgical specimen of a verruciform xanthoma affecting the tongue. (**a**) Gross specimen comprised a round tissue with a verrucous surface. (**b**) Cut surface showing a homogeneous aspect and a verrucous surface

28.2 Microscopic Findings

1. *Verruciform Xanthoma*
   - Presence of papillary or verrucous proliferation of the overlying squamous epithelium.
   - Elongated rete ridges, but usually with a uniform depth.
   - Thick parakeratin with a frayed surface and prominent "salmon or orange coloration" which shows a sharp demarcation.
   - The parakeratin may extend into the epithelial crypts to form parakeratin plugs.
   - Presence of variable degrees of acanthosis.
   - Parakeratin clefting into the underlying spinous layer.
   - Lipid-laden foamy macrophages (xanthoma cells) are the hallmark cells of this condition.
   - Aggregates of foamy macrophages are predominantly located within the elongated connective tissue papillae.
   - They usually do not extend below the tips of the rete ridges.
   - These macrophages exhibit large granular to foamy cytoplasm and a central nucleus.
   - Mild to moderate sub-epithelial chronic inflammation in the lamina propria is often present.
   - Nowparast et al. (1981) suggested a microscopic classification of verruciform xanthomas as *verrucous* type, *papillary* type and *flat* type according to the epithelial growth pattern and resemblance to other lesions like verruca vulgaris and oral papilloma.
2. *Intraosseous Xanthoma*
   - Diffuse aggregates of foamy cells.
   - The stroma consists of a delicate fibrous component.
   - Fragments of lamellar and woven bone or dystrophic calcifications can be found surrounded by foamy histiocytes.
   - -The presence of cholesterol clefts may be present and associated with foreign body-type multinucleated giant cell reaction, which, however, is only rarely described.
   - Hyaline globules (thanatosomes), which appear as round or ovoid eosinophilic structures, may be seen. They can be found intracellularly or extracellularly, and range from light pink to strong red in color.
   - Macrophages appear as large, round, or ovoid foamy cells, with vesicular or hyperchromatic nuclei.
   - Mild-to-moderate reactive chronic inflammatory infiltrate containing lymphocytes and plasma cells is also usually observed.
   - Spindle-cells, represented by a fibroblastic population, are found surrounding the periphery of the xanthomatous population.
   - The occurrence of a more prominent spindle cell population arranged in a storiform growth pattern favors the diagnosis of a benign fibrous histiocytoma of the bone (Figs. 28.3, 28.4, 28.5, 28.6, 28.7, 28.8, and 28.9).

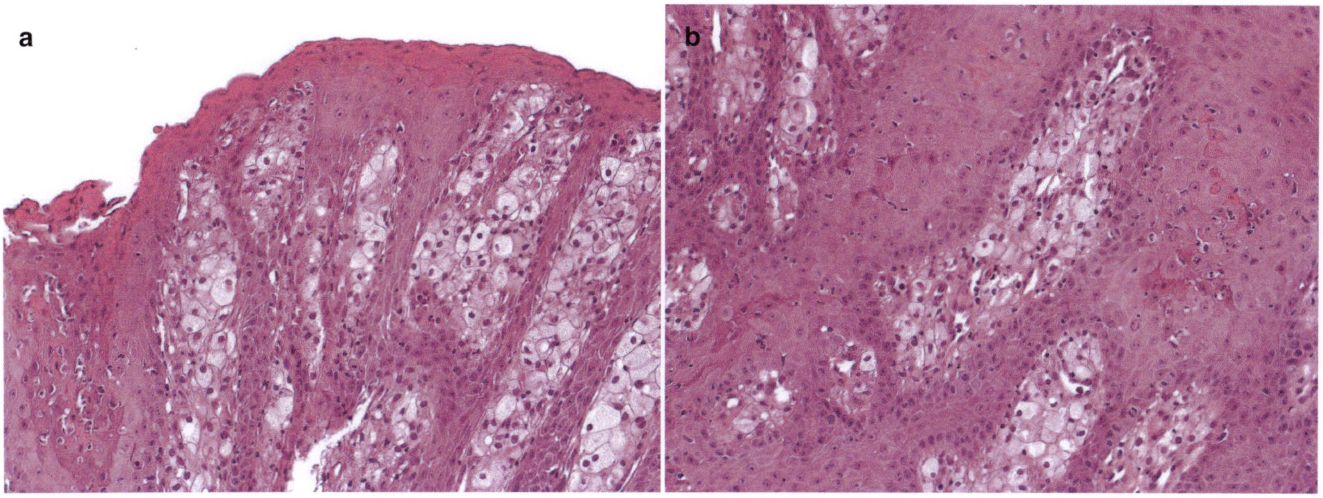

Fig. 28.3 Microscopic features of oral verruciform xanthoma. (**a**) Presence of xanthomatous histiocytes in the lamina propria (H&E; 200X). (**b**) Observe the xanthomatous histiocytes located between the epithelial ridges (H&E; 200X)

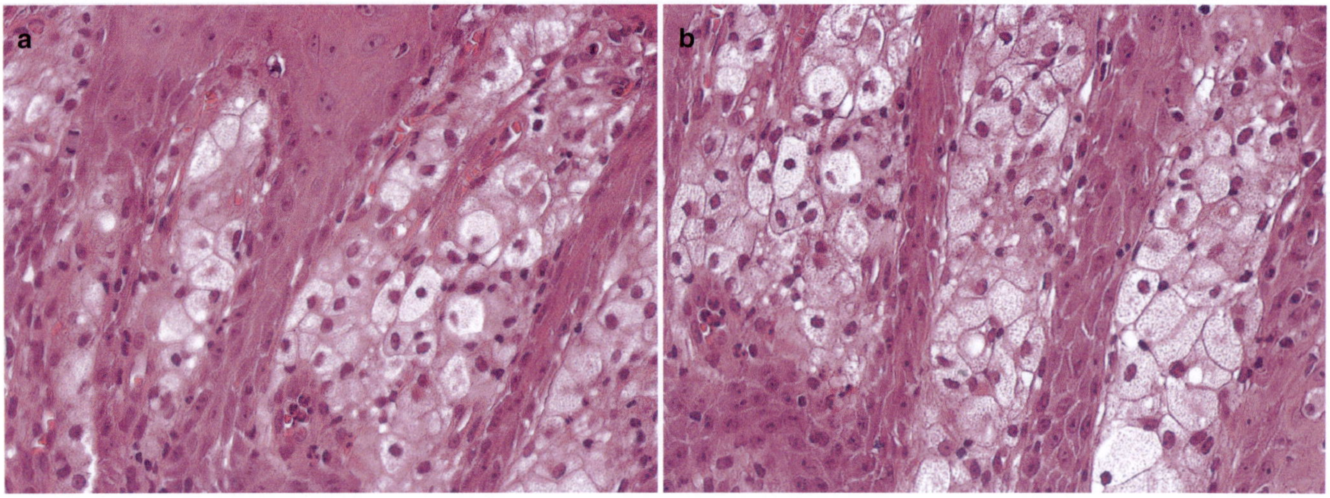

Fig. 28.4 Microscopic features of oral verruciform xanthoma. (**a**) The xanthomatous histiocytes are large cells with granular cytoplasm and hyperchromatic round nuclei (H&E; 400X). (**b**) Observe the xanthomatous histiocytes with their large granulomatous cytoplasm (H&E; 400X)

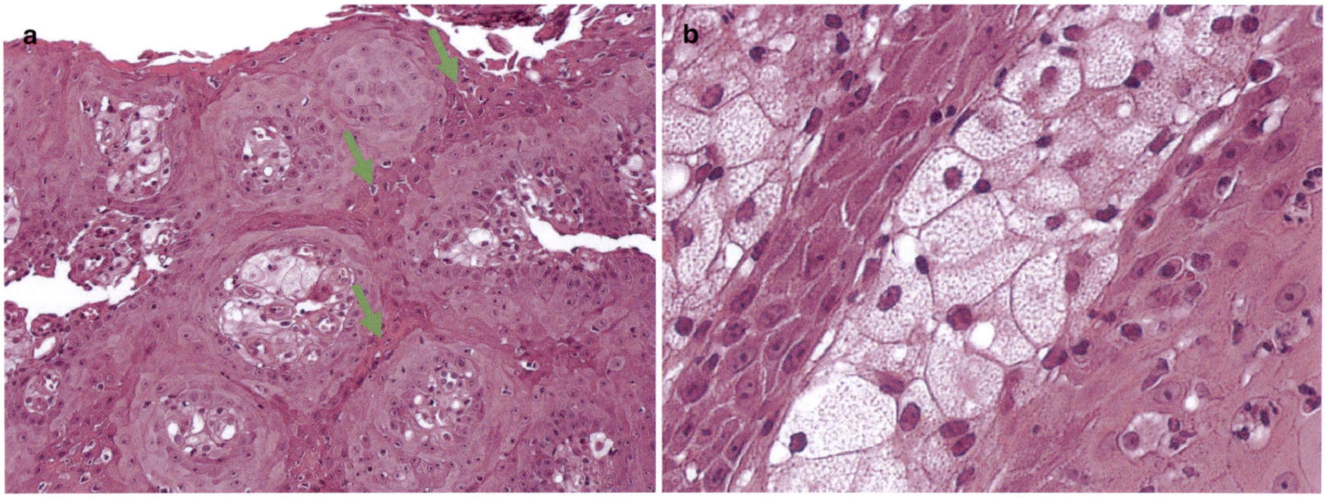

Fig. 28.5 Microscopic features of oral verruciform xanthoma. (**a**) The overlying epithelium often demonstrates regions with a more reddish to orange-colored appearance (green arrows) (H&E; 200X). (**b**) Under high power, observe the xanthomatous histiocytes with their large granulomatous cytoplasm round nuclei located between the epithelial ridges (H&E; 600X)

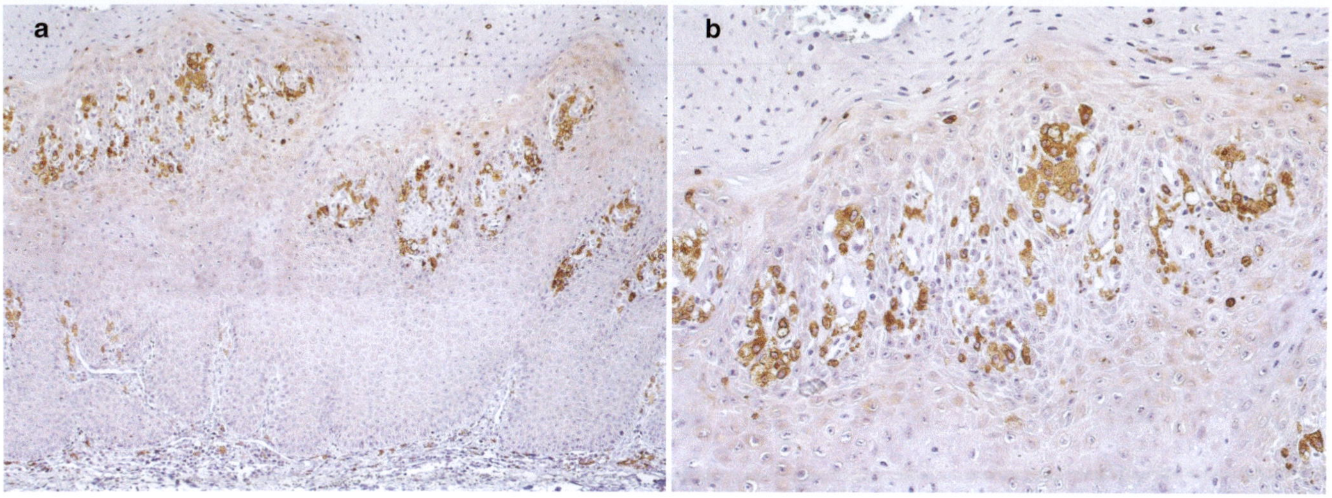

Fig. 28.6 Immunohistochemical features of verruciform xanthoma in the oral cavity. (**a**) Foamy histiocytes are strongly positive for histiocytic markers like CD68 (DAB; 50X), (**b**) and CD163. These markers can be useful to demonstrate the presence of the histiocytes in those cases where their microscopic recognition using H&E staining is not easily observed (DAB; 100X)

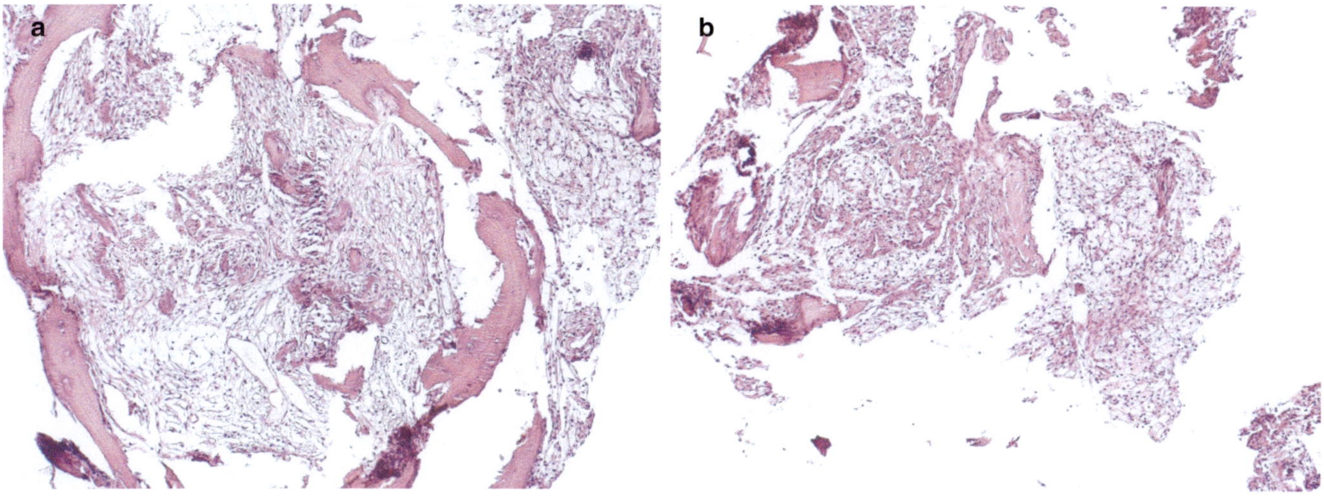

Fig. 28.7 Microscopic features of intraosseous xanthoma affecting the mandible. (**a**) The presence of residual normal bone trabeculae surrounded by foamy histocytes (H&E; 50X). (**b**) Mature foamy histiocytes permeating the bone trabeculae of the mandible (H&E; 50X)

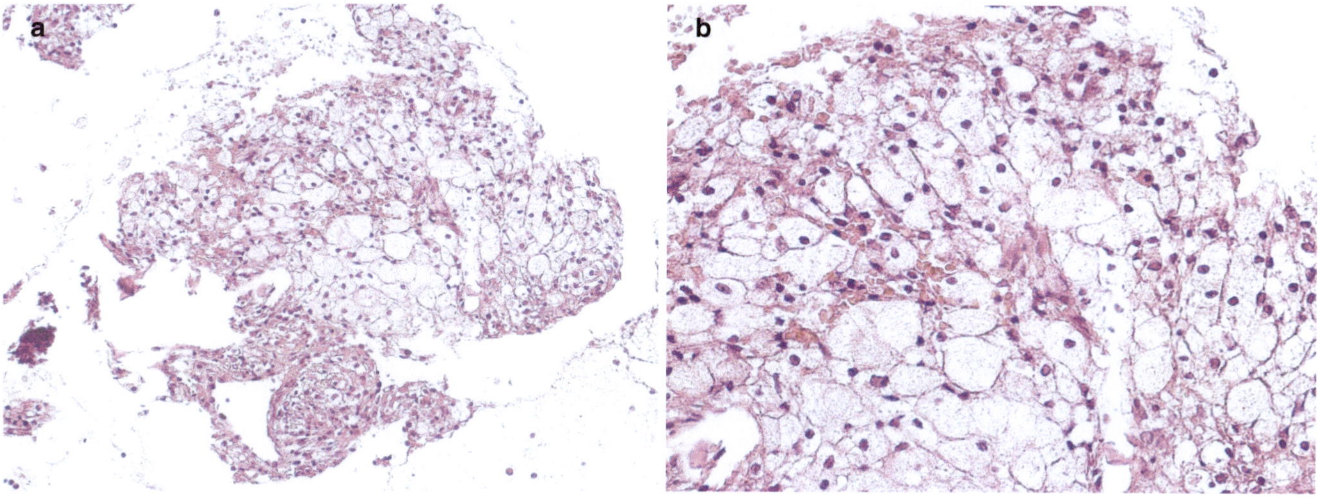

Fig. 28.8 Microscopic features of intraosseous xanthoma affecting the mandible. (**a**) The stroma of the lesion consists of a slight connective tissue (H&E; 100X). (**b**) Mature foamy histiocytes show a large granular cytoplasm and hyperchromatic nuclei (H&E; 200X)

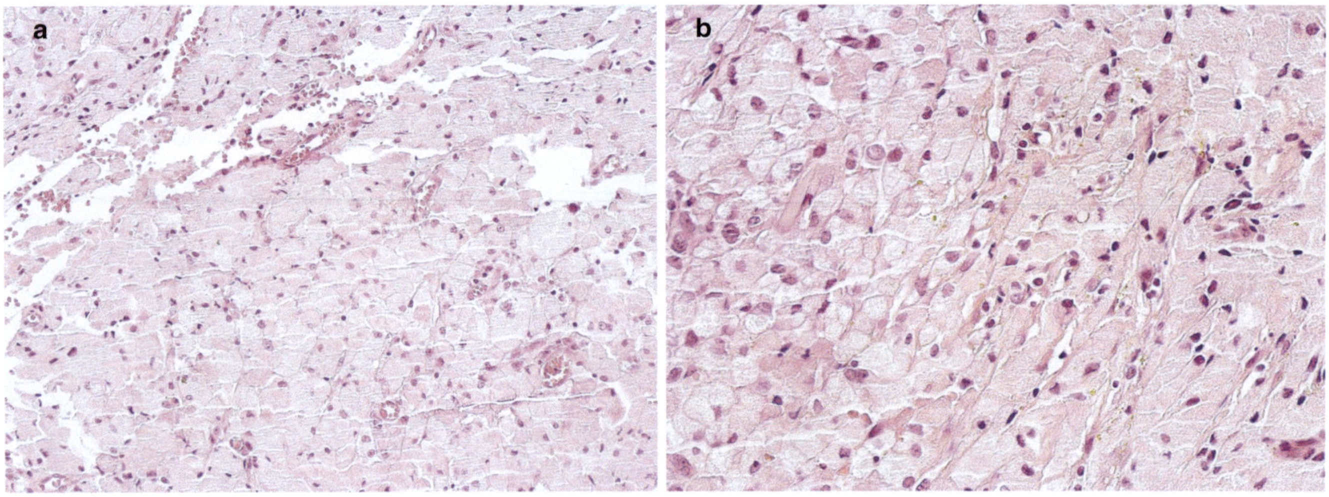

Fig. 28.9 Microscopic features of intraosseous xanthoma affecting the mandible. (**a**) Closely packed mature foamy histiocytes in an intraosseous xanthoma affecting the posterior region of the mandible (H&E; 100X). (**b**) Observe the granular aspect of the cytoplasm and the hyperchromatic, round nuclei (H&E; 200X)

Table 28.1 Summary of the main immunohistochemical reactions that can be used for verruciform xanthoma and intraosseous xanthoma diagnosis

Antibody/probe	Most frequent results	Pattern	Objective
CD20	Negative	Membrane	To exclude a B-cell origin of the lesion
CD3	Negative	Membrane	To exclude a T-cell origin of the lesion
CD68 (KP1)	Positive	Cytoplasm	To demonstrate the histiocytic differentiation
CD68 (PGM1)	Positive	Cytoplasm	To demonstrate the histiocytic differentiation
CD163	Positive	Membrane	To demonstrate the histiocytic differentiation
S100	Negative	Cytoplasm/Nucleus	To exclude the diagnosis of extranodal Rosai-Dorfman disease
CD1a	Negative	Membrane	To exclude a Langerhans cell histiocytosis
Ki67	Very low	Nucleus	To demonstrate the proliferative index of the lesions

These results are considered in the macrophages. CD163 is considered a more specific marker to demonstrate the histiocytic differentiation than CD68

28.3 Immunohistochemistry and/or Genetics

The diagnosis of verruciform xanthomas is almost always done under H&E evaluation; however, when immunohistochemistry is done, the macrophages located in the lamina propria near the squamous epithelium usually express S100, CD68 and CD163 proteins, with no staining for CD1a and CD207 markers. A very low proliferative index is observed. Intraosseous xanthomas also have a similar immunohistochemical pattern, with the expression of mature histiocytic markers. The occurrence of mutations in the *NSDHL* gene has been described in rare cases of sporadic verruciform xanthomas (Table 28.1; Fig. 28.10).

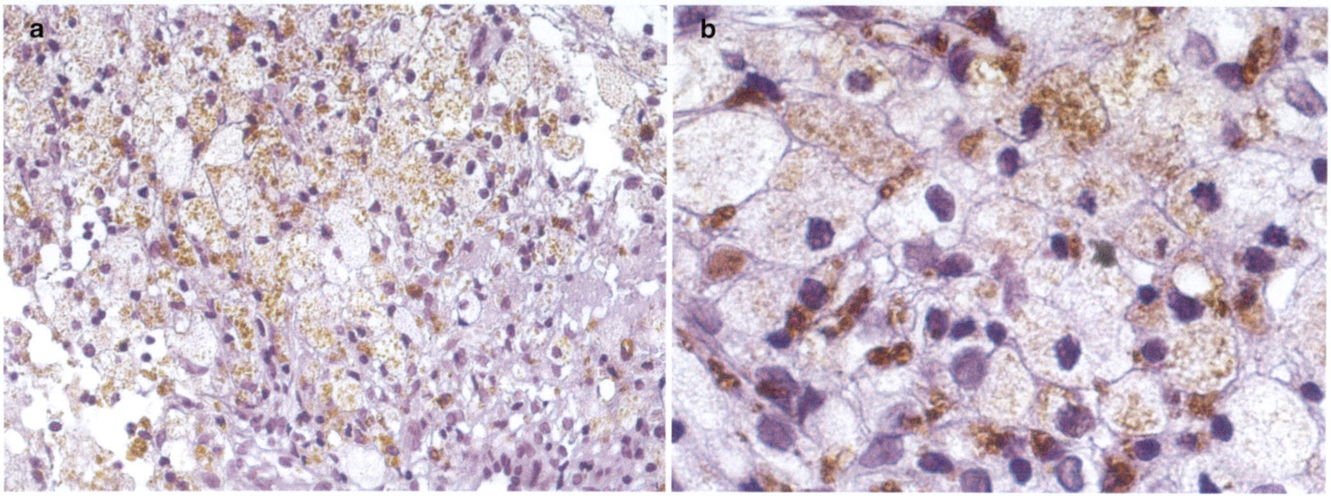

Fig. 28.10 Immunohistochemical features of intraosseous xanthoma affecting the mandible. (**a**) Foamy histiocytes are positive for the histiocytic marker CD68 (DAB; 200X). (**b**) Note the granular staining pattern of CD68 in the foamy histiocytes (DAB; 1000X)

Sources

1. Shafer WG. Verruciform xanthoma. Oral Surg Oral Med Oral Pathol. 1971;31(6):784–9.
2. Nowparast B, Howell FV, Rick GM. Verruciform xanthoma: a clinicopathologic review and report of fifty-four cases. Oral Surg Oral Med Oral Pathol. 1981;51(6):619–25.
3. Philipsen HP, Reichart PA, Takata T, Ogawa I. Verruciform xanthoma—biological profile of 282 oral lesions based on a literature survey with nine new cases from Japan. Oral Oncol. 2003;39(4):325–36. https://doi.org/10.1016/s1368-8375(02)00088-x.
4. Mehra S, Li L, Fan CY, Smoller B, Morgan M, Somach S. A novel somatic mutation of the 3beta-hydroxysteroid dehydrogenase gene in sporadic cutaneous verruciform xanthoma. Arch Dermatol. 2005;141(10):1263–7. https://doi.org/10.1001/archderm.141.10.1263.
5. Ide F, Obara K, Yamada H, Mishima K, Saito I, Kusama K. Cellular basis of verruciform xanthoma: immunohistochemical and ultrastructural characterization. Oral Dis. 2008;14(2):150–7. https://doi.org/10.1111/j.1601-0825.2007.01362.x.
6. Shahrabi Farahani S, Treister NS, Khan Z, Woo SB. Oral verruciform xanthoma associated with chronic graft-versus-host disease: a report of five cases and a review of the literature. Head Neck Pathol. 2011;5(2):193–8. https://doi.org/10.1007/s12105-011-0246-2.
7. de Andrade BA, Agostini M, Pires FR, Rumayor A, Carlos R, de Almeida OP, et al. Oral verruciform xanthoma: a clinicopathologic and immunohistochemical study of 20 cases. J Cutan Pathol. 2015;42(7):489–95. https://doi.org/10.1111/cup.12500.
8. Rawal YB, Chandra SR, Hall JM. Central xanthoma of the jaw bones: a benign tumor. Head Neck Pathol. 2017;11(2):192–202. https://doi.org/10.1007/s12105-016-0764-z.
9. Tamiolakis P, Theofilou VI, Tosios KI, Sklavounou-Andrikopoulou A. Oral verruciform xanthoma: report of 13 new cases and review of the literature. Med Oral Patol Oral Cir Bucal. 2018;23(4):e429–35. https://doi.org/10.4317/medoral.22342.
10. de Arruda JAA, Almeida TFA, Abreu LG, do Amaral MBF, Anbinder AL, Flores RM, et al. Intraosseous xanthoma of the mandible: a multi-institutional case series with a literature review. J Oral Pathol Med. 2019;48(10):935–42. https://doi.org/10.1111/jop.12940.
11. Mainville GN. Non-HPV papillary lesions of the oral mucosa: clinical and histopathologic features of reactive and neoplastic conditions. Head Neck Pathol. 2019;13(1):71–9. https://doi.org/10.1007/s12105-019-01001-9.
12. Barrett AW, Boyapati RP, Bisase BS, Norris PM, Shelley MJ, Collyer J, et al. Verruciform xanthoma of the oral mucosa: a series of eight typical and three anomalous cases. Int J Surg Pathol. 2019;27(5):492–8. https://doi.org/10.1177/1066896919827374.
13. Belknap AN, Islam MN, Bhattacharyya I, Cohen DM, Fitzpatrick SG. Oral verruciform xanthoma: a series of 212 cases and review of the literature. Head Neck Pathol. 2020;14(3):742–8. https://doi.org/10.1007/s12105-019-01123-0.
14. Wilkinson PE, Merkourea S, Gopalakrishnan R, Argyris PP. Primary intraosseous xanthomas of the jaws: a series of six cases including an example with formation of apoptosis-related hyaline globules, so-called "Thanatosomes". Head Neck Pathol. 2020;14(4):859–68. https://doi.org/10.1007/s12105-020-01126-2.
15. Javadi T, Saeed F, Parker DC, Magliocca KR. Verruciform xanthoma: clinical and morphologic spectrum across oral, genital, and cutaneous sites. Head Neck Pathol. 2023;17(3):673–8. https://doi.org/10.1007/s12105-023-01568-4.
16. Mewar P, Foss RD. Benign fibrohistiocytic jaw lesions: a 48-year clinicopathologic analysis and review of the literature. Oral Surg Oral Med Oral Pathol Oral Radiol. 2023. https://doi.org/10.1016/j.oooo.2023.04.002.
17. Venkat S, Islam MN, Bhattacharyya I, Cohen DM, Kratochvil FJ, Woods TR, et al. Xanthoma of the jaw bones: cases series and review of literature. Head Neck Pathol. 2024;18(1):19. https://doi.org/10.1007/s12105-024-01615-8.

Juvenile Xanthogranuloma

29

Tatiana Nayara Libório Kimura, Ana Lia Anbinder, and Felipe Paiva Fonseca

29.1 General Overview and Clinical Presentation

Histiocytosis includes different disorders characterized by the proliferation of mononuclear phagocytic cells, like dendritic cells, monocytes, and macrophages. According to the last classification of histiocytosis proposed by Emile et al. in 2016, five different groups were recognized based on cellular origin, molecular pathology, and clinical features: The L group (Langerhans histiocytosis), C group (cutaneous and mucocutaneous histiocytosis), M group (malignant histiocytosis), R group (Rosai-Dorfman disease and histiocytosis not otherwise specified), and H group (hemophagocytic lymphohistiocytosis and macrophage activation syndrome).

Juvenile xanthogranuloma is a benign non-Langerhans cell histiocytosis classified in the C group histogenetically associated with dermal macrophages that more often appears as papules or yellow-red nodules in the skin (76.8%) or soft tissues (15.7%). The disease was initially recognized in 1905 as single or multiple cutaneous nodules in the infant, and during the following decades, it received different terminologies, including nevoxanthoendothelioma, juvenile xanthoma, and congenital tuberous xanthoma. The exact etiology of juvenile xanthogranuloma is still unknown, and its self-limiting clinical nature suggests that it is more likely a reactive rather than neoplastic process, although some clonality analyses have favored a neoplastic origin.

Similar to other types of histiocytosis including Langerhans cell histiocytosis, Rosai-Dorfman disease and Edheran-Chester Disease, the presence of mutations in members of the *MAPK-ERK* pathway, although rare, suggests that alterations in these genes may play some role in the pathogenesis of a subset of cases. Mutations in members of the *PI3K* pathway have also been described in some juvenile xanthogranulomas. Some cases were shown to develop in the context of neurofibromatosis type 1 and juvenile myelomonocytic leukemia; however, the true pathogenetic association with these conditions remains to be fully validated, especially those cases in the oral cavity.

Non-soft tissue, extracutaneous manifestations of the disease are also well known and many locations can be affected, including the eye, liver and spleen, brain, lungs, intestines, pancreas, testis, bone, and heart. Juvenile xanthogranuloma mainly affects people during the first years of life with a mean age of 4.5 years old at diagnosis; however, many cases affecting adults have been described. Approximately 45%–50% of juvenile xanthogranulomas are diagnosed at or before 1 year of age and may also be noted at birth. Congenital cases are typically large (>3 cm), solitary, firm, ill-defined subcutaneous plaque(s) or firm nodules, and the head and neck region is one of the most affected sites. Juvenile xanthogranuloma may develop synchronically or metacronically with other histiocytosis, and may also evolve from a previous histiocytic condition like Langerhans cell histiocytosis. Approximately 5% of the cases are systemic and frequently associated with the occurrence of numerous skin lesions, systemic symptoms, abnormal laboratory test alterations, or ophthalmological alterations, and these patients should be differentiated from Erdheim-Chester disease that presents similar histologic features and is characterized by frequent activating somatic mutations of *MAPK* pathway genes, including *BRAF-V600E* mutation.

Juvenile xanthogranulomas may also affect the oral mucosa, with the cheek mucosa, tongue and gingiva being the most affected locations, followed by the palate. In accordance

T. N. Libório Kimura (✉)
Department of Pathology and Legal Medicine, School of Medicine, Federal University of Amazonas, Manaus, AM, Brazil
e-mail: tliborio@ufam.edu.br

A. L. Anbinder
Department of Biosciences and Oral Diagnosis, Institute of Science and Technology, São Paulo State University (UNESP), São José dos Campos, Brazil
e-mail: ana.anbinder@unesp.br

F. P. Fonseca
Department of Oral Surgery and Pathology, School of Dentistry, Universidade Federal de Minas Gerais, Belo Horizonte, Brazil

© The Author(s), under exclusive license to Springer Nature Switzerland AG 2025

F. P. Fonseca et al. (eds.), *Lymphoproliferative and Granulomatous Disorders of the Oral Cavity*,
https://doi.org/10.1007/978-3-031-98844-8_29

with cutaneous cases, most oral lesions affect children in their first and second decades of life (mean 14 years old), with a slight male predominance. Less than 10% of cases have co-existing cutaneous lesions, usually with no visceral involvement. Oral lesions commonly present as painless mucosal nodules of normal-colored to yellowish to brownish aspect. These lesions are usually small, soft and non-ulcerated, and surgical specimen analysis often depicts a yellowish appearance of the cut surface. Oral lesions usually do not regress spontaneously, although they frequently follow an indolent clinical course. Clinical differential diagnosis of oral juvenile xanthogranuloma involves a wide spectrum of lesions, including verruciform xanthoma, lipoma, lymphoid aggregate, pyogenic granuloma, peripheral ossifying fibroma, and salivary gland neoplasms, among others.

Juvenile xanthogranuloma is a self-limited condition, and some cutaneous lesions may undergo spontaneous regression. On the other hand, systemic juvenile xanthogranuloma may have a more aggressive clinical course, especially in those cases with liver and/or central nervous system involvement in infants. Conservative surgical removal is the most common therapeutic choice and recurrences are uncommon, ranging from 15% to 17% of the cases.

29.2 Microscopic Findings

- Unencapsulated, circumscribed, widespread proliferation of foamy or eosinophilic histiocytic cells.
- Proliferation of eosinophilic mononuclear spindle cells with histiocytic differentiation.
- Presence of multinucleated giant cells (Touton cells and foreign body type cells); The presence of Touton cells is generally considered a hallmark histologic feature, although not present in all cases.
- Infiltrated lymphocytes and eosinophils are present in different grades.
- Two less common histologic variants are described: Those with absence of foamy cells (non-lipid variant) and those with absence of multinucleated giant cells (mononuclear variant).
- Given the variable morphology and cellular composition of the disease, juvenile xanthogranuloma has also been classified according to four patterns: (1) xanthomatous (consisting of dense sheets of monomorphous, mononuclear histiocytes with variable lipid content, few lymphocytes and/or eosinophils, absence of Touton cells and mitotic figures), (2) xanthogranulomatous (consisting of diffuse infiltrate of foamy or xanthomatized histiocytes, varying numbers of Touton and non-Touton giant cells, and interspersed lymphocytes and/or eosinophils), (3) fibrohistiocytic (variable amount of mononuclear cells, presenting Touton and non-Touton giant cells, spindled morphology interspersed with collagen deposition), and a less common (4) combined subtype.
- Foamy histiocytes are usually large with clear and granular cytoplasm, and round to oval nuclei.
- Spindle cells have an eosinophilic cytoplasm and elongated nuclei.
- Multinucleated giant cells that contain multiple peripherally located nuclei have an external clear halo that surrounds an eosinophilic cytoplasm. These cells are named Touton cells.
- Mitotic figures are generally absent or rare (Figs. 29.1, 29.2, 29.3, 29.4, 29.5, 29.6, and 29.7).

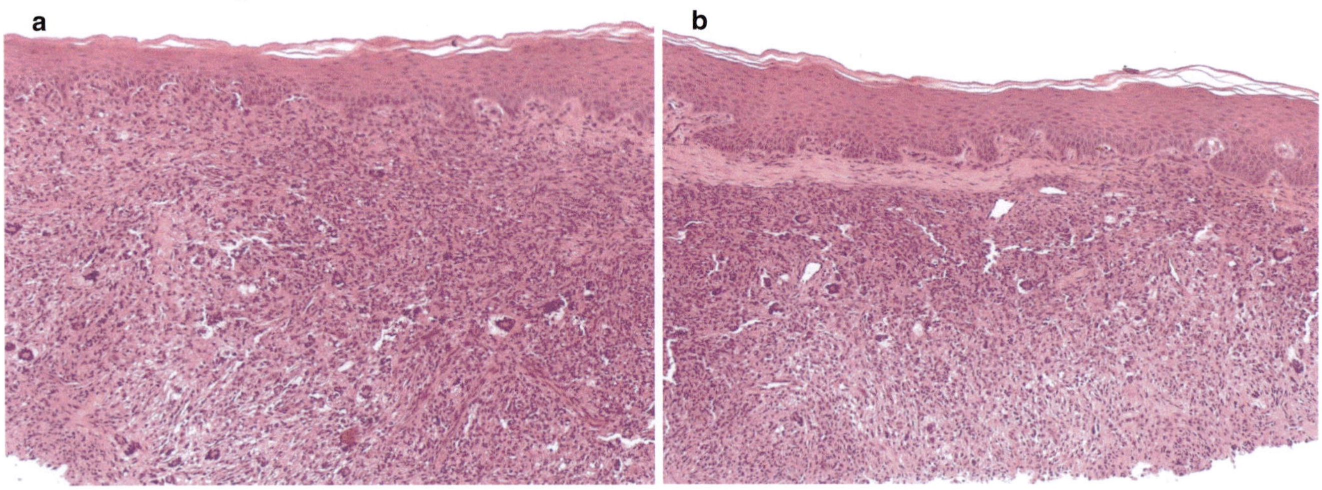

Fig. 29.1 Microscopic features of juvenile xanthogranuloma affecting the oral cavity. (**a**) Proliferation of histiocytic cells in the lamina propria of oral mucosa (H&E; 50X). (**b**) The cells are round to oval, with epithelioid aspect in some instances and the presence of Touton cells is a strong clue for the diagnosis (H&E; 50X)

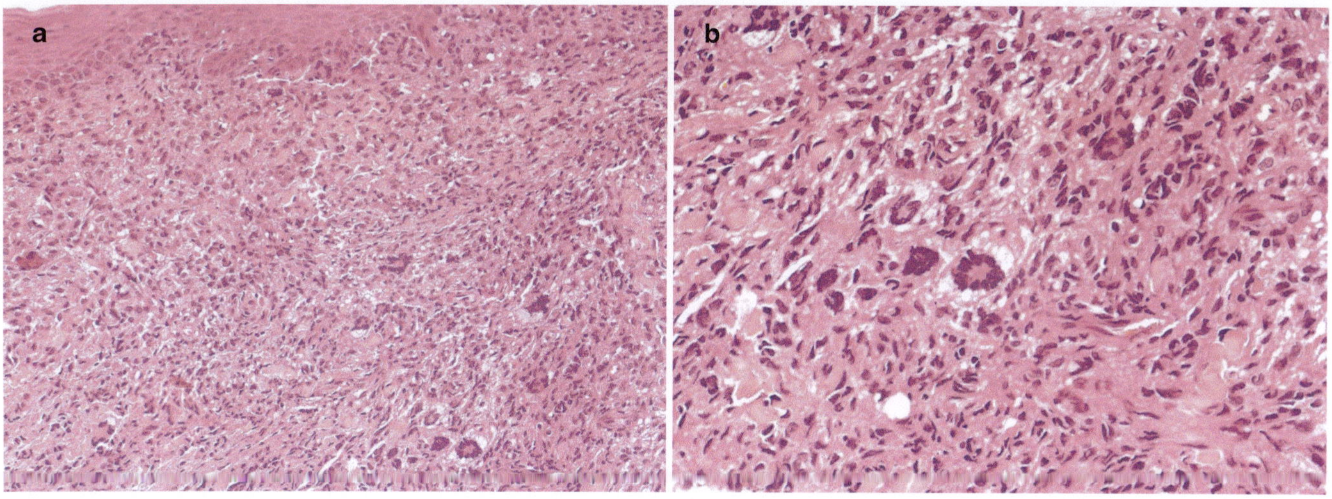

Fig. 29.2 Microscopic features of juvenile xanthogranuloma affecting the oral cavity. (**a**) In addition to epithelioid cells, juvenile xanthogranuloma may also exhibit spindle cell proliferation. The stroma of the lesion is fibrotic and a variable inflammatory infiltrate may be present (H&E; 50X). (**b**) Touton cells are commonly observed in juvenile xanthogranulomas, although their amount varies significantly from case to case (H&E; 100X)

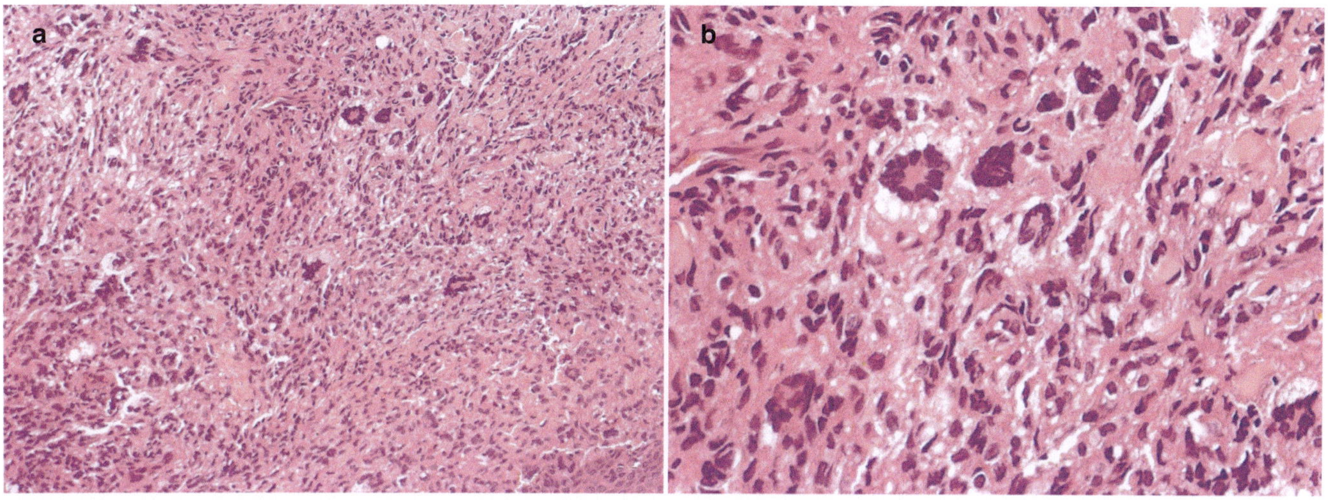

Fig. 29.3 Microscopic features of juvenile xanthogranuloma affecting the oral cavity. (**a**) Example of juvenile xanthogranuloma exhibiting a large number of multinucleated giant cells of the Touton type (H&E; 50X). (**b**) The Touton cells are large cells with multiple peripherally-located nuclei, showing an external clear rim containing adipocytic content (H&E; 200X)

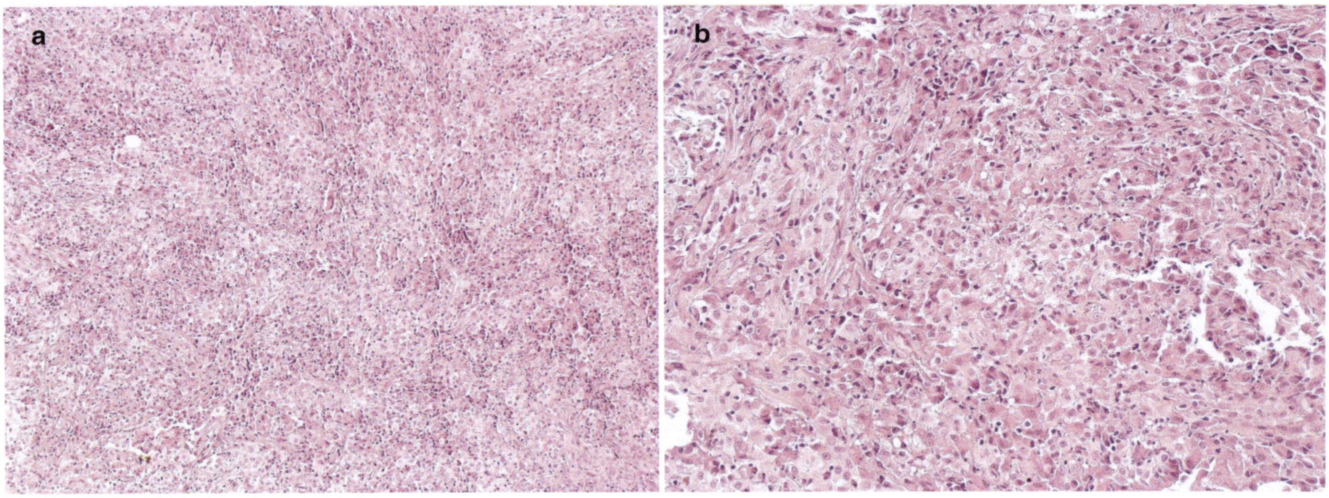

Fig. 29.4 Microscopic features of juvenile xanthogranuloma affecting the oral cavity. (**a**) Juvenile xanthogranuloma cases not exhibiting foamy macrophages are described as a non-lipid variant, as illustrated in this example (H&E; 50X). (**b**) Observe the diffuse proliferation of histiocytic cells. Few multinucleated giant cells are present (H&E; 100X)

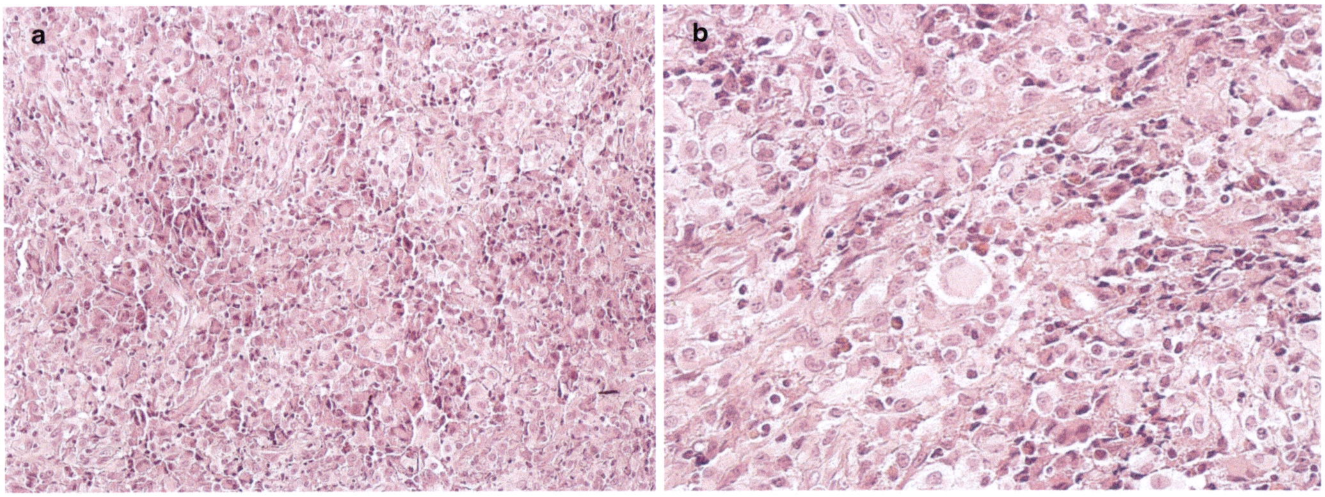

Fig. 29.5 Microscopic features of juvenile xanthogranuloma affecting the oral cavity. (**a**) The histiocytic cells predominantly exhibit a large eosinophilic cytoplasm. Multinucleated giant cells are present throughout the specimen (H&E; 100X). (**b**) Scattered Touton cells (example located in the center of the image) could also be found (H&E; 200X)

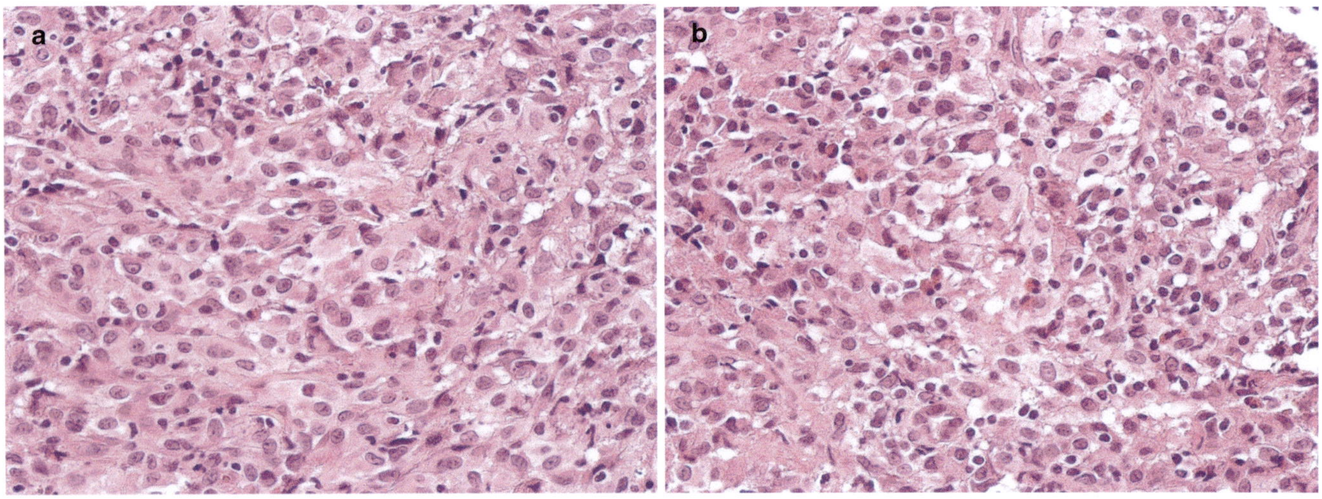

Fig. 29.6 Microscopic features of juvenile xanthogranuloma affecting the oral cavity. (**a**) A few inflammatory cells exhibiting round, more hyperchromatic nuclei are present among the histiocytic proliferation (H&E; 200X). (**b**) The presence of eosinophils is also a frequent finding (H&E; 200X)

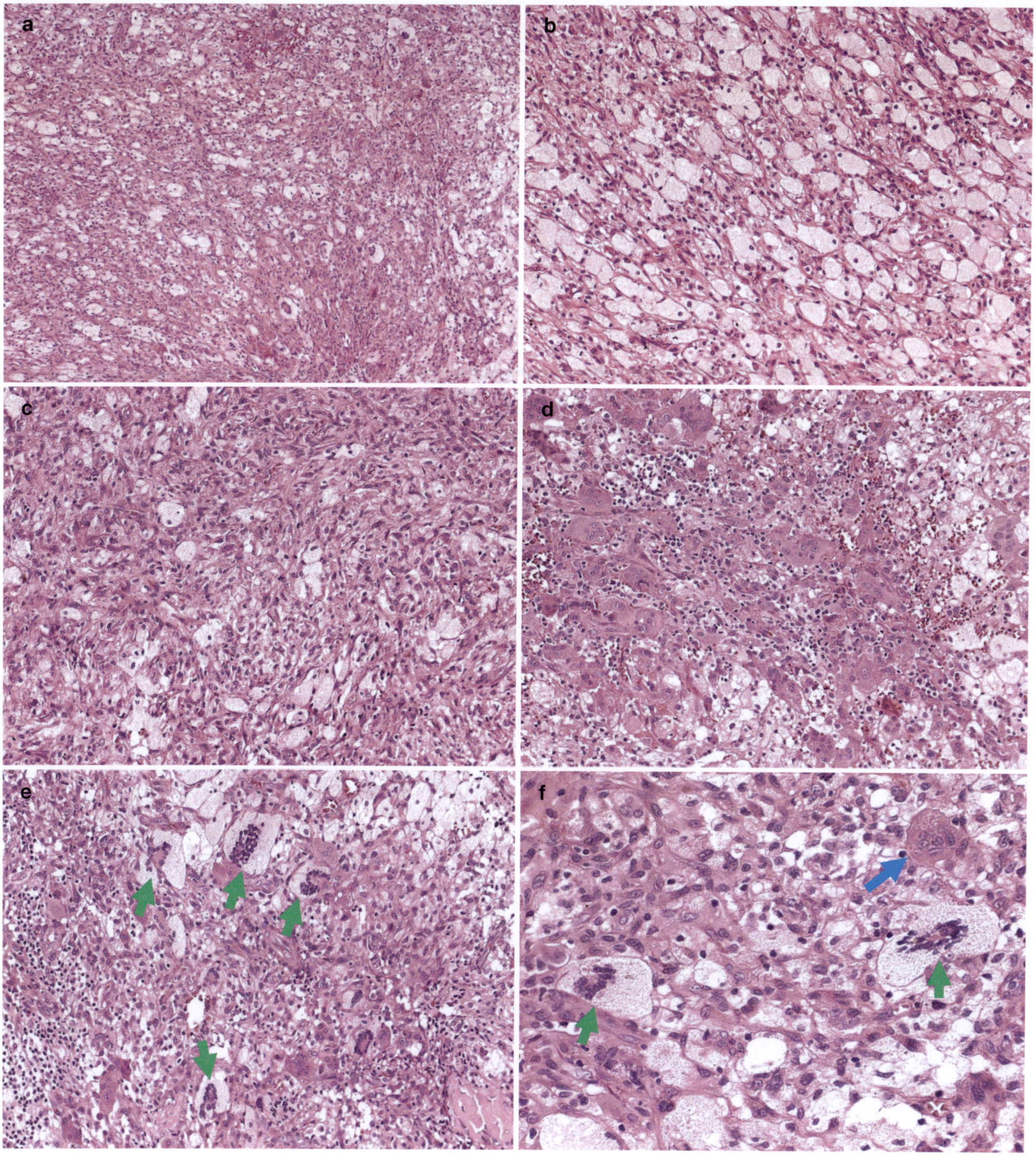

Fig. 29.7 Microscopic features of a juvenile xanthogranuloma affecting the buccal mucosa of a 27-year-old male patient. (**a**) Diffuse proliferation of mononuclear cells, xanthomatous cells and multinucleated giant cells. A reactive mononuclear inflammatory infiltrate with a predominance of lymphocytes is also observed (H&E; 100X). (**b**) In some areas of the lesion there was a predominance of foamy, xanthomatous cells (H&E; 200X). (**c**) In some regions there was a predominance of spindle cells with eosinophilic cytoplasm (H&E; 200X). (**d**) Langhans-type and Foreign body-type multinucleated giant cells (non-Touton-type giant cells) are also present in this case (H&E; 200X). (**e**) The presence of Touton-type multinucleated giant cells (green-arrows) is a microscopic hallmark of juvenile xanthogranuloma, although it may be absent in some cases (H&E; 200X). (**f**) These giant cells are characterized by a central eosinophilic region containing multiple nuclei, and a clear to foamy peripheral halo (green arrows). However, an example of a Foreign body-type multinucleated giant cell can also be observed in this image (blue arrow) (H&E; 400X)

29.3 Immunohistochemistry and/or Genetics

Immunohistochemistry is useful to demonstrate the histiocytic nature of the disease with expression of CD68 and CD163 and to demonstrate that the lesion is a non-Langerhans's disorder, with lack of CD207 and CD1a expression. Other markers also support the histiocytic lineage of the disease like Factor XIIIa expressed in 89.7%–100% of the cases and lysozyme expressed in 50%–100% of the cases. CD11c is present in almost 100% of the cases and is supportive of a hematopoietic nature of the disease. The S100 protein shows a variable and usually a focal positivity in about 30% of the cases. ALK protein is negative. CD4 is present in 78%–100% of the cases and it has been advocated as a useful tool to differentiate juvenile xanthogranuloma from benign fibrohistiocytoma, an important differential diagnosis frequently negative for CD4 expression. The proliferative index is variable, but more often considered low. The occurrence of genetic abnormalities in the *MAPK* and *PIK3K* pathways, including *BRAF-V600E*, although not observed in oral cavity lesions, was reported in a few cases of systemic juvenile xanthogranulomas. Shen et al. (2024) recently described a case of disseminated juvenile xanthogranuloma harboring *GAB2::BRAF* fusion successfully treated with trametinib, a *MEK* inhibitor drug (Table 29.1; Figs. 29.8 and 29.9).

Table 29.1 Summary of the main immunohistochemical reactions used for juvenile xanthogranuloma diagnosis. Important genetic features are also described

Antibody/probe	Most frequent results	Pattern	Objective
CD20	Negative	Membrane	To exclude a B-cell lymphoma
CD3	Negative	Membrane	To exclude a T-cell lymphoma
S100	Negative[a]	Cytoplasm/Nucleus	To exclude a Langerhans cell histiocytosis
CD68 (KP1 and PGM1)	Positive	Cytoplasm	To demonstrate the histiocytic origin of the lesion
CD11c	Positive	Cytoplasm	To characterize the disorder. Hematopoietic marker.
CD163	Positive	Membrane	To demonstrate the histiocytic origin of the lesion
CD1a	Negative	Membrane	To exclude a Langerhans cell histiocytosis
CD207	Negative	Cytoplasm	To exclude a Langerhans cell histiocytosis
Factor XIIIa	Positive	Cytoplasm	To demonstrate the histiocytic origin of the lesion
Lysozyme	Positive	Cytoplasm	To demonstrate the histiocytic origin of the lesion
CD21/CD23/CD35	Negative	Membrane	To exclude a follicular dendritic cell neoplasm
Ki67	Low	Nucleus	To demonstrate the proliferative index of the lesion
MAPK-ERK[b]	Rare cases	–	To characterize the molecular basis of the lesion
PI3K[b]	Rare cases	–	To characterize the molecular basis of the lesion

[a]It can be focally positive in some cases
[b]Investigated by PCR

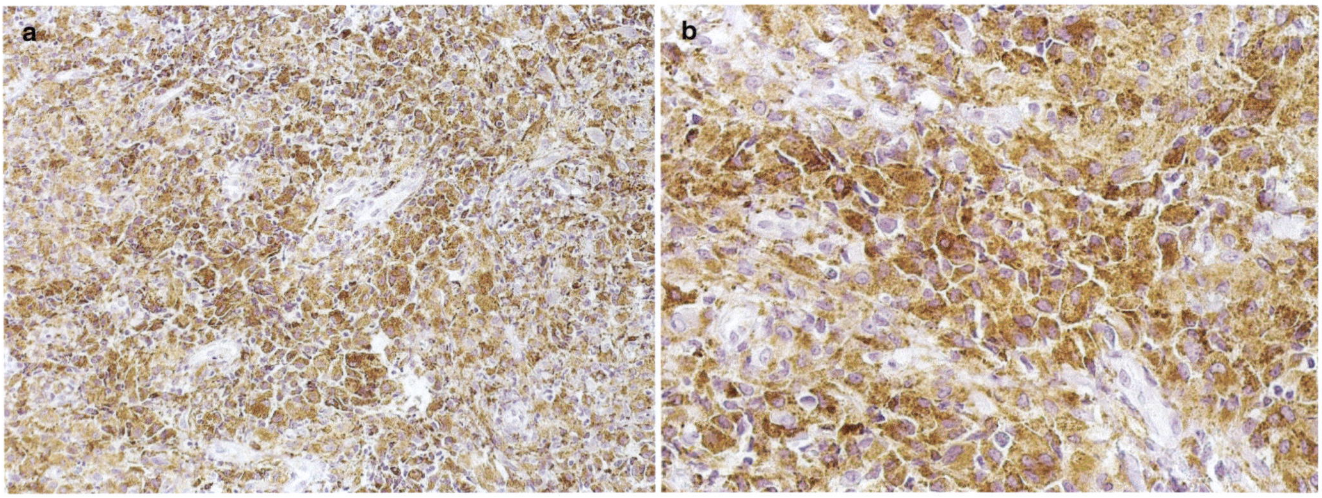

Fig. 29.8 Immunohistochemical features of juvenile xanthogranuloma. (**a**) The cells of the lesion reveal a diffuse cytoplasmic expression of CD68 (DAB; 100X). (**b**) Observe the strong and diffuse expression of CD68 in the histiocytic proliferation (DAB; 200X)

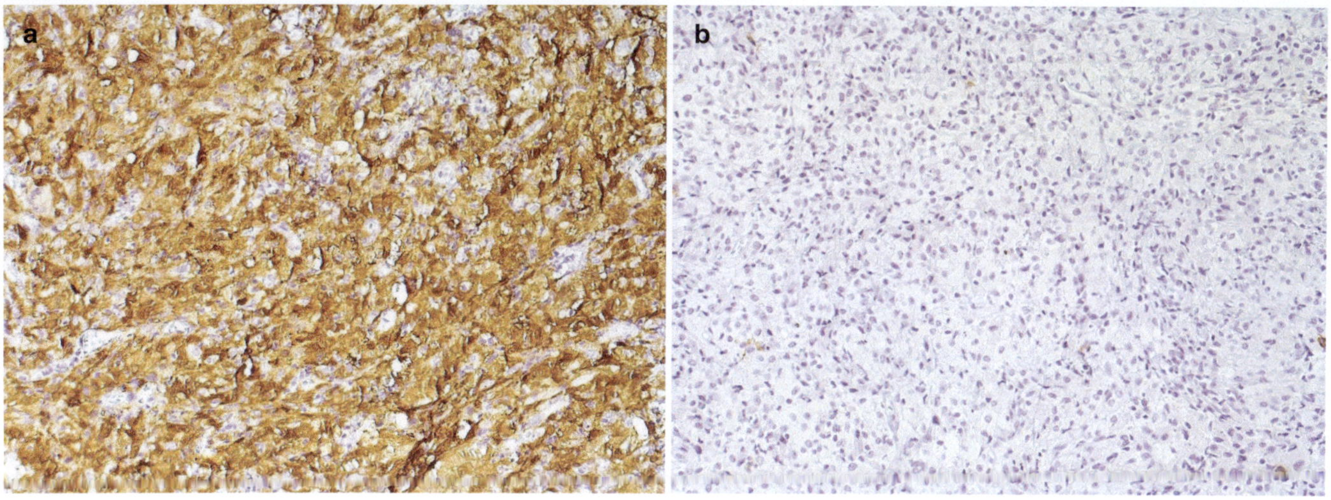

Fig. 29.9 Immunohistochemical features of juvenile xanthogranuloma. (a) Factor XIIIa is also observed in most cases, as exemplified in this image. Observe the strong and diffuse expression of this protein (DAB; 100X). (b) Juvenile xanthogranuloma cells are negative for Langerhans cell markers like CD1a (DAB; 100X)

Sources

1. Flaitz C, Allen C, Neville B, Hicks J. Juvenile xanthogranuloma of the oral cavity in children: a clinicopathologic study. Oral Surg Oral Med Oral Pathol Oral Radiol Endod. 2002;94(3):345–52. https://doi.org/10.1067/moe.2002.122340.
2. Batista AC, Mendonça EF, Arantes Elias LS, Andrade BA, Almeida OP. Nonlipidized juvenile xanthogranuloma: an unusual variant with a potential diagnostic pitfall. Int J Pediatr Otorhinolaryngol. 2012;76:295–9. https://doi.org/10.1016/j.ijporl.2011.11.010.
3. Baik FM, Andeen NK, Schmechel SC, Futran ND. A large juvenile xanthogranuloma within the tongue. Otolaryngol Head Neck Surg. 2014;150(2):332–3. https://doi.org/10.1177/0194599813514534.
4. Collins L, Banks R, Robinson M. Juvenile xanthogranuloma: unusual intraoral finding. Br J Oral Maxillofac Surg. 2015;53(1):86–8. https://doi.org/10.1016/j.bjoms.2014.09.014.
5. Emile JF, Abla O, Fraitag S, Horne A, Haroche J, Donadieu J, Histiocyte Society, et al. Revised classification of histiocytoses and neoplasms of the macrophage-dendritic cell lineages. Blood. 2016;127(22):2672–81. https://doi.org/10.1182/blood-2016-01-690636.
6. Frater JL. The histiocytoses: as easy as ABC (or LCMRH). Blood. 2016;127(22):2655–6. https://doi.org/10.1182/blood-2016-03-706267.
7. Israel MS, Carlos R, Pires FR. Oral juvenile xanthogranuloma: report of two cases. Pediatr Dent. 2017;39(3):238–40.
8. Sánchez-Romero C, Cuenca Arriaga AI, Paes de Almeida O, Gutiérrez CE. Oral juvenile xanthogranuloma in a child: clinical, histological and immunohistochemical profile of a rare entity. J Cutan Pathol. 2018;45(7):515–21. https://doi.org/10.1111/cup.13152.
9. Picarsic J, Pysher T, Zhou H, Fluchel M, Pettit T, Whitehead M, et al. BRAF V600E mutation in Juvenile Xanthogranuloma family neoplasms of the central nervous system (CNS-JXG): a revised diagnostic algorithm to include pediatric Erdheim-Chester disease. Acta Neuropathol Commun. 2019;7(1):168. https://doi.org/10.1186/s40478-019-0811-6.
10. Gioco G, Rupe C, Basco A, Contaldo M, Gallenzi P, Lajolo C. Oral juvenile xanthogranuloma: an unusual presentation in an adult patient and a systematic analysis of published cases. Oral Surg Oral Med Oral Pathol Oral Radiol. 2022;133(1):42–9. https://doi.org/10.1016/j.oooo.2021.09.015.
11. Salari B, Dehner LP. Juvenile and adult xanthogranuloma: a 30-year single-center experience and review of the disorder and its relationship to other histiocytoses. Ann Diagn Pathol. 2022;58:151940. https://doi.org/10.1016/j.anndiagpath.2022.151940.
12. Mota CP, Silva Cunha JL, Magalhães MCSV, Israel MS, Freire NA, Dos Santos ERC, et al. Oral juvenile xanthogranuloma: a clinicopathological, immunohistochemical and BRAF V600E study of five new cases, with literature review. Head Neck Pathol. 2022;16(2):407–15. https://doi.org/10.1007/s12105-021-01373-x.
13. Hélias-Rodzewicz Z, Donadieu J, Terrones N, Barkaoui MA, Lambilliotte A, Moshous D, et al. Molecular and clinicopathologic characterization of pediatric histiocytoses. Am J Hematol. 2023;98(7):1058–69. https://doi.org/10.1002/ajh.26938.
14. Seidel MG, Brcic L, Hoefler G, Hutter C, Minkov M, Steffen LS, et al. Concurrence of a kinase-dead BRAF and an oncogenic KRAS gain-of-function mutation in juvenile xanthogranuloma. Pediatr Blood Cancer. 2023;70(4):e30060. https://doi.org/10.1002/pbc.30060.
15. Shaker N, Sangueza OP. Langerhans cell histiocytosis evolving into juvenile xanthogranuloma: two linked entities. Am J Dermatopathol. 2023;45(4):259–63. https://doi.org/10.1097/DAD.0000000000002394.
16. Xu J, Ma H, Yao X, Han X, Wen Y, Wang S, et al. Frequent detection of genetic aberrations reveals novel pathogenesis and treatment modalities in systemic juvenile xanthogranuloma. Pediatr Investig. 2023;7(3):212–5. https://doi.org/10.1002/ped4.12398.
17. Shen KN, Lin H, Chang L, Cao XX. Disseminated juvenile xanthogranuloma harbouring a GAB2::BRAF fusion successfully treated with trametinib: a case report. Br J Dermatol. 2024;192(1):169–71. https://doi.org/10.1093/bjd/ljae328.

Langerhans Cell Histiocytosis

30

Jean Nunes dos Santos,
Sara Ferreira dos Santos Costa, Fábio Luiz Coracin,
and Felipe Paiva Fonseca

30.1 General Overview and Clinical Presentation

Langerhans cell histiocytosis is a clonal neoplastic proliferation of bone marrow-derived histiocytes (Langerhans-type cells) characterized by unifocal, multifocal single-system, or multisystem disease that occurs in all age groups, but with most cases occurring during childhood, more often during the first and third decades of life. The incidence of Langerhans cell histiocytosis is estimated to range from three to five cases per million children and from one to two cases per million adults.

Historically, the first clinical cases were initially recognized in the early 1900s in children with unusual constellations of lesions involving the bone isolated or together with the involvement of other organs, when Langerhans cell histiocytosis used to be classified as three different variants depending on the clinical presentation of the disease: Letterer-Siwe disease (subacute or acute disseminated form), Hand-Schüller-Christian disease (disseminated chronic form), and eosinophilic granuloma (localized chronic form). In 1953, based on the presence of cytoplasmic structures known as X bodies, these conditions were grouped together as histiocytosis X and later renamed to Langerhans cell histiocytosis following the observation of Birbeck granules and their histiocytic/Langerhans cell nature. Currently, considering the last proposed classification of histiocytic disorders, Langerhans cell histiocytosis belongs to the "L group (Langerhans-related)" of diseases together with intermediate-cell histiocytosis, Erdheim-Chester disease, and Mixed Langerhans cell histiocytosis/Erdheim-Chester disease.

The etiology of Langerhans cell histiocytosis remains unclear and different theories like the dysfunction of the immune system, an inflammatory, bacteriological or viral origin have been advocated. In 2010, the genetic basis of the disease was better understood and the occurrence of *BRAF-V600E* mutations was demonstrated in approximately 50% of the cases. Mutations in other members of the *MAPK* family of genes and in other molecular pathways were later demonstrated and are believed to be present in more than 85% of the cases, including *ARAF*, *ERBB3*, *PIK3CA*, *MAP2K1*, *KRAS* and *NRAS* genes.

The clinical course of Langerhans cell histiocytosis is considered highly variable and unpredictable. In the *single-system* form, the disease affects one organ or one system, and the disease can be unifocal or multifocal. The disorder more frequently involves the skin, pituitary, and the bone (80% of the cases), with adjacent soft tissue being usually affected as painful ulcerative lesions or swellings. The skull, femur, vertebra, pelvic bones, ribs, and the jaws are the most affected locations and bone manifestations frequently present as painless or painful osteolytic lesions of the bone cortex and/or vertebra plana of the spine. In its *multisystem* presentation, Langerhans cell histiocytosis is more disseminated, and a life-threatening condition may occur. Skin lesions can be found in up to 33% of the cases and manifest as seborrheic dermatitis or eczematous eruption on the scalp and trunk. The lung, liver and spleen are very often affected. The occurrence of lymphadenopathy (5%–10% of the cases), central nervous system involvement (2%–4% of the cases), and bone marrow involvement are also described. According to the

J. N. dos Santos (✉)
Department of Oral Pathology, School of Dentistry, Federal University of Bahia, Salvador, Brazil

S. F. dos Santos Costa
Department of Pathology and Parasitology, Institute of Biomedical Sciences, Federal University of Alfenas, Alfenas, Brazil
e-mail: sara.costa@unifal-mg.edu.br

F. L. Coracin
Department of Dentistry and Department of Pathology, Barretos Cancer Hospital, Barretos, São Paulo, Brazil

F. P. Fonseca
Department of Oral Surgery and Pathology, School of Dentistry, Universidade Federal de Minas Gerais, Belo Horizonte, Brazil

© The Author(s), under exclusive license to Springer Nature Switzerland AG 2025
F. P. Fonseca et al. (eds.), *Lymphoproliferative and Granulomatous Disorders of the Oral Cavity*,
https://doi.org/10.1007/978-3-031-98844-8_30

Histiocyte Society trials, Langerhans cell histiocytosis can be clinically divided into "high risk" (liver, spleen, and/or bone marrow involvement) or "low risk" (lesions anywhere else) disease, reflecting the relative risk of death of the patient.

The oral and maxillofacial are involved in about 20%–30% of the cases, more frequently the posterior region of the mandible and the surrounding gingival tissue. The palatine mucosa is also commonly affected. The gingival lesions are painful and frequently ulcerated and swollen, which may be frequently misdiagnosed as biofilm-related periodontal disease, and therefore frequently delay the correct diagnosis and treatment. More advanced staged diseases cause alveolar bone resorption that leads to the so-called floating teeth radiographic appearance, where teeth lose their periodontal support and present important levels of mobility, usually leading to premature dental loss. The posterior region of the jaws is more affected than the anterior regions. Gingival bleeding is also observed, and yellowish areas of tissue necrosis can also be described. Langerhans cell histiocytosis radiographically resembling inflammatory periapical lesions may also occur.

Treatment depends on the extent of the disease. For single-system Langerhans cell histiocytosis bone curettage, oral indomethacin and/or intra-lesional injections of corticosteroids are recommended. Multisystem diseases usually demand systemic chemotherapy and are usually treated with a combination of prednisone and vinblastine, with the use of mercaptopurine added for treating high-risk diseases. For patients who have relapsed or refractory Langerhans cell histiocytosis following frontline therapy, there seems to be no consensus about the best therapeutic approach, and the use of several drugs like cytarabine, cladribine, and clofarabine under different schemes has been proposed, as well as the use of hematopoietic stem cell transplantation. Patients affected in single organs such as skin and bone have an excellent prognosis, with a mortality rate of less than 10%. Those patients who develop lesions in multiple organs, particularly in organs such as the liver, lung, spleen, and hematopoietic system, have a considerable mortality rate, ranging from 30% to 50%.

Several studies attempted to investigate the prognostic significance of genetic mutations for Langerhans cell histiocytosis; however, results vary, and the clinical impact of the presence of abnormalities in members of the *MAPK* pathway remains to be better determined, and the effectiveness of targeted therapy using, for instance, *BRAF-V600E* and *MEK*

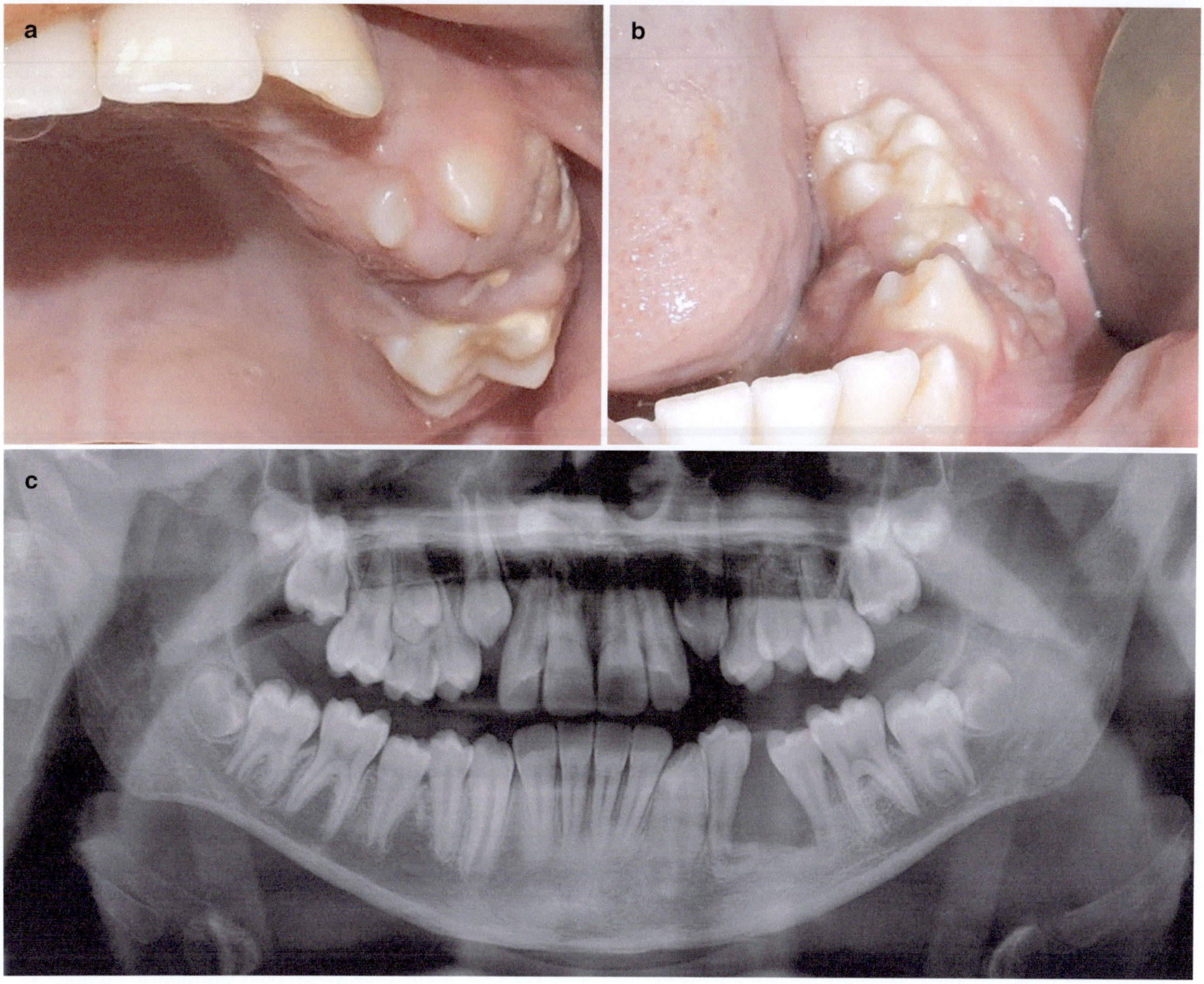

Fig. 30.1 Clinical presentation of Langerhans cell histiocytosis in the oral cavity. (**a**) Male child presented with multiple lesions affecting different areas of the gingival tissue. Observe in this image the irregular swelling affecting the upper left gingiva. There were some areas of ulceration in the vestibular aspect of the gingival tissue. (**b**) The same patient also had the lower gingiva affected by the disease. Observe the irregular gingival overgrowth with yellowish areas of necrosis. (**c**) Radiographically, the disease causes an ill-defined osteolytic destruction of the alveolar bone. Observe a more extensive radiolucid region in the mandible and an extensive periodontal defect in the gnathic bones

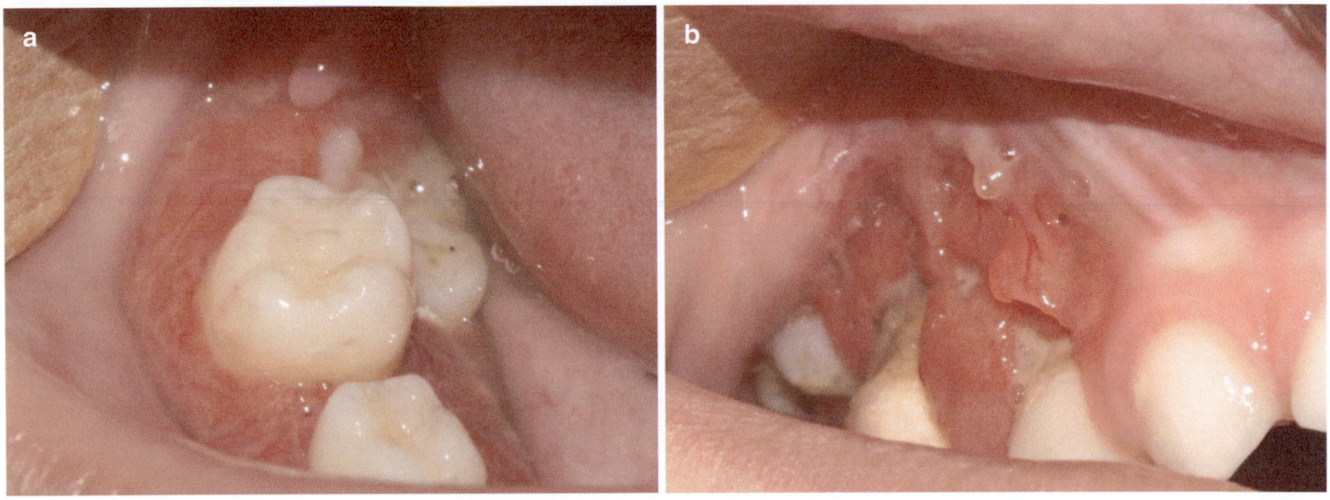

Fig. 30.2 Clinical presentation of Langerhans cell histiocytosis in the oral cavity. (**a**) Male child showing the presence of an asymptomatic gingival swelling in the mandible. (**b**) The same patient also had an ulcerative lesion in the upper right gingiva. Observe that the ulcer leads to the exposure of dental roots

inhibitors, still need to be better evaluated (Figs. 30.1 and 30.2).

30.2 Microscopic Findings

- The cells of Langerhans cell histiocytosis exhibit a diffuse growth pattern.
- There might be a variable degree of fibrosis with collagen deposition in the stroma that results from chronic inflammation and that can lead to changes in the tissue architecture.
- Tumor cells, also called Langerhans cell histiocytosis cells, present clearer nuclei than the surrounding reactive lymphocytes, which present a more hyperchromatic appearance.
- Predominance of medium-sized, oval to round Langerhans cell histiocytosis cells containing eosinophilic cytoplasm and fine nuclear chromatin.
- Langerhans cell histiocytosis cells typically show grooved, folded, indented (coffee bean aspect) or lobed nuclei.
- Atypia and pleomorphism are minimal, with no high-grade cytological features. In the presence of a neoplasm with high-grade morphology and a Langerhans cell immunophenotype, the diagnosis of Langerhans cell sarcoma is more likely.
- Scattered mitotic figures can be found.
- Reactive inflammatory infiltrate is variable, but eosinophils are prominent in most cases, sometimes leading to eosinophilic granulomas, which may demonstrate central areas of necrosis.
- Necrosis can be found.
- Multinucleated giant cells may be found.
- Charcot-Layden crystal can be occasionally found.

Note: On electron microscopy, Langerhans cell histiocytosis cells contain Birbeck granules, which are elongated rod-shaped or tennis racket-shaped organelles. These granules are a hallmark of Langerhans cell histiocytosis and are visible as dispersed structures throughout the cytoplasm, close to the cell membrane and are associated with cytoplasmic extensions. The exact function of the Birbeck granules is not completely understood, but they are thought to be

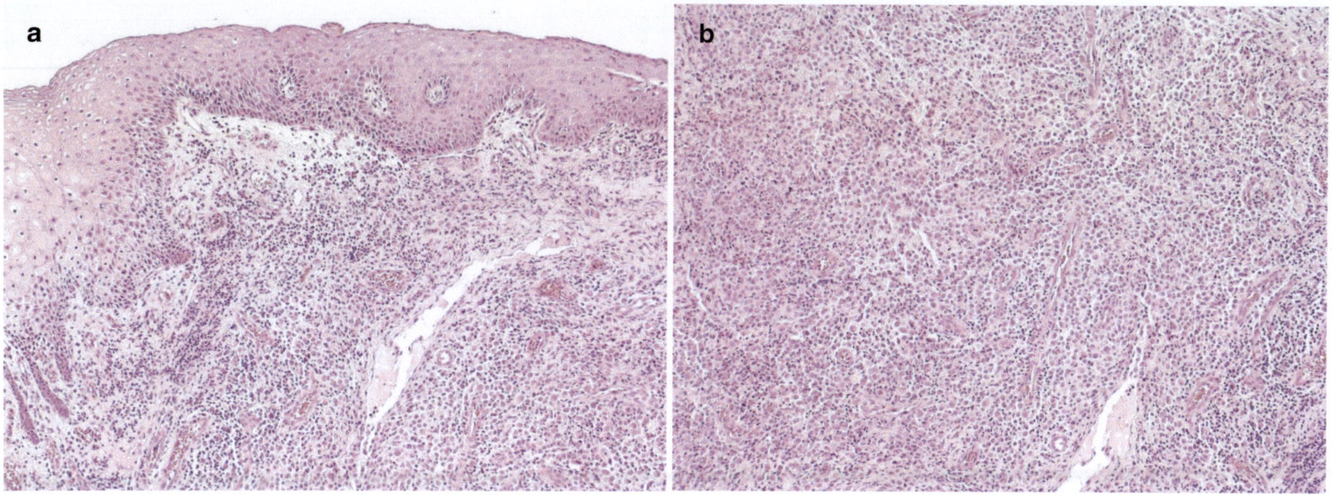

Fig. 30.3 Microscopic features of Langerhans cell histiocytosis affecting the periodontal tissue. (**a**) Tumor cells infiltrate the lamina propria (H&E; 50X). (**b**) A diffuse distribution of tumor cells in a fibrous stroma containing blood vessels of different sizes and shapes is observed (H&E; 50X)

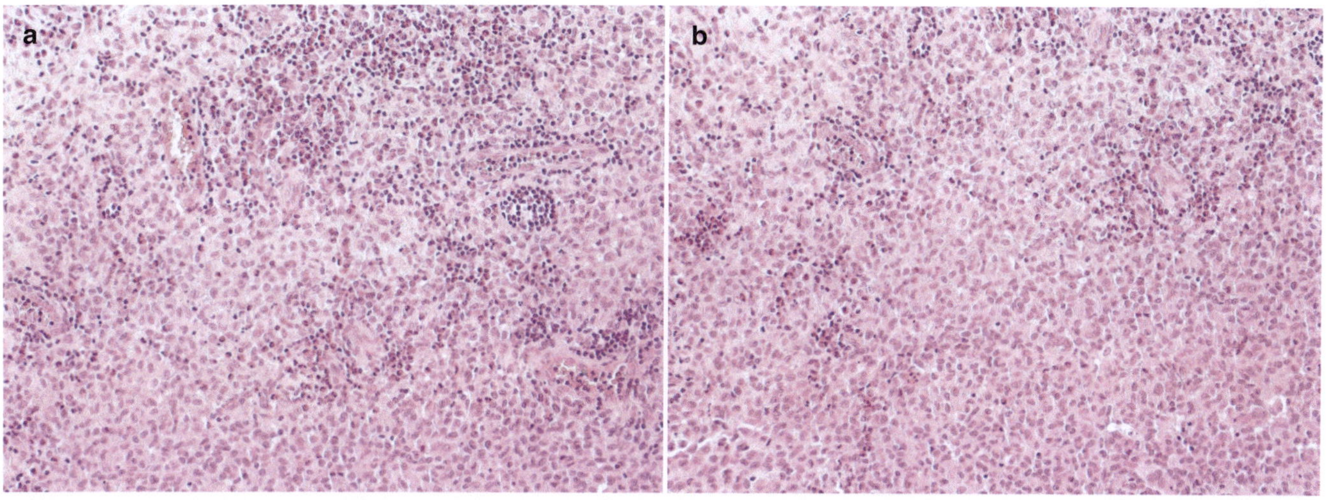

Fig. 30.4 Microscopic features of Langerhans cell histiocytosis affecting the gingiva. (**a**) The tumor cells predominantly present a bland-looking aspect with pale nuclei and abundant eosinophilic cytoplasm. Foci of small cells with hyperchromatic nuclei represent reactive lymphocytes (H&E; 100X). (**b**) In addition to reactive lymphocytes, the presence of eosinophils is a hallmark of Langerhans cell histiocytosis (H&E; 100X)

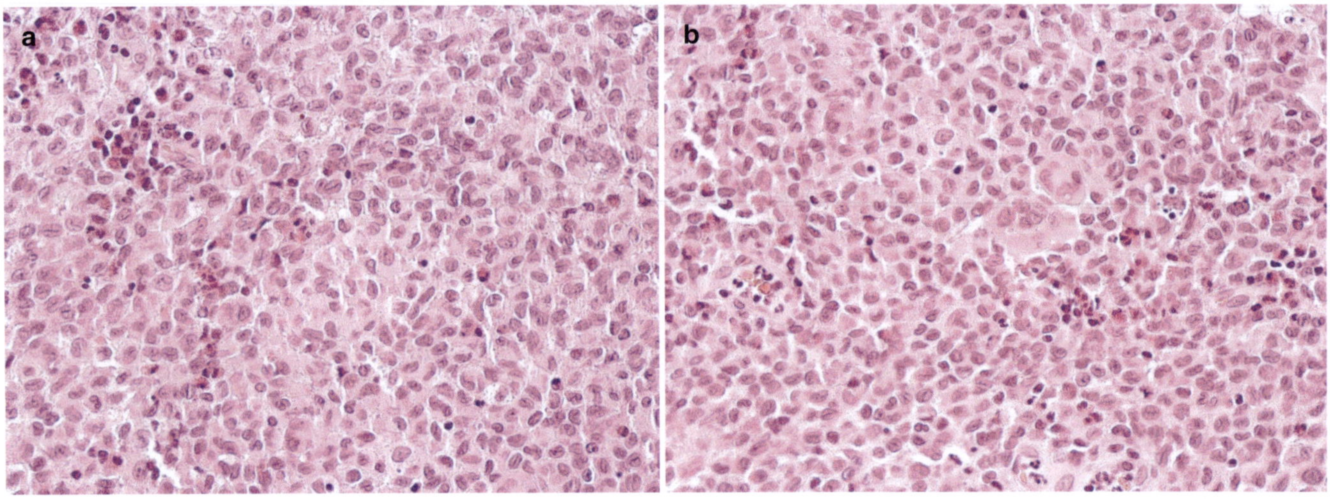

Fig. 30.5 Microscopic features of Langerhans cell histiocytosis affecting the gingiva. (**a**) Under higher magnification, it is possible to observe that tumor cells exhibit nuclear grooving and/or nuclear indentation. These cells are usually referred to as "kidney shaped" or "coffee bean" cells. Observe the presence of eosinophils throughout the specimen (H&E; 200X). (**b**) The presence of multinucleated giant cells is also frequently found. Tumor cells exhibit some pleomorphism, but they are usually not significant. Mitotic figures can be found, but not at a large frequency (H&E; 200X)

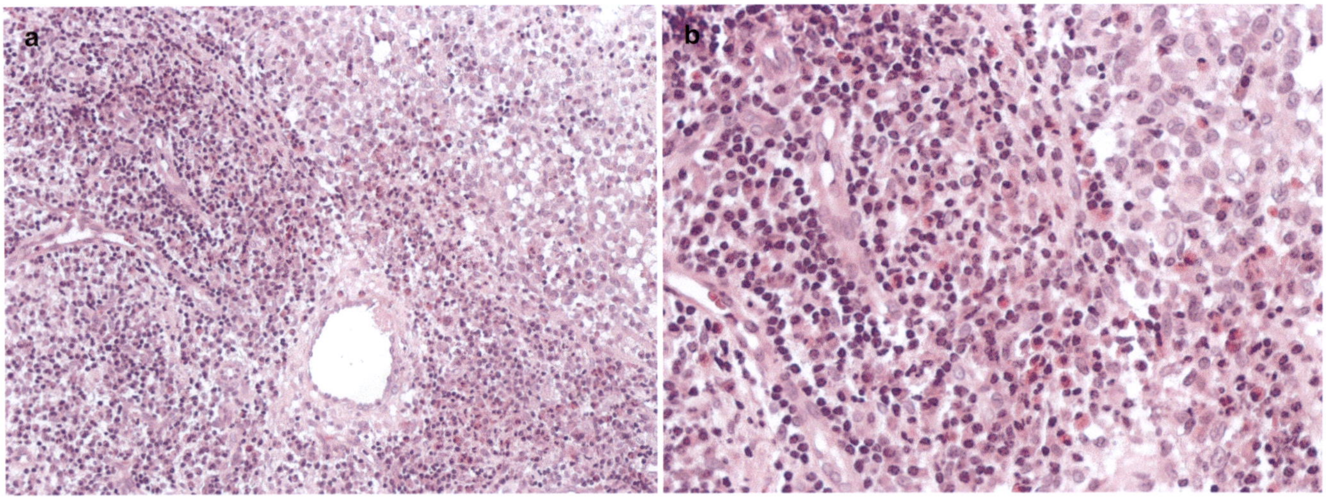

Fig. 30.6 Microscopic features of Langerhans cell histiocytosis affecting the gingiva. (**a**) Observe the presence of the reactive inflammatory infiltrate consisting of lymphocytes and plasma cells. The presence of eosinophils is a strong clue for the diagnosis. The Langerhans cell histiocytosis cells are located in the upper right corner of the image with a paler nucleus and eosinophilic cytoplasm (H&E; 100X). (**b**) Under higher magnification the eosinophils are more easily appreciated throughout the image, and the Langerhans cell histiocytosis cells are located on the right side of the image. Observe the nuclear grooves in some of the cells of the lesion, most of them presenting cleaved nuclei (H&E; 100X)

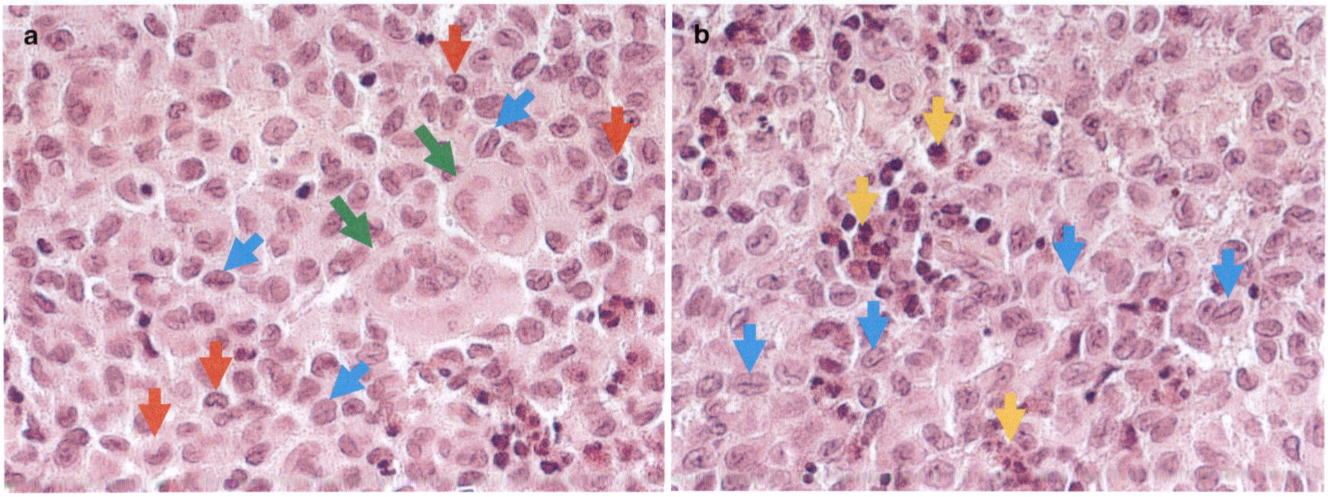

Fig. 30.7 Microscopic features of Langerhans cell histiocytosis affecting the gingiva. (**a**) Langerhans cell histiocytosis cells exhibit nuclear grooving as shown by the blue arrows, and/or nuclear indentation resembling "kidney shaped" or "coffee bean" appearance as exemplified by red arrows. Multinucleated giant cells are shown by green arrows (H&E; 400X). (**b**) Observe the Langerhans cell histiocytosis cells exhibiting nuclear grooving as shown by the blue arrows and the typical presence of eosinophils demonstrated by yellow arrows (H&E; 400X)

Table 30.1 Summary of the main immunohistochemical reactions used for Langerhans cell histiocytosis diagnosis. The main results for molecular findings are also described

Antibody/probe	Main result	Pattern	Objective
CD20	Negative	Membrane	To exclude the diagnosis of a B-cell lymphoma
CD3	Negative	Membrane	To exclude the diagnosis of a T-cell lymphoma
HLA-DR	Positive	Membrane	To confirm the LCH diagnosis
CD1a	Positive	Membrane	To confirm the LCH diagnosis
S100	Positive	Cytoplasm and nucleus	To confirm the LCH diagnosis
CD207 (Langerin)	Positive	Cytoplasm	To confirm the LCH diagnosis
CD68	Positive	Cytoplasm	To confirm the LCH diagnosis
CD163	Negative	Membrane	To exclude the diagnosis of other histiocytic neoplasms
Factor XIIIa	Negative	Cytoplasm	To exclude the diagnosis of other histiocytic neoplasms
Cyclin D1	Positive	Nucleus	Result of MAPK pathway activation
pERK	Positive	Nucleus	Result of MAPK pathway activation
ALK	Negative	Nucleus/Cytoplasm	To differentiate LCH from ALK-positive histiocytosis
Ki67	~10%–30%	Nucleus	To demonstrate the proliferative potential of the neoplasm
BRAF-V600E[a]	Positive in ~50% of the cases	–	To evaluate the genetic basis of the neoplasm
MAPK genes[a]	Positive in ~85% of the cases	–	To evaluate the genetic basis of the neoplasm

LCH Langerhans cell histiocytosis
[a]Investigated by PCR

involved in antigen processing and presentation, which is the key function of Langerhans cells in the immune response (Figs. 30.3, 30.4, 30.5, 30.6, and 30.7).

30.3 Immunohistochemistry and/or Genetics

Immunohistochemistry is used to demonstrate reactivity to Langerhans cells markers, which is mandatory to confirm the diagnosis of the disease. Langerhans cell histiocytosis is strongly and diffusely positive to CD1a and S100, and together with the observation of CD207 (Langerin) expression, this immunohistochemistry-based approach replaced the electron transmission microscopy evaluation of the cytoplasmic Birbeck granules, typical ultrastructural components of Langerhans cell histiocytosis. The absence of CD207 expression demands that the pathologist consider a diagnosis of *indeterminate cell histiocytosis*. ALK protein expression is negative. The positive expression of CD68 is variable and negativity to CD20 and CD3 helps to distinguish this lesion from lymphomas. Proliferative index is variable and Ki67 expression usually achieves 10% in most cases. *BRAF-V600E* mutation is present in approximately 50% of the cases; therefore, immunohistochemical expression for the mutated protein is also observed in these cases. *MAP2K1* represents the second most common mutation, and altera-

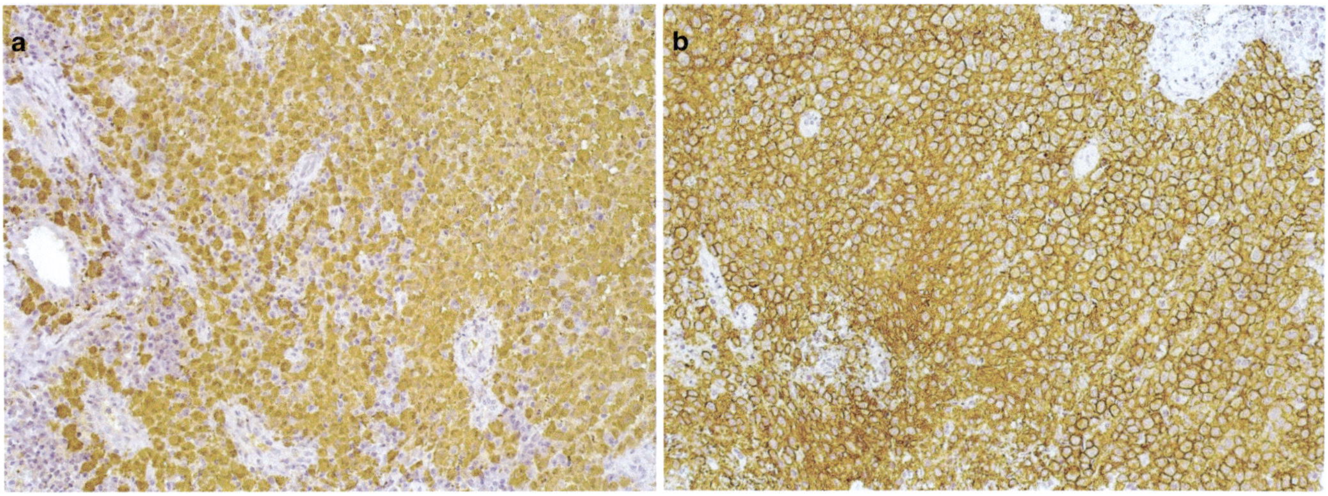

Fig. 30.8 Immunohistochemical features of Langerhans cell histiocytosis affecting the gingiva. (**a**) Tumor cells are strongly and diffusely positive for S100 (DAB; 100X). (**b**) The Langerhans cell marker CD1a is also strongly positive (DAB; 100X)

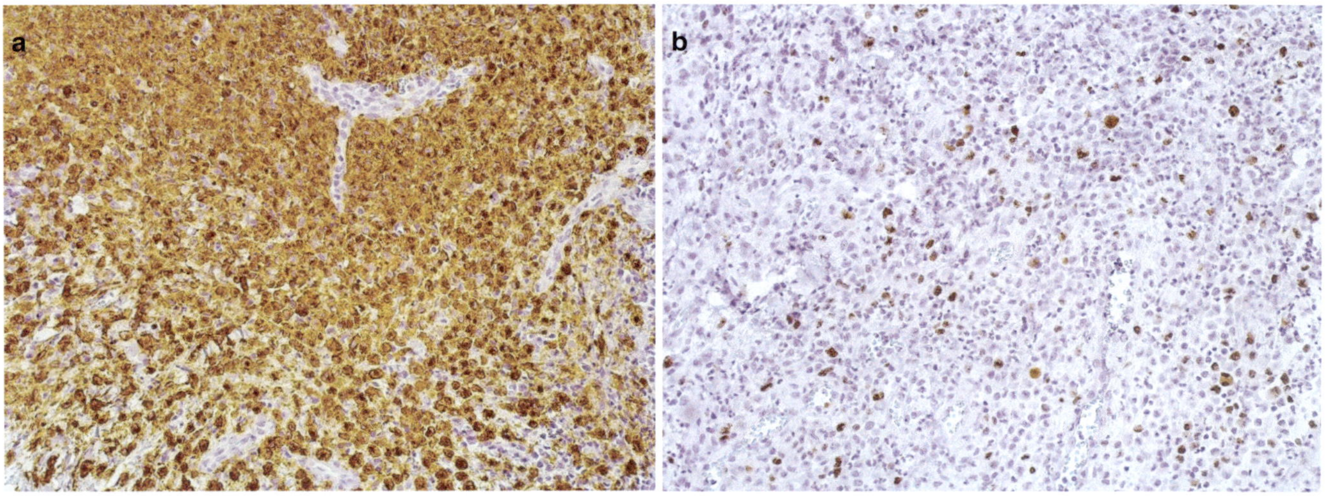

Fig. 30.9 Immunohistochemical features of Langerhans cell histiocytosis affecting the gingiva. (**a**) The cells of Langerhans cell histiocytosis exhibit a cytoplasmic expression for CD207 (Langerin) (DAB; 100X). (**b**) The proliferative index of Langerhans cell histiocytosis is variable, usually ranging from 20% to 30% in most cases (DAB; 100X)

tions in *ARAF*, *ERBB3*, *NRAS*, and *KRAS* have also been reported. As a consequence of *MAPK* pathway activation, phosphorylated ERK protein is expressed in almost all cases (Table 30.1; Figs. 30.8 and 30.9).

Sources

1. Hicks J, Flaitz CM. Langerhans cell histiocytosis: current insights in a molecular age with emphasis on clinical oral and maxillofacial pathology practice. Oral Surg Oral Med Oral Pathol Oral Radiol Endod. 2005;100(2 Suppl):S42–66. https://doi.org/10.1016/j.tripleo.2005.06.016.
2. Badalian-Very G, Vergilio JA, Degar BA, et al. Recurrent BRAF mutations in Langerhans cell histiocytosis. Blood. 2010;116(11):1919–23.
3. Mile JF, Abla O, Fraitag S, et al. Revised classification of histiocytoses and neoplasms of the macrophage-dendritic cell lineages. Blood. 2016;27:2672–81. https://doi.org/10.1182/blood-2016-01-690636.
4. Neves-Silva R, Fernandes DT, Fonseca FP, Rebelo Pontes HA, Brasileiro BF, Santos-Silva AR, et al. Oral manifestations of Langerhans cell histiocytosis: a case series. Spec Care Dentist. 2018;38(6):426–33. https://doi.org/10.1111/scd.12330.
5. McGinnis LM, Nybakken G, Ma L, Arber DA. Frequency of MAP2K1, TP53, and U2AF1 mutations in BRAF-mutated Langerhans cell histiocytosis: further characterizing the genomic landscape of LCH. Am J Surg Pathol. 2018;42(7):885–90. https://doi.org/10.1097/PAS.0000000000001057.
6. Bedran NR, Carlos R, de Andrade BAB, Bueno APS, Romañach MJ, Milito CB. Clinicopathological and immunohistochemical study of head and neck Langerhans cell histiocytosis from

Latin America. Head Neck Pathol. 2018;12(4):431–9. https://doi.org/10.1007/s12105-017-0867-1.
7. Krooks J, Minkov M, Weatherall AG. Langerhans cell histiocytosis in children: history, classification, pathobiology, clinical manifestations, and prognosis. J Am Acad Dermatol. 2018;78:1035–44.
8. Gulati N, Allen CE. Langerhans cell histiocytosis: version 2021. Hematol Oncol. 2021;39 Suppl 1(Suppl 1):15–23. https://doi.org/10.1002/hon.2857.
9. Faustino ISP, Fernandes PM, Pontes HAR, Mosqueda-Taylor A, Santos-Silva AR, Vargas PA, et al. Langerhans cell histiocytosis in the oral and maxillofacial region: an update. J Oral Pathol Med. 2021;50(6):565–71. https://doi.org/10.1111/jop.13207.
10. Goyal G, Tazi A, Go RS, Rech KL, Picarsic JL, Vassallo R, et al. International expert consensus recommendations for the diagnosis and treatment of Langerhans cell histiocytosis in adults. Blood. 2022;139(17):2601–21. https://doi.org/10.1182/blood.2021014343.
11. Sato A, Kobayashi M, Yusa N, et al. Clinical and prognostic features of Langerhans cell histiocytosis in adults. Cancer Sci. 2023. https://doi.org/10.1111/cas.15879.
12. Abagnale G, Schwentner R, Ben Soussia-Weiss P, van Midden W, Sturtzel C, Pötschger U, et al. BRAFV600E induces key features of LCH in iPSCs with cell type-specific phenotypes and drug responses. Blood. 2024. https://doi.org/10.1182/blood.2024026066.
13. Koh KN, Jun HR, Lee JY, Kim JY. Unraveling the genetic landscape of Langerhans cell histiocytosis in Korean patients: comprehensive insights from mutational profiles and clinical correlations. Cancer Res Treat. 2024. https://doi.org/10.4143/crt.2024.782.
14. Tang X, Gao J, Guo X, Wan Z, Sun JJ. Beyond BRAF(V600E): investigating the clinical and genetic spectrum of Langerhans cell histiocytosis in children. Cancer Med. 2024;13(24):e70532. https://doi.org/10.1002/cam4.70532.
15. Wongpattaraworakul W, Krongbaramee T, Lanzel EA, Hellstein JW, Teixeira FB. Hematolymphoid neoplasm mimicking endodontic lesions: case series and review of the literature. Oral Surg Oral Med Oral Pathol Oral Radiol. 2025;139(1):e1–e12. https://doi.org/10.1016/j.oooo.2024.07.011.

31 Histiocytic Sarcoma

Juan Manuel Arteaga Legarrea, Liam Robinson, Lucas Fabian Polti, and Felipe Paiva Fonseca

31.1 General Overview and Clinical Presentation

Histiocytic sarcoma, formerly designated as true histiocytic lymphoma, is a very rare malignant neoplasm that exhibits a morphological and immunophenotypic differentiation resembling mature histiocytes. It is an aggressive neoplasm that accounts for less than 1% of all hematological malignancies. Consequently, its correct diagnosis demands a high level of suspicion from pathologists and usually a large immunohistochemical panel. Some of the previously diagnosed pleomorphic or undifferentiated sarcomas would be better recognized as histiocytic sarcomas following more modern laboratory tests, including immunohistochemistry and molecular biology assays.

The etiology of histiocytic sarcoma is largely unknown, but its pathogenesis has more recently been investigated, with some studies demonstrating mutations in members of the *MAPK* pathway, including *NRAS, KRAS* and *MAP 2K1*. *BRAF-V600E* mutations have been reported in approximately 12% of the cases, and tumor-suppressor genes *CDKN2A* and *TP53* were mutated in many cases. Moreover, approximately 21% of the cases also show mutations in components of the *PI3K* signaling pathway (*PTEN, MTOR, PIK3R1* and *PIK3CA*). It is well known that although histiocytic sarcoma may arise as a primary neoplasm, it is also strongly associated with a pre-existing or concurrently diagnosed hematologic malignancy, more often a low-grade neoplasm like follicular lymphoma and chronic lymphocytic leukemia/small lymphocytic lymphoma, as well as B- or T-lymphoblastic leukemia/lymphoma. More rarely, cases associated with mediastinal germ cell tumors have also been documented. Exceptionally rare cases of double histiocytic and Langerhans cell components have been documented, with Langerhans cells presenting either as aggregates or scattered throughout the histiocytic sarcoma cells. In these instances, the distinction between histiocytic sarcoma and Langerhans cell neoplasms may be challenging, and the final diagnosis relies on the main cellular component.

The cases arising in the context of a lymphoid neoplasm are usually referred to as "secondary" histiocytic sarcomas and have been shown to be clonally and molecularly associated with the primary lymphoid malignancy. The mechanism by which a previous lymphoid malignancy transforms into a neoplasm with a different lineage, such as histiocytic sarcoma, is still poorly understood. Theories include an origin from a common neoplastic progenitor, a process described as the transdifferentiation of a mature lymphoid cell into a myeloid lineage, or possible dedifferentiation of a lymphoid cell to an immature progenitor with subsequent differentiation along the myeloid/dendritic differentiation.

Histiocytic sarcoma more commonly occurs in adulthood, but a wide age range is observed. There is no apparent sex predominance, and most of the cases affect the lymph nodes as asymptomatic or painful swellings. Extranodal manifestations also occur, usually involving the gastrointestinal tract, skin, lungs, central nervous system, and liver. The lesions are more frequently solitary, but multifocal disease may also be diagnosed. When cutaneous involvement is present, the neoplasm may manifest as plaques, nodules or tumors that may affect any part of the body. Intestinal obstruction and splenomegaly may also be reported, and systemic symptoms such as fever, fatigue, night sweats and weight loss may be reported by affected patients. The cervical lymph nodes are

J. M. A. Legarrea (✉) · F. P. Fonseca
Department of Oral Surgery and Pathology, School of Dentistry, Universidade Federal de Minas Gerais, Belo Horizonte, Brazil

L. Robinson
Department of Oral and Maxillofacial Pathology, School of Dentistry, University of Pretoria, Pretoria, South Africa
e-mail: liam.robinson@up.ac.za

L. F. Polti
Department of Oral Surgery and Pathology, School of Dentistry, Universidade Federal de Minas Gerais, Belo Horizonte, Brazil

Department of Pathology, School of Dentistry, University of Buenos Aires, Buenos Aires, Argentina

© The Author(s), under exclusive license to Springer Nature Switzerland AG 2025

F. P. Fonseca et al. (eds.), *Lymphoproliferative and Granulomatous Disorders of the Oral Cavity*,
https://doi.org/10.1007/978-3-031-98844-8_31

the most affected subsite in the head and neck region, followed by the tonsils. However, cases affecting different regions of the oral cavity have been reported, more commonly involving the soft and hard palate. However, in these cases, a local manifestation of a widespread disease should be ruled out. In the oral cavity, tumors more often manifest as ulcered swellings with or without necrotic regions. Bone invasion by tumor cells, causing an ill-defined radiolucent image that may infiltrate surrounding structures like the maxillary sinus and the nasal cavity, can occur.

There is no standardized treatment for histiocytic sarcoma, and affected patients are treated by complete surgical resection with or without accompanying radiotherapy and chemotherapy. A single case of histiocytic sarcoma, positive for *BRAF-V600E* mutation, involving the central nervous system, was reported to show significant remission following vemurafenib administration, raising the possibility of targeted therapy as an effective treatment option; however, this requires further validation with appropriate clinical studies. Overall, the prognosis of histiocytic sarcoma is poor, with unsatisfactory response to available chemotherapeutic regimens and a median overall survival of 6 months. Moreover, a previous study demonstrated that patients affected by *secondary* histiocytic sarcomas present an even poorer overall survival rate than those affected by de novo histiocytic sarcomas.

31.2 Microscopic Findings

- Neoplastic cells exhibit an infiltrative growth pattern into surrounding normal structures.
- A diffuse growth pattern of tumor cells is typically observed.
- Areas of tissue necrosis are very often observed.
- The neoplasm is comprised of large polygonal tumor cells that range from round to oval.
- Neoplastic cells are usually arranged in discohesive sheets.
- Focal or prominent areas of spindle cell differentiation may be seen.
- The large neoplastic cells frequently have a moderate to abundant eosinophilic cytoplasm.
- Clear cytoplasm or a granular, foamy-like appearance is common and represents a useful morphological clue to a pathologist to consider a possible histiocytic differentiation.
- Neoplastic cells have round to irregular nuclei with vesicular chromatin and one to several distinct nucleoli.
- Indented or grooved nuclei may be found.
- Varied cytologic atypia, but most cases exhibit a high-grade morphological phenotype.
- A varied number of anaplastic cells can be found.
- The presence of foreign-body multinucleated giant cells has already been described, but is rarely found.
- Frequent mitotic figures.
- Reactive neutrophils, lymphocytes, plasma cells and eosinophils are usually present (Figs. 31.1, 31.2, 31.3 and 31.4).

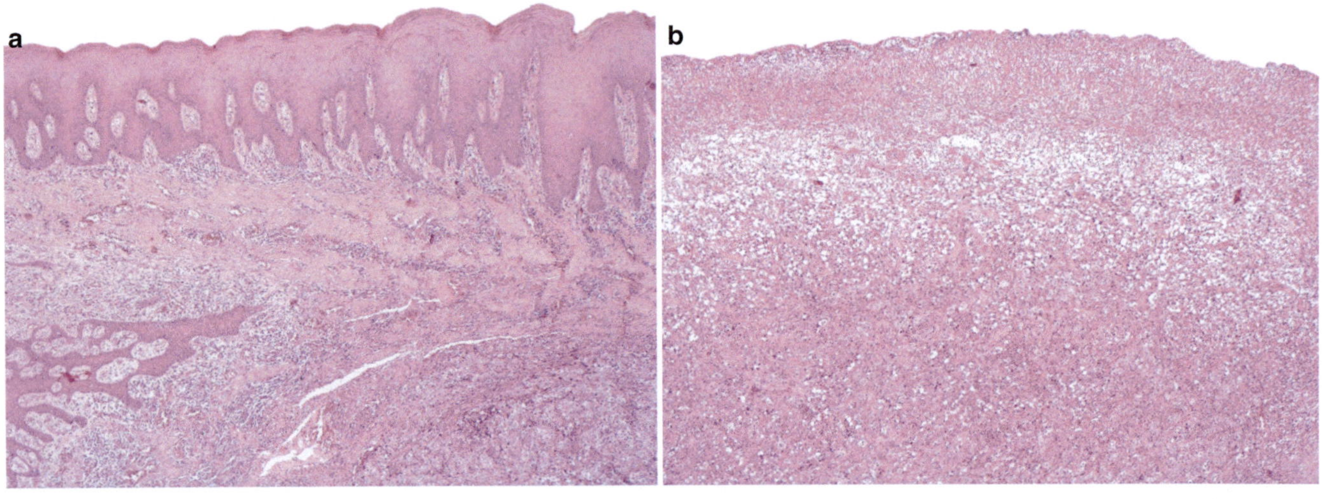

Fig. 31.1 Microscopic features of histiocytic sarcoma affecting the oral cavity. (**a**) Overlying squamous epithelium of the oral mucosa with a neoplasm present in the lower right corner of the lamina propria (H&E; 50X). (**b**) A fibrinopurulent membrane covered some areas of the tumor, with a diffuse proliferation of malignant cells (H&E; 50X)

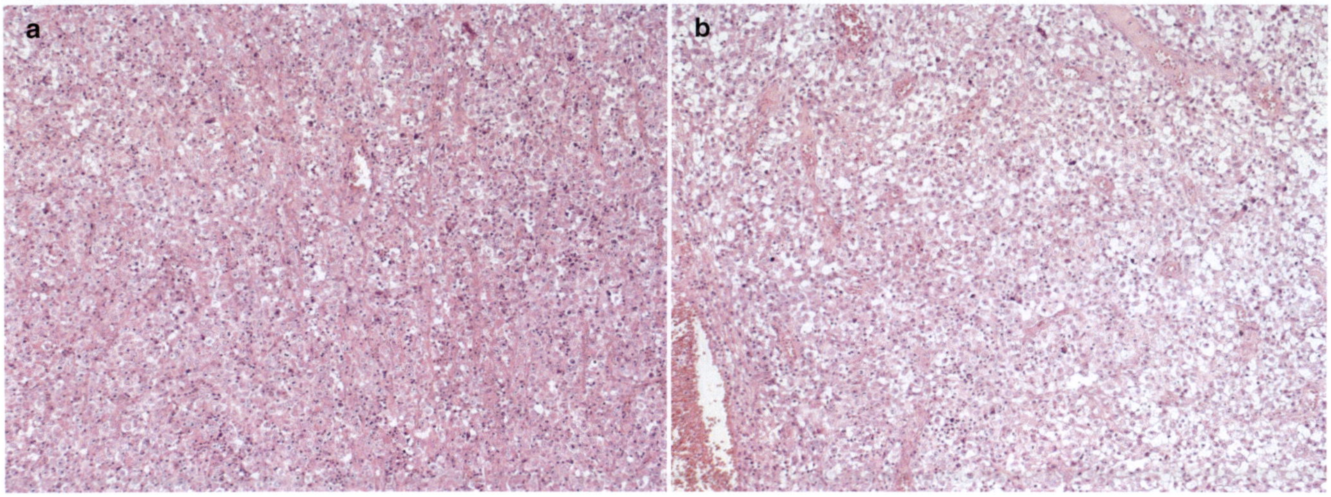

Fig. 31.2 Microscopic features of histiocytic sarcoma affecting the oral cavity. (**a**) Diffuse and discohesive proliferation of large neoplastic cells that exhibited abundant eosinophilic cytoplasm. Reactive smaller hyperchromatic lymphocytes may be appreciated (H&E; 50X). (**b**) In some tumor regions, the neoplastic cells exhibited a clear to foamy cytoplasm reminiscent of the histiocytic differentiation (H&E; 50X)

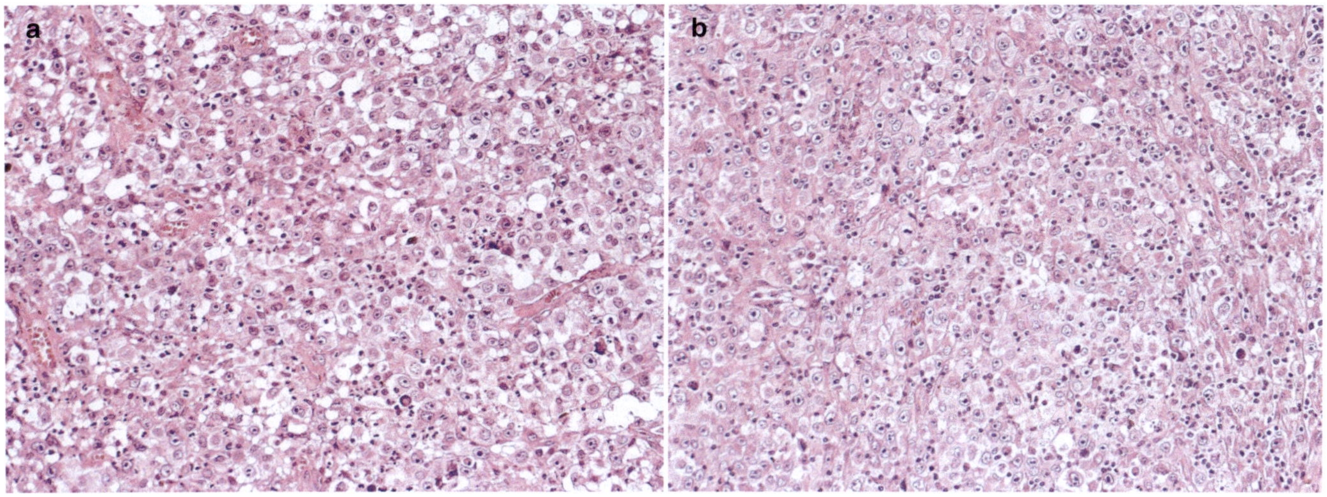

Fig. 31.3 Microscopic features of histiocytic sarcoma affecting the oral cavity. (**a**) The large neoplastic cells exhibited abundant eosinophilic cytoplasm and round to oval centrally located nuclei, most of which contain a prominent single nucleolus (H&E; 100X). (**b**) The neoplastic cells exhibited an abundant cytoplasm ranging from eosinophilic to clear to foamy. The large nuclei and prominent nucleoli may be easily observed (H&E; 100X)

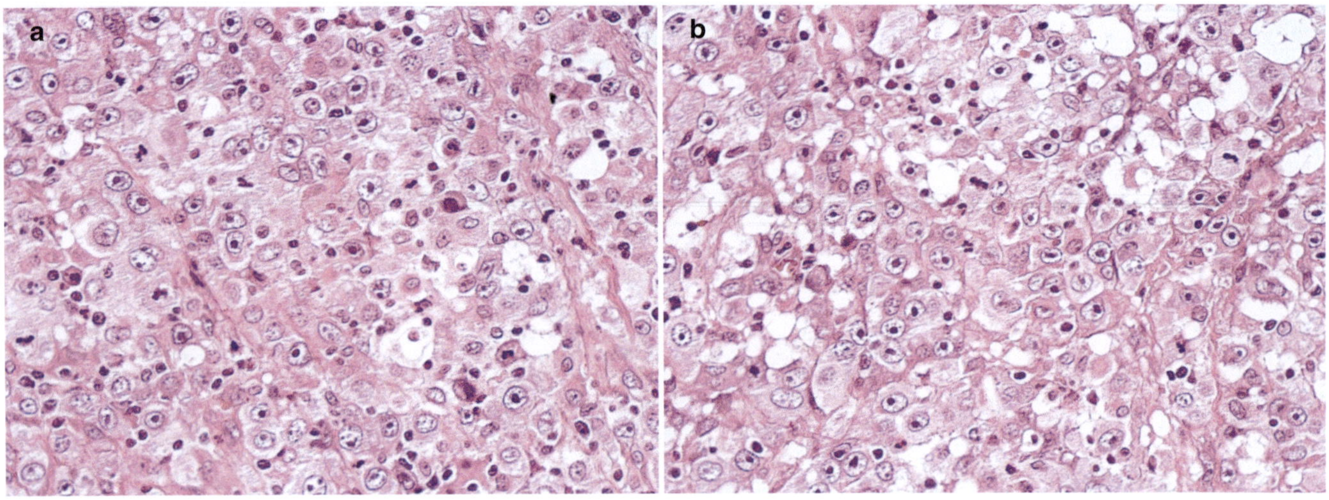

Fig. 31.4 Microscopic features of histiocytic sarcoma affecting the oral cavity. (**a**) Under high power magnification, the neoplastic cells are large with round to oval nuclei and prominent nucleoli. Reactive plasma cells and lymphocytes are present, and the limited stroma is fibrotic (H&E; 200X). (**b**) Many of the tumor cells exhibited a foamy cytoplasm, suggesting possible histiocytic differentiation (H&E; 200X)

31.3 Immunohistochemistry and/or Genetics

Immunohistochemistry helps to demonstrate the mature histiocytic differentiation of tumor cells, which will be negative for Langerhans cell markers such as CD1a and CD207, and follicular dendritic cell markers including CD21, CD23 and CD35. The tumor cells will express histiocytic markers such as CD68, CD163 and lysozyme, as well as CD4 and CD11c, but care must be taken not to misinterpret the expression of these proteins by stromal reactive cells. Focal staining for S100 is observed in some cases. Immunohistochemistry will also be useful to exclude other important differential diagnoses like mature B- and T-cell lymphomas (CD20/CD3), anaplastic large cell lymphoma (CD30), carcinoma (AE1/AE3), melanoma (HMB45/Melan A) and rhabdomyosarcoma (Desmin/Myogenin). Myeloid markers like myeloperoxidase and CD13 are negative, which are ancillary markers to differentiate histiocytic sarcoma from myeloid sarcoma. ALK protein is also negative. The proliferative index of histiocytic sarcomas is usually very high (Table 31.1; Figs. 31.5, 31.6, 31.7, and 31.8).

Table 31.1 Summary of the main immunohistochemical reactions used for histiocytic sarcoma diagnosis

Antibody/probe	Most frequent results	Pattern	Objective
CD20	Negative	Membrane	To exclude a B-cell nature of the tumor
CD3	Negative	Membrane	To exclude a T-cell nature of the tumor
HMB45 or Melan A	Negative	Cytoplasm	To exclude a melanoma
S100	Focally positive	Cytoplasm/nucleus	To demonstrate the histiocytic differentiation
Desmin or myogenin	Negative	Cytoplasm and nucleus, respectively	To exclude a rhabdomyosarcoma
CD30	Negative	Membrane/Golgi accentuation	To exclude an ALCL
AE1/AE3	Negative	Cytoplasm	To exclude the diagnosis of a carcinoma
CD68	Positive	Cytoplasm	To demonstrate the histiocytic differentiation
CD163	Positive	Membrane	To demonstrate the histiocytic differentiation
CD1a	Negative	Membrane	To exclude a Langerhans cell neoplasm
CD207	Negative	Cytoplasm	To exclude a Langerhans cell neoplasm
Lysozyme	Positive	Cytoplasm	To demonstrate the histiocytic differentiation
CD21	Negative	Membrane	To exclude the follicular dendritic cell differentiation
CD23	Negative	Membrane	To exclude the follicular dendritic cell differentiation
CD35	Negative	Membrane	To exclude the follicular dendritic cell differentiation
Myeloperoxidase	Negative	Cytoplasm	To exclude a myeloid sarcoma
Ki67	High	Nucleus	To investigate the proliferative potential of the tumor
BRAF-V600E[a]	0%–19%	–	To investigate the molecular basis of the neoplasm
MAPK pathway genes[a]	Most common event	–	To investigate the molecular basis of the neoplasm
PI3K pathway genes[a]	21%	–	To investigate the molecular basis of the neoplasm

Important genetic features are also described
ALCL anaplastic large cell lymphoma
[a]Investigated by PCR

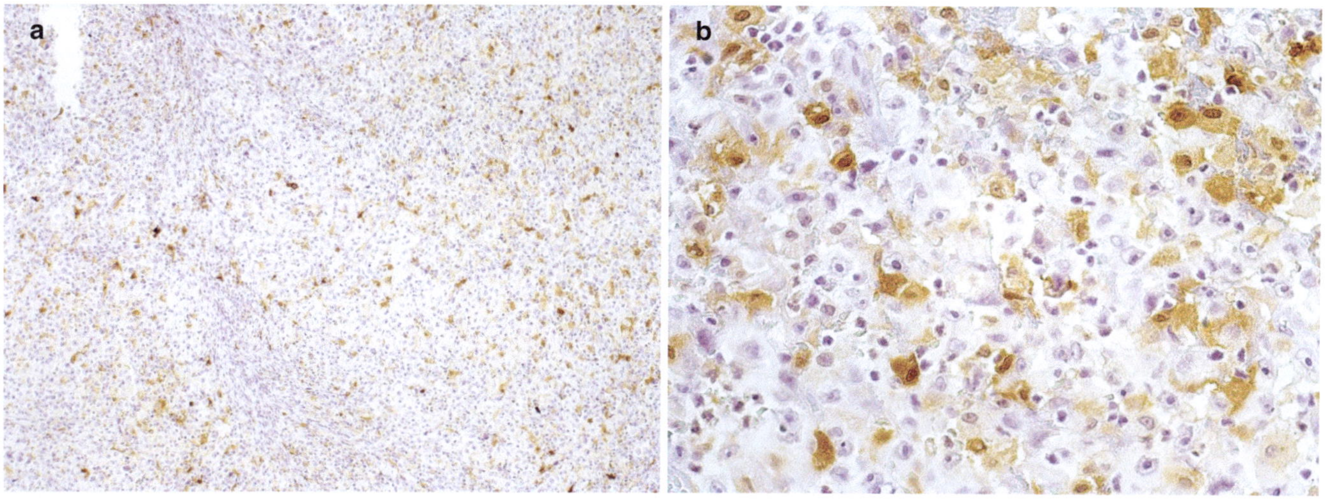

Fig. 31.5 Immunohistochemical features of histiocytic sarcoma. (**a**) Scattered tumor cells positive for S100 (DAB; 50X). (**b**) Observe the nuclear and cytoplasmic staining pattern of S100 in some of the larger neoplastic cells. Care must be taken to differentiate the staining in tumor cells from reactive cells (DAB; 200X)

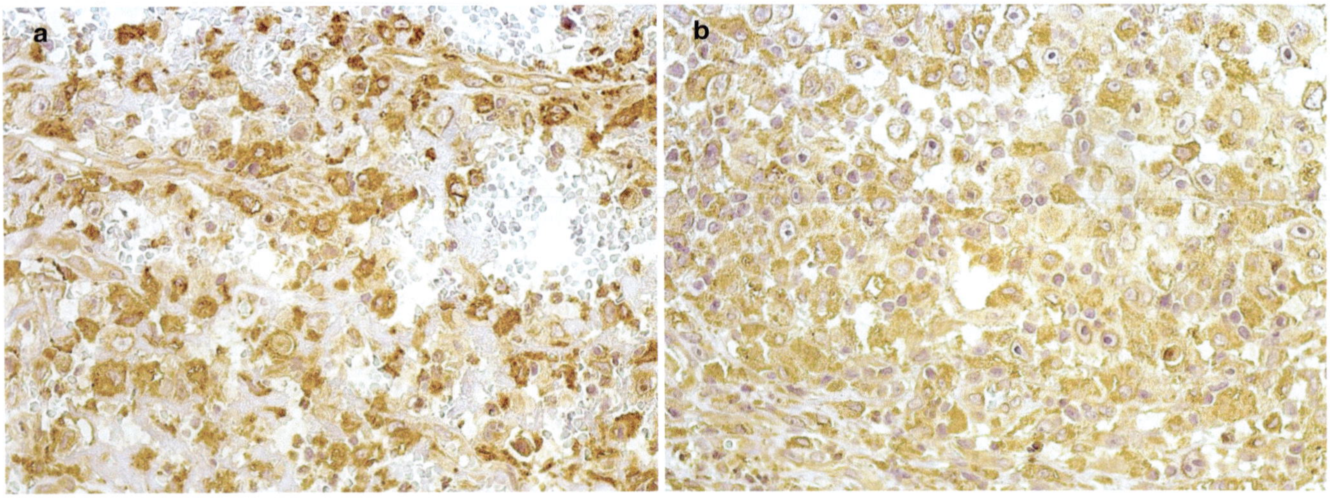

Fig. 31.6 Immunohistochemical features of histiocytic sarcoma. (**a**) Histiocytic marker CD68 is usually diffusely positive (DAB; 200X). (**b**) Observe the strong and diffuse cytoplasmic staining of CD68 in the neoplastic cells (DAB; 200X)

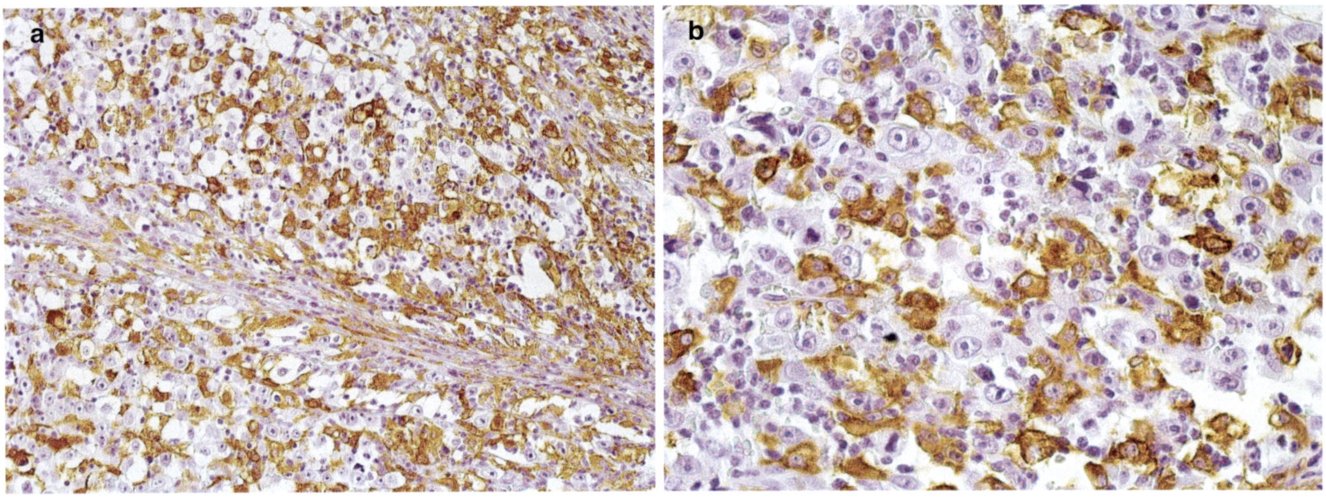

Fig. 31.7 Immunohistochemical features of histiocytic sarcoma. (**a**) CD163 is a more specific marker for histiocytic differentiation. This marker is diffusely expressed by tumor cells, although not all cells will express this marker (DAB; 100X). (**b**) Observe the strong cytoplasmic staining for CD163 in many large and pleomorphic neoplastic cells, although not all tumor cells are positive (DAB; 200X)

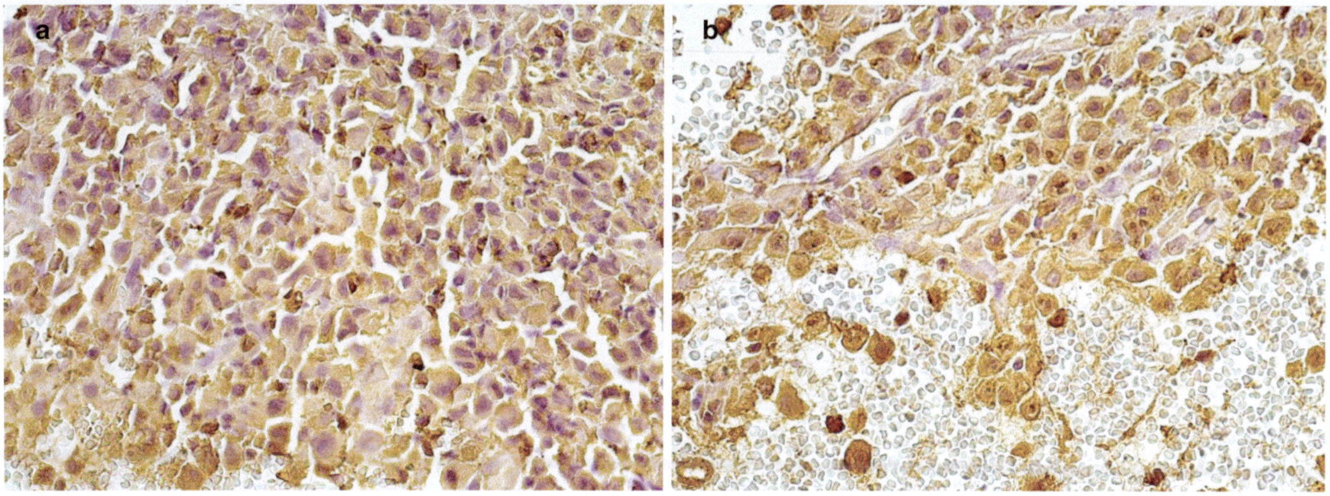

Fig. 31.8 Immunohistochemical features of histiocytic sarcoma. (**a**) Histiocytic marker lysozyme is also diffusely positive (DAB; 200X). (**b**) Observe the strong and diffuse cytoplasmic staining of lysozyme in the neoplastic cells (DAB; 200X)

Sources

1. Hornick JL, Jaffe ES, Fletcher CD. Extranodal histiocytic sarcoma: clinicopathologic analysis of 14 cases of a rare epithelioid malignancy. Am J Surg Pathol. 2004;28(9):1133–44. https://doi.org/10.1097/01.pas.0000131541.95394.23.
2. Go H, Jeon YK, Huh J, Choi SJ, Choi Y-D, Cha HJ, et al. Frequent detection of BRAFV600E mutations in histiocytic and dendritic cell neoplasms. Histopathology. 2014;65:261–72. https://doi.org/10.1111/his.12416.
3. Idbaih A, Mokhtari K, Emile JF, Galanaud D, Belaid H, de Bernard S, et al. Dramatic response of a BRAF V600E-mutated primary CNS histiocytic sarcoma to vemurafenib. Neurology. 2014;83:1478–80.
4. Facchetti F, Pileri SA, Lorenzi L, Tabanelli V, Rimsza L, Pittaluga S, et al. Histiocytic and dendritic cell neoplasms: what have we learnt by studying 67 cases. Virchows Arch. 2017;471(4):467–89. https://doi.org/10.1007/s00428-017-2176-1.
5. Broadwater DR, Conant JL, Czuchlewski DR, Hall JM, Wei S, Siegal GP, et al. Clinicopathologic features and clinical outcome differences in de novo versus secondary histiocytic sarcomas: a multi-institutional experience and review of the literature. Clin Lymphoma Myeloma Leuk. 2018;18(10):e427–35. https://doi.org/10.1016/j.clml.2018.07.286.
6. Shanmugam V, Griffin GK, Jacobsen ED, Fletcher CDM, Sholl LM, Hornick JL. Identification of diverse activating mutations of the RAS-MAPK pathway in histiocytic sarcoma. Mod Pathol. 2019;32(6):830–43. https://doi.org/10.1038/s41379-018-0200-x.
7. Aytekin A, Ozet A, Bilgetekin I, Ogut B, Ciltas A, Benekli M. A metastatic histiocytic sarcoma case with primary involvement of the tonsil. J Cancer Res Ther. 2020;16(3):665–7. https://doi.org/10.4103/0973-1482.188435.
8. Egan C, Nicolae A, Lack J, Chung HJ, Skarshaug S, Pham TA, et al. Genomic profiling of primary histiocytic sarcoma reveals two molecular subgroups. Haematologica. 2020;105(4):951–60. https://doi.org/10.3324/haematol.2019.230375.
9. Egan C, Lack J, Skarshaug S, Pham TA, Abdullaev Z, Xi L, et al. The mutational landscape of histiocytic sarcoma associated with lymphoid malignancy. Mod Pathol. 2021;34(2):336–47. https://doi.org/10.1038/s41379-020-00673-x.
10. Khoury JD, Solary E, Abla O. The 5th edition of the World Health Organization classification of haematolymphoid tumours: myeloid and histiocytic/dendritic neoplasms. Leukemia. 2022;36:1703–19. https://doi.org/10.1038/s41375-022-01613-1.
11. Kurimoto T, Goto T, Yasuda T, Yoshioka H. Histiocytic sarcoma of the palate: a case report. Int J Oral Maxillofac Surg. 2023:S0901-5027(23)00190-X. https://doi.org/10.1016/j.ijom.2023.08.003.
12. Chiu LJ, Huang WT, Wang MC, Medeiros LJ, Chang KC. Low-grade histiocytic sarcoma with aggressive clinical behaviour: an unusual case with novel genetic mutations identified by whole genome sequencing. Pathology. 2024;56(7):1064–6. https://doi.org/10.1016/j.pathol.2024.05.008.
13. Koh KN, Yoon SH, Kang SH, Kim H, Im HJ. Advancements in the understanding and management of histiocytic neoplasms. Blood Res. 2024;59(1):22. https://doi.org/10.1007/s44313-024-00022-w.
14. Legarrea JMA, Alves HS, Chaves RRM, Soares CD, Robinson L, van Heerden WFP, et al. Histiocytic sarcoma affecting the oral cavity: a clinical, pathologic and molecular study. Oral Surg Oral Med Oral Pathol Oral Radiol. 2024;S2212-4403(24):00368–7. https://doi.org/10.1016/j.oooo.2024.06.014.
15. Ruan GJ, Zanwar S, Ravindran A, Schram S, Abeykoon JP, Hazim A, et al. Clinical characteristics, molecular aberrations, treatments, and outcomes of malignant histiocytosis. Am J Hematol. 2024;99(5):871–9. https://doi.org/10.1002/ajh.27263.

Follicular Dendritic Cell Sarcoma

32

Liam Robinson and Felipe Paiva Fonseca

32.1 General Overview and Clinical Presentation

Follicular dendritic cell sarcoma is a rare neoplasm first reported in 1986 by Monda et al. It accounts for less than 1% of all head and neck neoplasms, characterized by the proliferation of tumor cells demonstrating immunohistochemical features of normal follicular dendritic cells. Follicular dendritic cells are antigen and immune-complex-presenting cells found in germinal centers of lymphoid follicles in lymph nodes and secondary lymphoid organs. This mesenchymal neoplasm is strongly associated with a high rate of misdiagnosis, which may range from 29% to 58% in different series, likely due to the unawareness of this entity linked to its rarity and its variable histopathologic features.

It is known that approximately 10%–20% of follicular dendritic cell sarcomas are diagnosed in the setting of hyaline-vascular Castleman disease. Additionally, an indolent T-lymphoblastic proliferation is observed in the lymphoid component of a subset of the cases. However, the exact etiology of this sarcoma is still poorly understood. On the other hand, the pathogenic basis of the disease has been better appreciated during the last years, with alterations in genes of the *NFκB* pathway, including *BIRC3, NFKBIA, TRAF3, SOCS3, CYLD*, and *TNFAIP3* occurring in almost 60% of the cases, and alterations in tumor suppressor genes like *CDKN2A*, *RB1*, and *TP53* occurring in approximately 20%–30% of the cases, and, less commonly, the occurrence of *BRAF-V600E* mutation. There does not seem to be a sex predilection, and patients are diagnosed over a wide age range, with a median of 50 years.

It is commonly diagnosed in the lymph nodes, especially in the cervical region; however, extranodal cases are also frequently reported, including the gastrointestinal tract, soft tissue and the lungs. Moreover, this neoplasm can also be diagnosed simultaneously in the lymph node and other extranodal sites. Regarding nodal presentation, the tumor is usually characterized by an asymptomatic swelling with an indolent course and long-term duration, non-ulcerated and more often without systemic manifestations. The rare patients who develop systemic complaints more often demonstrate fatigue, fever, and night sweats.

In the oral and maxillofacial region, the tonsils and the soft palate are the most commonly affected locations, with these manifestations first described by Chan et al. in 1994. In the tonsils and soft palate, follicular dendritic cell sarcoma is more often described as a unilateral ulcerated tumor, with or without associated pain. Rare cases affecting the parotid gland and in the submandibular region have also been described.

Since this malignant neoplasm is very rare, there is no standardized treatment for affected patients. Therefore, follicular dendritic cell sarcoma is usually treated by complete surgical resection followed by radiotherapy and chemotherapy. Overall survival is usually high and may achieve up to 80% among low to intermediate-risk patients in some studies, with poorer survival for high-risk patients. Local recurrences may be higher than 40%, and distant metastases may occur in up to 25% of the patients, usually in the lungs, liver, adrenal glands, and ribs. Important prognostic factors include tumor stage at diagnosis, high mitotic count (>5 mitoses/mm^2), significant nuclear atypia, and extensive necrosis.

In 2001, Cheuk et al. described a more indolent variant of the neoplasm and proposed classifying follicular dendritic cell sarcoma into classic and inflammatory pseudotumor-like types. According to the fifth edition of the World Health Organization classification of hematolymphoid tumors, the term Epstein-Barr virus-positive inflammatory follicular dendritic cell sarcoma (EBV+ IFDCS) is recommended, and this

L. Robinson (✉)
Department of Oral and Maxillofacial Pathology, School of Dentistry, University of Pretoria, Pretoria, South Africa
e-mail: liam.robinson@up.ac.za

F. P. Fonseca
Department of Oral Surgery and Pathology, School of Dentistry, Universidade Federal de Minas Gerais, Belo Horizonte, Brazil

© The Author(s), under exclusive license to Springer Nature Switzerland AG 2025

F. P. Fonseca et al. (eds.), *Lymphoproliferative and Granulomatous Disorders of the Oral Cavity*,
https://doi.org/10.1007/978-3-031-98844-8_32

disorder is now considered a distinct entity, rather than a subtype of follicular dendritic cell sarcoma. Microscopically, it exhibits spindle to oval cells organized in whorled fascicles and a dense lymphoplasmacytic infiltrate; however, the tumor is known to present a highly variable morphology. The expression of follicular dendritic cell markers is a hallmark of the neoplasm that is pathogenetically associated with EBV infection. It more commonly involves the liver and the spleen, although extrahepatosplenic reports are available in the literature. EBV+ inflammatory follicular dendritic cell sarcoma is usually asymptomatic, but it can be associated with systemic symptoms, and affected patients have a favorable outcome, despite the possible occurrence of local recurrences and rare distant metastases. Two cases of EBV+ inflammatory follicular dendritic cell sarcoma diagnosed in the palatine tonsils have recently been described, and therefore, pathologists should be aware of this rare entity to avoid misdiagnoses and inappropriate use of the recommended terminologies.

32.2 Microscopic Findings

- Microscopic diagnosis of follicular dendritic cell sarcoma usually demands an elevated degree of diagnostic suspicion in the initial histological evaluation.
- The neoplasm is characteristically composed of spindle-shaped cells distributed in variable patterns like small fascicles or whorls.
- It is also possible to observe growth patterns in the form of diffuse sheets or vague nodules.
- The neoplastic cells are predominantly oval to spindle-shaped with fine chromatin, prominent nucleoli and indistinct cell borders.
- Tumor cells have a moderate to abundant eosinophilic cytoplasm.
- Presence of cytologic atypia is observed.
- Nuclear pseudoinclusions may occur.
- Intermingled lymphocytes are common.
- Necrosis and atypical mitotic figures can also be found.
- Other less common features include: epithelioid cells, oncocytic cells, myxoid stroma, and multinucleated giant cells (Figs. 32.1, 32.2, and 32.3).

Note: Microscopically, EBV+ inflammatory follicular dendritic cell sarcoma is more often characterized by the presence of spindled to oval neoplastic cells with poorly-defined cell borders, which may form loosely arranged whorled fascicles. The presence of a dense lymphoplasma-cytic background is a common finding and may make the correct diagnosis difficult.

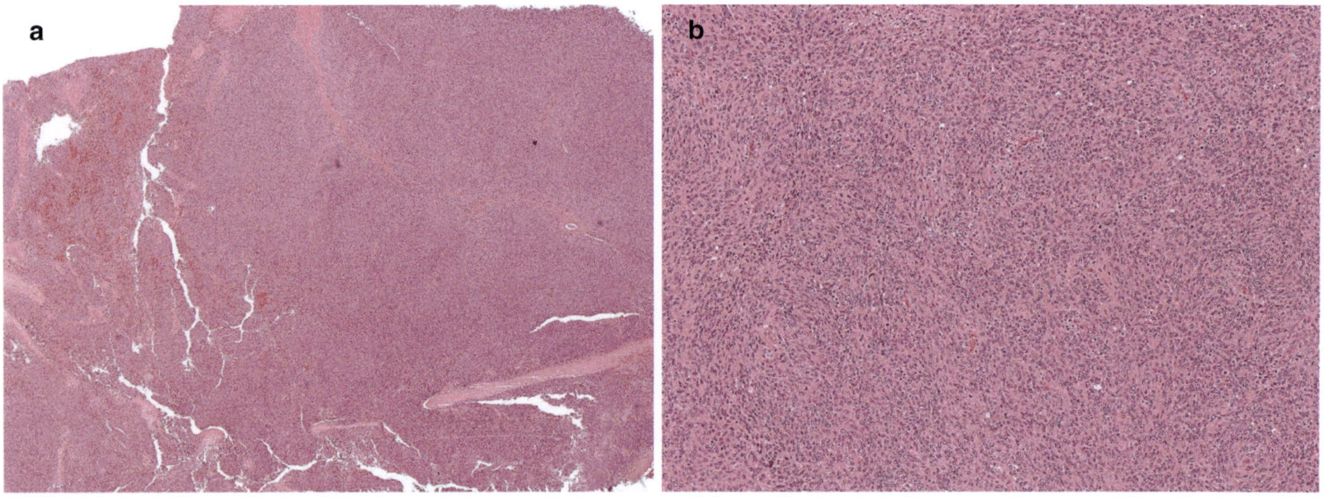

Fig. 32.1 Microscopic features of follicular dendritic cell sarcoma. (**a**) The neoplasm exhibits a diffuse proliferation of tumor cells (H&E; 25X). (**b**) The neoplastic cells appear monotonous, with a predominance of spindled nuclei with eosinophilic cytoplasms (H&E; 50X)

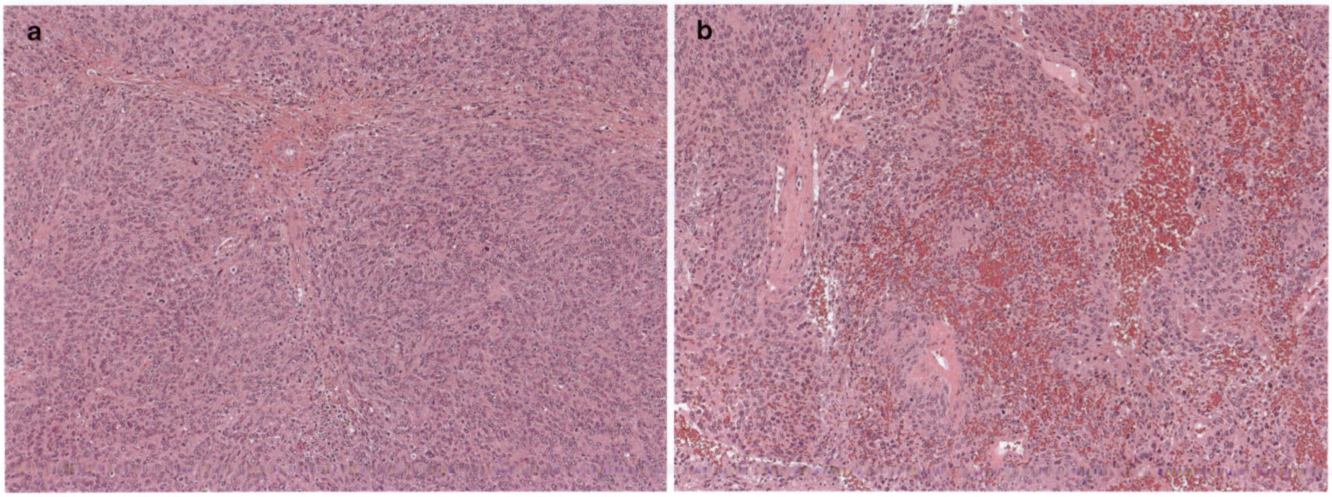

Fig. 32.2 Microscopic features of follicular dendritic cell sarcoma. (**a**) The neoplasm has a scant fibrous stroma and exhibits different growth patterns ranging from diffuse sheets to vaguely nodular proliferations (H&E; 50X). (**b**) More vascularized areas with erythrocyte extravasation may be found (H&E; 100X)

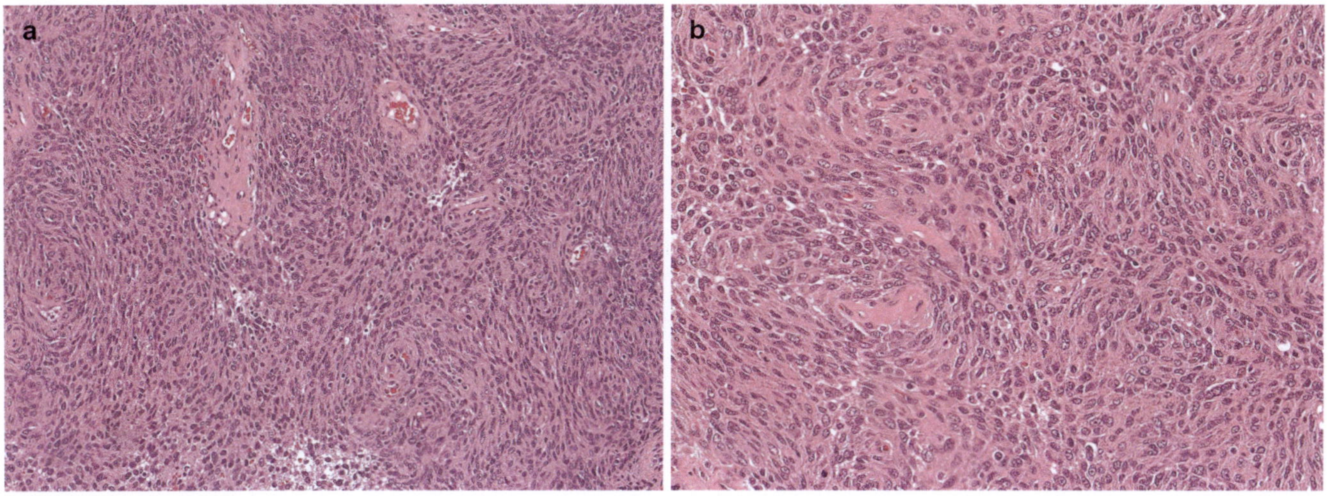

Fig. 32.3 Microscopic features of follicular dendritic cell sarcoma. (**a**) The tumor cells may also present with short fascicles or whorls (H&E; 100X). (**b**) Whorls of oval-to-spindle tumor cells with fine chromatin and eosinophilic cytoplasm (H&E; 200X)

32.3 Immunohistochemistry and/or Genetics

The microscopic diagnosis of follicular dendritic cell sarcoma is usually very challenging and therefore, immunohistochemistry is considered very useful to demonstrate the follicular dendritic cell differentiation of the tumor. The neoplastic cells will be negative for Langerhans cell markers such as CD1a and CD207, and only occasionally positive for histiocytic markers like CD68 and CD163. Diffuse positivity will be seen for CD21, CD23 and CD35, clusterin, CXCL13 and D2–40. The B-cell (CD20, CD79a) and T-cell (CD3, CD45RO) markers are negative. Uncommon expressions of other markers have been described, but with limited diagnostic significance. The simultaneous presence of indolent T-lymphoblastic proliferation is observed by TdT expression. The proliferative index is highly variable, ranging from as low as 5% up to 70% in some cases. EBV detection by immunohistochemistry (LMP1) or in situ hybridization is observed in EBV+ inflammatory follicular dendritic cell sarcoma (Table 32.1; Fig. 32.4).

Table 32.1 Summary of the main immunohistochemical reactions used for follicular dendritic cell sarcoma diagnosis

Antibody/probe	Most frequent results	Pattern	Objective
CD20	Negative	Membrane	To exclude a B-cell lymphoma
CD3	Negative	Membrane	To exclude a T-cell lymphoma
D2–40	Positive	Membrane	Positive in cases of FDCS
S100	Variably positive	Cytoplasm/nucleus	It can also be positive in a few cases of FDCS
EMA	Variably positive	Membrane/cytoplasm	It can also be positive in a few cases of FDCS
AE1/AE3	Negative	Cytoplasm	To exclude the diagnosis of a carcinoma
CD68	Rarely positive	Cytoplasm	It can also be positive in a few cases of FDCS
CD163	Rarely positive	Membrane	It can also be positive in a few cases of FDCS
CD1a and CD207	Negative	Membrane	To exclude a Langerhans cell neoplasm
Factor XIIIa	Negative	Cytoplasm	To exclude a histiocytic sarcoma
Lysozyme	Negative	Cytoplasm	To exclude a histiocytic sarcoma
CD21/CD23/CD35	Positive	Membrane	To demonstrate the follicular dendritic cell differentiation
Clusterin and Fascin	Positive	Cytoplasm	To demonstrate the follicular dendritic cell differentiation
CXCL13	Positive	Golgi-dot pattern	To demonstrate the follicular dendritic cell differentiation
SMMHC	Positive	Cytoplasm	Positive in cases of FDCS
Ki67	Variable	Nucleus	To investigate the proliferative potential of the tumor
NFkB pathway genes[a]	Approximately 60%	–	To investigate the molecular basis of the neoplasm
CDKN2A/RB1/TP53[a]	20%–30%	–	To investigate the molecular basis of the neoplasm
BRAF-V600E[a]	0%–19%	–	To investigate the molecular basis of the neoplasm

Important genetic features are also described
SMMHC smooth muscle myosin heavy chain, *FDCS* follicular dendritic cell sarcoma
[a]Investigated by PCR

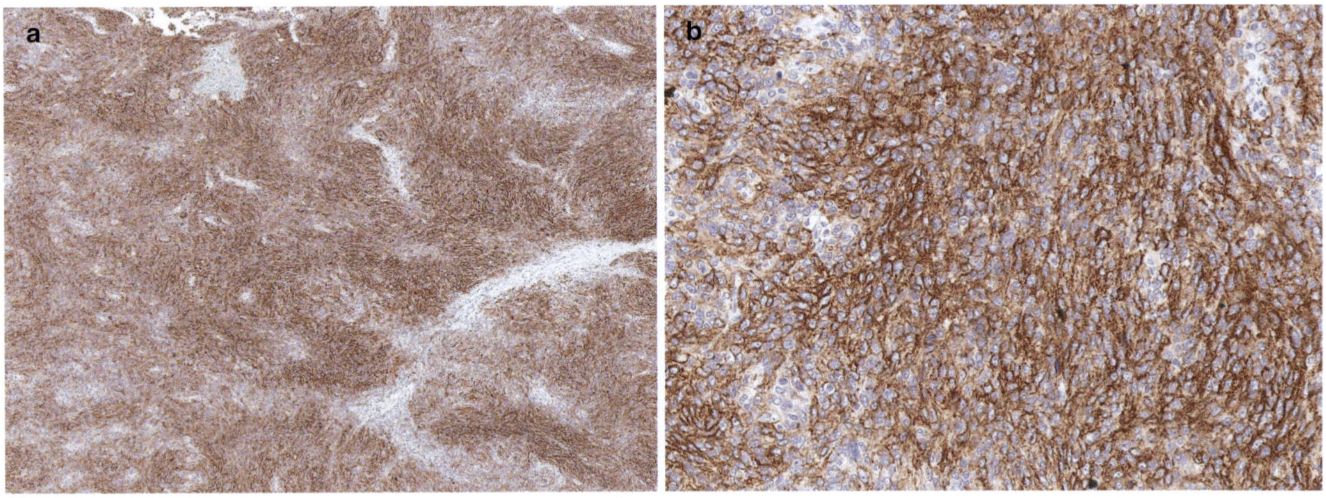

Fig. 32.4 Immunohistochemical features of follicular dendritic cell sarcoma. (**a**) Strong and diffuse expression of follicular dendritic cell marker CD23 (DAB; 50X). (**b**) Under high-power, observe the strong membrane staining of CD23 in the tumor cells (DAB; 200X)

Sources

1. Monda L, Warnke R, Rosai J. A primary lymph node malignancy with features suggestive of dendritic reticulum cell differentiation. A report of 4 cases. Am J Pathol. 1986;122(3):562–72.
2. Chan JK, Tsang WY, Ng CS, Tang SK, Yu HC, Lee AW. Follicular dendritic cell tumors of the oral cavity. Am J Surg Pathol. 1994;18:148–57. https://doi.org/10.1097/00000478-199402000-00004.
3. Araújo VC, Martins MT, Salmen FS, Araújo NS. Extranodal follicular dendritic cell sarcoma of the palate. Oral Surg Oral Med Oral Pathol Oral Radiol Endod. 1999;87:209–14. https://doi.org/10.1016/s1079-2104(99)70274-x.
4. Cheuk W, Chan JK, Shek TW, Chang JH, Tsou MH, Yuen NW, et al. Inflammatory pseudotumor-like follicular dendritic cell tumor: a distinctive low-grade malignant intra-abdominal neoplasm with consistent Epstein-Barr virus association. Am J Surg Pathol. 2001;25(6):721–31. https://doi.org/10.1097/00000478-200106000-00003.
5. Satoh K, Hibi G, Yamamoto Y, Urano M, Kuroda M, Nakamura S. Follicular dendritic cell tumor in the oro-pharyngeal region: report of a case and a review of the literature. Oral Oncol. 2003;39:415–9. https://doi.org/10.1016/s1368-8375(02)00138-0.

6. Tisch M, Hengstermann F, Kraft K, von Hinüber G, Maier H. Follicular dendritic cell sarcoma of the tonsil: report of a rare case. Ear Nose Throat J. 2003;82(7):507–9.
7. Go H, Jeon YK, Huh J, et al. Frequent detection of BRAF (V600E) mutations in histiocytic and dendritic cell neoplasms. Histopathology. 2014;65:261–72. https://doi.org/10.1111/his.12416.
8. Li J, Zhou ML, Zhou SH. Clinical and pathological features of head and neck follicular dendritic cell sarcoma. Hematology. 2015;20(10):571–83. https://doi.org/10.1179/1607845415Y.0000000008.
9. Griffin GK, Sholl LM, Lindeman NI, Fletcher CD, Hornick JL. Targeted genomic sequencing of follicular dendritic cell sarcoma reveals recurrent alterations in NF-κB regulatory genes. Mod Pathol. 2016;29:67–74. https://doi.org/10.1038/modpathol.2015.130.
10. Amirtham U, Manohar V, Kamath MP, Srinivasamurthy PC, Chennagiriyappa LK, Shenoy AM, et al. Clinicopathological profile and outcomes of follicular dendritic cell sarcoma of the head and neck region – a study of 10 cases with literature review. J Clin Diagn Res. 2016;10(8):XC08–11. https://doi.org/10.7860/JCDR/2016/19763.8386.
11. Wu B, Lim CM, Petersson F. Primary tonsillar epithelioid follicular dendritic cell sarcoma: report of a rare case mimicking undifferentiated carcinoma and a brief review of the literature. Head Neck Pathol. 2019;13:606–12. https://doi.org/10.1007/s12105-019-01015-3.
12. Bao L, Wang T, Liu M, Xing F. Follicular dendritic cell sarcoma of the tonsil: case report and review of literature. Int J Clin Exp Pathol. 2021;14(4):493–500.
13. Facchetti F, Simbeni M, Lorenzi L. Follicular dendritic cell sarcoma. Pathologica. 2021;113:316–29. https://doi.org/10.32074/1591-951X-331.
14. Jiang XN, Zhang Y, Xue T, Chen JY, Chan ACL, Cheuk W, et al. New clinicopathologic scenarios of EBV+ inflammatory follicular dendritic cell sarcoma: report of 9 extrahepatosplenic cases. Am J Surg Pathol. 2021;45(6):765–72. https://doi.org/10.1097/PAS.0000000000001632.
15. Din NU, Ahmad Z, Rahim S, Fritchie K, Tariq MU, Ahmed A. Extranodal follicular dendritic cell sarcoma of the head and neck region: a clinicopathological study of 7 cases. Int J Surg Pathol. 2022:10668969221133352. https://doi.org/10.1177/10668969221133352.
16. Aslam S, Ibe I, Zhang Y, Demianets R, Tran T, Gamayo A, et al. Follicular dendritic cell sarcoma involving the parotid gland with expression of the melanocytic marker PRAME. J Hematop. 2024;17(4):271–4. https://doi.org/10.1007/s12308-024-00605-7.
17. Oh KY, Hong SD. Follicular dendritic cell sarcoma in the submandibular region: a report of a rare case. J Dent Sci. 2024;19(4):2430–2. https://doi.org/10.1016/j.jds.2024.07.022.
18. Kelley JT, Amoth HM, Lopez-Hisijos N, Hrycaj S, Valdez R, Rottmann D. Smooth Muscle Myosin Heavy Chain expression in nodal and extranodal follicular dendritic cell sarcoma. Appl Immunohistochem Mol Morphol. 2025. https://doi.org/10.1097/PAI.0000000000001241.
19. Moe K, Maa HC, Lin ST, Kuo YJ. Follicular dendritic cell sarcoma of the parotid gland: a case report and review of literature. Head Neck Pathol. 2024;18(1):55. https://doi.org/10.1007/s12105-024-01659-w.

Part V

Leukemic Manifestations

33 Leukemic Myeloid Infiltrations and Myeloid Sarcoma

Tarcilia Aparecida da Silva, Mariana Villarroel-Dorrego, Javier Rendon Henao, and Felipe Paiva Fonseca

33.1 General Overview and Clinical Presentation

Leukemia is a neoplasm originating from different cellular components of the hematolymphoid complex that typically affects the bone marrow. The current World Health Organization classification of Hematolymphoid Tumors recognizes a large number of leukemia subtypes based on a complex analysis of clinical features, morphological findings, immunophenotype, genetic events and lineage of differentiation. Lymphoblastic leukemia/lymphoma derives from immature lymphoid cells, represents the most common leukemia subtype among infants and will be discussed in detail in Chap. 34, while chronic lymphocytic leukemia/small lymphocytic lymphoma is a leukemic disease derived from mature B lymphocytes; it is more prevalent among adults and will be discussed in Chap. 35. Acute myeloid leukemia (AML) is a highly heterogeneous clonal expansion of cells from the myeloid lineage, representing the most common form of acute leukemia in adults, with a median age at diagnosis of 68 years and is frequently associated with anemia, thrombocytopenia, and neutropenia.

AML is currently classified according to the presence of defining genetic abnormalities (acute promyelocytic leukemia with *PML::RARA* fusion; AML with *RUNX1::RUNX1T1* fusion; AML with *CBFB::MYH11* fusion; AML with *DEK::NUP214* fusion; AML with *RBM15::MRTFA* fusion; AML with *BCR::ABL1* fusion; AML with *KMT2A* rearrangement; AML with *MECOM* rearrangement; AML with *NUP98* rearrangement; AML with *NPM1* mutation; AML with *CEBPA* mutation; AML, myelodysplasia-related; AML with other defined genetic alterations) or by differentiation (AML with minimal differentiation; AML without maturation; AML with maturation; Acute basophilic leukemia; Acute myelomonocytic leukemia; Acute monocytic leukemia; Acute erythroid leukemia; Acute megakaryoblastic leukemia). Other myeloid neoplasms include chronic myeloproliferative neoplasms, mastocytosis, myelodysplastic neoplasms, myelodysplastic/myeloproliferative neoplasms, myeloid neoplasms secondary to predisposing conditions, myeloid/lymphoid neoplasms and acute leukemias of mixed or ambiguous lineage, all them carrying specific clinical, pathological and genetic features, encompassing a myriad of subtypes whose detailed description is beyond of the scope of this book and readers are encouraged to consult more specialized textbooks on leukemic diseases.

Leukemic infiltrations in the oral cavity are not rare and are well described in the literature, more frequently representing AML manifestations, although many reports available in the literature do not attempt to classify the type of myeloid neoplasm in detail. Clinically, oral leukemic infiltrations more commonly manifest as a diffuse, painless, reddish and swollen gingival tissue. The gingivae also show spontaneous bleeding in many cases, and not only can the free gingival margin and the interpapilae regions be affected, but also the adherent gingival tissue. The presence of petechiae and/or ecchymosis, more often diffusely distributed in different regions of the mucosa, has also been frequently described as indicative of leukemic manifestations in the oral cavity. In the gnathic bones myeloid leukemic infiltration may cause ill-defined radiolucent images in the maxilla or mandible, usually associated with tooth loosening.

Myeloid sarcoma, originally termed *chloroma* due to the green color of the tumor secondary to the oxidation of myeloperoxidase (MPO) within the granules of immature myeloid cells, and latter known as *myeloblastoma* and then

T. A. da Silva (✉) · F. P. Fonseca
Department of Oral Surgery and Pathology, School of Dentistry, Universidade Federal de Minas Gerais, Belo Horizonte, Brazil

M. Villarroel-Dorrego
Instituto de Investigaciones Odontológicas, Universidad Central de Venezuela, Caracas, Venezuela
e-mail: mariana.villarroel@ucv.ve

J. R. Henao
Department of Hematopathology and Flow Cytometry, Ayudas Diagnósticas Sura Center, Cartagena, Colombia

© The Author(s), under exclusive license to Springer Nature Switzerland AG 2025
F. P. Fonseca et al. (eds.), *Lymphoproliferative and Granulomatous Disorders of the Oral Cavity*,
https://doi.org/10.1007/978-3-031-98844-8_33

granulocytic sarcoma, is defined as a solid mass consisting of myeloblasts, with or without maturation, that develops in extramedullary sites, including the oral and maxillofacial region. It more commonly coincides with AML or it may also constitute a (leukemic) transformation at an extramedullary site of myelodysplastic or myeloproliferative neoplasms. However, it may also present as an isolated neoplasm without concomitant bone marrow involvement, although the majority of these cases will develop metachronous medullary disease with a median latency period of a few months. Myeloid sarcoma occurs in 5%–12% of post-allogeneic hematopoietic stem cell transplanted patients.

Considering the biological heterogeneity of AML and of the other myeloid neoplasms, it is reasonable to understand myeloid sarcoma as a set of heterogeneous diseases, rather than a homogeneous entity, and molecular and cytogenetic analyses may be done as an attempt to refine the diagnosis. The nutational landscape of myeloid sarcoma parallels those abnormalities with bone marrow AML, and chromosomal abnormalities have been shown in approximately 50% of the cases. Moreover, some evidence points to the occurrence of specific molecular events depending on the anatomical site affected by the neoplasm. Any region of the body can be affected, more frequently the skin, soft tissue, lymph nodes, gastrointestinal tract, bones, and the head and neck region. Male patients in the sixth decade of life are the most affected individuals. Morphologically, myeloid sarcoma can be very difficult to diagnose when there is no clinical data suggestive of a myeloid malignancy, demanding a high level of diagnostic suspicion from pathologists.

In the oral cavity, myeloid sarcoma also more frequently affects the gingival tissue, manifesting as nodules or tumors that range in size, usually presenting with a reddish to purple-colored aspect. Moreover, patients presenting asymptomatic, non-ulcerated swellings that can affect any region of the oral cavity, as well as cases exhibiting a more aggressive clinical behavior illustrated by painful and ulcerated tumors with areas of tissue necrosis, have also been described. Myeloid sarcomas may be clinically misdiagnosed as pyogenic granuloma, peripheral giant cell granuloma or other reactive oral lesions. Intraosseous involvement of the mandible and maxilla can also be found, and the occurrence of multiple simultaneous lesions in the oral cavity has also been reported.

The prognosis of patients affected by leukemic infiltrations or myeloid sarcoma varies significantly depending on several prognostic factors, including its mutational landscape, but it is usually considered poor. Moreover, different chemotherapeutic schemes can be applied, and once again, the presence of specific mutations will impact the selection of the most effective regimen (Figs. 33.1, 33.2, 33.3, and 33.4).

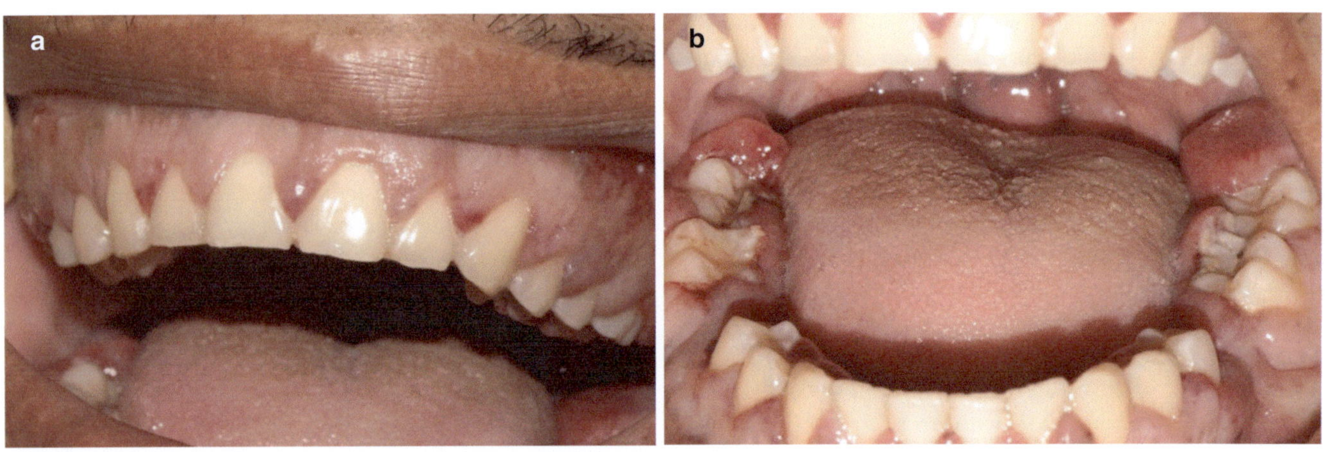

Fig. 33.1 Clinical presentation of leukemic infiltration/myeloid sarcoma affecting the oral cavity. (**a**) Diffuse asymptomatic swelling in the upper gingiva. Observe that the gingival tissue is diffusely erythematous, especially in the gingival papillae. (**b**) The same patient also exhibited a diffuse infiltration in the lower gingiva. In the retromolar region, the patient exhibited solid growths bilaterally

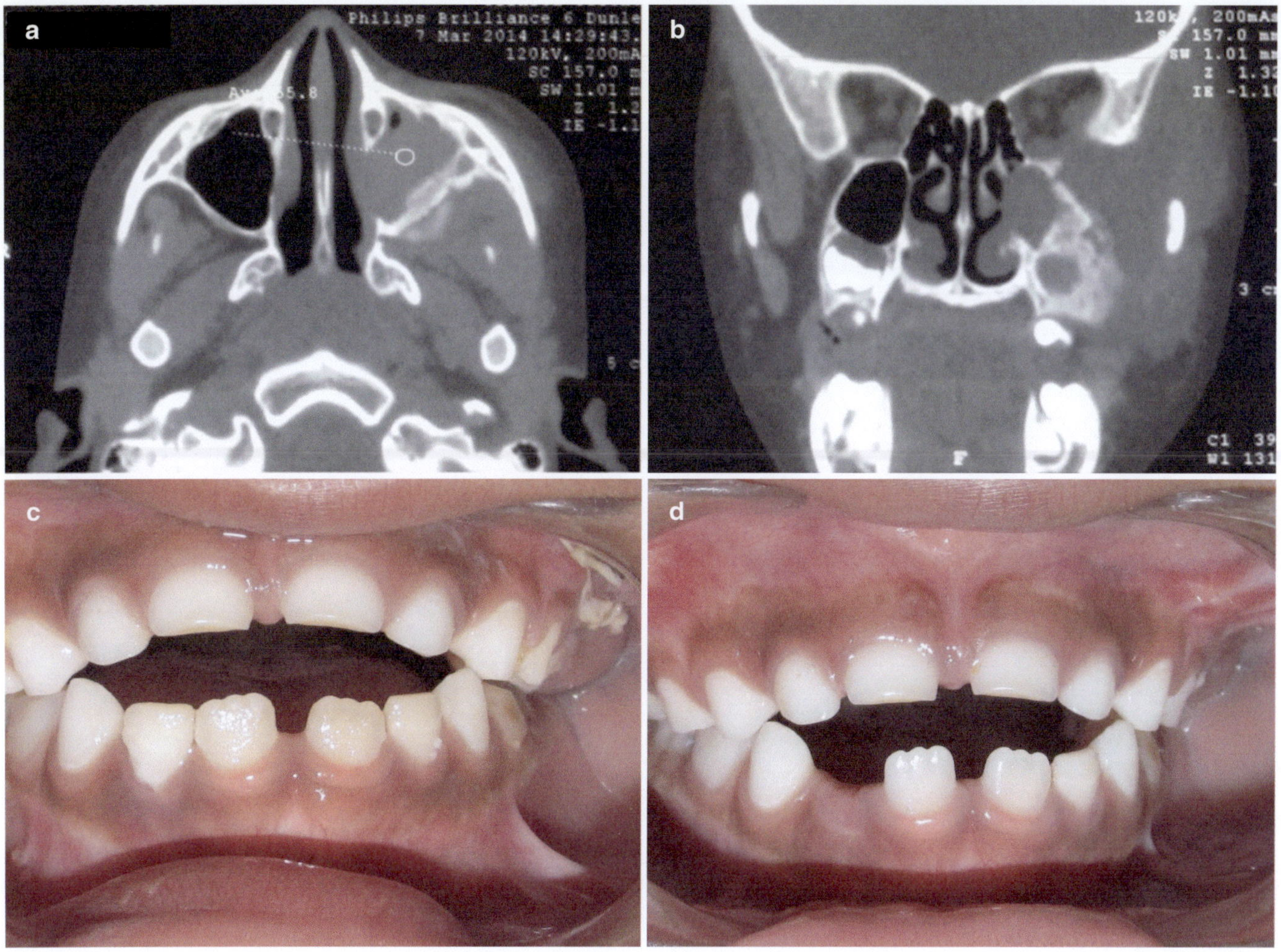

Fig. 33.2 Clinical presentation of acute myeloid leukemia infiltration in the facial region extending towards the oral cavity in a 6-year-old male patient. (**a**) Computed tomography exam, axial section, showing the infiltration of the left side of the maxillary sinus by the neoplasm. (**b**) In the coronal section it is possible to observe the very extensive infiltration of the tumor affecting the left side of the patients' craniofacial bones and soft tissues, leading to a significant facial asymmetry. (**c**) The neoplasm extended towards the oral cavity, causing an ulcerative and necrotic lesion in the maxillary vestibular mucosa. (**d**) After chemotherapy, the oral lesion disappeared

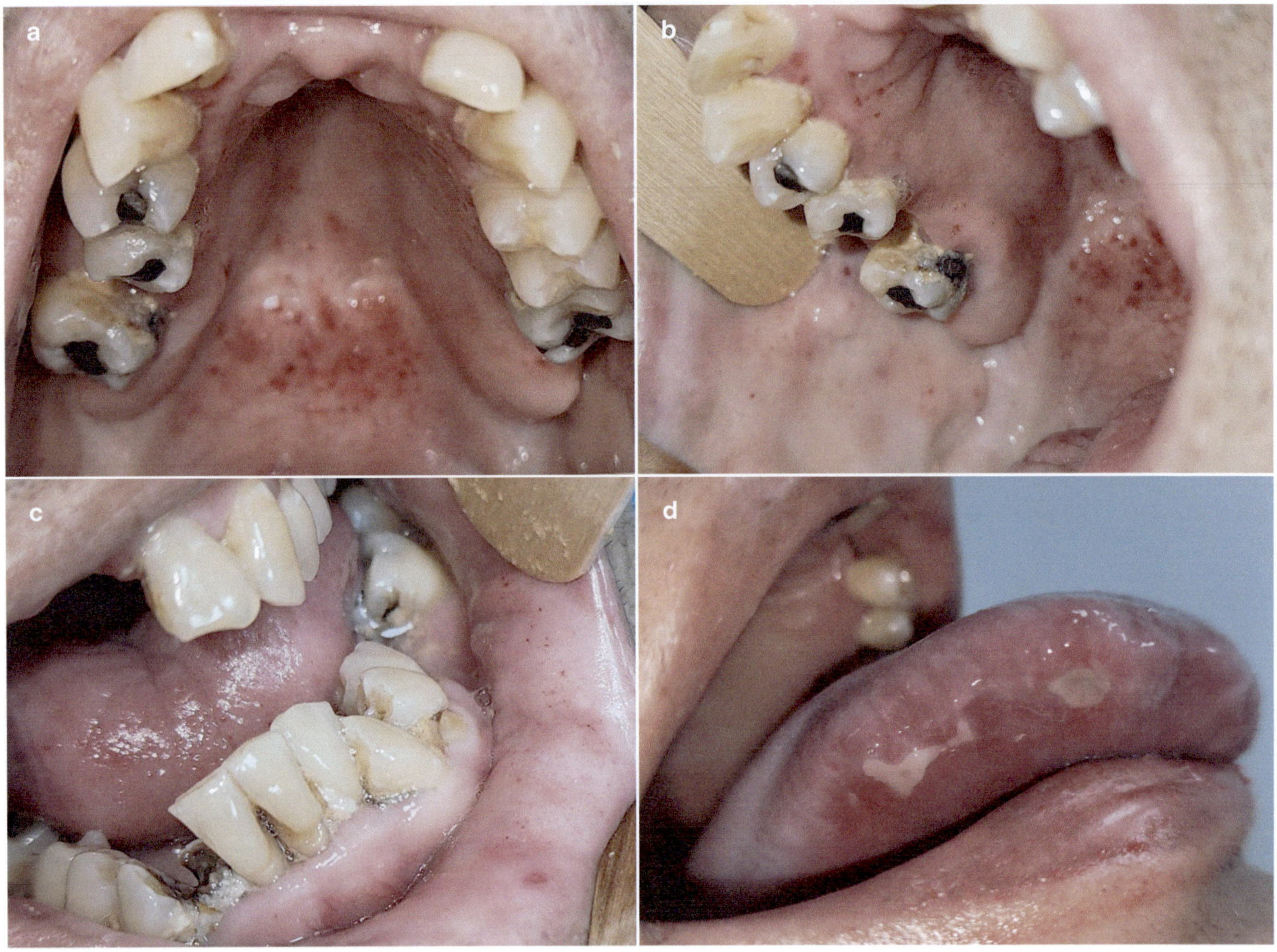

Fig. 33.3 Clinical presentation of acute myeloid leukemia oral manifestations in two different adult patients. (**a**) Observe the diffuse erythematous lesions in the form of multiple petechiae distributed in the palate of a male patient. (**b**) Similar lesions were found in the vestibular mucosa of the right side, and (**c**) in the lower lip. (**d**) The second patient had multiple ulcerative lesions affecting the tongue

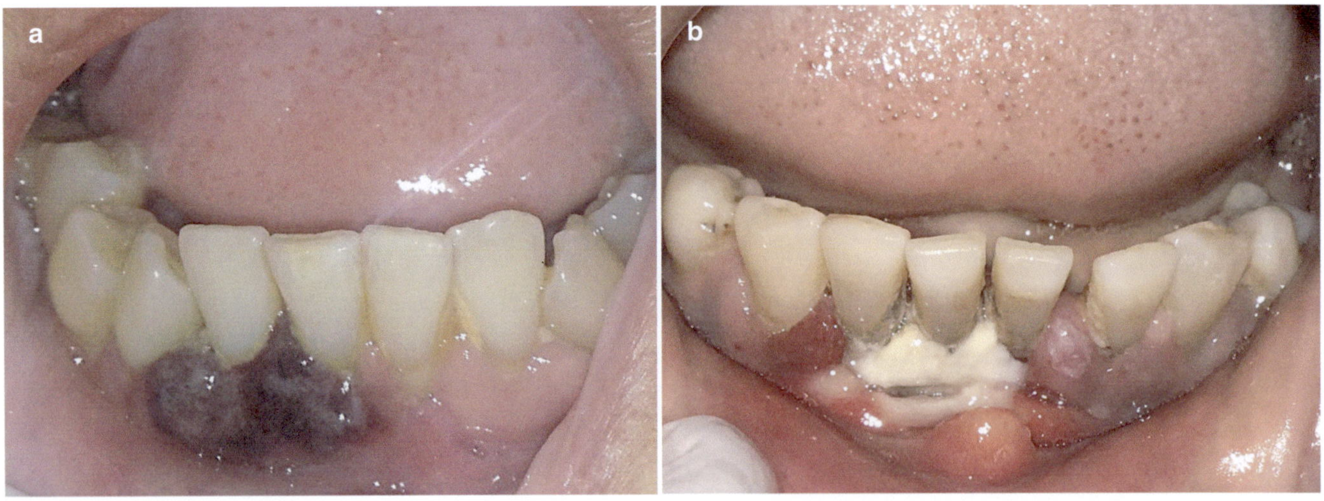

Fig. 33.4 Clinical presentation of acute myeloid leukemia affecting the oral cavity. (**a**) Female patient exhibiting a purple-colored swelling in the lower gingival tissue. (**b**) Female patient with a diffuse involvement of the lower gingival tissue with extensive areas of necrosis

33.2 Microscopic Findings

- The morphological aspect of myeloid sarcoma/leukemic infiltrations varies depending on the degree of differentiation of myeloblasts.
- A solid proliferation of poorly differentiated blast-like cells is usually observed.
- Intermingled with chronic inflammatory infiltrate.
- Presence of extravasated erythrocytes.
- A starry sky pattern can be found in a few cases.
- Tumor cells vary in size from small to large, round to oval, with mild to moderately basophilic cytoplasm.
- Mitotic figures are common.
- Neoplastic cells may have features of promyelocytic or granulocytic maturation, while many cases show a myelomonocytic or a pure monoblastic morphology.
- Myeloid blasts may have round to oval, or irregular nuclei, fine (blastic) chromatin, and inconspicuous to small nucleoli; hyperchromatic nuclei are also present.
- The presence of eosinophilic precursors is found in many cases.
- It can be seen as solitary infiltrating neoplastic cells or they can be found arranged in a linear or "Indian file" growth pattern.
- Tumor cells may also show acinus-like, cord-like, nested, cobblestone-like and patchy arrangements.
- The presence of signet ring-like or plasmacytoid cells is uncommon, but has been described in a few cases (Figs. 33.5, 33.6, and 33.7).

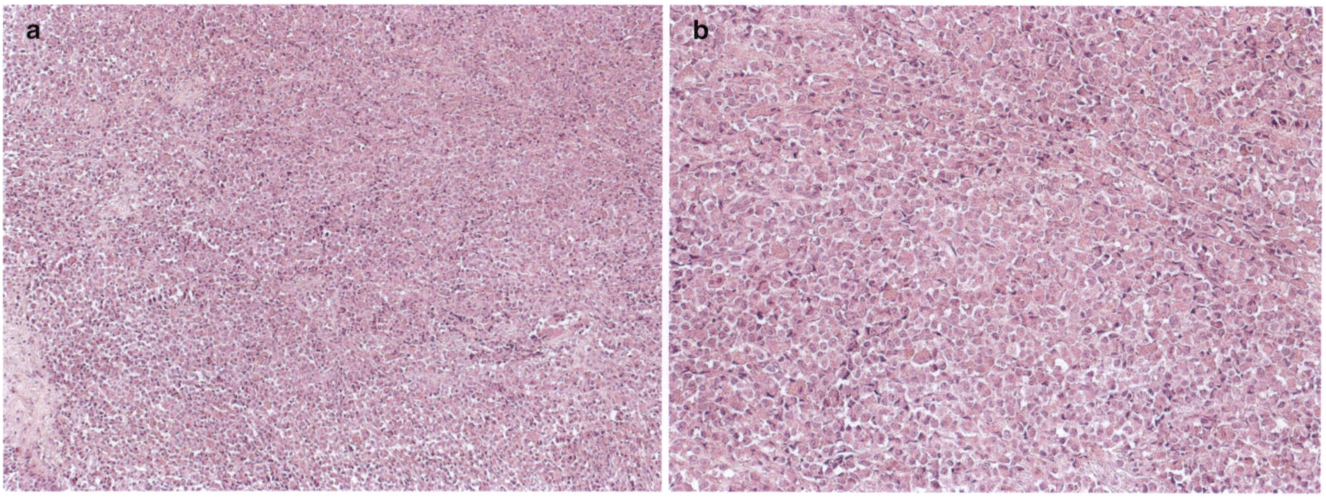

Fig. 33.5 Microscopic features of myeloid sarcoma affecting the oral mucosa. (**a**) Neoplastic cells proliferate in the lamina propria of the oral mucosa, exhibiting a diffuse growth pattern (H&E; 50X). (**b**) Neoplastic cells are predominantly medium-sized and some of them exhibit an abundant eosinophilic cytoplasm (H&E; 100X)

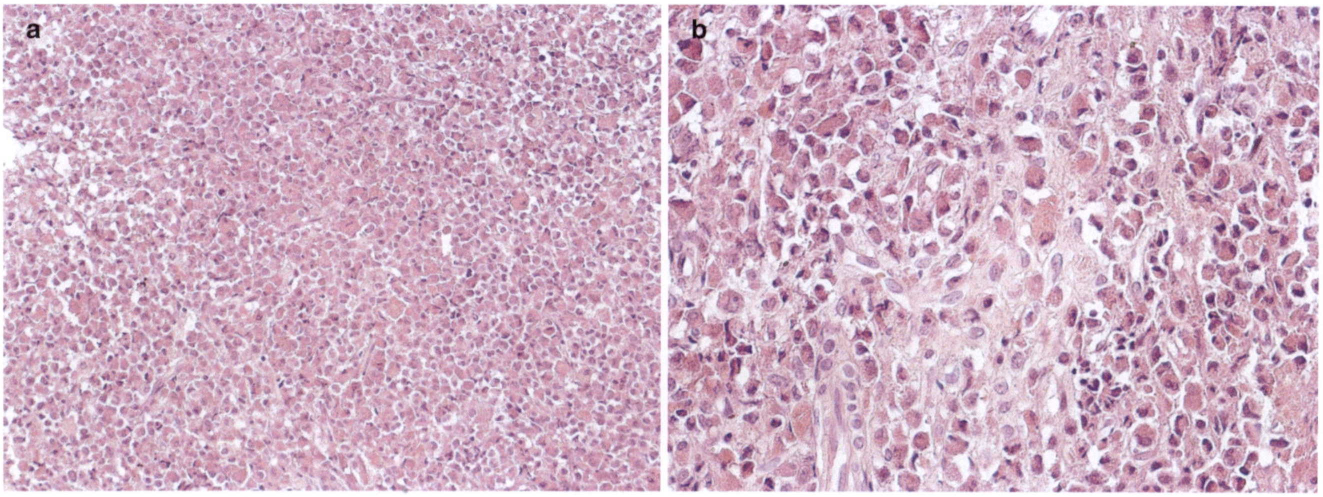

Fig. 33.6 Microscopic features of myeloid sarcoma affecting the oral mucosa. (**a**) Diffuse proliferation of neoplastic myeloid cells (H&E; 100X). (**b**) The presence of various eosinophils is a common finding in myeloid sarcoma/leukemic infiltration (H&E; 200X)

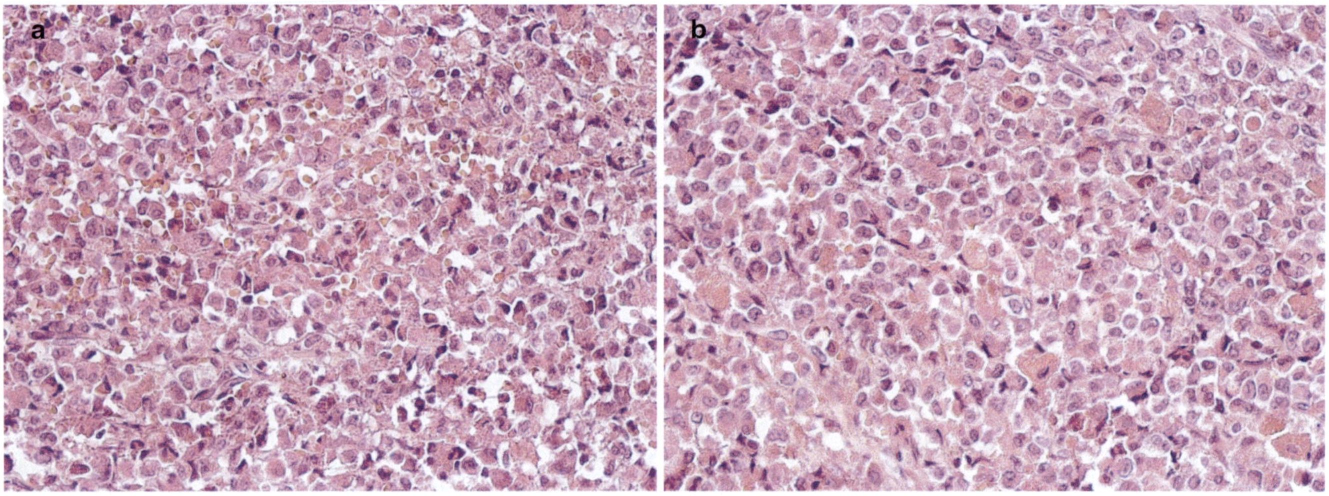

Fig. 33.7 Microscopic features of myeloid sarcoma affecting the oral mucosa. (**a**) Myeloid sarcoma usually exhibits erythrocyte extravasation. The presence of pleomorphic cells is common. Some of them may show plasmacytic morphology (H&E; 200X). (**b**) Large cells with abundant eosinophilic cytoplasm are present in this image. Some cells are binucleated (H&E; 200X)

Table 33.1 Summary of the main immunohistochemical reactions used for myeloid sarcoma diagnosis

Antibody	Most frequent results	Pattern	Objective
CD20	Negative	Membrane	To exclude a B-cell nature of the tumor
CD3	Negative	Membrane	To exclude a T-cell nature of the tumor
TdT	Negative[a]	Nucleus	To investigate a possible lymphoblastic leukemia
CD33	Positive	Cytoplasm	To demonstrate the myeloid nature of the neoplasm
MPO	Positive	Cytoplasm	To demonstrate the myeloid nature of the neoplasm
CD99	Positive	Membrane	To demonstrate the myeloid nature of the neoplasm
CD117	Positive	Membrane	To demonstrate the myeloid nature of the neoplasm
CD34	Positive	Membrane	To demonstrate the myeloid nature of the neoplasm
CD68 (KP1/PGM1)[b]	Positive	Cytoplasm	To demonstrate the myeloid nature of the neoplasm
CD43	Positive	Membrane	To demonstrate the myeloid nature of the neoplasm
Lysozyme	Positive	Cytoplasm	To demonstrate the myeloid nature of the neoplasm
Ki67	High	Nucleus	To demonstrate the proliferative index of tumor cells

MPO myeloperoxidase
[a]It can be positive in approximately 30% of the cases
[b]KP1 is more commonly positive than PG-M1

33.3 Immunohistochemistry and/or Genetics

Immunohistochemistry is used to demonstrate the myeloid nature of the tumor cells, which, however, can be of different myeloid lineages and present different grades of maturation. Therefore, many different markers can be used to specify both differentiation and maturation features of the neoplasm. The most frequently used markers that lead to a myeloid sarcoma diagnosis are myeloperoxidase (MPO), CD68/KP1, CD68/PGM1 (The KP1 clone is reported in 90% of the cases, whereas the PG-M1 clone that is considered to carry a higher macrophage specificity is reported in 50% of the cases), CD99, CD34, CD43 and lysozyme, with negativity to mature lymphoid markers like CD20 and CD3. The expression of TdT is commonly negative, but positivity can be found in some cases. Approximately 80% of the cases are positive for BCL2, and the proliferative index is usually high. Diagnosis must always be followed by systemic evaluation, and genetic investigation is frequently necessary to determine the specific subtype, the most appropriate chemotherapeutic approach and the prognostic determination. Molecular studies of myeloid sarcomas have shown a large number of molecular abnormalities, including mutations in *NPM1*, *KMT2A* and members of the *RAS* pathway (Table 33.1; Figs. 33.8, 33.9, 33.10, 33.11, 33.12, and 33.13).

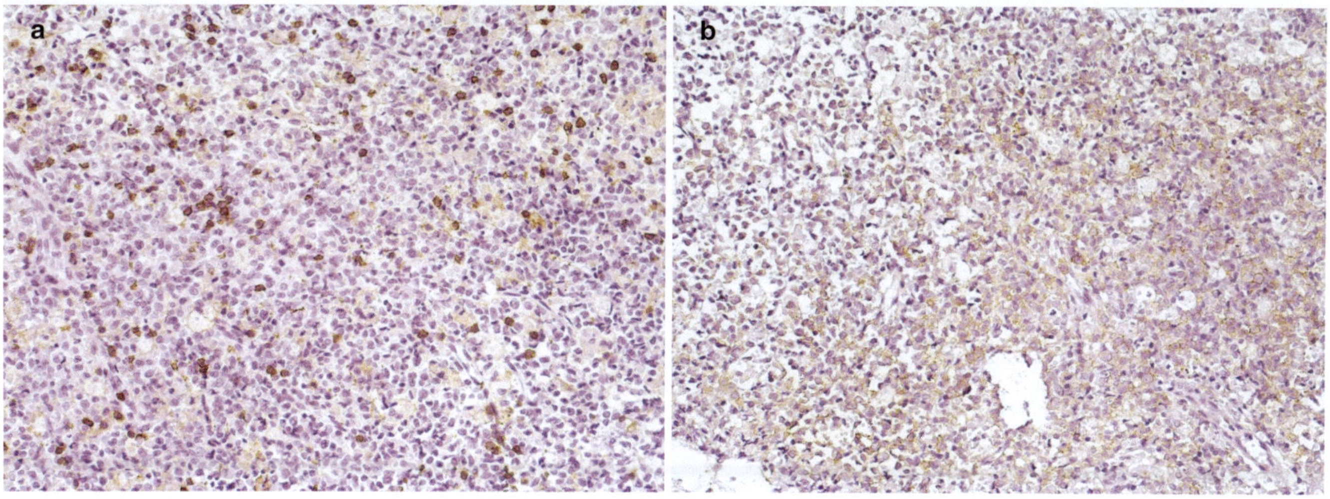

Fig. 33.8 Immunohistochemical findings of myeloid sarcoma affecting the oral mucosa. (**a**) LCA expression is stronger in reactive lymphoid cells (DAB; 100X). (**b**) The diffuse expression of CD99 can be seen in neoplastic cells (DAB; 100X)

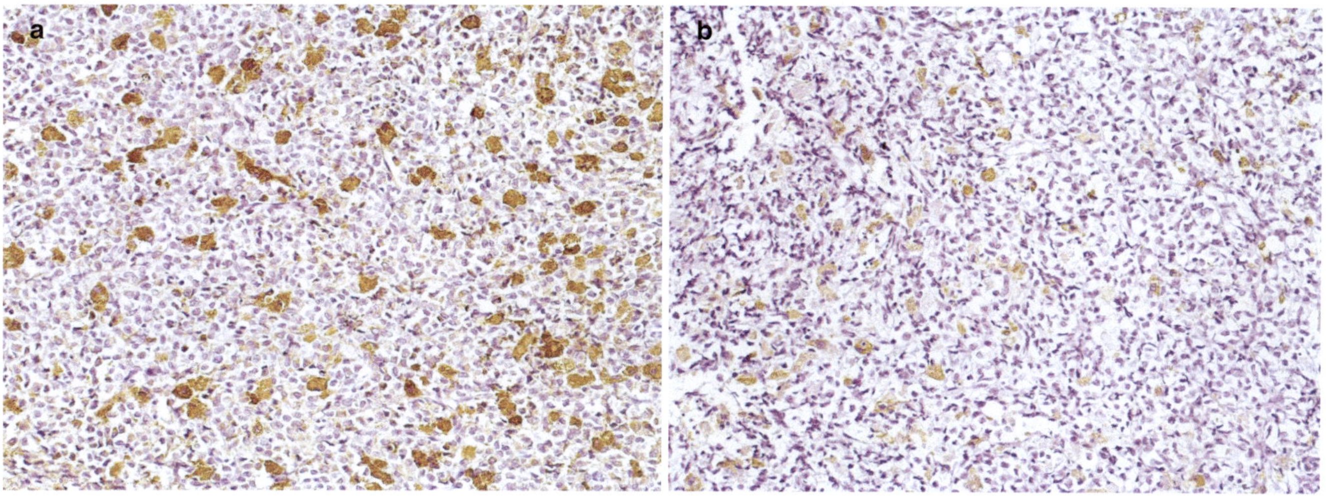

Fig. 33.9 Immunohistochemical findings of myeloid sarcoma affecting the oral mucosa. (**a**) Diffuse expression of CD68 using the KP1 clone (DAB; 100X). (**b**) The expression of CD68 using the PGM1 clone is also found, but in a more focal pattern (DAB; 100X)

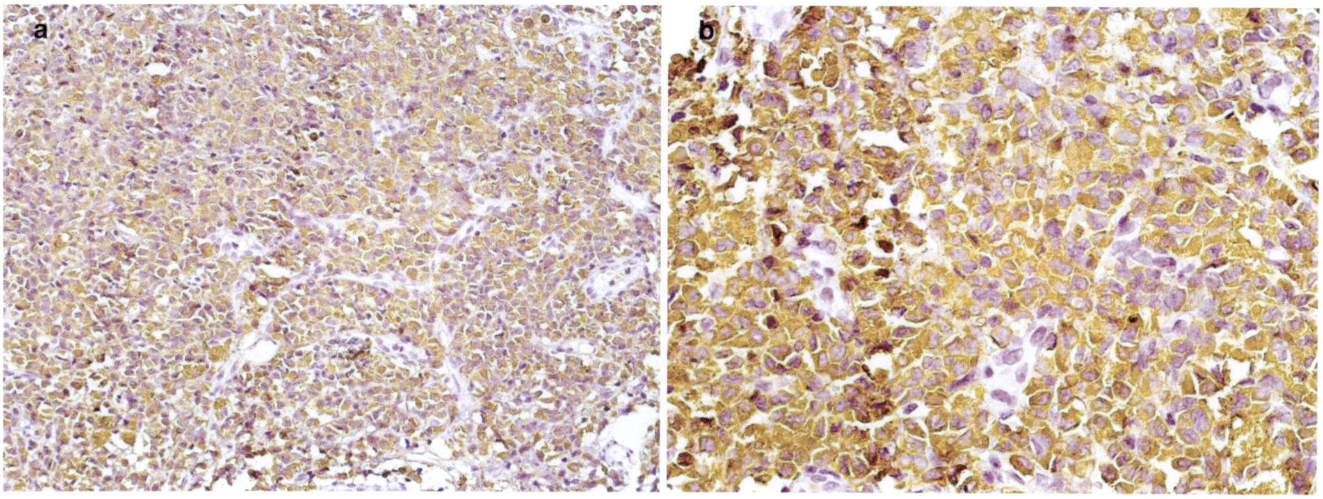

Fig. 33.10 Immunohistochemical findings of myeloid sarcoma affecting the oral mucosa. (**a**) Diffuse expression of MPO in tumor cells (DAB; 100X). (**b**) Observe the strong cytoplasmic expression of MPO in neoplastic cells (DAB; 200X)

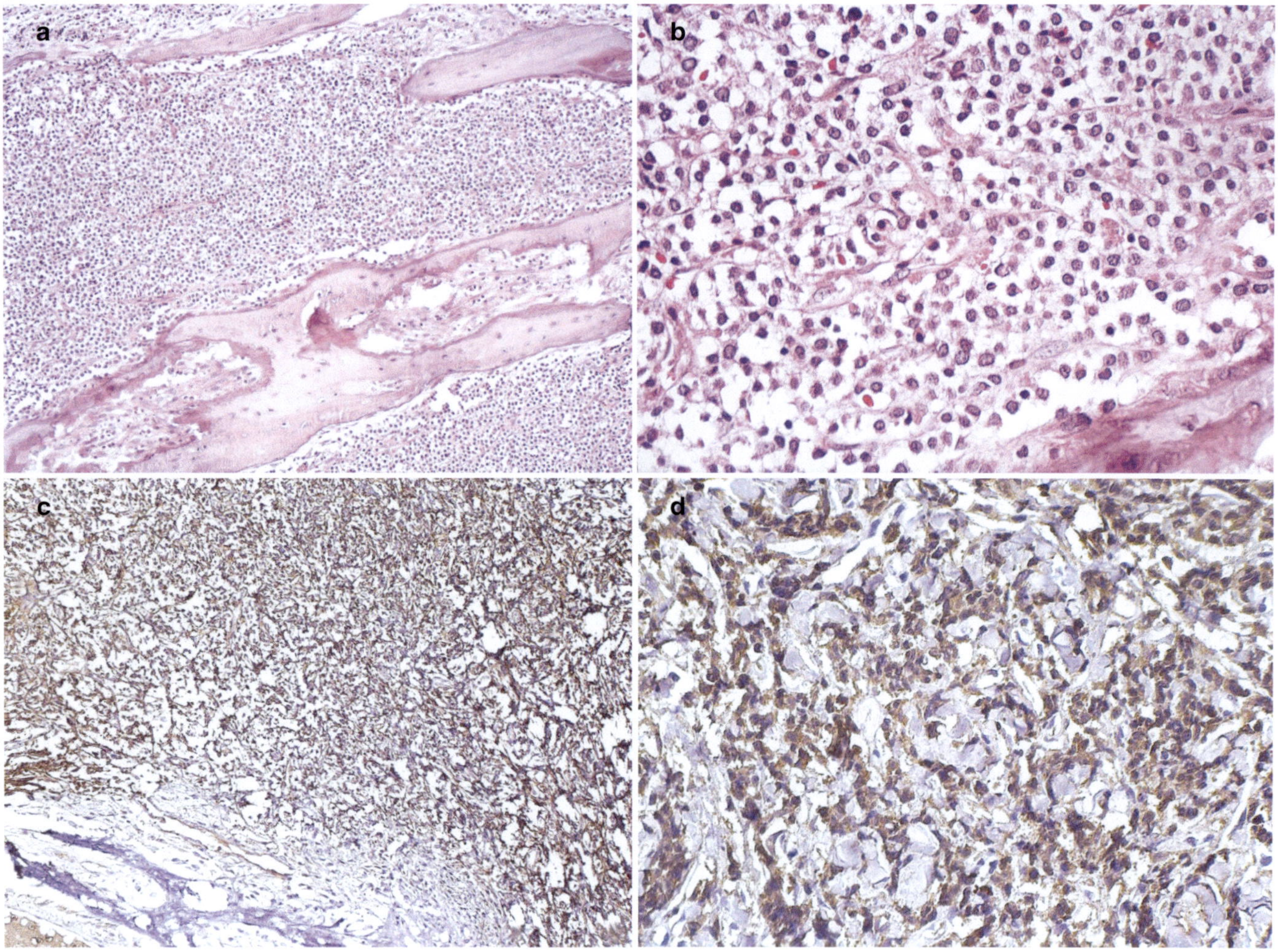

Fig. 33.11 Microscopic and immunohistochemical features of myeloid sarcoma affecting the oral mucosa and the mandible. (**a**) Diffuse proliferation of neoplastic myeloid cells infiltrates the bone tissue of the mandible of a child (H&E; 50X). (**b**) A discohesive feature is observed among tumor cells that are predominantly small to medium-sized, with a variable cytological pattern (H&E; 100X). (**c**) Tumor cells were diffusely positive for CD99 (DAB; 50X), (**d**) and exhibited a strong cytoplasmic expression of MPO (DAB; 100X)

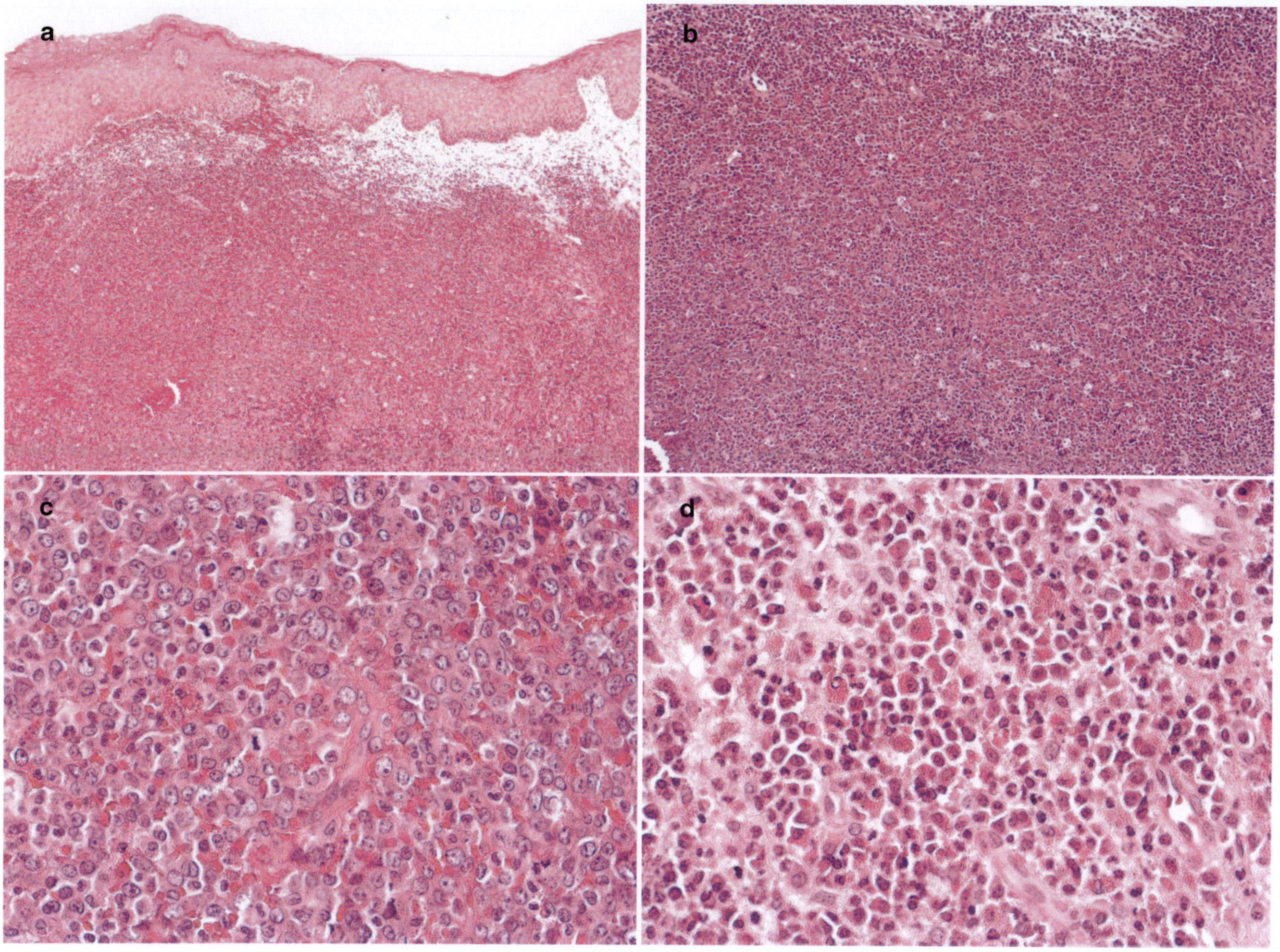

Fig. 33.12 Microscopic features of myeloid sarcoma affecting the gingiva. (**a**) Overlying squamous epithelium with diffuse proliferation of neoplastic cells in the lamina propria. There are scattered tingible body macrophages (H&E; 50X). (**b**) Tumor cells with abundant eosinophilic cytoplasm, mitotic figures and tingible body macrophages that impart a starry sky appearance (H&E; 100X). (**c**) The neoplastic cells have a large eosinophilic cytoplasm and a round-to-oval nucleus, with prominent nucleoli (H&E; 400X). (**d**) Some cells exhibit a plasmacytoid appearance with eosinophilic cytoplasm (H&E; 400X)

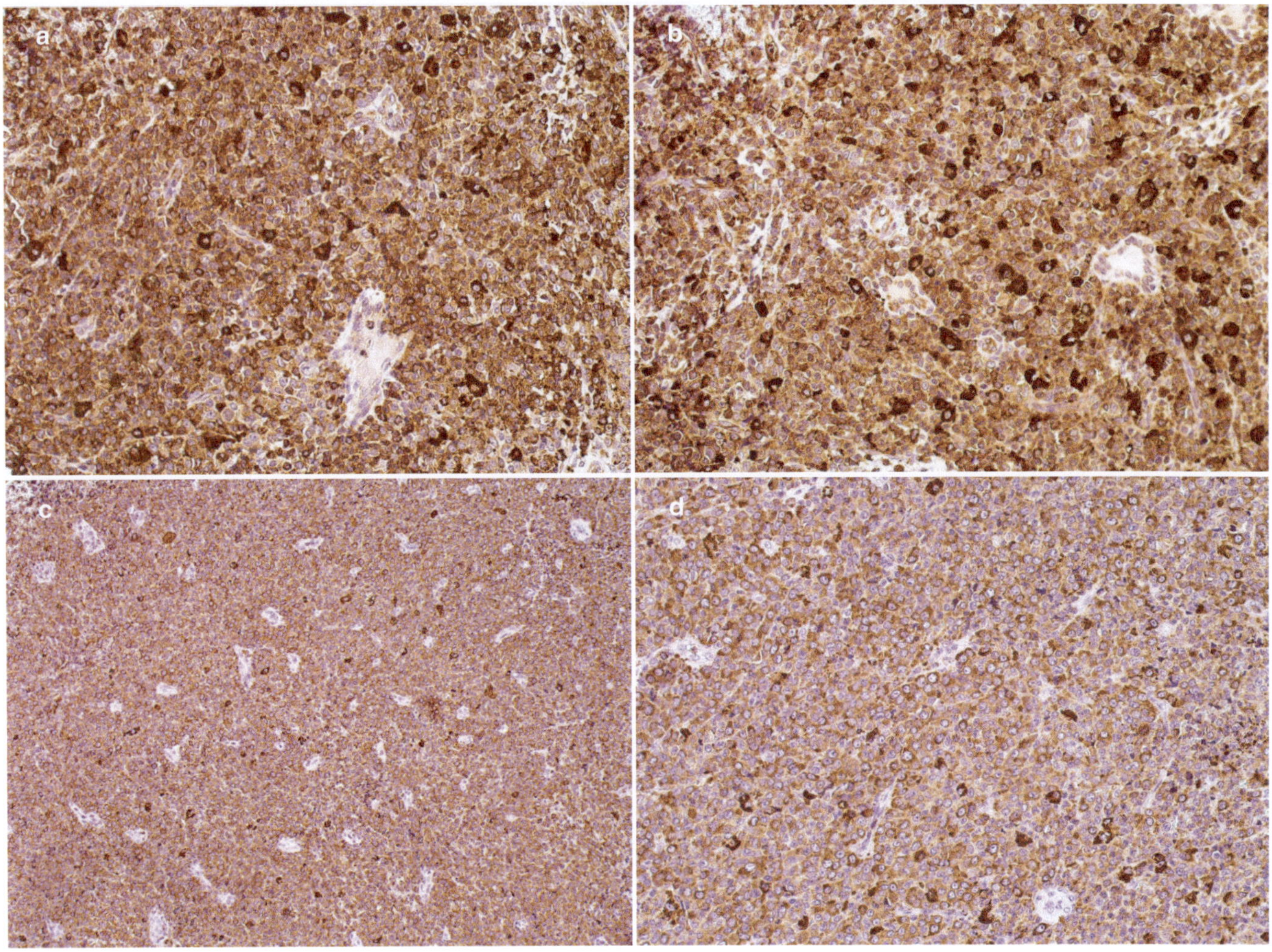

Fig. 33.13 Immunohistochemical findings of myeloid sarcoma affecting the gingiva. (**a**) Diffuse expression of CD68 in tumor cells (DAB; 100X). (**b**) Note the strong cytoplasmic expression in the tumor cells (DAB; 200X). (**c**) Diffuse expression of MPO in the cytoplasm of tumor cells (DAB; 100X). (**d**) Note the strong cytoplasmic expression of MPO in the cytoplasm of the tumor cells. (DAB; 200X)

Sources

1. Guan G, Firth N. Oral manifestations as an early clinical sign of acute myeloid leukaemia: a case report. Aust Dent J. 2015;60(1):123–7. https://doi.org/10.1111/adj.12272.
2. Wang HQ, Li J. Clinicopathological features of myeloid sarcoma: report of 39 cases and literature review. Pathol Res Pract. 2016;212:817–24.
3. Andrade BA, et al. Myeloid sarcoma of the oral cavity: a case report and review of 89 cases from the literature. J Clin Exp Dent. 2017;9(9):e1167–71.
4. Kashofer K, Gornicec M, Lind K, Caraffini V, Schauer S, Beham-Schmid C, et al. Detection of prognostically relevant mutations and translocations in myeloid sarcoma by next generation sequencing. Leuk Lymphoma. 2018;59:501–4. https://doi.org/10.1080/10428194.2017.1339879.
5. Watson E, Wood RE, Maxymiw WG, Schimmer AD. Prevalence of oral lesions in and dental needs of patients with newly diagnosed acute leukemia. J Am Dent Assoc. 2018;149(6):470–80. https://doi.org/10.1016/j.adaj.2018.01.019.
6. Benites BM, Fonseca FP, Miranda-Silva W, Bruno JS, Tucunduva L, Fregnani ER. Myeloid sarcoma in the tongue. Autops Case Rep. 2020;10:e2020160. https://doi.org/10.4322/acr.2020.160.
7. de Sena ACVP, de Arruda JAA, Costa FPD, Lemos APV, Kakehasi FM, Travassos DV, et al. Leukaemic infiltration in the oral and maxillofacial region: an update. J Oral Pathol Med. 2021;50:558–64. https://doi.org/10.1111/jop.13206.
8. Wang D, He K, Sroussi H, Treister N, Luskin M, Villa A, et al. Oral myeloid sarcoma as an uncommon manifestation of acute myeloid leukemia: a case series and review of the literature. J Am Dent Assoc. 2021;152(5):393–400.e8. https://doi.org/10.1016/j.adaj.2021.01.017.
9. Barros P, Islam MN, Fitzpatrick SG, Cohen DM, Bhattacharyya I, Alramadhan SA. Essentials of oral manifestations of leukemia for the dental practitioner. Gen Dent. 2022;70(2):33–6.
10. de Sena ACVP, de Arruda JAA, Bemquerer LM, Pantuzzo ES, Kakehasi FM, Fonseca FP, et al. Leukemia/lymphoma oral infiltration and its impact on disease outcomes: a Brazilian study. Oral Dis. 2022. https://doi.org/10.1111/odi.14452.
11. Falini B, Martelli MP. Comparison of the International Consensus and 5th WHO edition classifications of adult myelodysplastic syndromes and acute myeloid leukemia. Am J Hematol. 2023. https://doi.org/10.1002/ajh.26812.

12. Shimony S, Stahl M, Stone RM. Acute myeloid leukemia: 2023 update on diagnosis, risk-stratification and management. Am J Hematol. 2023. https://doi.org/10.1002/ajh.26822.
13. Loscocco GG, Vannucchi AM. Myeloid sarcoma: more and less than a distinct entity. Ann Hematol. 2023. https://doi.org/10.1007/s00277-023-05288-1.
14. Demir D, Hekimgil M, Karaca E, Ulusoy Y, Özdemir HH, Saydam G, et al. Clinicopathological characteristics, genetics and prognosis of patients with myeloid sarcoma: a single-center study. J Clin Pathol. 2023;76:244–51. https://doi.org/10.1136/jclinpath-2021-208000.
15. Pamukcu U, Dal MS, Yaman S, Aslan Candır B, Bozan E, Secilmis S, et al. Evaluation of oral manifestations and head and neck lymphadenopathy in newly diagnosed acute leukemia patients. Spec Care Dentist. 2024;44(3):911–8. https://doi.org/10.1111/scd.12941.

Lymphoblastic Leukemia/Lymphoma

34

Javier Rendon Henao, Pablo Agustin Vargas,
Hélder Antônio Rebelo Pontes,
and Felipe Paiva Fonseca

34.1 General Overview and Clinical Presentation

Lymphoblastic leukemia is the most common malignant neoplasm of childhood, while lymphoblastic lymphoma comprises approximately 2% of all cases of non-Hodgkin lymphoma. Lymphoblastic leukemia/lymphoma derives from precursor B or T lymphocytes, and the term lymphoma is used for solid lesions with no or minimal involvement of peripheral blood and/or bone marrow, with a threshold value of <25% bone marrow blasts being usually used to define lymphoma. Although the etiology of this neoplasm is unknown, a better understanding on its pathogenesis was achieved and a series of genetic mutations have been recognized to have prognostic significance for B-lymphoblastic leukemia/lymphoma, being used to subclassify this entity depending on the presence of specific chromosomal abnormalities by molecular tests, while genetic events in the T-cell variant have also been better demonstrated, but still need to be further investigated according to their potential to determine patients' survival and prognosis.

The occurrence of chromosomal imbalances in B-lymphoblastic leukemia/lymphoma may be associated with clinical manifestations, carry important therapeutic implications and demonstrate significant prognostic determination. The World Health Classification recommends that the term B-lymphoblastic leukemia/lymphoma not otherwise specified (NOS) be applied for those cases cytogenetially and/or molecularly investigated and that were shown not to carry any of the currently recognized cytogenetic and molecular abnormalities. Those cases not submitted to molecular analysis should be followed by the "no further classified (NFC)" statement. The following B-lymphoblastic leukemia/lymphoma subtypes are currently recognized: those with high hyperdiploidy, with hypodiploidy, with iAMP21, with *BCR::ABL1* fusion, with *BCR::ABL1*-like features, with *KMT2A* rearrangement, with *ETV6::RUNX1* fusion, with *ETV6::RUNX1*-like features, with *TCF3::PBX1* fusion, with *IGH::IL3* fusion, with *TCF3::HLF* fusion, and with other defined genetic alterations. Important genetic mutations that may occur in T-lymphoblastic leukemia/lymphoma affect *TAL1, TAL2, TLX1, TLX3, HOXA, LMO1/LMO2, LMO2/LYL1, NKX2-1*, among other genes.

Young children are the patients most commonly affected by B-lymphoblastic leukemia/lymphoma, representing the most common malignancy in childhood, whereas adolescents and young adults are the most commonly affected individuals when the neoplasm manifests as a lymphoma, of either B- or T-cell phenotype. It is more common in males, and in its solid presentation, the lymph nodes and the skin represent the most involved sites. In the oral and maxillofacial region, extranodal lymphoblastic leukemia/lymphoma is more commonly derived from the immature B-cell lineage, whereas the T-cell variant is very rare. The mandible and the surrounding mucosa are the most affected locations, presenting as a painful swelling often associated with teeth displacement or mobility, and patients are usually young adults.

J. R. Henao
Department of Hematopathology and Flow Cytometry, Ayudas Diagnósticas Sura Center, Cartagena, Colombia

P. A. Vargas
Oral and Maxillofacial Division, Piracicaba Dental School, State University of Campinas (UNICAMP), Piracicaba, Brazil
e-mail: pavargas@fop.unicamp.br

H. A. R. Pontes
Service of Oral Pathology, João de Barros Barreto University Hospital, Federal University of Pará, Belém, Brazil
e-mail: harp@ufpa.br

F. P. Fonseca (✉)
Department of Oral Surgery and Pathology, School of Dentistry, Universidade Federal de Minas Gerais, Belo Horizonte, Brazil

© The Author(s), under exclusive license to Springer Nature Switzerland AG 2025

F. P. Fonseca et al. (eds.), *Lymphoproliferative and Granulomatous Disorders of the Oral Cavity*,
https://doi.org/10.1007/978-3-031-98844-8_34

B-symptoms are common and patients usually complain of fever, weight loss and night sweats. The occurrence of numb chin syndrome in the absence of a solid tumor can also represent an oral manifestation of the disease. The presence of the lymphomatous tumor in the oral cavity demands from clinicians a systemic analysis, and in many cases, a leukemic disease is already present.

Indolent B-lymphoblastic proliferation (haematogone hyperplasia) and indolent T-lymphoblastic proliferation represent rare benign cellular expansions of TdT-positive immature cells known to occur in lymph nodes and tonsils. These reactive cells may also be associated with other lesions like Castleman disease and some types of neoplasms. It may be randomly found, or it may manifest as asymptomatic swellings. In the oral cavity, only rare reports are available, more often as gingival localized swelling.

Outcome of affected patients improved significantly during the last years, but relapsed and refractory disease remains a therapeutic challenge. Lymphoblastic leukemia/lymphoma is associated with a more favorable prognosis among pediatric patients than among adult individuals, with a long-term remission rate of >90% among children. The prognosis of patients affected by B-lymphoblastic leukemia/lymphoma is variable and depends on several prognostic factors, including age, elevated white blood cell count, slow blast clearance, the presence of central nervous system disease at diagnosis, and minimal residual disease positive at the end of induction or consolidation. The occurrence of specific translocations in each case also has important prognostic significance, especially for B-lymphoblastic leukemia/lymphoma, while genetic abnormalities do not seem to carry the same prognostic importance for patients affected by the T-cell variant. Consequently, different chemotherapeutic schemes are used to treat patients.

The occurrence of late side effects of oncological treatment in childhood includes several systemic disturbances like neurocognitive, musculoskeletal, and endocrine alterations, among others. Moreover, the occurrence of irreversible alterations in tooth development, which includes microdontia, hypodontia, abnormal root development, taurodontism, and enamel hypoplasia has also been well demonstrated in approximately 39%–51% of the young patients treated for lymphoblastic leukemia/lymphoma, and the severity of these alterations will depend on different determinant factors like the stage of odontogenesis, age when receiving chemotherapy and type and intensity of oncological treatment employed (Fig. 34.1).

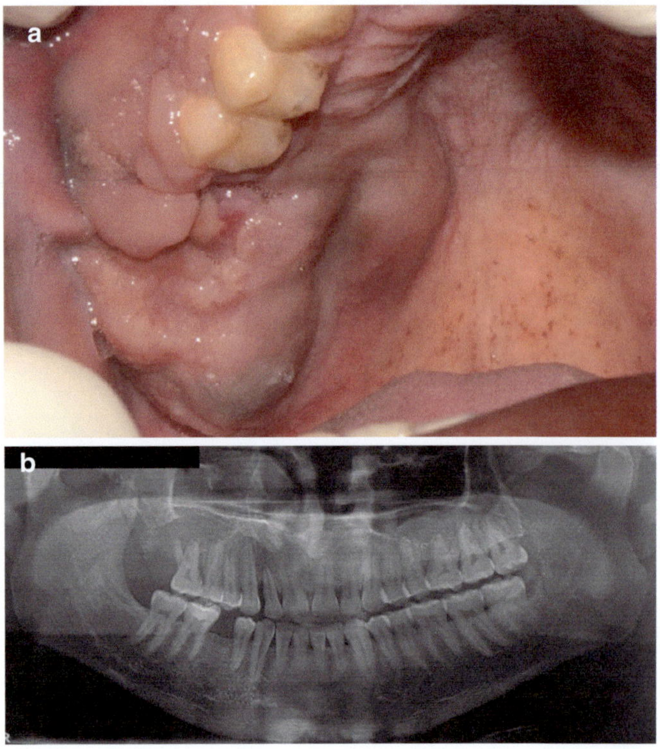

Fig. 34.1 Clinical features of lymphoblastic leukemia/lymphoma affecting the oral cavity. (**a**) Expansive swelling affecting the upper alveolar ridge causes expansion towards the vestibular aspect and also in the hard palate. (**b**) In the panoramic radiograph an ill-defined radiolucent image is observed in the posterior region of the maxilla, right side, associated with the loss of alveolar bone around the first molar

34.2 Microscopic Findings

- Microscopic presentation of B and T-lymphoblastic leukemia/lymphoma is similar.
- There is a diffuse infiltration of small to moderate-sized immature cells.
- The presence of a single-file growth pattern is a frequent finding.
- Tumor cells have a propensity to invade the overlying epithelium (resembling Pautrier microabscess).
- The presence of tingible body macrophages leading to a starry sky pattern can be frequently found.
- Since the tumor cells are predominantly small to medium-sized with a very high proliferative rate, the diagnosis of Burkitt lymphoma should always be ruled out, representing an important differential diagnosis for lymphoblastic leukemia/lymphoma;
- The "puzzle-like" aspect of adjacent cells that seem to fit each other may also be found.
- The immature neoplastic cells have a uniform appearance.
- The cells present a blastoid aspect with scant cytoplasm, round to oval nuclei, finely dispersed chromatin and inconspicuous nucleoli.
- The blastoid appearance of the cells should be especially differentiated from other lymphomas with similar features like mantle cell lymphoma (blastoid variant), high-grade B-cell lymphoma and Burkitt lymphoma (Figs. 34.2, 34.3, 34.4, and 34.5).

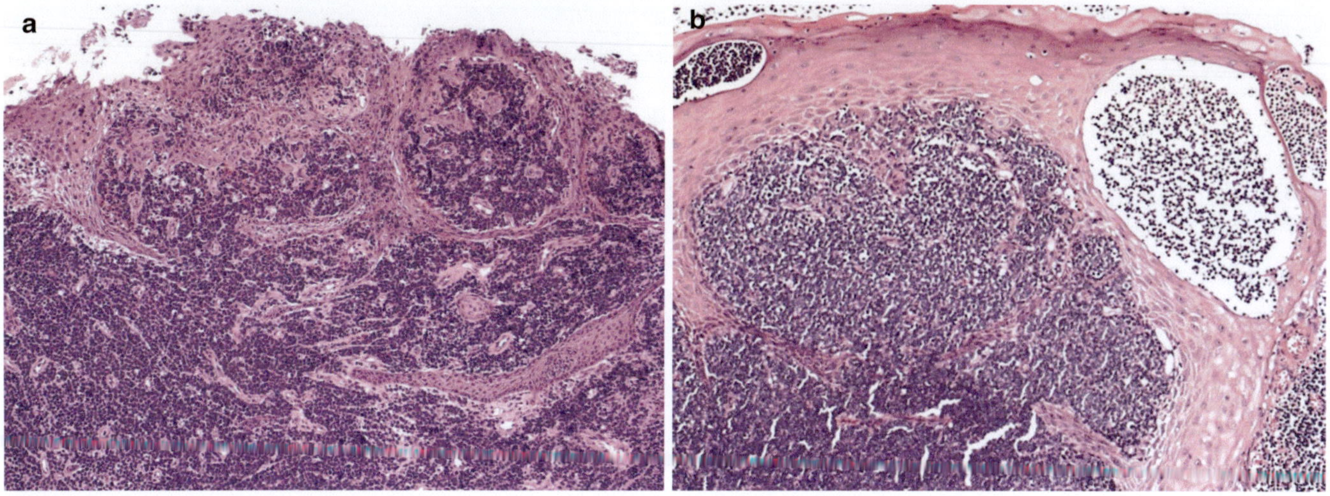

Fig. 34.2 Microscopic features of lymphoblastic leukemia/lymphoma affecting the oral cavity. (**a**) Tumor cells frequently proliferate towards the overlying epithelium. A reactive hyperplastic proliferation of the epithelium is usually observed (H&E; 50X). (**b**) In some regions, the presence of neoplastic cells around the squamous epithelium resembles Pautrier microabscess (H&E; 50X)

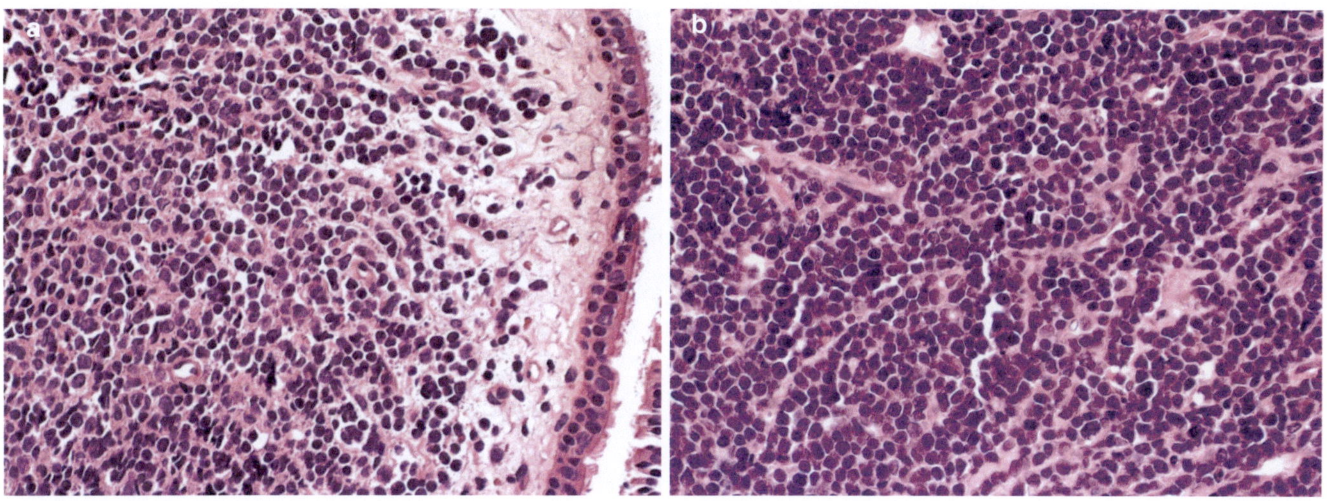

Fig. 34.3 Microscopic features of lymphoblastic leukemia/lymphoma affecting the maxilla. (**a**) Tumor cells infiltrated the maxillary bone and are located near the respiratory epithelium of the maxillary sinus (H&E; 200X). (**b**) The neoplastic cells are small to medium-sized, with hyperchromatic nuclei and scant cytoplasm. The cells exhibit a more monotonous aspect (H&E; 200X)

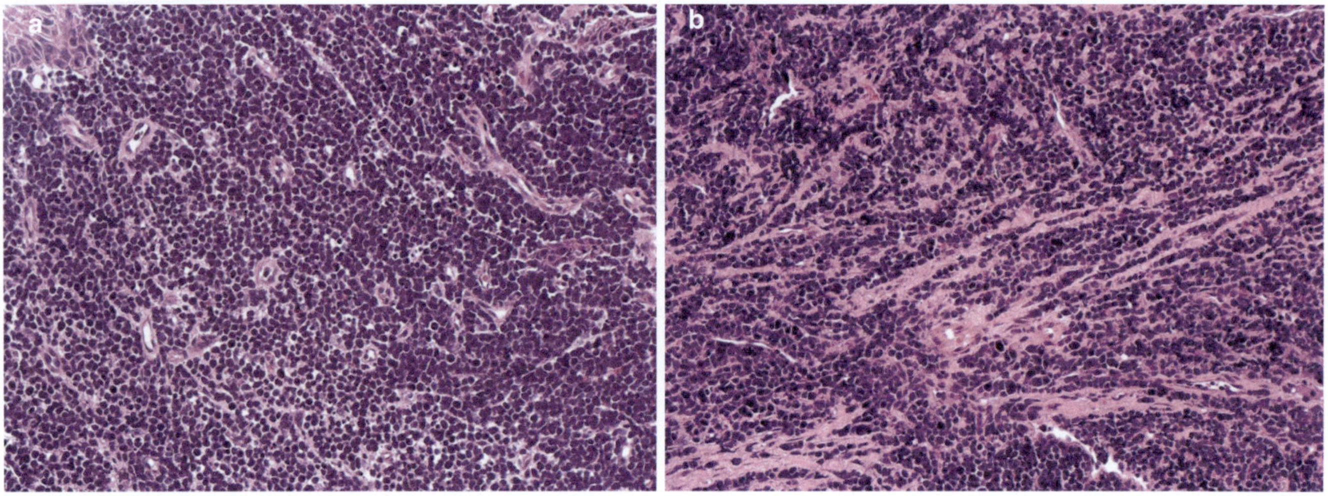

Fig. 34.4 Microscopic features of lymphoblastic leukemia/lymphoma affecting the oral cavity. (**a**) Neoplastic cells of lymphoblastic leukemia/lymphoma exhibit a diffuse growth pattern and reveal a monotonous aspect. The cells are predominantly small to medium-sized (H&E; 100X). (**b**) The "single line" growth pattern of some cells can be frequently observed in lymphoblastic leukemia/lymphoma and is exemplified in this image (H&E; 100X)

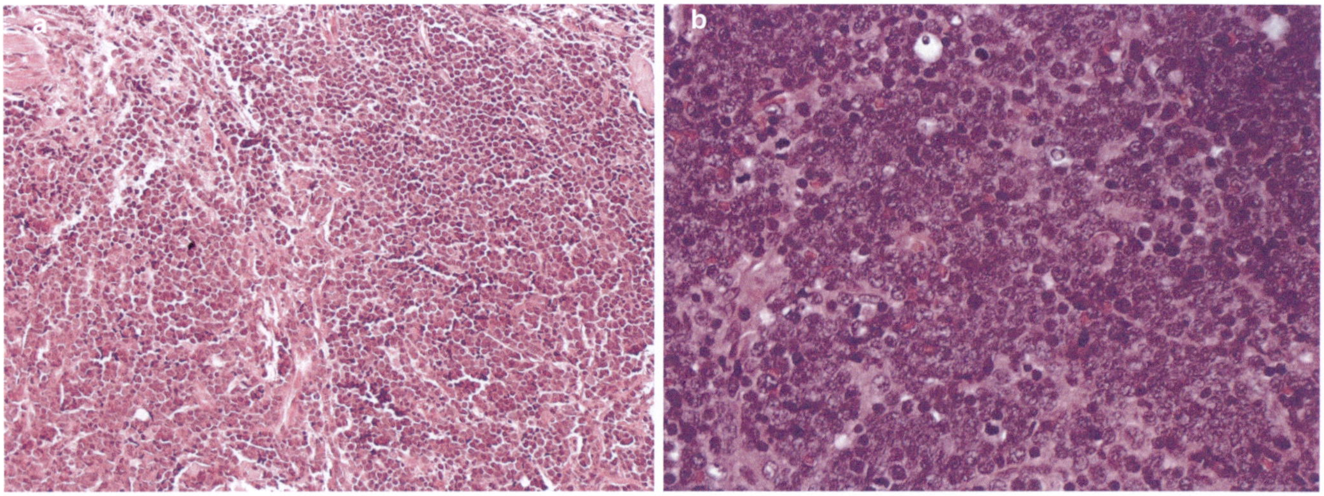

Fig. 34.5 Microscopic features of lymphoblastic leukemia/lymphoma affecting the oral cavity. (**a**) Diffuse proliferation of tumor cells with a scant fibrous stroma (H&E; 100X). (**b**) The neoplastic cells exhibit a blastoid aspect with multiple small pinpoint nucleoli. Mitotic figures are common, and the presence of tingible body macrophages is often observed (H&E; 200X)

34.3 Immunohistochemistry and/or Genetics

Immunohistochemistry should demonstrate the immature nature of the neoplastic cells. The nuclear expression of TdT has long been used to show the precursor origin of the cells; however, it is now recognized that TdT can also be expressed by high-grade B-cell lymphoma and diffuse large B-cell lymphoma, at the same time that TdT-negative lymphoblastic leukemia/lymphoma has also been reported. Therefore, the diagnosis of this neoplasm should not be based solely on the expression of this protein, but rather in a combination of markers that, taken together, indicate the immature nature of the disease, like low expression to absence of CD20 and the expression of other proteins indicative of cellular immaturity like CD10, CD99, CD34 and CD1a. To demonstrate the B-cell lineage differentiation, CD19, CD22, CD79a, and PAX5 are often the most used antibodies, although CD79a can also be aberrantly expressed in T-lymphoblastic lymphoma/leukemia, which usually express CD3, CD7, cCD3 and CD45RO. This neoplasm exhibits a high proliferative potential measured by

Ki67, achieving up to 90% positivity. The pan-lymphocyte marker LCA (or CD45) is usually dim or negative. The molecular basis of lymphoblastic lymphoma is complex, and different abnormalities have been described for B and T-lymphoblastic lymphoma. A more detailed discussion about the molecular basis of this lymphoma is beyond the scope of this book, and readers are encouraged to refer to more specialized textbooks to better understand the significance of each molecular abnormality (Table 34.1; Figs. 34.6, 34.7, 34.8, 34.9, and 34.10).

Table 34.1 Summary of the main immunohistochemical reactions used for lymphoblastic lymphoma/leukemia diagnosis

Antibody/probe	Most frequent results	Pattern	Objective
CD20	Dim or Negative	Membrane	To exclude a mature B-cell lymphoma
CD3	Positive	Membrane	To demonstrate the T-cell lineage of ALL
TdT	Positive	Nucleus	To demonstrate the immature nature of the tumor cells
CD79a	Positive	Membrane	To demonstrate the B-cell lineage of ALL
PAX5	Positive	Nucleus	To demonstrate the B-cell lineage of ALL
CD45RO	Positive	Membrane	To demonstrate the T-cell lineage of ALL
CD10	Positive	Membrane	To demonstrate the immature nature of the tumor cells
CD99	Positive	Membrane	To demonstrate the immature nature of the tumor cells
CD34	Positive	Membrane	To demonstrate the immature nature of the tumor cells
BCL2	Positive	Cytoplasm	Frequently positive in ALL cases
Ki67	High (~90%)	Nucleus	To demonstrate the proliferative index of the neoplasm

ALL lymphoblastic leukemia/lymphoma

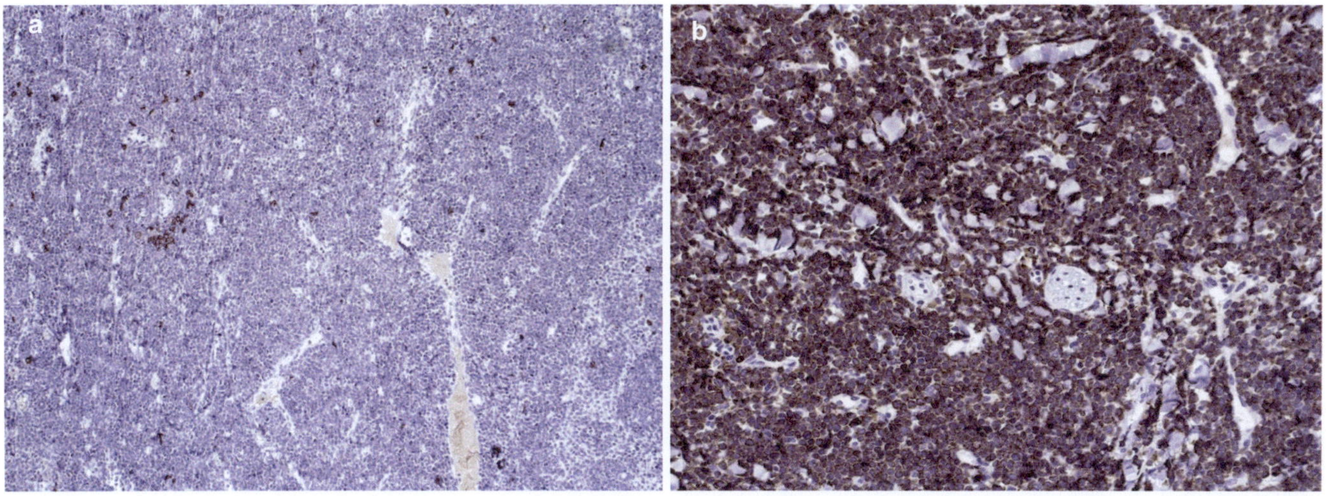

Fig. 34.6 Immunohistochemical features of lymphoblastic leukemia/lymphoma. (**a**) As a consequence of the immaturity of tumor cells, mature B-cell marker CD20 is absent (DAB; 50X). (**b**) The B-cell differentiation commitment is demonstrated by other markers like CD79a (DAB; 100X)

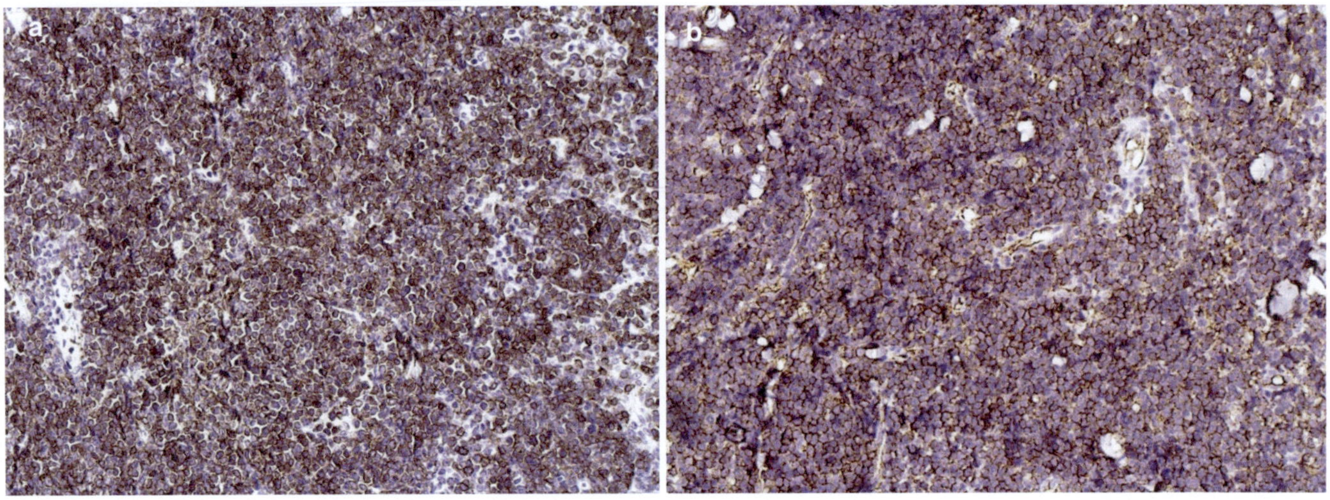

Fig. 34.7 Immunohistochemical features of lymphoblastic leukemia/lymphoma. (**a**) The expression of CD10 is evidence of the immature nature of tumor cells (DAB; 100X). (**b**) CD34 is also used to demonstrate this immaturity. Uncommon TdT negative cases are known, and the presence of other markers like CD10 and CD34 together with the loss of CD20 is useful to the diagnosis (DAB; 100X)

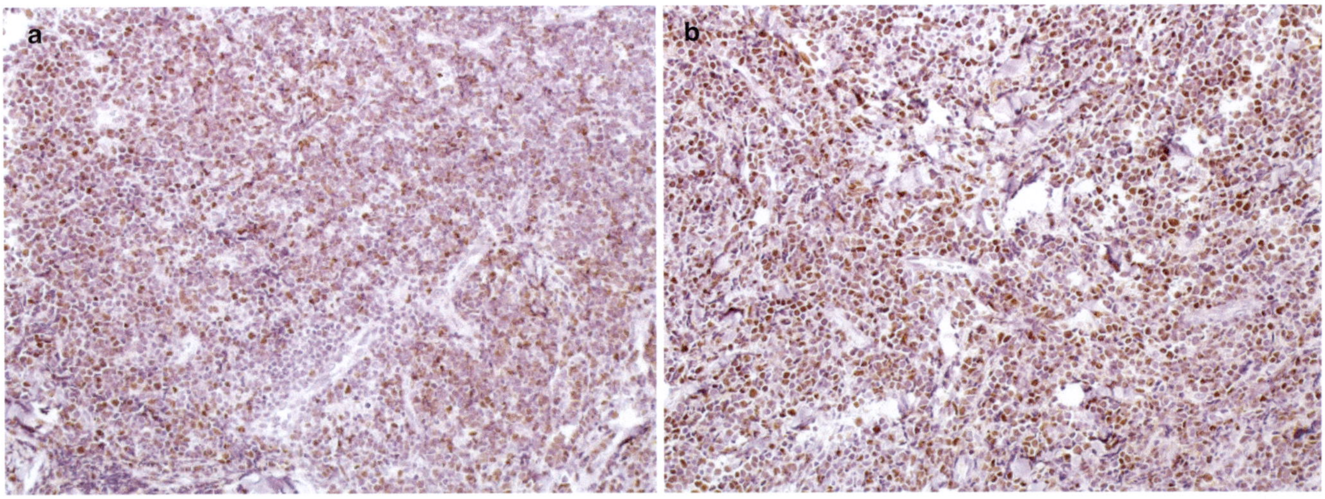

Fig. 34.8 Immunohistochemical features of lymphoblastic leukemia/lymphoma. (**a**) The expression of TdT is the most important marker to determine the diagnosis of the neoplasm (DAB; 100X). (**b**) TdT usually demonstrates a strong and diffuse nuclear expression pattern. It is accepted that rare cases of high-grade B-cell lymphoma and diffuse large B-cell lymphoma may focally express TdT, but the simultaneous expression of mature B-cell markers like CD20 helps to differentiate these cases from lymphoblastic leukemia/lymphoma (DAB; 100X)

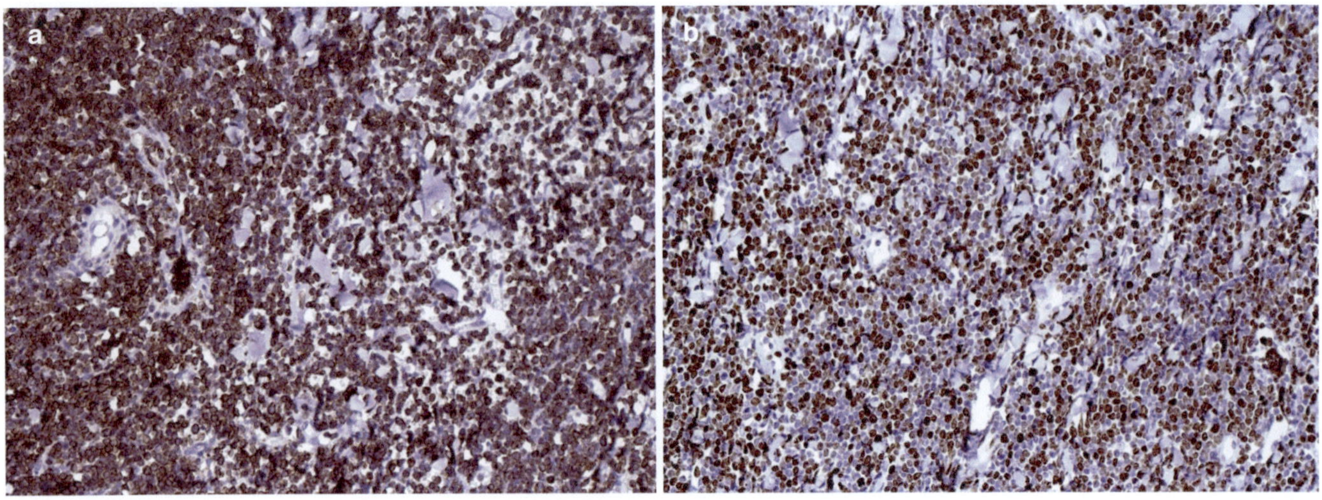

Fig. 34.9 Immunohistochemical features of lymphoblastic leukemia/lymphoma. (**a**) The tumor cells frequently express BCL2 protein (DAB; 100X). (**b**) The proliferative index of the neoplasm is usually very high with Ki67, achieving approximately 80%–90% in most cases (DAB; 100X)

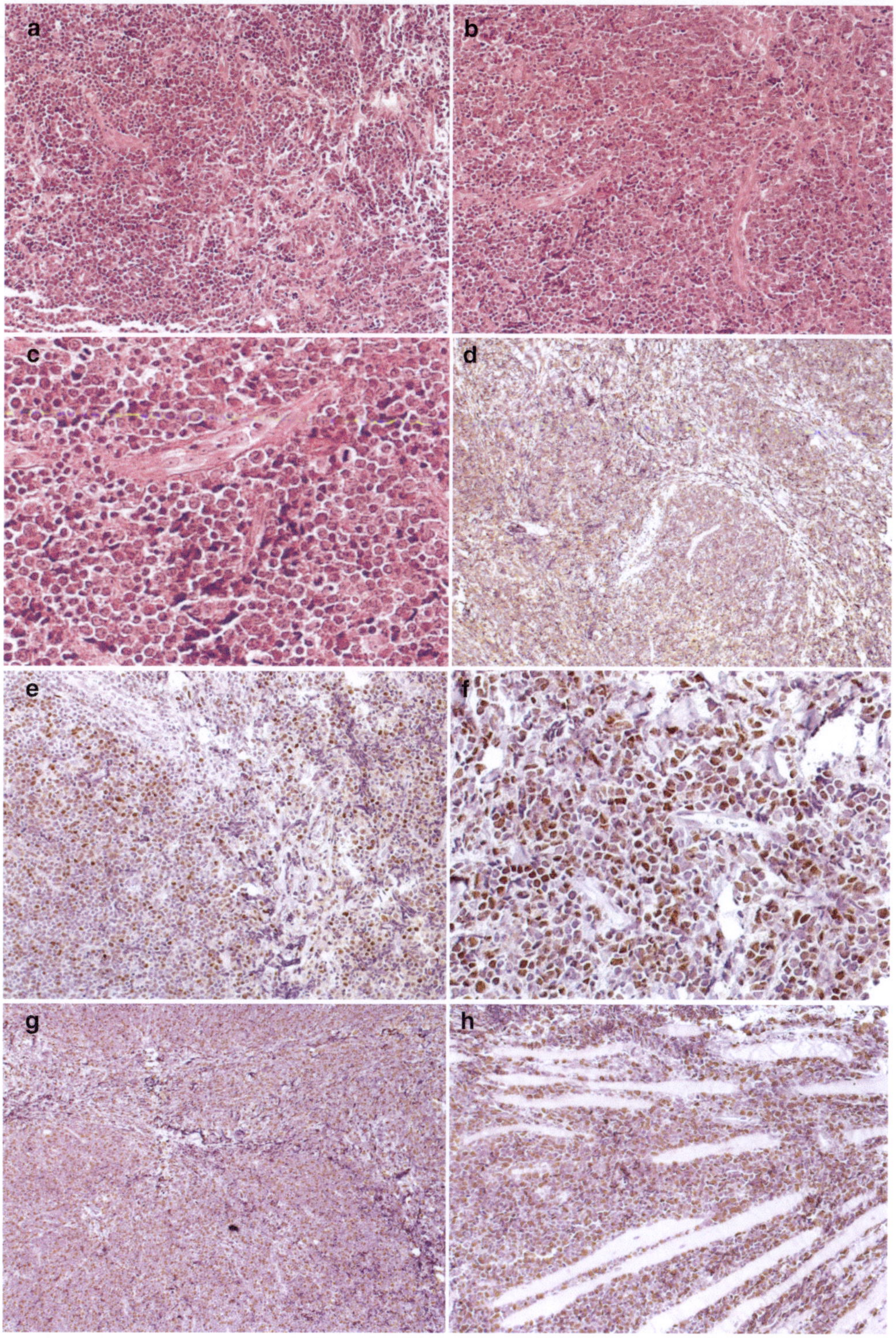

Fig. 34.10 Microscopic and immunohistochemical features of lymphoblastic leukemia/lymphoma affecting the oral cavity of a female patient. (**a**) Diffuse proliferation of tumor cells with a monotonous appearance (H&E; 100X). (**b**) Apoptotic debris is surrounded by neoplastic cells (H&E; 100X). (**c**) Tumor cells predominantly demonstrate a medium size morphology, with small nucleoli and scant cytoplasm (H&E; 200X). (**d**) Diffuse expression of CD10 (DAB; 100X). (**e**) Diffuse expression of TdT by neoplastic cells (DAB; 100X). (**f**) Strong nuclear expression of TdT in the nucleus of most of the neoplastic cells (DAB; 400X). (**g**) Lymphoblastic leukemia/lymphoma characteristically shows a high proliferative rate using Ki67 protein (DAB; 100X). (**h**) Note that most of the cells are positive for Ki67 (DAB; 200X)

Sources

1. Cavalcante ASR, Anbinder AL, Pontes EM, Carvalho YR. B-cell lymphoblastic lymphoma in the maxilla of a child: a rare case report. Int J Oral Maxillofac Surg. 2009;38:1326–30.
2. Bakathir AA, Al-Hamdani AS. Relapse of acute lymphoblastic leukemia in the jaw. Oral Surg Oral Med Oral Pathol Oral Radiol Endod. 2009;107:E14–6.
3. Lopes da Silva R, Fernandes T, Lopes A, Santos S, Mafra M, Rodrigues AS, et al. B lymphoblastic lymphoma presenting as a tumor of the nasopharynx in an adult patient. Head Neck Pathol. 2010;4(4):318–23. https://doi.org/10.1007/s12105-010-0206-2.
4. Dalirsani Z, Ghazi A. T-cell lymphoblastic lymphoma in the maxilla and mandible of a child: a rare case report. J Clin Diagn Res. 2015;9:ZD22–4.

5. Talreja KL, Barpande SR, Bhavthankar JD, Mandale MS. Precursor B-cell lymphoblastic lymphoma of oral cavity: a case report with its diagnostic workup. J Oral Maxillofac Pathol. 2016;20:133–6.
6. Lam PD, Kuribayashi A, Sakamoto J, Nakamura S, Harada H, Kurabayashi T. Imaging findings of childhood B-cell lymphoblastic lymphoma in the mental region: a case report. Dentomaxillofac Radiol. 2017;46:20160313.
7. Sánchez-Romero C, Pontes HAR, Pontes FSC, Rocha AC, Carlos R, Rendón JC, et al. Acute lymphoblastic leukemia/lymphoma of the oral and maxillofacial region. Oral Surg Oral Med Oral Pathol Oral Radiol. 2018;126:152–64.
8. Chen J, Feng J, Xiao H, Ma Q, Chen Z. Indolent T-lymphoblastic proliferation associated with Castleman disease and low grade follicular dendric cell sarcoma: report of a case and review of literature. Int J Clin Exp Pathol. 2019;12(4):1497–505.
9. Goutzanis L, Apostolidis J, Giatra C, Chrysomali E, Deskos D. A case of systemic precursor T-cell lymphoblastic lymphoma presenting with single tooth mobility. SAGE Open Med Case Rep. 2020;8:2050313X20927961. https://doi.org/10.1177/2050313X20927961.
10. Immonen E, Nikkilä A, Peltomäki T, Aine L, Lohi O. Late adverse effects of childhood acute lymphoblastic leukemia treatment on developing dentition. Pediatr Blood Cancer. 2021;68(9):e29200. https://doi.org/10.1002/pbc.29200.
11. Yuanyuan Z, Jianlan X, Yanlin Z, Xiaoge Z. Indolent T-lymphoblastic proliferation: a report of three cases. Virchows Arch. 2022;480(5):1121–6. https://doi.org/10.1007/s00428-021-03184-5.
12. Alghandour R, Sakr DH, Shaaban Y. Philadelphia-like acute lymphoblastic leukemia: the journey from molecular background to the role of bone marrow transplant-review article. Ann Hematol. 2023;102(6):1287–300. https://doi.org/10.1007/s00277-023-05241-2.
13. Boutin C, Huynh N, Rompré P, Laverdière C, Asselin MÈ. Prevalence, severity, and description of dental anomalies in children treated for acute lymphoblastic leukemia. Pediatr Dent. 2023;45(6):465–8.
14. Kara İ, Ramadan S, Şenkal E, Koçdor P. Pediatric T-cell lymphoblastic leukemia/lymphoma diagnosed at routine adenoidectomy specimen. Int J Surg Pathol. 2023;31(5):846–51. https://doi.org/10.1177/10668969221142044.
15. Hughes AD, Pölönen P, Teachey DT. Relapsed childhood T-cell acute lymphoblastic leukemia and lymphoblastic lymphoma. Haematologica. 2025. https://doi.org/10.3324/haematol.2024.285643.

Chronic Lymphocytic Leukemia/Small Lymphocytic Lymphoma

35

Guilherme Rossi Assis de Mendonça, Javier Rendon Henao, Vanessa Santiago-Pacheco, Ciro Dantas Soares, and Felipe Paiva Fonseca

35.1 General Overview and Clinical Presentation

Chronic lymphocytic leukemia is an indolent mature B-cell neoplasm characterized by the proliferation of small monomorphic cells, representing the most frequent type of leukemia in Western countries, accounting for approximately 25%–35% of all leukemia cases in the United States and Europe, with an estimated annual incidence ranging from 5 to 15/100,000 cases. Approximately 20,700 patients are expected to be diagnosed with chronic lymphocytic leukemia, and approximately 4440 deaths are expected to occur in 2024 in the USA. Small lymphocytic lymphoma is considered to be the same entity, comprised of neoplastic cells demonstrating the same morphology and immunophenotype, but in the presence of $<5 \times 10^9$/L circulating neoplastic B cells and a solid tissue involvement, representing approximately 7% of all non-Hodgkin lymphoma biopsies.

A possible inherited genetic contribution to chronic lymphocytic leukemia/small lymphocytic lymphoma onset is speculated, but its exact etiology still needs to be better understood. The exact cell of origin for this lymphoma remains debatable, although some molecular evidences point towards a memory-like B-cell origin. The molecular basis of chronic lymphocytic leukemia/small lymphocytic lymphoma is very heterogeneous and many different events have been demonstrated, including chromosomal aberrations involving the deletions in the long arm of chromosome 13 [del(13q)] and 11 [del(11q)], the short arm of 17 [del(17p)], and the gain of chromosome 12. Moreover, the genes that are more often mutated in this neoplasm include *NOTCH1* (10%–15%), *ATM* (10%–15%), *SF3B1* (10%), *TP53* (5%–10%), and *BIRC3* (5%), with the presence or absence of somatic hypermutation of IGHV. The genetic landscape of diffuse large B-cell lymphoma arising from a previous chronic lymphocytic leukemia/small lymphocytic lymphoma is highly heterogeneous and complex, and differs from the molecular features observed in de novo diffuse large B-cell lymphomas.

Despite the mature B-cell differentiation of this neoplasm, chronic lymphocytic leukemia/small lymphocytic lymphoma is well known for the aberrant expression of the T-cell marker CD5, in addition to the expression of CD23 and CD200 proteins. Therefore, the use of these markers is very important for the diagnosis of this entity. The majority of the affected patients are older adults aged 50–70 years, with a slight predominance of females. Although some patients remain asymptomatic during the course of the disease, in the presence of a leukemic presentation, clinical manifestations are related to bone marrow involvement, being associated with the suppression of production of blood cell types commonly leading to anemia, higher infection susceptibility, spontaneous bleeding, fatigue, autoimmune hemolytic anemia, hepatomegaly, splenomegaly, or lymphadenopathy. Following the bone marrow and the peripheral blood, the liver, spleen, and lymph nodes are the most commonly affected sites.

The involvement of the oral cavity by this disorder may rarely represent the first manifestation of the disease and clinically present as an asymptomatic expansive swelling, but in most cases the oral cavity involvement represents the manifestation of an already disseminated chronic

G. R. A. de Mendonça
Department of Pathology, School of Medical Sciences, University of Campinas, Campinas, Brazil

J. R. Henao
Department of Hematopathology and Flow Cytometry, Ayudas Diagnósticas Sura Center, Cartagena, Colombia

V. Santiago-Pacheco
Department of Pathology, Hematopathology, University of Antioquia, Medellin, Colombia
e-mail: vanessa.santiago@udea.edu.co

C. D. Soares
Laboratório de Patologia Getúlio Sales, Natal, Brazil

F. P. Fonseca (✉)
Department of Oral Surgery and Pathology, School of Dentistry, Universidade Federal de Minas Gerais, Belo Horizonte, Brazil

© The Author(s), under exclusive license to Springer Nature Switzerland AG 2025
F. P. Fonseca et al. (eds.), *Lymphoproliferative and Granulomatous Disorders of the Oral Cavity*,
https://doi.org/10.1007/978-3-031-98844-8_35

lymphocytic leukemia/small lymphocytic lymphoma. Some epidemiological studies describing the distribution of lymphoma subtypes in the oral cavity claim that chronic lymphocytic leukemia/small lymphocytic lymphoma accounts for approximately 5% of all cases in this location. Older adults are also the most affected population, and most of the patients have a previous medical history positive for chronic lymphocytic leukemia/small lymphocytic lymphoma diagnosed some years before. The tonsils, palate, and gingival tissue are the most commonly affected locations, but cases affecting the lips, tongue, floor of the mouth and salivary glands have already been described. Rare cases have been described as multiple erythematous papules in the palate. Petechial hemorrhages of the posterior hard and soft palate are also common findings. Moreover, gingival diffuse swelling and bleeding are frequent manifestations of the leukemic infiltration of the gums, and the presence of ulcerated tumors and pain may also occur and should raise suspicion for high-grade transformation.

Richter transformation represents the occurrence of high-grade transformation in a previous chronic lymphocytic leukemia/small lymphocytic lymphoma, more often a diffuse large B-cell lymphoma. The prevalence of Richter transformation in patients with chronic lymphocytic leukemia/small lymphocytic lymphoma varies from as low as 0.7%, increasing with time to up to 16.2% after 10 years of follow-up. This high-grade transformation is more frequently reported among males who are more than 60 years old, and different clinical, laboratorial and molecular features are believed to increase the risk for transformation. In the oral cavity, although very rare, some cases have been reported, usually describing painful swellings that may be ulcerated and affect different oral locations.

Chronic lymphocytic leukemia/small lymphocytic lymphoma remains an incurable disease, despite the development of novel targeted therapies like Bruton tyrosine kinase (BTK) inhibitors, BCL2 inhibitors, and CD20 monoclonal antibodies, which have improved the therapeutic management of patients. The clinical behavior and patients' prognosis are variable depending on many clinical, morphological, laboratorial and molecular determinants. In the presence of Richter transformation, the median survival of patients is approximately 2 years, but many prognostic determinants also impact the survival rate of these individuals.

35.2 Microscopic Findings

- Diffuse infiltration of small and monomorphous neoplastic cells.
- Tumor cells are predominantly small, round and monomorphous, with hyperchromatic nucleus and scant cytoplasm.
- The prolymphocytes are medium-sized neoplastic cells with visible nucleoli.
- The paraimmunoblasts are larger cells, with a round-to-oval nucleus, dispersed chromatin, centrally located nucleolus and scant pale cytoplasm;
- The presence of pale-staining regions in the neoplasm is termed proliferation centers.
- Proliferation centers contain larger cells, predominantly paraimmunoblasts, but also some prolymphocytes.
- Mitosis is uncommon.
- Areas of Richter transformation for diffuse large B-cell lymphoma exhibit larger, more pleomorphic neoplastic cells with one or more prominent nucleoli and dispersed chromatin. Atypical mitotic figures are common and areas of necrosis can be found (Figs. 35.1, 35.2, and 35.3).

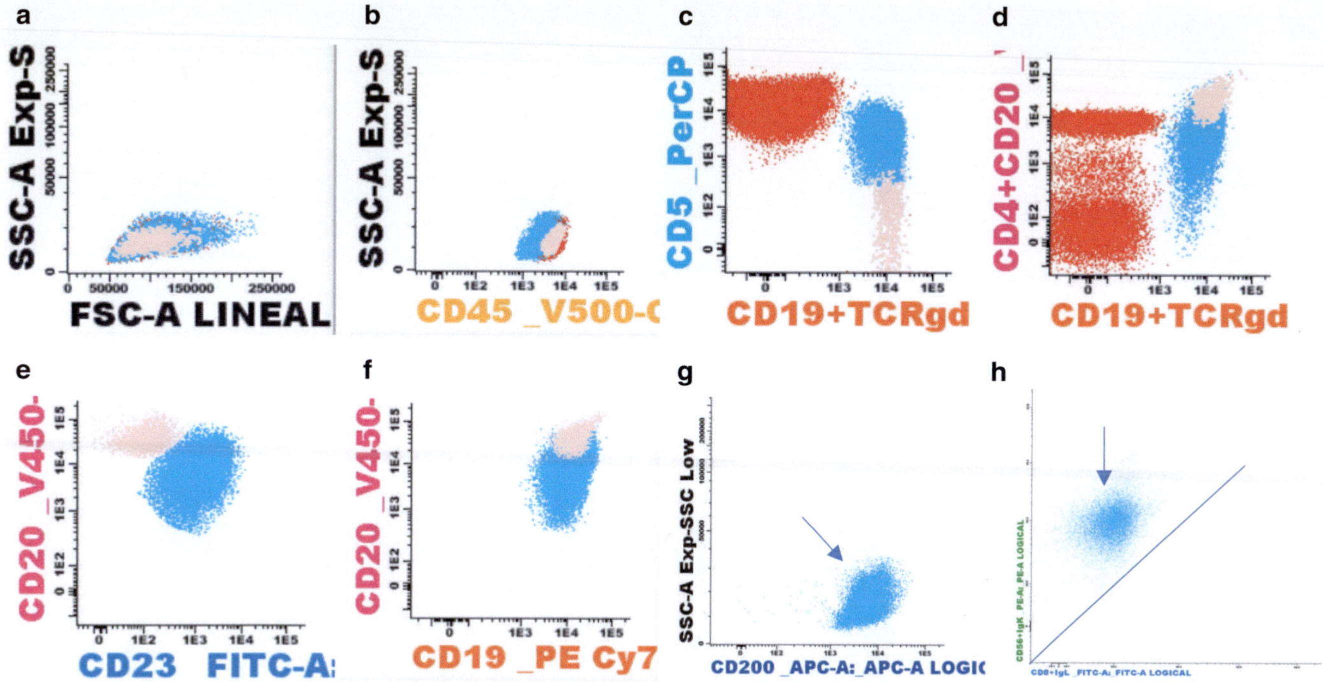

Fig. 35.1 Immunophenotype of chronic lymphocytic leukemia/small lymphocytic lymphoma is more often determined using flow cytometry of peripheral body sample approach, given the leukemic presentation of the disease that is more frequent than its lymphomatous presentation. (**a**) Normal B cells (pink dots), T cells (red dots) and neoplastic B cells (blue dots), (**b**) expressing CD45, (**c**) CD5 (aberrant expression) and CD19, and (**d**) CD20 dim positive. (**e**) The neoplastic cells (blue dots) are CD23 positive, (**f**) CD19 and CD20 positive, (**g**) and CD200 positive. (**h**) Observe a Kappa light chain restriction (dim expression)

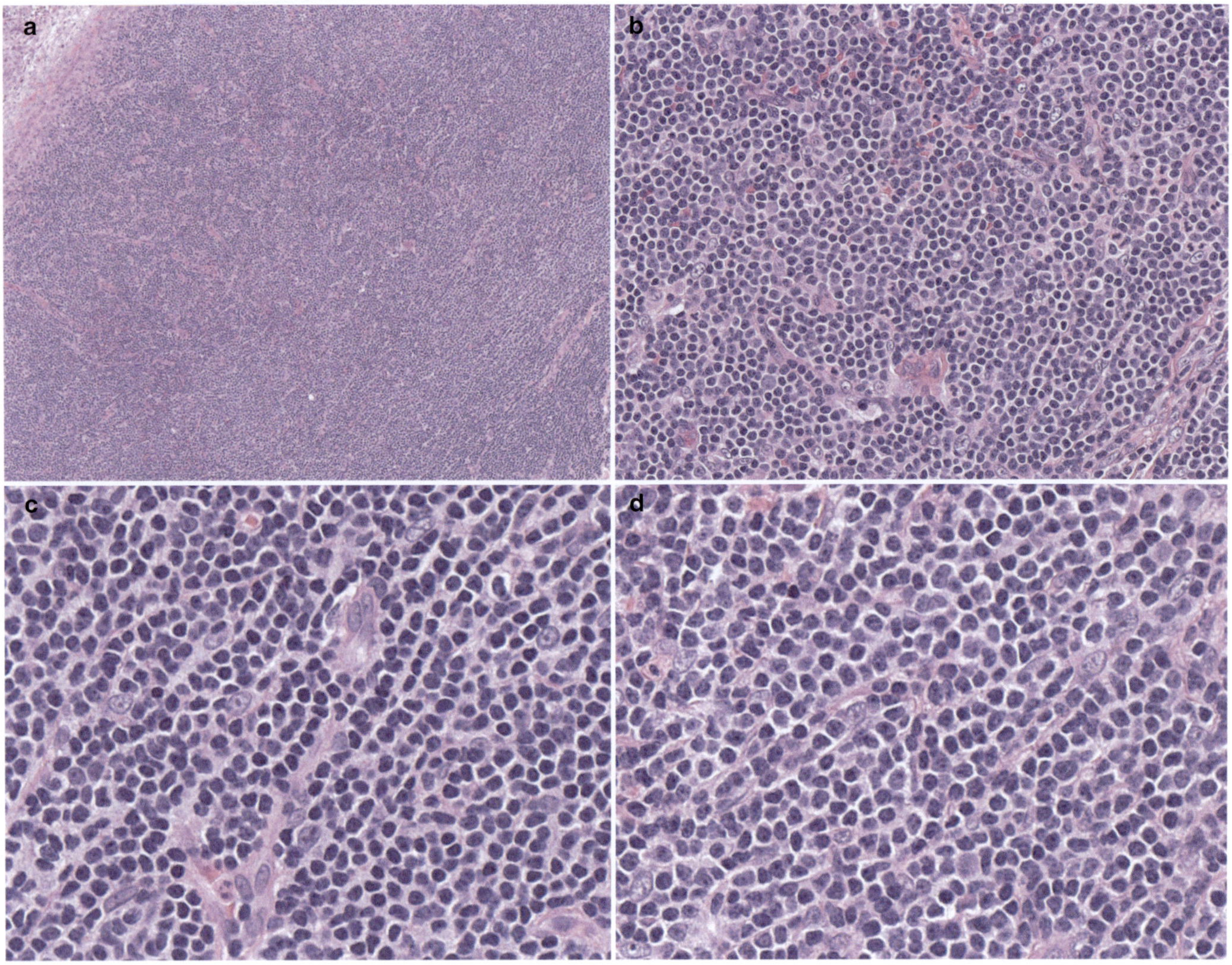

Fig. 35.2 Microscopic features of chronic lymphocytic leukemia/small lymphocytic lymphoma affecting the buccal mucosa of a 54-year-old male patient. (**a**) Diffuse proliferation of small neoplastic cells (H&E; 25X). (**b**) Note the monotonous histologic appearance of tumor cells, predominantly exhibiting a round nuclear contour and scant cytoplasm (H&E; 100X). (**c**) Under high magnification, observe the presence of small neoplastic cells (H&E; 200X). (**d**) Tumor cells exhibit a monotonous microscopic appearance (H&E; 200X)

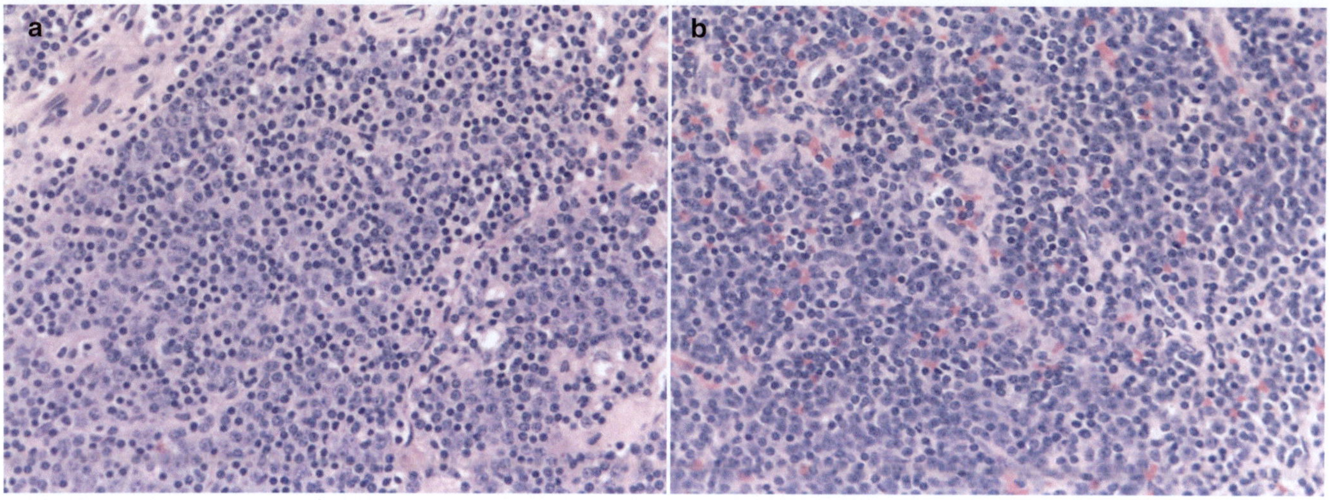

Fig. 35.3 Microscopic features of chronic lymphocytic leukemia/small lymphocytic lymphoma. (**a**) Diffuse proliferation of round, small neoplastic cells that represent the majority of the cell types present in this image. The prolymphocytes represent another population of neoplastic cells characterized by a medium size, containing only visible nucleoli. The last population is represented by the paraimmunoblasts that are larger cells with a more prominent centrally located nucleolus. Aggregates of paraimmunoblasts lead to the formation of proliferation centers (H&E; 100X). (**b**) Observe in this image all three cellular populations that typically characterize chronic lymphocytic leukemia/small lymphocytic lymphoma (H&E; 100X)

Table 35.1 Summary of the main immunohistochemical reactions used for chronic lymphocytic leukemia/small lymphocytic lymphoma diagnosis

Antibody	Most frequent results	Pattern	Objective
CD20	Positive	Membrane	To demonstrate the mature B-cell differentiation
PAX5	Positive	Nucleus	To demonstrate the mature B-cell differentiation
CD79a	Positive	Membrane	To demonstrate the mature B-cell differentiation
CD3	Negative	Membrane	To exclude a T-cell lineage lymphoma
CD5	Positive	Membrane	Characteristically positive in CLL/SLL cases
CD23	Positive	Membrane	Characteristically positive in CLL/SLL cases
CD200	Positive	Membrane	Characteristically positive in CLL/SLL cases
LEF1	Positive	Nucleus	Characteristically positive in CLL/SLL cases
MUM1	Positive	Nucleus	Positive in the proliferation centers
BCL2	Positive	Cytoplasm	Characteristically positive in CLL/SLL cases
TdT	Negative	Nucleus	To exclude a lymphoblastic lymphoma
CD10	Negative	Membrane	To exclude a follicular lymphoma
BCL6	Negative	Nucleus	To exclude a follicular lymphoma
Cyclin D1	Negative	Nucleus	To exclude a mantle cell lymphoma
SOX11	Negative	Nucleus	To exclude a mantle cell lymphoma
Ki67	Low (~10%), but higher in proliferative centers and in Richter transformation	Nucleus	To demonstrate the proliferative index of the neoplasm

CLL/SLL chronic lymphocytic leukemia/small lymphocytic lymphoma

35.3 Immunohistochemistry and/or Genetics

Immunohistochemistry is very useful for the diagnosis of chronic lymphocytic leukemia/small lymphocytic lymphoma. Tumor cells are strongly positive for mature B-cell markers like CD20, CD79a and PAX5, but they also aberrantly express the T-cell marker CD5, similar to mantle cell lymphoma. However, chronic lymphocytic leukemia/small lymphocytic lymphoma also expresses CD23, CD200 and lacks Cyclin D1 and SOX11 expression. Chronic lymphocytic leukemia/Small lymphocytic lymphoma typically lacks germinal center markers like CD10 and Bcl6. LEF1 is present in most cases and represents a useful diagnostic marker to differentiate chronic lymphocytic leukemia/small lymphocytic lymphoma from other small B-cell lymphomas. Proliferative index is low, but Ki67 expression is usually higher in proliferative centers, and it is much higher in cases of Richter transformation. The molecular basis of chronic lymphocytic leukemia/small lymphocytic lymphoma is very heterogeneous and complex, with multiple genetic abnormalities occurring in this neoplasm (Table 35.1; Fig. 35.4).

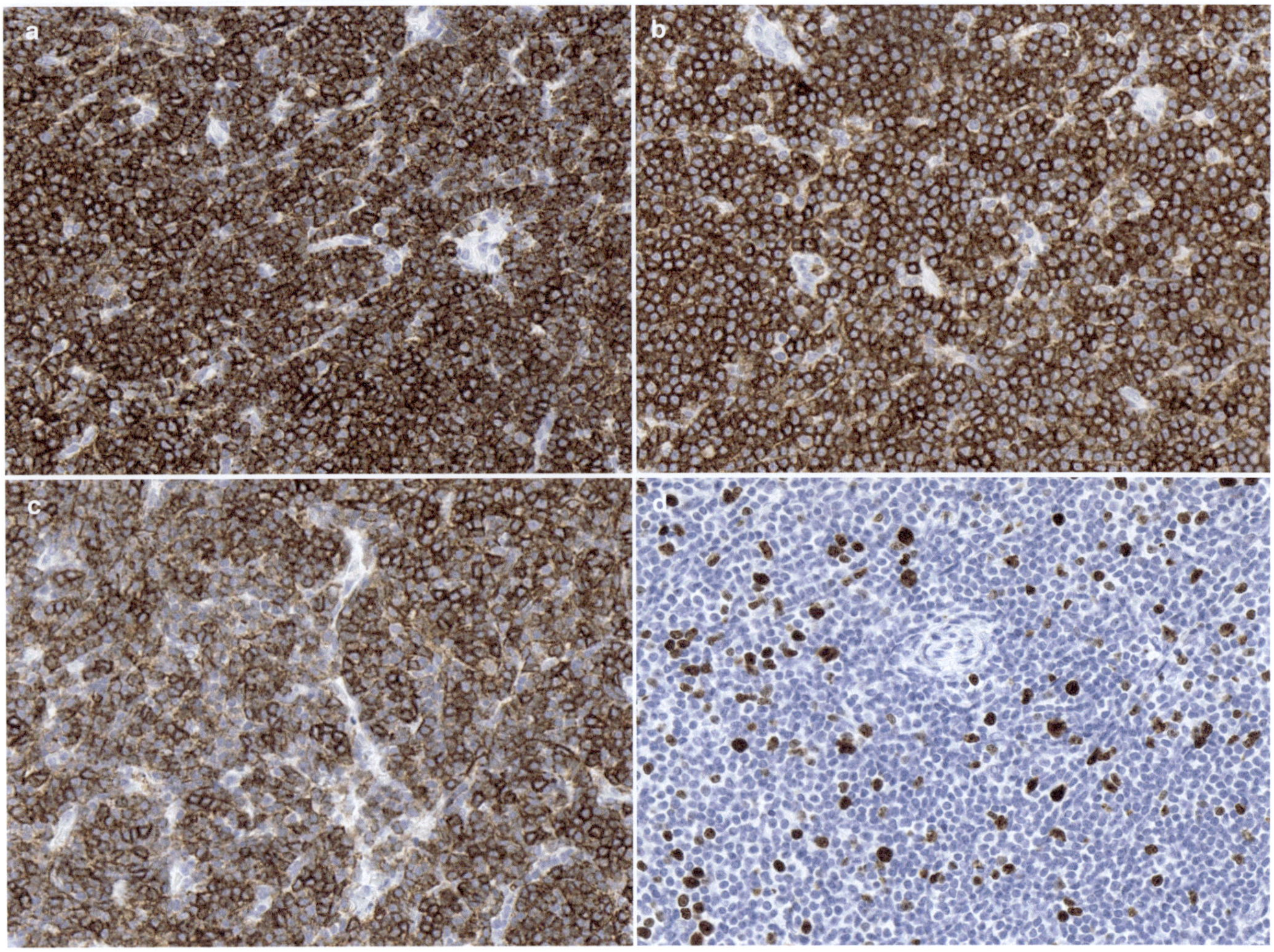

Fig. 35.4 Immunohistochemical features of chronic lymphocytic leukemia/small lymphocytic lymphoma. (**a**) Tumor cells are diffusely and strongly positive for CD20 protein, denoting its B-cell origin (DAB; 200X). (**b**) The neoplastic cells typically demonstrate the aberrant expression of CD5 protein (DAB; 200X). (**c**) Another hallmark of this neoplasm is the expression of CD23 (DAB; 200X). (**d**) Proliferative index is often low as demonstrated in this image using Ki67 expression (H&E; 200X)

Sources

1. Porter SR, Matthews RW, Scully C. Chronic lymphocytic leukaemia with gingival and palatal deposits. J Clin Periodontol. 1994;21(8):559–61. https://doi.org/10.1111/j.1600-051x.1994.tb01173.x.
2. Vibhute P, Carneiro E, Genden E, Som PM. Palatal enlargement in chronic lymphocytic leukemia. AJNR Am J Neuroradiol. 2006;27(8):1649–50.
3. Alessandrini M, Micarelli A, Mugnaini F, De Padova A, Pavone I, Bruno E. Unusual case of oral chronic lymphocytic leukemia presenting as recurrent epistaxis and asymptomatic intraoral swelling. Rev Stomatol Chir Maxillofac. 2012;113(6):455–7. https://doi.org/10.1016/j.stomax.2012.10.001.
4. Peters SM, Han C, Yoon AJ, Philipone EM. Chronic lymphocytic leukemia in association with a ranula: a report and review of the literature. Oral Surg Oral Med Oral Pathol Oral Radiol. 2017;123(5):e160–3. https://doi.org/10.1016/j.oooo.2016.11.006.
5. Theofilou VI, Katsoulas N, Tosios KI, Sklavounou A, Nikitakis NG. Richter transformation in the oral and maxillofacial area: report of 2 cases and literature review. Oral Surg Oral Med Oral Pathol Oral Radiol. 2021;131(1):e14–20. https://doi.org/10.1016/j.oooo.2020.02.016.
6. Wagner VP, Rodrigues-Fernandes CI, Carvalho MVR, Dos Santos JN, Barra MB, Hunter KD, et al. Mantle cell lymphoma, malt lymphoma, small lymphocytic lymphoma, and follicular lymphoma of the oral cavity: an update. J Oral Pathol Med. 2021;50(6):622–30. https://doi.org/10.1111/jop.13214.
7. Barros P, Islam MN, Fitzpatrick SG, Cohen DM, Bhattacharyya I, Alramadhan SA. Essentials of oral manifestations of leukemia for the dental practitioner. Gen Dent. 2022;70(2):33–6.
8. Yeh JE, Lorenzo ME, Larocca C, Fisher DC, Foreman RK. Small lymphocytic lymphoma presenting as chronic diffuse lip swelling. Dermatol Online J. 2022;28(5). https://doi.org/10.5070/D328559249.
9. Ottinger AM, Singh R, Chen D, Parham K. Unilateral tonsillar enlargement as initial presentation of bilateral chronic lymphocytic leukemia/small lymphocytic lymphoma.

Ear Nose Throat J. 2023:1455613231214634. https://doi.org/10.1177/01455613231214634.
10. Deodato M, Frustaci AM, Zappaterra A, Rapella A, Gambacorti-Passerini C, Cairoli R, et al. Advances in the understanding of molecular genetics and therapy of Richter transformation in chronic lymphocytic leukemia. Leuk Lymphoma. 2024;65(14):2096–107. https://doi.org/10.1080/10428194.2024.2398660.
11. Jain N, Wierda WG, O'Brien S. Chronic lymphocytic leukaemia. Lancet. 2024;404(10453):694–706. https://doi.org/10.1016/S0140-6736(24)00595-6.
12. Sobczyńska-Konefał A, Jasek M, Karabon L, Jaskuła E. Insights into genetic aberrations and signalling pathway interactions in chronic lymphocytic leukemia: from pathogenesis to treatment strategies. Biomark Res. 2024;12(1):162. https://doi.org/10.1186/s40364-024-00710-w.
13. Tausch E, López C, Stilgenbauer S, Siebert R. Genetic alterations in chronic lymphocytic leukemia and plasma cell neoplasms – a practical guide to WHO HAEM5. Med Genet. 2024;36(1):47–57. https://doi.org/10.1515/medgen-2024-2006.
14. Lodolo M, Jordan R, Villa A. An unusual oral manifestation of chronic lymphocytic leukemia: a case report and review of the literature. J Am Dent Assoc. 2025;156(1):68–73.e1. https://doi.org/10.1016/j.adaj.2024.10.009.
15. McKeague S, Tam C. Prognostic factors in chronic lymphocytic leukaemia – the old, the new and the future. Leuk Lymphoma. 2025:1–11. https://doi.org/10.1080/10428194.2024.2449214.

Part VI

Mature B Cell Lymphomas and Multiple Myeloma

Marginal Zone Lymphoma of the Mucosa-Associated Lymphoid Tissue (Malt Lymphoma)

36

Manoela Domingues Martins, Javier Rendon Henao, and Felipe Paiva Fonseca

36.1 General Overview and Clinical Presentation

Marginal zone lymphoma is a group of low-grade B-cell neoplasms that account for approximately 7%–8% of all non-Hodgkin lymphomas, representing the third most common subtype following diffuse large B-cell lymphoma and follicular lymphoma. Based on data from the United States Surveillance, Epidemiology, and End Results Program (US SEER), the age-standardized incidence rate for marginal zone lymphoma is 19.6 cases per 1,000,000 person-years, with an increasing trend of +1.0% in the USA. Marginal zone lymphomas are believed to originate from post-germinal center cells that can usually be found in the peripheral (marginal) zone of the germinal centers and according to the 5th edition of the World Health Organization classification of hematolymphoid tumors, five different marginal zone lymphomas are recognized: the well-known splenic marginal zone lymphoma, nodal marginal zone lymphoma and extranodal marginal zone lymphoma of the mucosa-associated lymphoid tissue (MALT lymphoma), as well as the newly recognized pediatric nodal marginal zone lymphoma and primary cutaneous marginal zone lymphoma. These entities have a similar morphology and immunophenotype, but different clinical manifestations and different etiopathogenesis, with autoimmune diseases like Sjögren disease, systemic lupus erythematosus and Hashimoto's thyroiditis representing important risk factors for the onset of some subtypes. Moreover, the strong association of some marginal zone lymphomas with specific microorganisms is also well established, which makes this neoplasm an important model of antigen-driven malignancy that carries significant implications for its prevention. The overall prognosis of patients affected by marginal zone lymphoma is usually good, with a 5-year survival rate achieving 89.8% in the USA.

Considering the scope of this textbook dedicated to oral and maxillofacial lymphoproliferative disorders, a more detailed discussion will be done for extranodal marginal zone lymphomas of the mucosa-associated lymphoid tissue, and readers are encouraged to consult specialized references to obtain additional data on the other types of this complex group of lymphomas. However, when dealing with intraoral marginal zone lymphomas, pathologists should always take into account the systemic condition of the patient and rule out the possibility of an oral manifestation of an otherwise primary nodal, splenic or cutaneous disorder.

MALT lymphoma represents the most common subtype of marginal zone lymphomas, accounting for approximately 61% of all cases diagnosed, while 9% represent the splenic subtype and 30% the nodal variant. This extranodal subtype is more commonly diagnosed among adults in their fifth to sixth decades of life, with a female predominance. It may affect many different extranodal locations, especially those where the presence of lymphocytes is acquired in response to chronic infectious conditions or autoimmune processes, like the stomach, ocular adnexa, lung, and salivary glands. The pathogenesis of this neoplasm is associated with chronic inflammatory stimulation due to exposure to different etiologic factors and autoimmune disorders depending on the primary site of the disease. For instance, in the gastrointestinal tract MALT lymphoma is strongly associated with *Helicobacter pylori* infection, while in the ocular adnexa it is associated with *Chlamydophila psittaci* and the primary cutaneous type may be associated with *Borrelia burgdorferi*. In the salivary glands, MALT lymphoma is associated with Sjögren disease in approximately 34% of the cases, which contributes to making this neoplasm the most commonly

M. D. Martins (✉)
Department of Oral Pathology, School of Dentistry, Federal University of Rio Grande do Sul, Porto Alegre, Brazil

J. R. Henao
Department of Hematopathology and Flow Cytometry, Ayudas Diagnósticas Sura Center, Cartagena, Colombia

F. P. Fonseca
Department of Oral Surgery and Pathology, School of Dentistry, Universidade Federal de Minas Gerais, Belo Horizonte, Brazil

© The Author(s), under exclusive license to Springer Nature Switzerland AG 2025
F. P. Fonseca et al. (eds.), *Lymphoproliferative and Granulomatous Disorders of the Oral Cavity*, https://doi.org/10.1007/978-3-031-98844-8_36

found in major salivary glands, while thyroid MALT lymphoma is commonly associated with Hashimoto's thyroiditis. Systemic lupus erythematosus, arthritis rheumatoid and other rheumatological disturbances have also been associated with an increased risk of MALT lymphoma development.

The molecular landscape of MALT lymphoma is being better appreciated and several recurrent genetic abnormalities seem to be important for the pathogenesis of the disease. Different chromosomal translocations have already been described including t(11;18)(q21;q21)/*BIRC3::MALT1*, t(1;14)(p22;q32)/*IGH::BCL10*, t(14;18)(q32;q21)/*IGH::MALT1*, and t(3;14)(p14;q32)/*IGH::FOXP1*, whose frequency varies depending on the anatomical site affected. In addition, a number of genes are known to be somatically mutated in MALT lymphomas like *TNFAIP3*, *GPR34*, *TET2*, *CD274(PD-L1)*, *TBL1XR1* and *TNFRSF14*, while the NF-kB molecular pathway is also frequently activated in these tumors.

In the head and neck, MALT lymphomas are more common in the major salivary glands, most often in the parotid glands (74.6% of all salivary gland MALT lymphomas), where they manifest as painless swellings. In the oral cavity, adult females in their seventh decade of life, but with a wide age range, are the most affected group of patients. The palate and the lips are the most affected locations, followed by the cheek mucosa. Most of the cases present as a solitary, asymptomatic and non-ulcerated nodule. Superficial telangiectasia is a common finding. The occurrence of B-symptoms is frequently absent, and most cases are diagnosed at initial Ann Arbor stages (I/II). In the oral cavity, the differential diagnosis between a MALT lymphoma and reactive lymphoid processes like lymphoepithelial sialadenitis (LESA), which exhibits very similar clinical and microscopic manifestations, is always very difficult, and in some cases the correct diagnosis can only be reliably established with genetic investigation.

The treatment approach is based on various factors related to the patient: age, comorbidities, performance status, and life expectancy; to the disease: tumor size, location, related symptoms, and ocular impairment; and to the treatment itself: objective, side effects, sequelae, and drug availability. In consideration of these variables, chemotherapy, surgery, immunotherapy, radiotherapy, or a watch-and-wait approach can be selected or combined. Surgery is considered therapeutic for patients with localized disease. *Helicobacter pylori* should be eradicated in all patients with gastric MALT lymphoma; approximately 75% respond to the eradication therapy, leading to tumor regression in localized disease; however, the effectiveness of antibiotic therapy for non-gastric MALT lymphoma is not clear. The prognosis of MALT lymphoma is usually good, achieving up to 94.1% of survival rates and a median survival exceeding 10 years. However, high-grade transformation to diffuse large B-cell lymphoma may occur, leading to a poorer prognosis (Figs. 36.1 and 36.2).

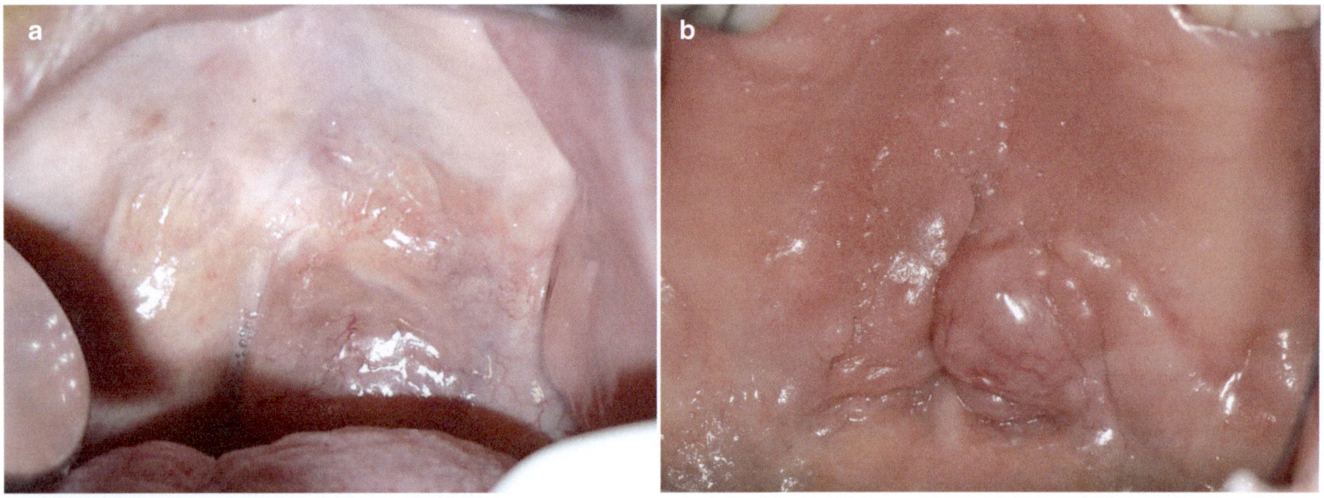

Fig. 36.1 Clinical presentation of MALT lymphoma affecting the oral cavity. (**a**) Asymptomatic, non-ulcerated, swelling in the soft palate. (**b**) Well-defined, asymptomatic, nodule affecting the transition of soft and hard palate

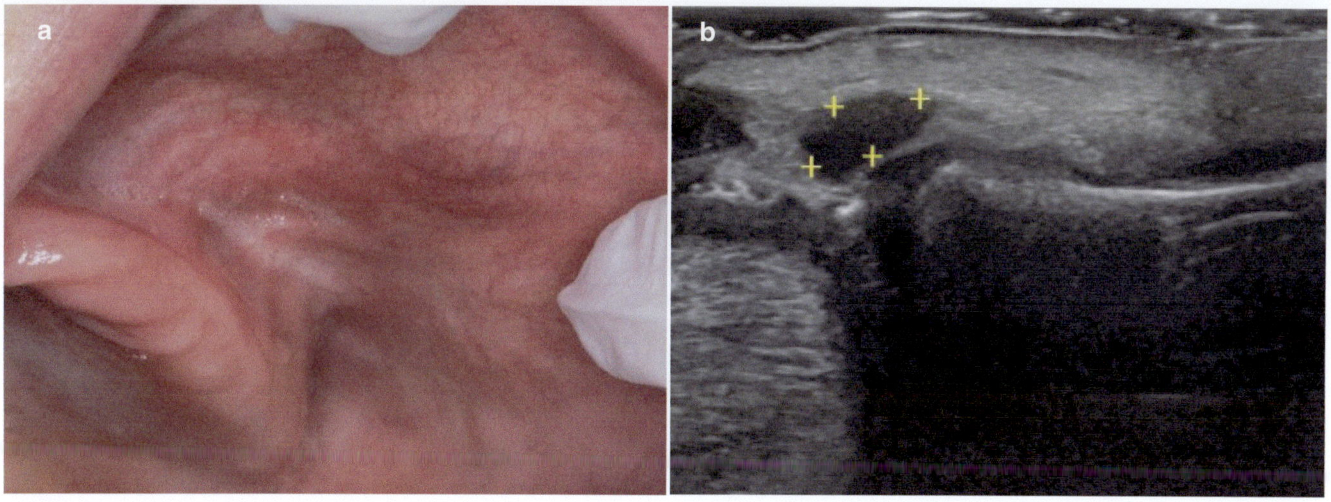

Fig. 36.2 Clinical and ultrasonographic presentation of MALT lymphoma affecting the oral cavity. (**a**) An 80-year-old female patient presenting with an asymptomatic nodule in the upper lip. (**b**) The ultrasonographic exam of the same patient revealed the presence of a well-defined hypoechoic image in the upper lip

36.2 Microscopic Findings

- There is a diffuse proliferation of small to medium-sized neoplastic cells with pale eosinophilic cytoplasm.
- Tumor cells very often infiltrate glandular ducts, leading to the development of lymphoepithelial lesions.
- Tumor cells are characteristically small to medium size.
- Most of the cells have irregular nuclei, dispersed chromatin, and inconspicuous nucleoli (centrocytes-like cells).
- Scarce transformed, larger cells with prominent nucleoli are also usually found.
- Some cells exhibit abundant light eosinophilic to clear cytoplasm and are called monocytoid B cells.
- The presence of aggregates of monocytoid cells may lead to regions with a lighter-stained aspect.
- Plasma cells are frequent and may be numerous in MALT lymphoma, more commonly exhibiting a monotypic light chain restriction.
- Other reactive inflammatory cells are also frequently present, like T lymphocytes and macrophages.
- Residual germinal centers that are infiltrated by neoplastic cells are common.
- Amyloid deposition may occur in a few cases.
- When solid, sheet-like or cluster proliferations (>20 cells) of large cells are present, the tumor should rather be diagnosed as diffuse large B-cell lymphoma transformation.
- In the microscopic differential diagnosis, the presence of residual germinal centers infiltrated by tumor cells demands attention to exclude a follicular lymphoma, while the large number of plasma cells may simulate a lymphoplasmacytic lymphoma or an extramedullary plasmacytoma.
- Differentiating an oral MALT lymphoma from a reactive lymphoepithelial sialadenitis (LESA) is usually very difficult, and sometimes it is not possible solely on the basis of H&E and immunohistochemistry. The presence of light chain immunoglobulin monoclonality investigated by immunohistochemistry or by in situ hybridization favors the diagnosis of a neoplastic condition, but this interpretation may be difficult in some cases (Figs. 36.3, 36.4, 36.5, and 36.6).

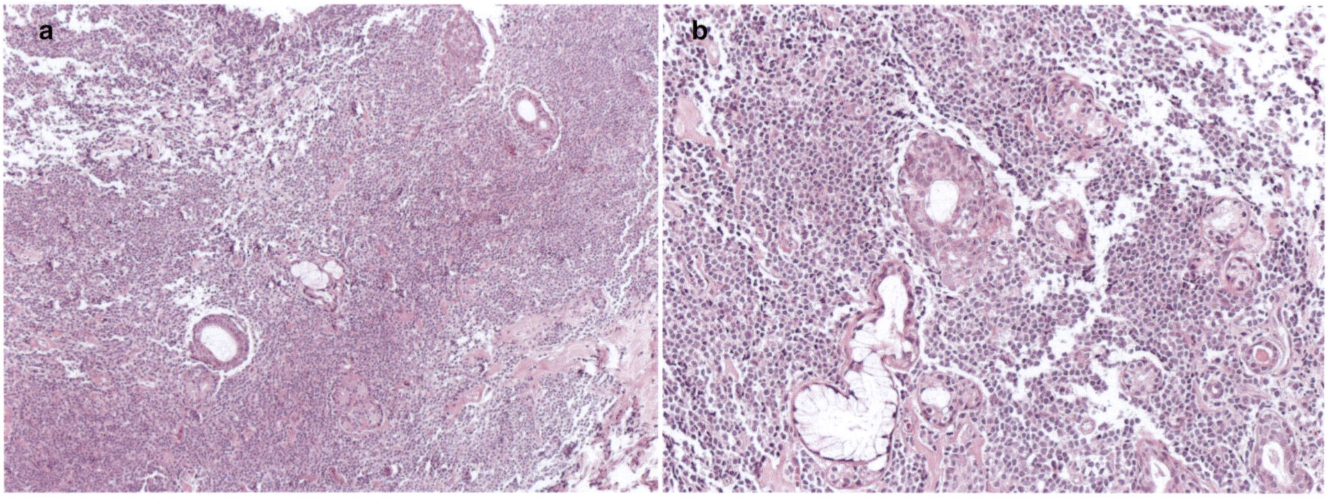

Fig. 36.3 Microscopic features of MALT lymphoma. (**a**) Diffuse proliferation of predominantly small cells that infiltrate adjacent normal tissues and surround the salivary gland structures (H&E; 25X). (**b**) Observe the close association between the neoplastic B cells of MALT lymphoma and the salivary gland ducts leading to the development of lymphoepithelial lesions (H&E; 50X)

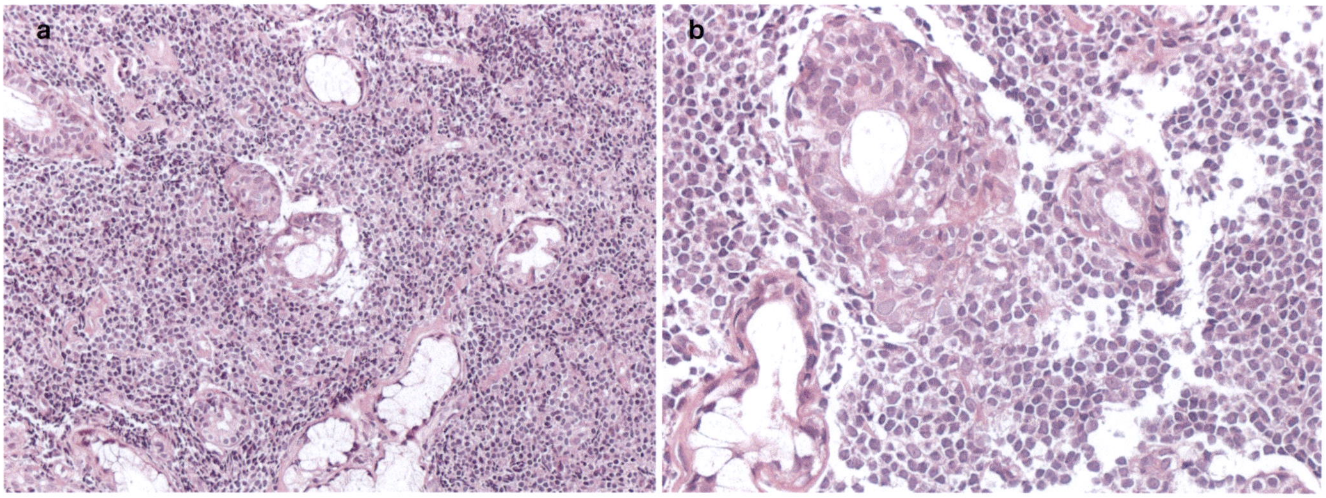

Fig. 36.4 Microscopic features of MALT lymphoma. (**a**) The neoplastic cells infiltrate the salivary gland structures (H&E; 50X). (**b**) In this image it is possible to observe the infiltration of neoplastic cells in the salivary gland ducts, giving rise to the lymphoepithelial lesions (H&E; 100X)

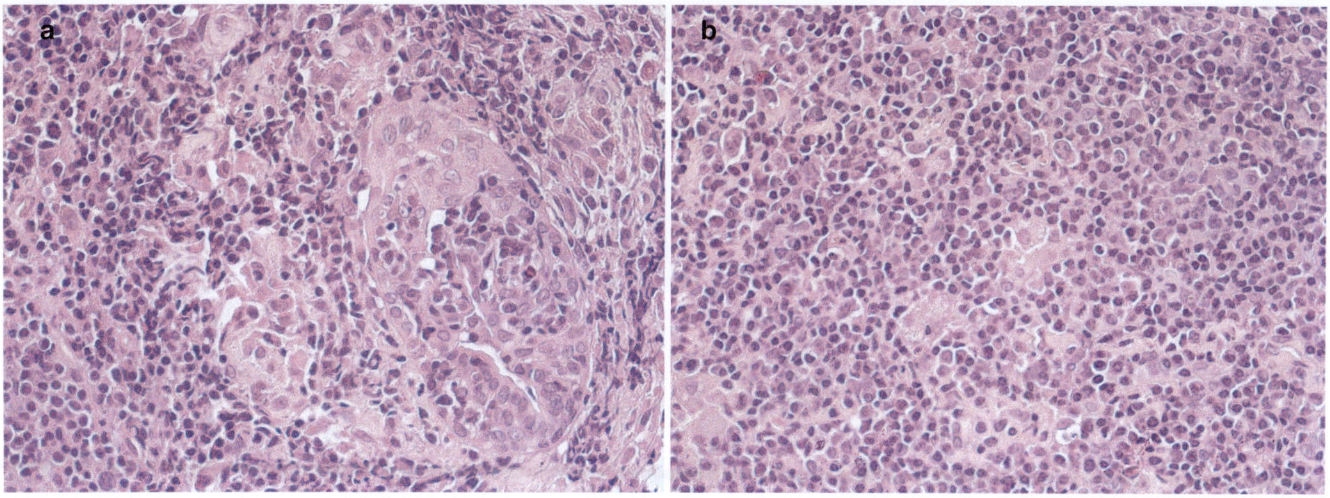

Fig. 36.5 Microscopic features of MALT lymphoma. (**a**) Despite the predominance of small cells in the neoplastic infiltrate of MALT lymphoma, it is possible to find scattered larger cells (H&E; 200X). (**b**) The presence of many plasma cells is a common microscopic feature of MALT lymphoma (H&E; 200X)

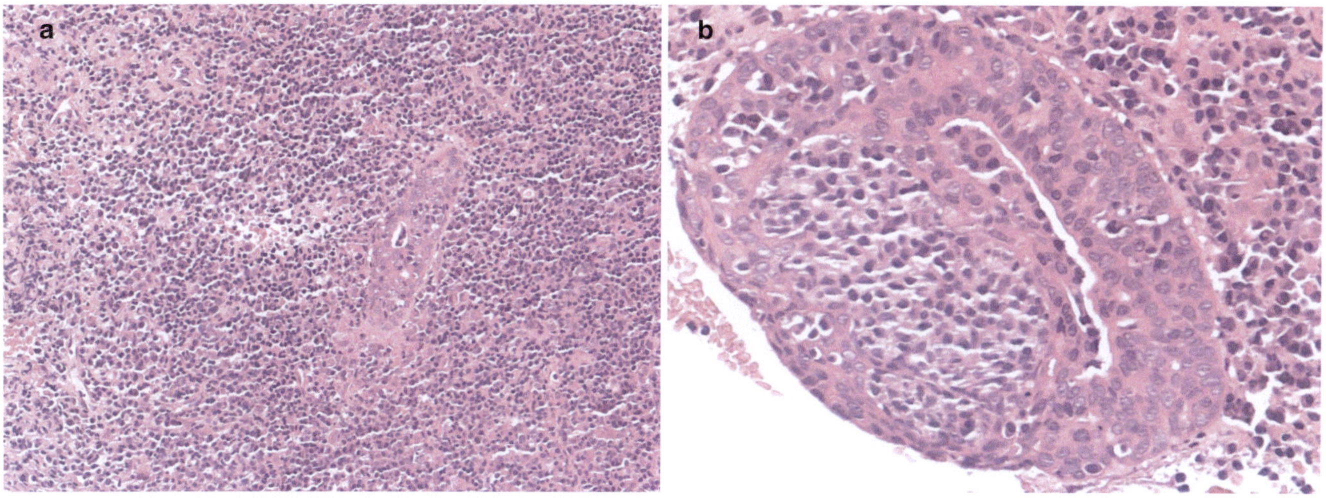

Fig. 36.6 Microscopic features of MALT lymphoma. (**a**) Observe the diffuse infiltrate of small cells in MALT lymphoma with a residual salivary gland duct in the center of the image (H&E;100X). (**b**) The occurrence of neoplastic cells with larger eosinophilic cytoplasm known as monocytoid cells, in this image located on the left side of the photo associated with the lymphoepithelial lesion, is a frequent finding in MALT Lymphomas. Observe the presence of plasma cells in the right side of the image (H&E; 200X)

36.3 Immunohistochemistry and/or Genetics

MALT lymphoma does not have specific immunohistochemical markers, and its diagnosis must be done after exclusion of other small B cell lymphomas and its distinction from reactive conditions like lymphoepithelial sialadenitis and IgG4-related disease, which may demand molecular analysis for confirmation. Tumor cells diffusely and strongly express B-cell markers like CD20, CD19, CD79, PAX-5; however, MALT lymphoma commonly has an abundant reactive T-cell component, demonstrated by CD3 stain. The expression of BCL2 is also strong and diffuse. Plasma cell markers like MUM1, CD138, and plasma cell (VS38c) are useful to highlight the plasma cell component, which is frequently monoclonal to kappa or lambda light chain and therefore contributes to demonstrating the neoplastic nature of the disease. However, monoclonality cannot always be assessed by immunohistochemistry or in situ hybridization. Other newer markers like MNDA and IRTA may be useful. To rule out mantle cell lymphoma and chronic lymphocytic leukemia/small lymphocytic lymphoma, cyclin D1, SOX-11, CD5, and CD23 negative results are mandatory, while the lack of BCL6 and CD10 expression contributes to excluding the diagnosis of follicular lymphoma. Cytokeratin (AE1/AE3) is useful to highlight the lymphoepithelial lesions and Ki67 is usually low. EBV is not present in MALT lymphoma cells. In addition to the recurrent translocations described above, the occurrence of trisomy of chromosomes 3 and 18 is a common molecular event observed in MALT lymphomas. Moreover, immunoglobulin heavy and light chains are usually rearranged and demonstrate somatic hypermutation of variable regions (Table 36.1; Figs. 36.7, 36.8, 36.9, 36.10, and 36.11).

Table 36.1 Summary of the main immunohistochemical reactions used for MALT lymphoma diagnosis

Antibody/probe	Most frequent results	Pattern	Objective
CD20	Positive	Membrane	To demonstrate the B-cell origin of the neoplasm
CD3	Negative	Membrane	To exclude the T-cell nature of the neoplasm
MUM1	Negative	Nucleus	To demonstrate the presence of plasma cells
BCL2	Positive	Cytoplasm	Characteristic of MALT lymphoma
BCL6	Negative	Nucleus	To exclude a follicular lymphoma
CD10	Negative	Membrane	To exclude a follicular lymphoma
CD5	Negative	Membrane	To exclude a MCL and a CLL/SLL
CD23	Negative	Membrane	To exclude a CLL/SLL
Cyclin D1/SOX11	Negative	Nucleus	To exclude a MCL
AE1/AE3	Negative	Cytoplasm	To demonstrate the presence of lymphoepithelial lesions
Ki67	Low (~5%)	Nucleus	To demonstrate the proliferative index of the neoplasm
BIRC3::MALT1[a]	Variably positive (lung/intestine)	–	To characterize the genetic landscape of the neoplasm
IGH::BCL10[a]	Variably positive (lung/intestine)	–	To characterize the genetic landscape of the neoplasm
IGH::MALT1[a]	Variably positive (lung/ocular/SG/skin)	–	To characterize the genetic landscape of the neoplasm
IGH::FOXP1[a]	Variably positive (thyroid/skin/ocular)	–	To characterize the genetic landscape of the neoplasm
+3[a]	Variably positive (intestine/SG/ocular)	–	To characterize the genetic landscape of the neoplasm
+18[a]	Variably positive (intestine/SG/ocular)	–	To characterize the genetic landscape of the neoplasm

The main results for molecular findings are also described

MALT mucosa-associated lymphoid tissue, *CLL/SLL* chronic lymphocytic leukemia/small lymphocytic lymphoma, *MCL* mantle cell lymphoma, *SG* salivary glands

[a]Investigated by fluorescent in situ hybridization or PCR

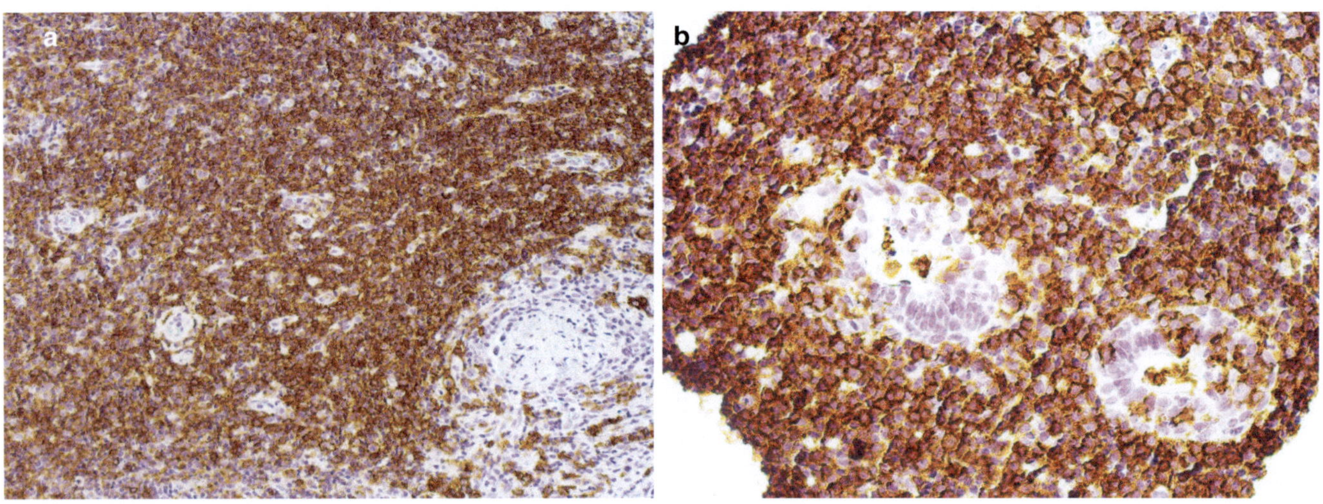

Fig. 36.7 Immunohistochemical features of MALT lymphoma. (**a**) As a mature B-cell lymphoma, MALT lymphoma cells strongly express CD20 protein (DAB; 100X). (**b**) Observe the presence of neoplastic B cells inside the salivary gland ducts, giving rise to lymphoepithelial lesions (DAB; 200X)

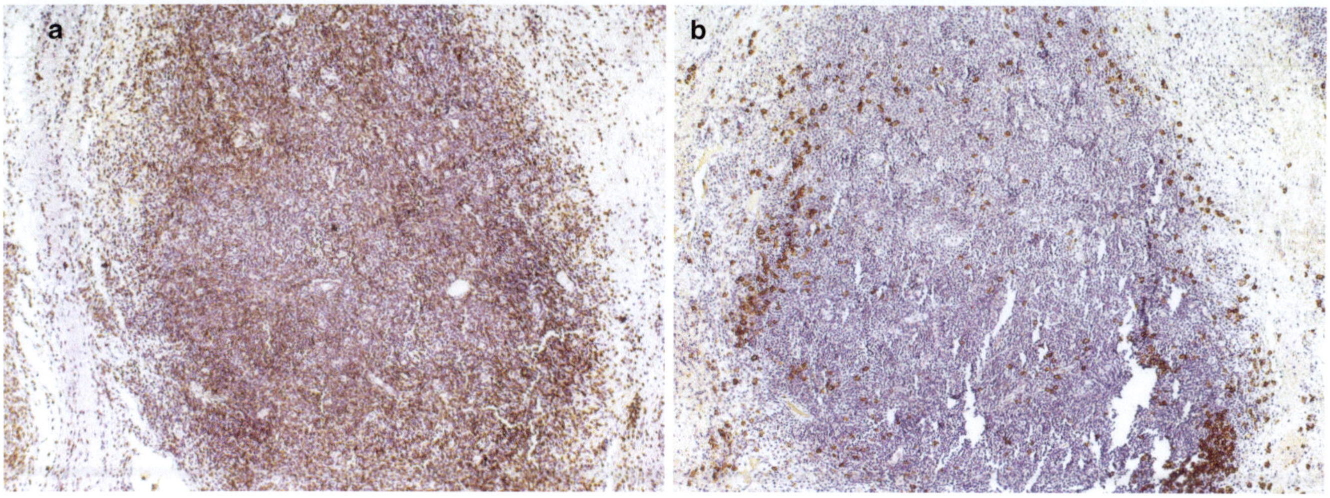

Fig. 36.8 Immunohistochemical features of MALT lymphoma. (**a**) MALT lymphoma usually demonstrates a large reactive component of T lymphomas, as demonstrated in this image using CD3 expression. Differentiating a reactive from a neoplastic condition may be difficult because of this feature of the tumor. The presence of immunoglobulin light chain restriction is very helpful in determining the neoplastic nature of the disorder (DAB; 50X). (**b**) The presence of plasma cells in the tumor is highlighted by CD138 expression (DAB; 50X)

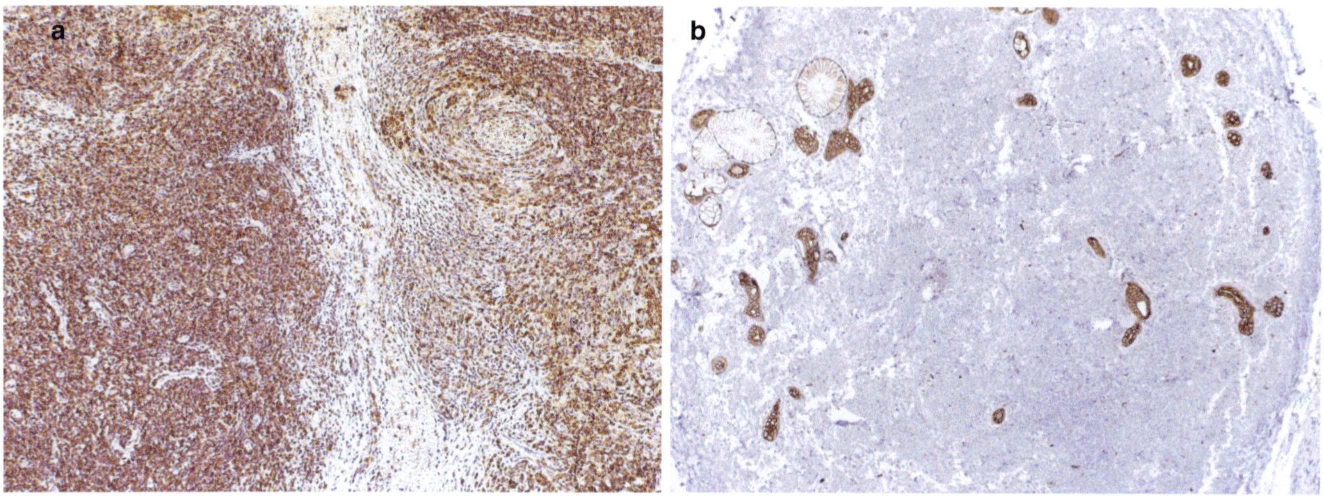

Fig. 36.9 Immunohistochemical features of MALT lymphoma. (**a**) Tumor cells are strongly positive for Bcl2 expression (DAB; 50X). (**b**) The residual salivary gland ducts can be better appreciated using cytokeratin (AE1/AE3) antibody (DAB; 50X)

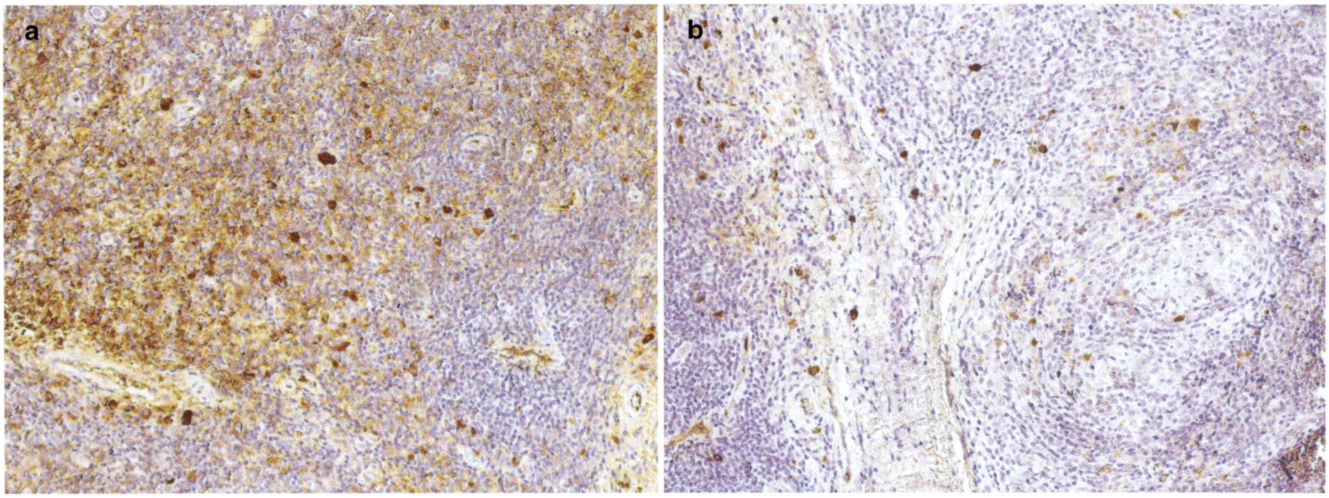

Fig. 36.10 Immunohistochemical features of MALT lymphoma to demonstrate the monoclonality of tumor cells. (**a**) In this example, neoplastic cells were monotypic for Kappa immunoglobulin light chain. Observe the diffuse expression of the protein (DAB; 100X). (**b**) Meanwhile, only scattered cells were positive for Lambda light chain (DAB; 100X)

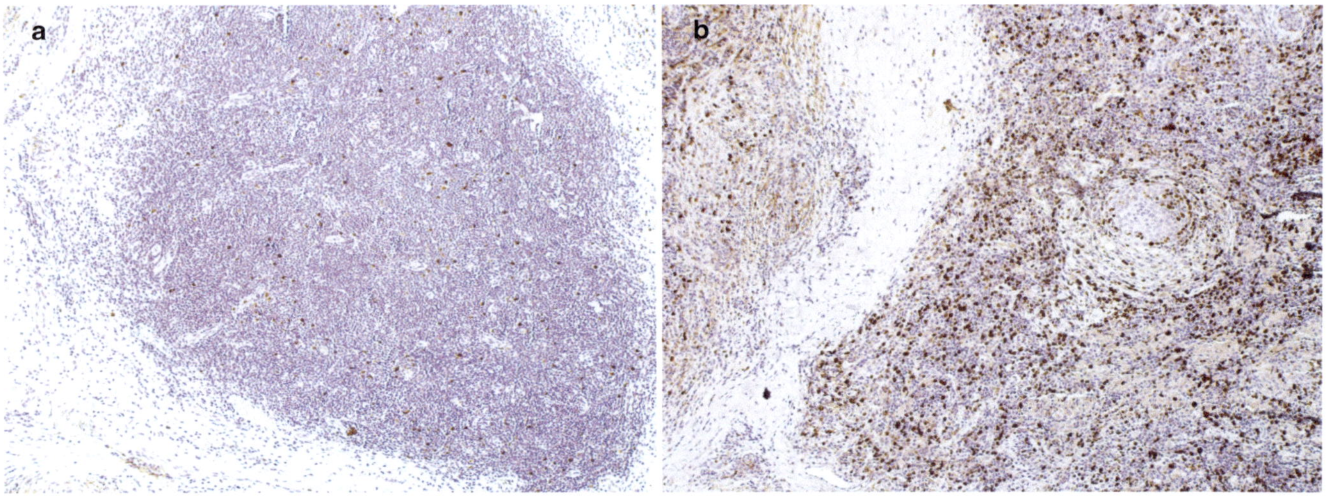

Fig. 36.11 Immunohistochemical features of MALT lymphoma. (**a**) Tumor cells usually exhibit a low proliferative index measured by the expression of Ki67 protein and exemplified in this case (DAB; 50X). (**b**) However, in some areas of the tumor, as exemplified in this image, there might be a higher proliferative rate, which should be evaluated with caution by pathologists to rule out a possible high-grade transformation into a diffuse large B-cell lymphoma. Focal areas with a higher proliferative rate may also represent a possible residual germinal center, which can be better appreciated using follicular dendritic cell markers like CD21, CD23 or CD35 (DAB; 50X)

Sources

1. Thieblemont C, Berger F, Dumontet C, Moullet I, Bouafia F, Felman P, et al. Mucosa-associated lymphoid tissue lymphoma is a disseminated disease in one third of 158 patients analyzed. Blood. 2000;95(3):802–6.
2. Zhang T, Wu Y, Ju H, Meng J, Guo W, Ren G. Extranodal marginal zone B-cell lymphoma of mucosa-associated lymphoid tissue in the oromaxillofacial head and neck region: a retrospective analysis of 105 patients. Cancer Med. 2020;9(1):194–203. https://doi.org/10.1002/cam4.2681.
3. Wagner VP, Rodrigues-Fernandes CI, Carvalho MVR, Dos Santos JN, Barra MB, Hunter KD, et al. Mantle cell lymphoma, malt lymphoma, small lymphocytic lymphoma, and follicular lymphoma of the oral cavity: an update. J Oral Pathol Med. 2021;50(6):622–30. https://doi.org/10.1111/jop.13214.
4. Zhang C, Xia R, Gu T, Wang L, Tian Z, Zhu L, et al. Clinicopathological aspects of primary mucosa-associated lymphoid tissue lymphoma of the salivary gland: a retrospective single-center analysis of 72 cases. J Oral Pathol Med. 2021;50(7):723–30. https://doi.org/10.1111/jop.13168.
5. Cerhan JR, Habermann TM. Epidemiology of marginal zone lymphoma. Ann Lymphoma. 2021;5. https://doi.org/10.21037/aol-20-28.
6. Zhou MX, Chen YY, Liu L, Wang GG, Zhang JQ, Zhao K, Li SQ. Mucosa-associated lymphoid tissue lymphoma in thymus: a SEER analysis. Expert Rev Anticancer Ther. 2022;22(12):1349–55. https://doi.org/10.1080/14737140.2022.2146582.

7. Kaur R, Shetty D, Bagal BP, Gujral S, Sengar M, Laskar S, et al. Extranodal MALT lymphoma in the oral cavity: a series of three cases with review of literature. Head Neck Pathol. 2022;16(4):1242–50. https://doi.org/10.1007/s12105-022-01461-6.
8. Lyapichev KA, Medeiros LJ, Ivashkevich Y, Thakral B, Dabaja BS, Lin P, et al. MALT lymphoma of the tongue: an unusual site that may present a diagnostic challenge. Ann Diagn Pathol. 2022;56:151841. https://doi.org/10.1016/j.anndiagpath.2021.151841.
9. Cook JR, Amador C, Czader M, Duffield A, Goodlad J, Ott G, et al. Transformations of marginal zone lymphomas and lymphoplasmacytic lymphomas: report from the 2021 SH/EAHP Workshop. Am J Clin Pathol. 2023:aqad034. https://doi.org/10.1093/ajcp/aqad034.
10. Zucca E, Rossi D, Bertoni F. Marginal zone lymphomas. Hematol Oncol. 2023;41(Suppl 1):88–91. https://doi.org/10.1002/hon.3152.
11. Peters A, Keating MM, Nikonova A, Doucette S, Prica A. Management of marginal zone lymphoma: a Canadian perspective. Curr Oncol. 2023;30(2):1745–59. https://doi.org/10.3390/curroncol30020135.
12. Qi S, Liu X, Noy A, Lee J, Teckie S, Hajj C, et al. Predictors of survival in patients with MALT lymphoma: a retrospective, case-control study. Blood Adv. 2023;7(8):1496–506. https://doi.org/10.1182/bloodadvances.2022007772.
13. Laurent C, Cook JR, Yoshino T, Quintanilla-Martinez L, Jaffe ES. Follicular lymphoma and marginal zone lymphoma: how many diseases? Virchows Arch. 2023;482(1):149–62. https://doi.org/10.1007/s00428-022-03432-2.
14. Chi Y, Zhang Q, Qin Z, Bai J, Yan J, Liu C, et al. Molecular pathology assists the diagnosis of lymphoepithelial sialadenitis, Sjögren's syndrome and extranodal marginal zone lymphoma of mucosa-associated lymphoid tissue. J Dent Sci. 2024;19:130–8. https://doi.org/10.1016/j.jds.2023.05.018.
15. Araújo GR, Morais-Perdigão AL, Lopez-de-Cáceres CV, Almeida OP, Vargas PA, Roman-Tager EM, et al. Lymphomas affecting the submandibular glands. Med Oral Patol Oral Cir Bucal. 2024;29(1):e78–86. https://doi.org/10.4317/medoral.26065.
16. Segura-Rivera R, Pina-Oviedo S. Marginal zone lymphoma of extranodal sites: a review with an emphasis on diagnostic pitfalls and differential diagnosis with reactive conditions. Hum Pathol. 2024:105683. https://doi.org/10.1016/j.humpath.2024.105683.
17. Watanabe Y, Fujii H, Yamamoto S, Masuoka S, Kobayashi R, Fujii N, et al. Parotid gland MALT lymphoma with amyloid deposition, challenges in preoperative diagnosis: a case report. Radiol Case Rep. 2024;19(12):6141–6. https://doi.org/10.1016/j.radcr.2024.09.083.
18. Legarrea JMA, Santos ML, Rodrigues NG, Gomez RS, Mesquita RA, Souza SF et al. MALT lymphoma affecting the oral cavity: a clinical, pathologic and genetic study of MALT 1 gene translocation. Oral Surg Oral Med Oral Pathol Oral Radiol. https://doi.org/10.1016/j.oooo.2025.07.016.

Follicular Lymphoma

37

Bruno Augusto Benevenuto de Andrade,
Renata Gonçalves de Resende,
Guilherme Rossi Assis de Mendonça,
and Felipe Paiva Fonseca

37.1 General Overview and Clinical Presentation

Follicular lymphoma represents the second most common subtype of non-Hodgkin lymphomas, accounting for approximately 20%–25% of all cases diagnosed in Western countries. It is a neoplasm derived from germinal center B-cells, consisting of a mixture of small-sized cleaved centrocytes and a variable amount of large-sized non-cleaved centroblasts. Follicular lymphoma most often affects the lymph nodes as asymptomatic swellings, and it usually manifests as a disseminated disease at the moment of diagnosis, although the occurrence of B-symptoms is considered uncommon. Extranodal involvement is frequently described, but primary extranodal neoplasms are uncommonly found, more often in the gastrointestinal tract, soft tissue, breast, and ocular adnexa.

The etiology of follicular lymphoma remains to be determined, but its molecular landscape is now better understood, and the genetic abnormality involving chromosomes 14 and 18 that leads to the translocation between *IGH* and *BCL2* genes is considered the genetic hallmark of the neoplasm and is present in approximately 85%–90% of the cases. The presence of this translocation causes the overexpression of BCL2 protein by the tumor cells and it is used as a key diagnostic feature, although high-grade follicular lymphomas may lose the expression of BCL2 protein in approximately 50% of the cases, which is believed to be consequence of the mutational event involving *BCL2* gene that leads to conformational changes in the protein that it is not recognized by some commercially available antibodies.

Follicular lymphoma affecting the oral cavity demands from diagnosticians a systemic analysis of the patient to rule out a disseminated disease. The palate and the cheek mucosa are the most affected locations. Males and females are equally affected, and adults with a wide age range from the third to the seventh decades of life can be affected. The tumors usually present as expansive, non-ulcerated, painless swellings with a long evolution, sometimes achieving more than 1 year of duration. Some cases may show superficial telangiectasia. Tumors affecting the palate must be investigated for maxillary sinus involvement. In the oral cavity, the most important differential diagnosis for follicular lymphoma is follicular lymphoid hyperplasia, which may also manifest as painless expansive swellings and microscopically also demonstrates a follicular growth pattern. A detailed discussion about follicular lymphoid hyperplasia is available in Chap. 11. A careful histological and immunohistochemical study, sometimes also including molecular analyses, is necessary to differentiate both entities.

In addition to its classic presentation, an associated lesion called "in situ follicular B-cell neoplasm" is also known, which is diagnosed by BCL2 and CD10 positivity in normally looking germinal centers. Furthermore, some other follicular lymphoma-related entities are recognized and must be taken into account when dealing with any lymphoid proliferation exhibiting a follicular and/or diffuse growth pattern with a mix of centrocytes and centroblasts. BCL2-rearrangement-negative CD23-positive follicle center lymphoma was recently proposed as a follicular lymphoma variant by the International Consensus Classification (ICC) of myeloid and lymphoid neoplasms in 2022. Of note, this variant exhibits some overlap with the so-called "diffuse variant" of follicular

B. A. B. de Andrade (✉)
Department of Oral Diagnosis and Pathology, School of Dentistry, Universidade Federal do Rio de Janeiro, Rio de Janeiro, Brazil

R. G. de Resende
Department of Oral Medicine, Hospital Metropolitano Odilon Behrens (Odilon Behrens Metropolitan Hospital), Belo Horizonte, Brazil

G. R. A. de Mendonça
Department of Pathology, School of Medical Sciences, University of Campinas, Campinas, Brazil

F. P. Fonseca
Department of Oral Surgery and Pathology, School of Dentistry, Universidade Federal de Minas Gerais, Belo Horizonte, Brazil

© The Author(s), under exclusive license to Springer Nature Switzerland AG 2025

F. P. Fonseca et al. (eds.), *Lymphoproliferative and Granulomatous Disorders of the Oral Cavity*,
https://doi.org/10.1007/978-3-031-98844-8_37

lymphoma, described in 2009. Other neoplasms are also described in this setting according to the World Health Organization classification, such as pediatric follicular lymphoma, duodenal follicular lymphoma, testicular follicular lymphoma, follicular lymphomas with uncommon features like those with "blastoid" or "large centrocyte" cytological features, primary cutaneous follicle center lymphoma, and large B-cell lymphoma with IRF4 rearrangement (LBCL-IRF4), however, they are currently better classified as distinct entities compared with conventional follicular lymphoma.

The use of rituximab with the CHOP scheme represents the most commonly used approach for treating follicular lymphomas, sometimes followed by rituximab maintenance. However, other schemes can also be applied, as well as a watchful wait approach. The prognosis varies significantly and may be predicted by indexes such as the Follicular Lymphoma International Prognostic Index (FLIPI), which encompasses both clinical and laboratory findings (age, stage, number of affected nodal sites, hemoglobin levels, and lactate dehydrogenase levels). The prognostic role of histological factors, such as grade or proliferation index (Ki67), is somewhat controversial. However, individuals affected by follicular lymphoma grade 3B usually present a worse prognosis and an aggressive clinical course. The histological transformation of low-grade follicular lymphomas into a high-grade disease like diffuse large B-cell lymphoma may occur, and it is associated with a poorer survival (Fig. 37.1).

37.2 Microscopic Findings

- Follicular lymphoma typically exhibits a follicular growth pattern. Some cases may also show some areas of diffuse proliferation, and attention must be paid when only small biopsies are available for analysis.
- Sometimes immunohistochemical reactions for follicular dendritic cells using CD21, CD23 and/or CD35 are necessary to demonstrate the follicular growth pattern not easily identifiable during H&E evaluation.
- Fibrous stroma with the presence of fibrotic bands is a common histological finding.
- The lack of tingible body macrophages in the lymphoid follicles of the follicular lymphomas is a clue for the neoplastic nature of the process, as these cells are normally present in reactive germinal centers.
- The zonation pattern of germinal centers is also lost, and light and dark zones cannot be differentiated from each other, also contributing to differentiating the lymphoma from a reactive follicular hyperplasia.
- The mantle zone is frequently altered. It can be irregular, decreased or even completely lost.
- Neoplastic follicles are frequently displayed very near to each other, leading to the "back-to-back" growth pattern.
- Most of the follicular lymphomas exhibit a mixture of small and large cells.

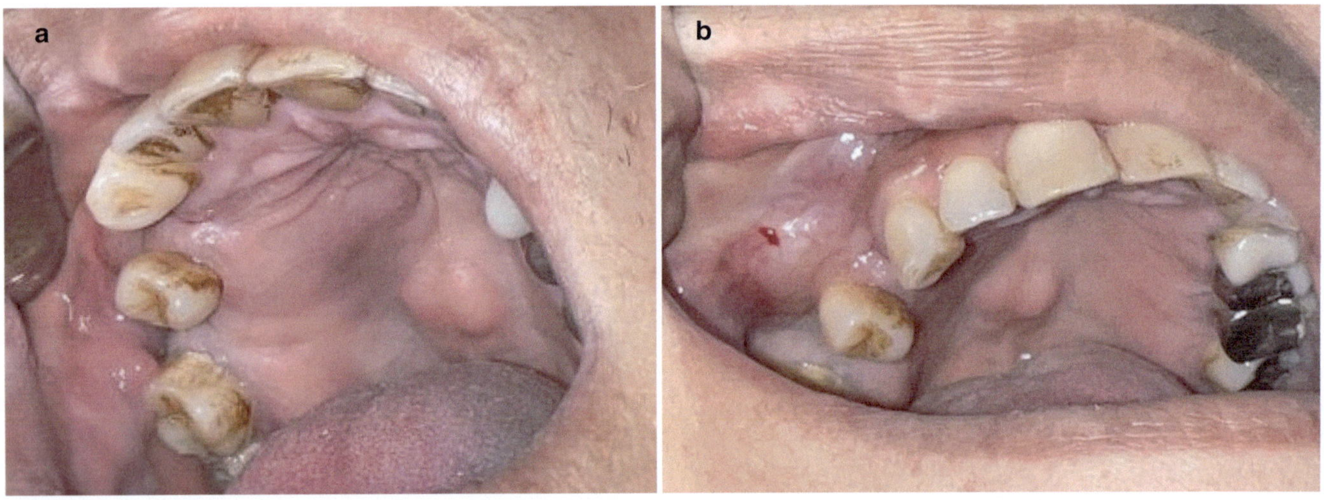

Fig. 37.1 Clinical presentation of follicular lymphoma affecting the oral cavity. (**a**) It usually manifests as an asymptomatic, non-ulcerated swelling in the palate. (**b**) The vestibular mucosa was also affected in this case. The involvement of the maxillary sinus by the tumor must be evaluated when palatine lesions are diagnosed

- The small to medium-sized neoplastic cells have hyperchromatic and irregular nuclear contour, and scant cytoplasm, consistent with centrocytes.
- The large cells represent centroblasts or immunoblasts and present a vesiculated nucleus with one or more evident nucleoli.
- Atypical cells can be found, especially in higher-grade follicular lymphomas.
- Mitotic figures can also be observed and are more frequent in high-grade follicular lymphomas.
- Microscopic grading of follicular lymphomas takes into account the proportion of large-sized centroblasts per high-power field (HPF).
- Grade 1 follicular lymphoma has fewer than 5 centroblasts/HPF.
- Grade 2 follicular lymphoma has between 5 and 15 centroblasts/HPF.
- Grade 3A follicular lymphoma has more than 15 centroblasts/HPF, but still has centrocytes.
- Grade 3B follicular lymphoma (also termed follicular large B-cell lymphoma) is composed entirely of centroblasts.
- Grades 1 and 2 follicular lymphomas are considered low-grade diseases. Grade 3A is considered a high-grade tumor, but with a better prognosis than cases classified as Grade 3B, which behave more similarly to diffuse large B-cell lymphoma. Of note, the grading system was recently revisited by the ICC group and World Health Organization classifications. The ICC group advocates grading for all follicular lymphoma cases, whereas the WHO considers grading as an optional approach. Both classifications, however, agree that follicular lymphoma grade 3B has a clinical course more similar to aggressive lymphomas (Figs. 37.2, 37.3, and 37.4).

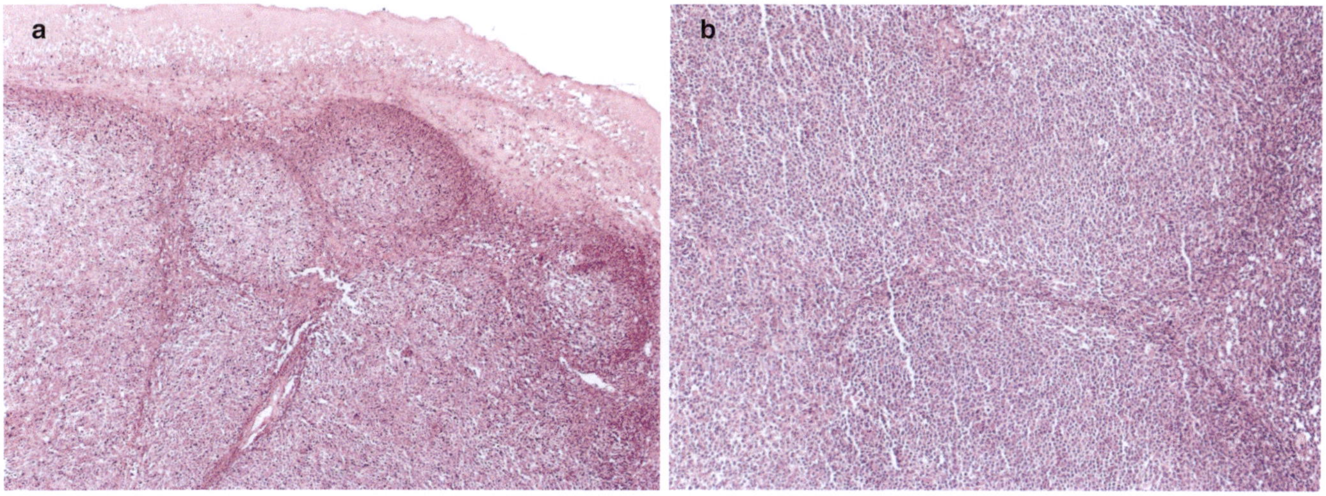

Fig. 37.2 Microscopic features of follicular lymphoma. (**a**) Neoplastic cells proliferate in the lamina propria of the oral mucosa, exhibiting a follicular growth pattern (H&E; 50X). (**b**) Neoplastic follicles exhibit the back-to-back aspect, do not show tingible body macrophages or the zonation of clear and dark zones. The mantle zone is disorganized and occasionally absent in some regions of the follicles (H&E; 50X)

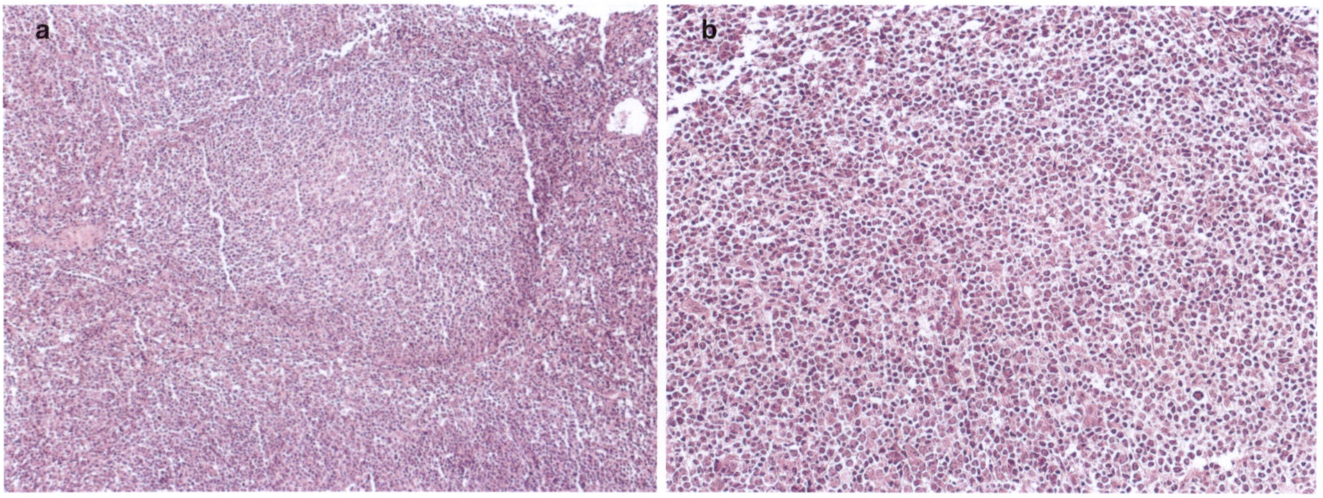

Fig. 37.3 Microscopic features of follicular lymphoma. (**a**) Irregular-shaped neoplastic follicle without tingible body macrophages (H&E; 50X). (**b**) In the center of this neoplastic follicle, a mixture of centrocytes (small cells) and centroblast (large cells) can be found. The presence of more than 15 centroblasts/HPF denotes a Grade 3A follicular lymphoma (H&E; 100X)

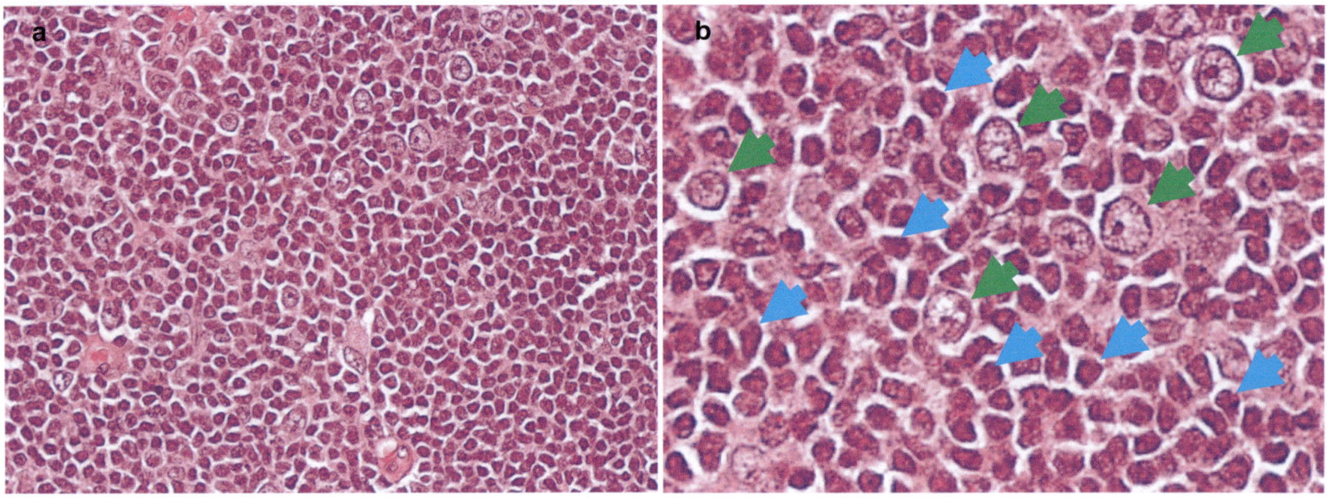

Fig. 37.4 Microscopic features of follicular lymphoma. (**a**) Under high magnification, observe the predominance of small cells with the presence of several large cells (H&E; 200X). (**b**) The green arrows illustrate some of the large cells (centroblasts) in this follicular lymphoma, while the blue arrows illustrate some of the small cells (centrocytes) that are predominant in this tumor (H&E; 400X)

37.3 Immunohistochemistry and/or Genetics

The immunohistochemical reactions are important to demonstrate that the follicular proliferation is neoplastic or reactive, and to reveal the presence of a follicular growth pattern in those cases where such an architectural pattern is not clearly observable under H&E analysis. Tumor cells in the follicles will be positive for B-cell markers like CD20, CD79a and PAX5, while reactive T cells will stain for CD3 mostly in the interfollicular region, but also inside the neoplastic follicles. To demonstrate that tumor cells have a germinal center phenotype CD10 and BCL6 are useful markers, although high-grade follicular lymphomas may partially or totally lose the expression of these markers. In these cases, the diagnosis becomes very difficult and distinction from other small B-cell lymphomas, especially marginal zone lymphoma, may demand careful microscopic interpretation and genetic evaluation or may not be possible to be done with a high level of reliability.

The expression of CD21, CD23 and/or CD35 may be very helpful to show follicular dendritic cells meshworks and highlight the follicular pattern when this feature is not observed using routine staining. Of note, diffuse areas usually lose these meshworks but remain with the same cellular composition as the neoplastic follicles. The expression pattern of Ki67 is variable depending on the grade of the tumor, but it usually loses its zonation, contributing to differentiating a neoplasm from a reactive process. The expression of BCL2 inside the follicles leads to the diagnosis of follicular lymphoma, while its expression only in the interfollicular area and in the reactive helper T cells located in the germinal center favors the diagnosis of follicular hyperplasia. However, caution should be made because in some cases, especially in high-grade tumors, they may also lose BCL2 expression. This may happen as a consequence of a modification in the protein structure following the occurrence of a genetic mutation in the *BCL2* gene. The use of different antibodies for the BCL2 protein may contribute to identifying these false-negative cases (Table 37.1; Figs. 37.5, 37.6, 37.7, 37.8, and 37.9).

Table 37.1 Summary of the main immunohistochemical reactions used for follicular lymphoma diagnosis

Antibody/probe	Most frequent results	Pattern	Objective
CD20	Positive	Membrane	To demonstrate the B-cell origin of the neoplasm
CD3	Negative	Membrane	To exclude a possible T-cell origin of the neoplasm
CD5	Negative	Membrane	To exclude a CLL/SLL diagnosis
MUM1	Negative	Nucleus	To exclude an IRF4-positive LBCL
CD10	Positive	Membrane	To demonstrate the germinal center origin of the neoplasm
BCL6	Positive	Nucleus	To demonstrate the germinal center origin of the neoplasm
CD23	Positive in the FDC and sometimes in the lymphoma cells	Membrane	To demonstrate the presence of FDC. There may be expression in lymphoma cells in some cases
CD21	Positive in the FDC and sometimes in the lymphoma cells	Membrane	To demonstrate the presence of FDC. There may be expression in lymphoma cells in some cases
BCL2	Positive in the follicles	Cytoplasm	To help determining the neoplastic or reactive nature of the disease
Cyclin D1	Negative	Nucleus	To exclude a mantle cell lymphoma
Ki67	Variable	Nucleus	To demonstrate the proliferative index of tumor cells
BCL2[a]	Positive in 90% of the cases	–	To demonstrate the genetic hallmark of the neoplasm

The main results for molecular findings are also described

FDC follicular dendritic cells, *CLL/SLL* chronic lymphocytic leukemia/small lymphocytic lymphoma, *IRF4-positive LBCL* IRF4-positive large B-cell lymphoma

[a]Investigated by fluorescent in situ hybridization or PCR

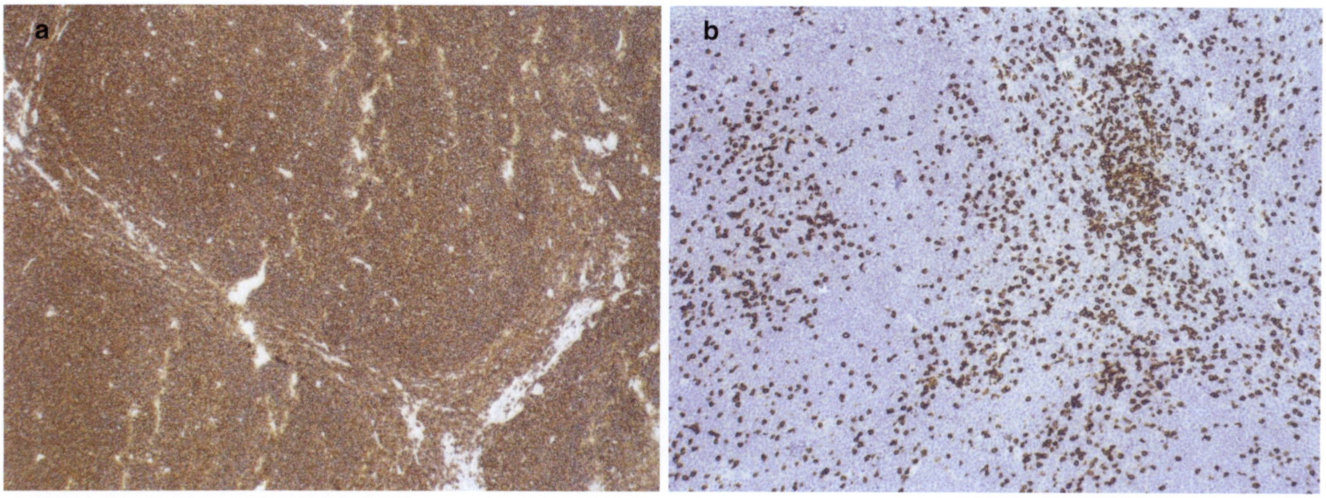

Fig. 37.5 Immunohistochemical features of follicular lymphoma. (**a**) Strong expression of CD20 demonstrates the mature B-cell origin of the tumor (DAB; 50X). (**b**) Expression of CD3 in the reactive T cells located in the interfollicular region and inside the neoplastic follicles (DAB; 50X)

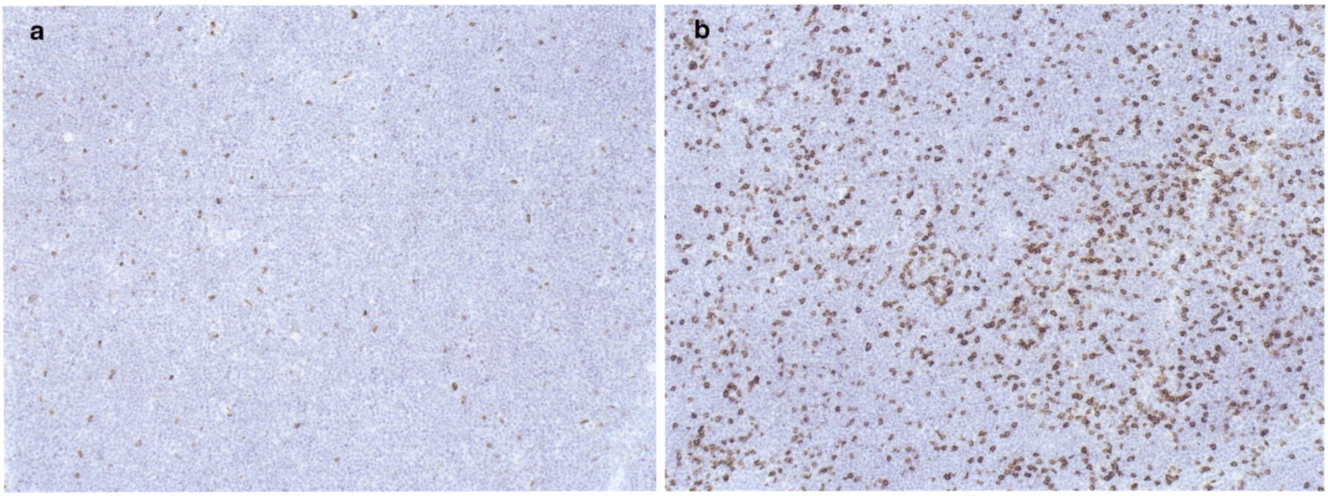

Fig. 37.6 Immunohistochemical features of follicular lymphoma. (**a**) Negative expression of Cyclin D1 rules out the diagnosis of mantle cell lymphoma (DAB; 50X). (**b**) Negative expression of CD5, which stains reactive T cells, helps to undermine the diagnosis of chronic lymphocytic leukemia/small lymphocytic lymphoma (DAB; 50X)

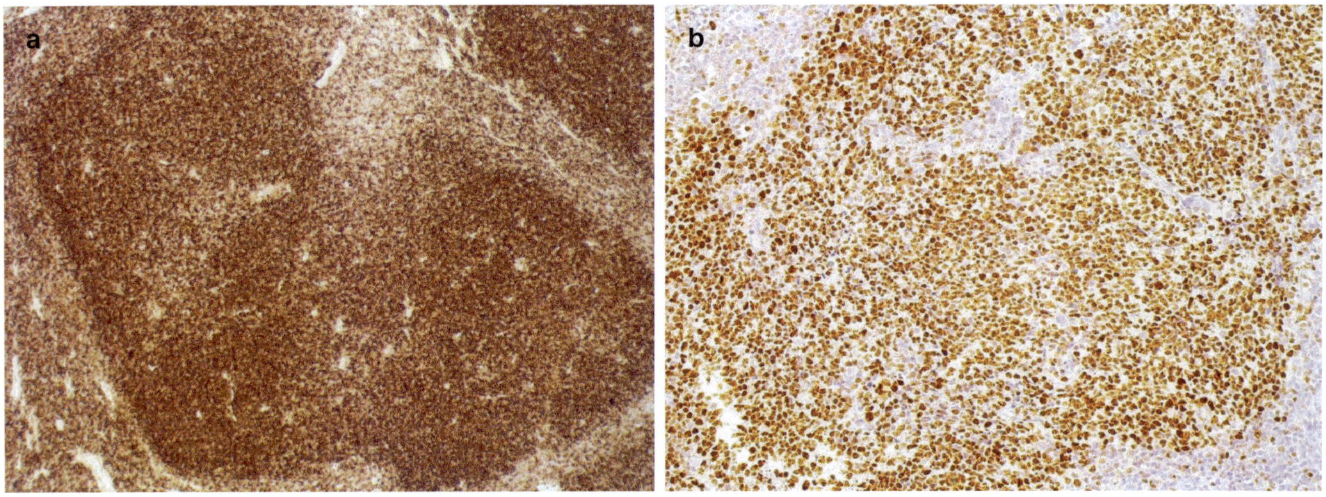

Fig. 37.7 Immunohistochemical features of follicular lymphoma. (**a**) Strong expression of CD10 demonstrates the germinal center origin of neoplasm (DAB; 100X), (**b**) the positive expression of BCL6 further confirms this origin (DAB; 100X)

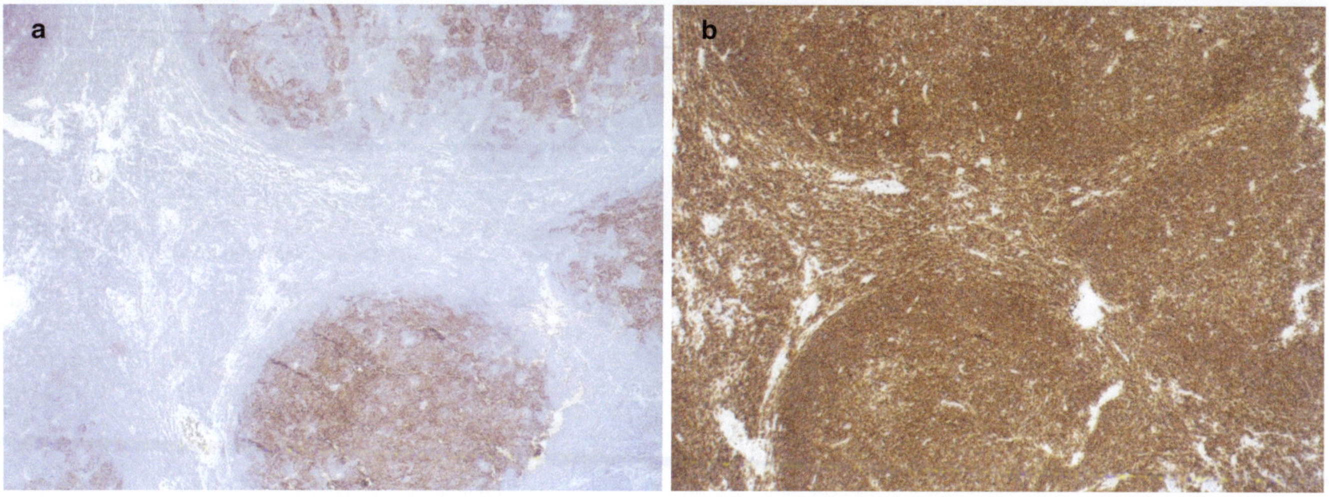

Fig. 37.8 Immunohistochemical features of follicular lymphoma. (**a**) The expression of CD23 in the follicular dendritic cells demonstrates the follicular proliferation (DAB; 50X). (**b**) The strong expression of BCL2 in the follicles confirms the neoplastic nature of the disease. Observe that BCL2 is also expressed by reactive T cells and neoplastic cells located in the interfollicular zone (DAB; 100X)

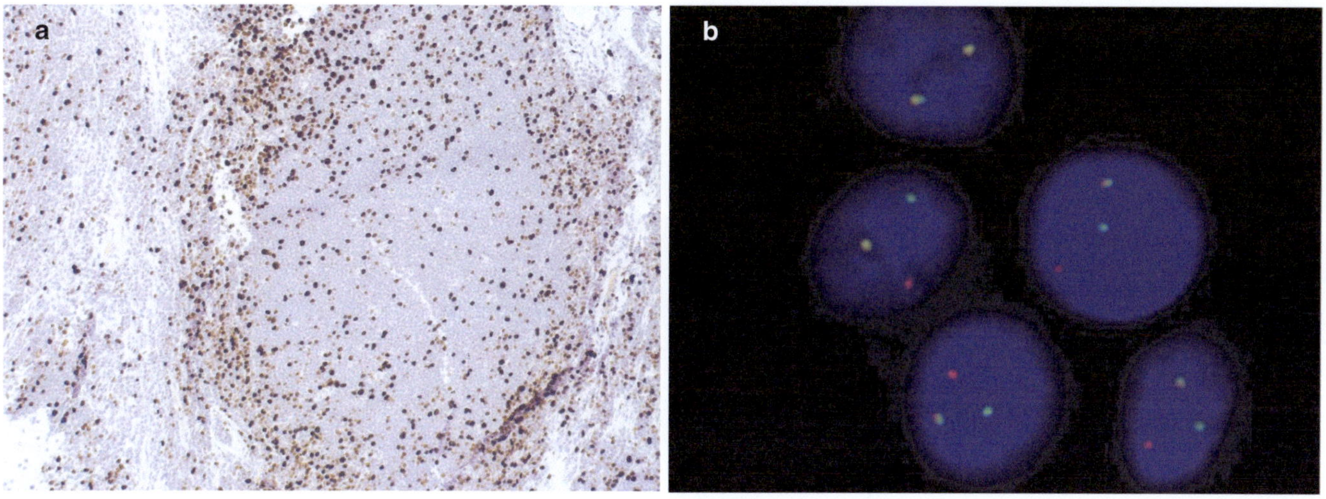

Fig. 37.9 Immunohistochemical and genetic features of follicular lymphoma. (**a**) Proliferative index varies according to tumor grade. In this case of a follicle lymphoma Grade 3A, a high Ki67 expression was achieved, with approximately 30% positivity. The zonation pattern is lost (DAB; 100X). (**b**) Translocation involving the *BCL2* gene is the genetic hallmark of this neoplasm. Observe the green and the red signals illustrating the mutation in *BCL2* using a break-apart probe (FISH; 1000X)

Sources

1. Katzenberger T, Kalla JJ, Leich E, et al. A distinctive subtype of t(14;18)-negative nodal follicular non-Hodgkin lymphoma characterized by a predominantly diffuse growth pattern and deletions in the chromosomal region 1p36. Blood. 2009;113:1053–61.
2. Horn H, Schmelter C, Leich E, Salaverria I, Katzenberger T, Ott MM, et al. Follicular lymphoma grade 3B is a distinct neoplasm according to cytogenetic and immunohistochemical profiles. Haematologica. 2011;96(9):1327–34.
3. Argyris PP, Dolan M, Piperi E, Tosios KI, Pambuccian SE, Koutlas IG. Oral follicular lymphomas. A short report of 8 cases with assessment of the IGH/BCL2 gene fusion with fluorescence in situ hybridization. Oral Surg Oral Med Oral Pathol Oral Radiol. 2013;116(3):343–7.
4. Miyaoka M, Kikuti YY, Carreras J, Ikoma H, Hiraiwa S, Ichiki A, et al. Clinicopathological and genomic analysis of double-hit follicular lymphoma: comparison with high-grade B-cell lymphoma with MYC and BCL2 and/or BCL6 rearrangements. Mod Pathol. 2018;31(2):313–26.
5. Montaner S, Weingertner N, Ledoux MP, Chenard MP, Lutz JC, Bornert F. Follicular lymphomas of oral region treated by rituximab monotherapy: about two cases. J Hematol. 2018;7(1):23–8. https://doi.org/10.14740/jh346w.
6. Carbone A, Roulland S, Gloghini A, Younes A, von Keudell G, López-Guillermo A, et al. Follicular lymphoma. Nat Rev Dis Primers. 2019;5(1):83.
7. Freedman A, Jacobsen E. Follicular lymphoma: 2020 update on diagnosis and management. Am J Hematol. 2020;95(3):316–27.

8. Fratoni S, Zanelli M, Zizzo M, Sanguedolce F, Aimola V, Cerrone G, Ricci L, Filosa A, Martino G, Ascani S. The broad landscape of follicular lymphoma: part I. Pathologica. 2020;112(1):1–16.
9. Wagner VP, Rodrigues-Fernandes CI, Carvalho MVR, Dos Santos JN, Barra MB, Hunter KD, et al. Mantle cell lymphoma, malt lymphoma, small lymphocytic lymphoma, and follicular lymphoma of the oral cavity: an update. J Oral Pathol Med. 2021;50:622–30.
10. Kumar E, Pickard L, Okosun J. Pathogenesis of follicular lymphoma: genetics to the microenvironment to clinical translation. Br J Haematol. 2021;194(5):810–21.
11. Jóna Á, Kenyeres A, Barna S, Illés Á, Simon Z. Clinical and biological prognostic factors in follicular lymphoma patients. PLoS One. 2022;17(8):e0272787.
12. Alaggio R, Amador C, Anagnostopoulos I, Attygalle AD, Araujo IBO, Berti E, et al. The 5th edition of the World Health Organization classification of haematolymphoid tumours: lymphoid neoplasms. Leukemia. 2022;36(7):1720–48.
13. Campo E, Jaffe ES, Cook JR, Quintanilla-Martinez L, Swerdlow SH, Anderson KC, et al. The international consensus classification of mature lymphoid neoplasms: a report from the Clinical Advisory Committee. Blood. 2022;140(11):1229–53.
14. Lin Z, Zha J, Yi S, Li Z, Ping L, He X, et al. Clinical characteristics and outcomes of follicular lymphoma patients with extranodal involvement: analysis of a series of 1090 cases in China. Clin Transl Oncol. 2023;25(6):1821–9.
15. Laurent C, Cook JR, Yoshino T, Quintanilla-Martinez L, Jaffe ES. Follicular lymphoma and marginal zone lymphoma: how many diseases? Virchows Arch. 2023;482(1):149–62.
16. de Araújo GR, Morais-Perdigão AL, de Cáceres CVBL, Lopes MA, Aguirre-Urizar JM, Carlos R, et al. Lymphomas affecting the sublingual glands: a clinicopathological study. Head Neck Pathol. 2023;17(1):154–64. https://doi.org/10.1007/s12105-022-01489-8.
17. Vageli DP, Doukas PG, Batrakouli O, Tsangari V, Zacharouli K, Pouliou E, et al. Head and neck follicular lymphoma with marginal zone differentiation and BCL2 translocation t(14;18) in both nodular and extranodular sites: a case report with mini-review. Oral Surg Oral Med Oral Pathol Oral Radiol. 2023;136(4):e139–48. https://doi.org/10.1016/j.oooo.2023.05.005.
18. Shi Y, Li X, Lai Y, Jia L. CD21 and CD23 expression differences in small B-cell lymphomas: comparative analysis in follicular dendritic cells and tumor cells. Int J Clin Exp Pathol. 2016;9(8):8395–405.

Mantle Cell Lymphoma

38

Cinthia Veronica Bardalez Lopez de Caceres,
Renata Gonçalves de Resende,
Guilherme Rossi Assis de Mendonça,
and Felipe Paiva Fonseca

38.1 General Overview and Clinical Presentation

Mantle cell lymphoma is a heterogeneous neoplasm believed to originate from naïve-like or memory-like mature B cells that accounts for approximately 5 to 10% of all non-Hodgkin lymphomas (NHLs). This tumor is biologically heterogeneous, exhibiting a clinical behavior that may vary from an aggressive tumor to an indolent disease, although it is still considered an incurable disorder. The etiology of this tumor is unknown, but pathogenesis of mantle cell lymphoma has been better understood during the last decades and the occurrence of the chromosomal translocation t(11;14)(q13;q32) that juxtaposes the *CCND1* gene to the *IGH* gene resulting in constitutive overexpression of cyclin D1 is considered the genetic hallmark of the disease. However, approximately 5% of the cases lack *CCND1* mutation, and in these cases the translocations of *CCND2* or *CCND3* can be frequently demonstrated. Moreover, abnormalities in the *CCND1* itself are not considered enough to cause the disease, and the occurrence of secondary genetic events like mutations in the *ATM, TP53, CDKN2A, CARD11, BTK, NOTCH*, among other genes, is necessary to promote tumor development.

Mantle cell lymphoma has been subclassified as either conventional mantle cell lymphoma or non-nodal leukemic mantle cell lymphoma, the latter being characterized by minimal lymphadenopathy, presence of lymphocytosis, bone marrow involvement and splenomegaly, accounting for 10% of all mantle cell lymphoma cases and representing a less aggressive clinical variant of the disease, more often an asymptomatic disorder. The in situ mantle cell neoplasia is considered a very rare and indolent entity that can be incidentally found in the lymph nodes, which represent the most commonly affected location, although very rare examples affecting extranodal tissues have also been reported. Older adults are the most affected individuals without a clear sex predominance. In situ mantle cell neoplasia contains some cells in the inner layer of the mantle zone surrounding reactive germinal centers that express Cyclin D1 and carry the t(11;14) mutation, but it only infrequently progresses to an overt lymphoma.

Mantle cell lymphoma more often affects elderly males, usually in their seventh decade of life, and the lymph nodes are the most affected locations, but splenomegaly and bone marrow involvement by tumor cells are also considered common findings. Extranodal manifestations of the disease can be found in approximately 25% of the cases, especially in the gastrointestinal tract, ocular adnexal region, lungs, pleurae, skin, brain and Waldeyer's ring. This lymphoma usually manifests as an advanced stage (Stage IV) and a disseminated disease, and therefore, any oral involvement necessarily demands from clinicians a complete systemic evaluation of the patient. The head and neck region is the second most affected extranodal site, and the oropharynx and the nasopharynx seem to be the most affected locations, where mantle cell lymphoma seems to be diagnosed in earlier stages. In the oral cavity the tumor usually affects the palate and the lips, causing an asymptomatic, ill-defined non-ulcerated swelling. Multiple simultaneous lesions or bilateral lesions affecting different sites of the oral cavity can be found. The overlying mucosa may be normal-colored or may show a bluish to purple color, with or without superficial telangiectasia.

The prognosis and the median overall survival of patients affected by mantle cell lymphoma have improved significantly over the last years. However, mantle cell lymphoma is still considered a very heterogeneous disease regarding its clinical behavior. A subgroup of patients does not require

C. V. B. L. de Caceres (✉) · F. P. Fonseca
Department of Oral Surgery and Pathology, School of Dentistry, Universidade Federal de Minas Gerais, Belo Horizonte, Brazil

R. G. de Resende
Department of Oral Medicine, Hospital Metropolitano Odilon Behrens (Odilon Behrens Metropolitan Hospital), Belo Horizonte, Brazil

G. R. A. de Mendonça
Department of Pathology, School of Medical Sciences, University of Campinas, Campinas, Brazil

© The Author(s), under exclusive license to Springer Nature Switzerland AG 2025

F. P. Fonseca et al. (eds.), *Lymphoproliferative and Granulomatous Disorders of the Oral Cavity*,
https://doi.org/10.1007/978-3-031-98844-8_38

treatment for several years, whereas the majority of the individuals affected by the neoplasm will demonstrate an aggressive disease. Therefore, treatment may vary from a watch-and-wait strategy to intensive chemotherapy followed by bone-marrow transplantation in eligible patients. There is currently no gold standard therapeutic approach for mantle cell lymphoma, which is most often treated with R-CHOP and cytarabine-containing regimens. Radiation and bone marrow transplant are variably used.

Stratifying patients according to their risk of death has become more important over the last years, and many different clinical and histological parameters may influence patients' prognosis, including cell proliferation (Ki67 expression) and aggressive histological variants (blastoid and pleomorphic). The mantle cell lymphoma International Prognostic Index (MIPI) score is used to stratify patients according to their prognostic risk and includes clinical parameters such as patient age, Eastern Cooperative Oncology Group (ECOG) performance score, lactate dehydrogenase level, and white blood cell count. Mutations involving the *TP53* gene with subsequent p53 immunoexpression, as well as a high Ki67 proliferative index, are also associated with a worse overall prognosis. (Fig. 38.1).

38.2 Microscopic Findings

- The neoplasm exhibits a diffuse growth pattern in most cases.
- A nodular growth pattern may be found in a few cases, as well as a "mantle zone" pattern surrounding germinal centers.
- Rare cases may exhibit a marginal zone growth pattern with cells containing a clear cytoplasm.
- The presence of tingible body macrophages in the blastoid and pleomorphic variants may focally give rise to the so-called "starry sky" pattern.
- In most cases, tumor cells present a more monomorphic appearance.
- The presence of scattered epithelioid macrophages is a common finding in mantle cell lymphoma.
- Mantle cell lymphoma can be cytologically classified as small cell [chronic lymphocytic leukemia/small lymphocytic lymphoma (CLL/SLL)-like], classic (centrocytic-like), blastoid or pleomorphic subtypes.
- The classic subtype is the most common and is characterized by the presence of small cells with irregular and cleaved nuclear contour, inconspicuous nucleoli and scant cytoplasm, resembling centrocytes.
- The small cell subtype is characterized by a monotonous proliferation of small round lymphoid cells that resemble those found in CLL/SLL.
- The blastoid subtype is characterized by the presence of medium-sized cells with inconspicuous nucleoli in a hyperchromatic nucleus, resembling lymphoblasts. This variant should be distinguished from lymphoblastic leukemia/lymphoma.
- The pleomorphic subtype shows a variable cellular morphology, with the presence of larger and atypical neoplastic cells, with prominent nucleoli. This variant must be distinguished from diffuse large B-cell lymphoma (Figs. 38.2, 38.3, and 38.4).

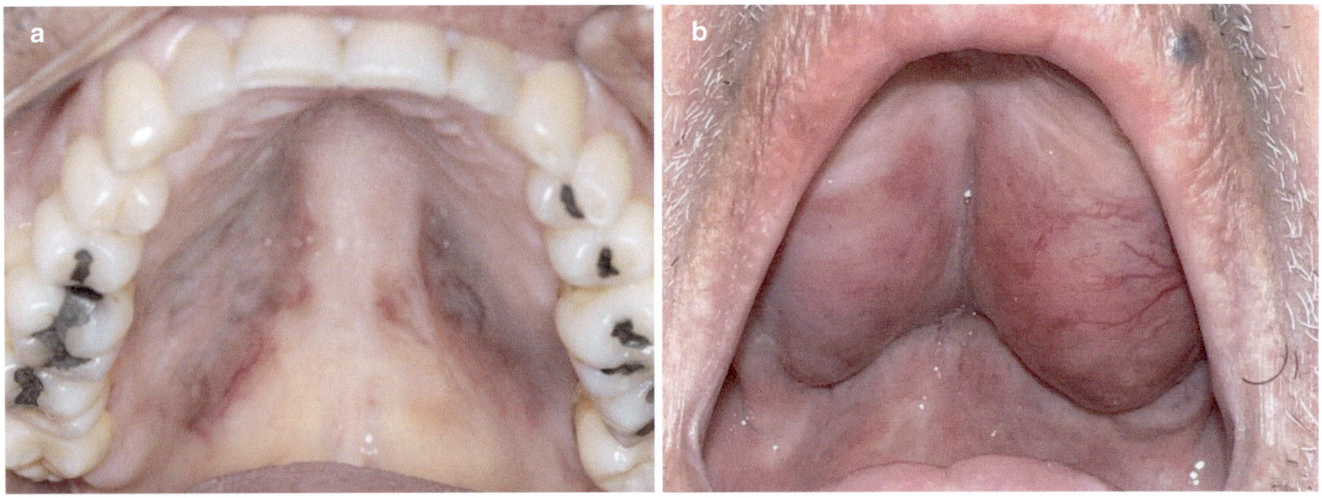

Fig. 38.1 Clinical presentation of mantle cell lymphoma in the oral cavity. (**a**) Male patient with bilateral involvement of the palate. Observe that the lesions present a bluish color with superficial telangiectasis. The patient already had a medical diagnosis of mantle cell lymphoma. (**b**) A male patient showing asymptomatic swellings affecting both sides of the palate

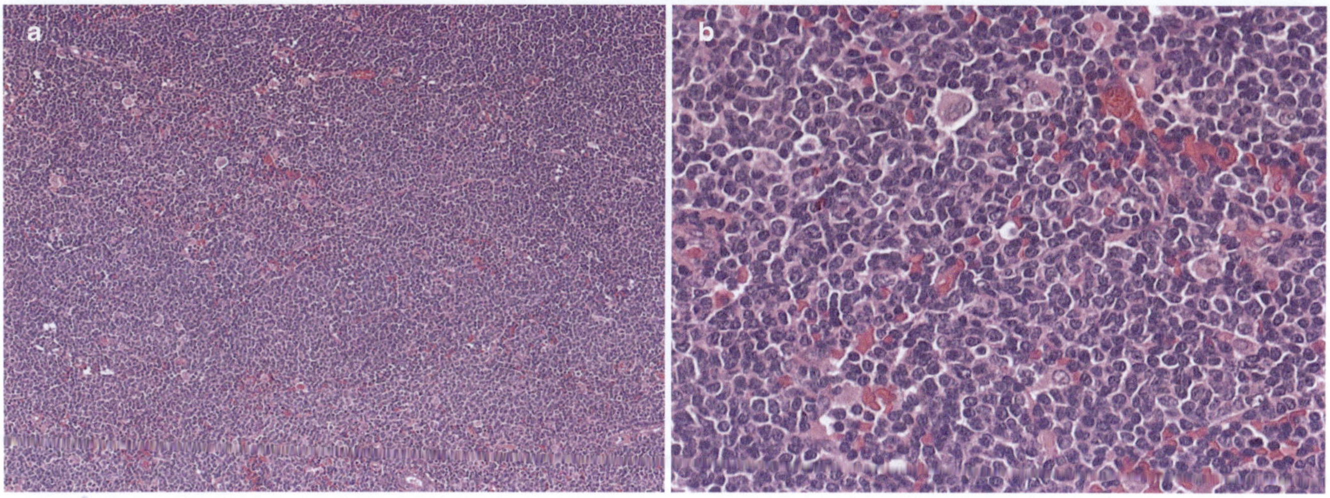

Fig. 38.2 Microscopic features of mantle cell lymphoma. (**a**) Tumor cells exhibit a diffuse and monotonous proliferation (H&E; 50×). (**b**) The neoplasm consists of small cells with hyperchromatic nuclei, inconspicuous nucleoli, scant cytoplasm. The nucleus often shows an irregular and cleaved morphology, resembling centrocytes. The presence of epithelioid macrophages exhibiting an eosinophilic cytoplasm and oval nucleus is a common finding (H&E; 100×)

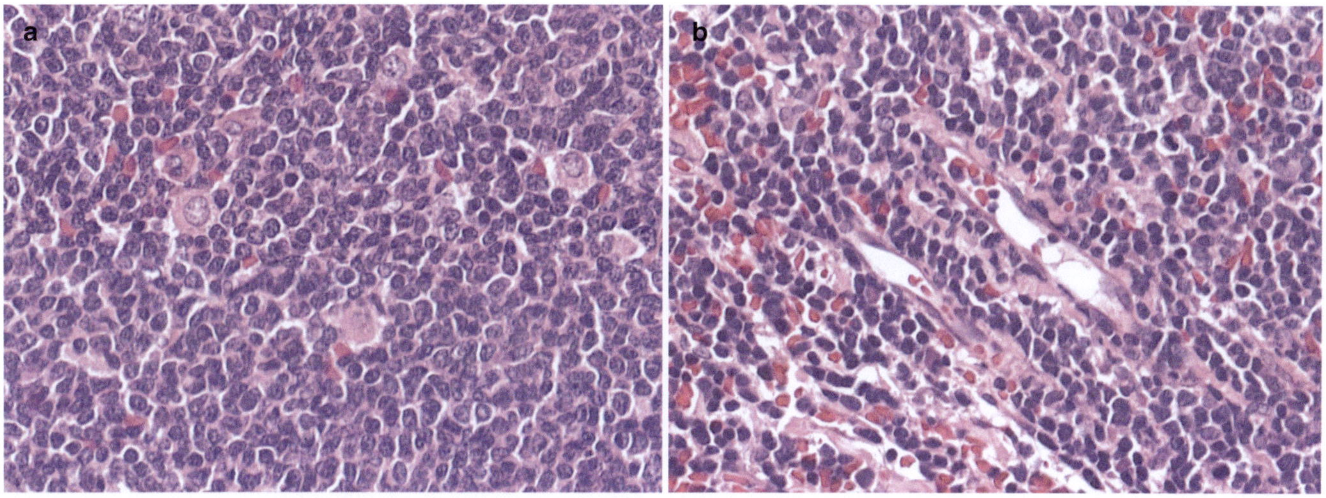

Fig. 38.3 Microscopic features of mantle cell lymphoma. (**a**) The tumor cell size can be measured by comparing the nucleus of the neoplastic cells with the nucleus of the macrophage. The tumor cells in mantle cell lymphoma are smaller (H&E; 200×). (**b**) However, because identifying a macrophage is often very difficult, the cell size can also be measured using endothelial cells as a reference. The small cells of mantle cell lymphoma exhibit a smaller to similar size of normal endothelial cells (H&E; 200×)

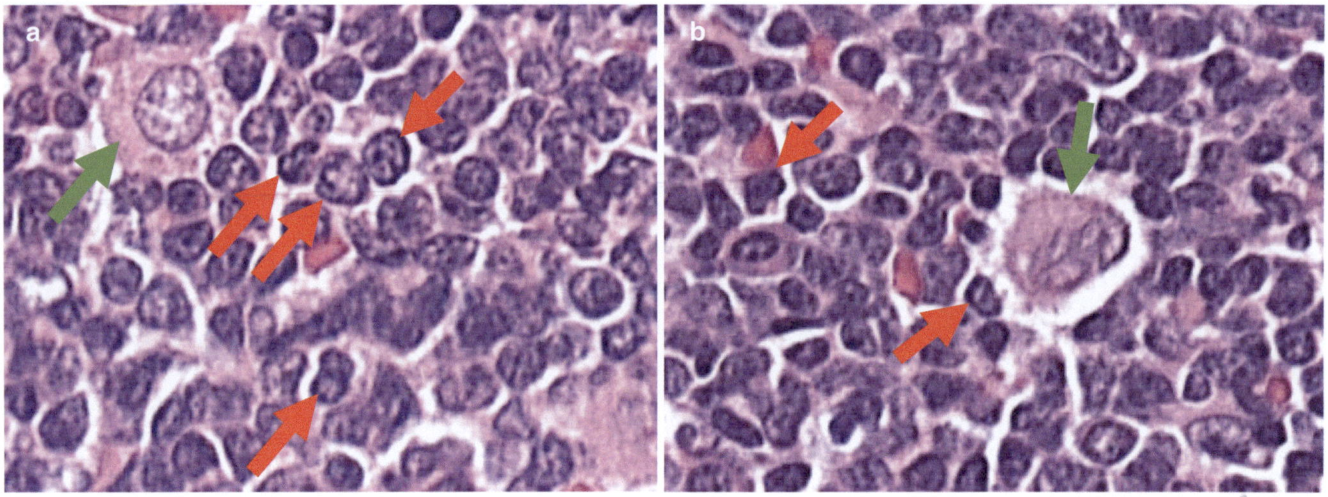

Fig. 38.4 Microscopic features of mantle cell lymphoma. (**a**) Tumor cells are predominantly small with irregular nuclear contour (red arrows). An epithelioid macrophage can be observed in this image (green arrow) (H&E; 400×). (**b**) Note the characteristic irregular or cleaved nuclear contour of tumor cells that are predominantly small and resemble centrocytes (red arrows). An epithelioid macrophage with large eosinophilic cytoplasm is also present in this image (green arrow) (H&E; 400×)

38.3 Immunohistochemistry and/or Genetics

Mantle cell lymphoma demonstrates the expression pattern observed in the normal mantle zone, with the expression of IgD and BCL2, but without the expression of germinal center markers like CD10 and BCL6, although these markers can be found in rare cases. Tumor cells are uniformly CD20 positive, but also aberrantly express, in the majority of cases, the T-cell marker CD5, like in chronic lymphocytic leukemia/small lymphocytic lymphoma; however, the lack of CD23 contributes to differentiating both neoplasms. Lymphoblastic leukemia/lymphoma should be distinguished from blastoid mantle cell lymphoma, and the lack of TdT/CD10 expression helps to differentiate these entities. The tumor is EBV negative, and the presence of the chromosomal translocation involving the *CCND1::IGH* genes leads to the overexpression of Cyclin D1 protein that is diffusely found in the nuclei of tumor cells. The nuclear expression of SOX11, a protein that is not expressed by normal lymphoid tissues nor by progenitor cells, is present in most of the mantle cell lymphomas, and it is also a very useful diagnostic marker, especially in those cases negative for *CCND1* mutation and Cyclin D1 expression. However, SOX11 is usually negative in leukemic non-nodal mantle cell lymphoma variant and may also be expressed by other lymphoma subtypes. Ki67 expression varies significantly depending on the histological subtype and represents an important prognostic marker, as well as *TP53* mutation and p53 protein expression. (Table 38.1; Figs. 38.5, 38.6, 38.7, 38.8, 38.9, 38.10, 38.11, and 38.12).

Table 38.1 Summary of the main immunohistochemical reactions used for mantle cell lymphoma diagnosis. The main molecular findings are also described

Antibody/ probe	Most frequent results	Pattern	Objective
CD20	Positive	Membrane	To demonstrate the B-cell origin of the neoplasm
CD3	Negative	Membrane	To exclude a possible T-cell origin of the neoplasm
CD5	Positive	Membrane	Aberrantly expressed in most cases. Negative cases occur.
BCL2	Positive	Cytoplasm	To characterize the neoplasm
CD10	Negative	Membrane	To exclude other small B-cell lymphomas originating from the germinal center
BCL6	Negative	Nucleus	To exclude other small B-cell lymphomas originating from the germinal center
CD23	Negative	Membrane	To exclude a CLL/SLL
Cyclin D1	Positive	Nucleus	To confirm the diagnosis of mantle cell lymphoma
SOX11	Positive	Nucleus	To confirm the diagnosis of mantle cell lymphoma
Ki67	Variable	Nucleus	To demonstrate the proliferative index of tumor cells
p53	Variable	Nucleus	Associated with prognostic determination
CCND1[a]	Present in 95% of the cases	–	To genetically characterize the neoplasm
CCND2[a]	Present in rare cases	–	To genetically characterize the neoplasm
CCND3[a]	Present in rare cases	–	To genetically characterize the neoplasm
TP53[a]	Variably present	–	To genetically characterize the neoplasm (prognostic importance)

[a]Investigated by fluorescent in situ hybridization or PCR. CLL/SLL: chronic lymphocytic leukemia /small lymphocytic lymphoma

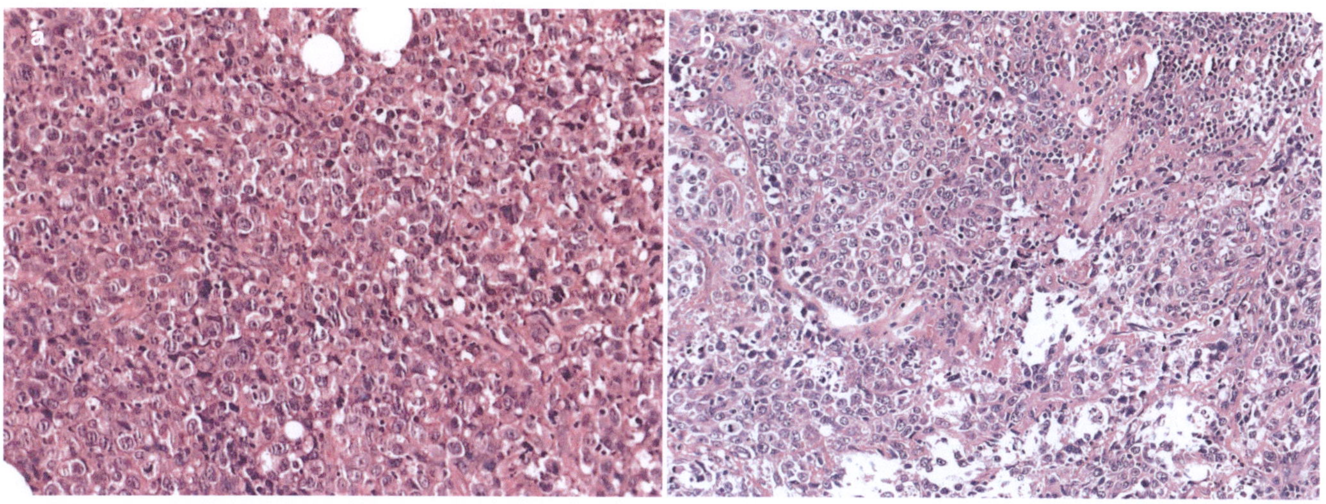

Fig. 38.5 Microscopic features of mantle cell lymphoma. (**a**) Mantle cell lymphoma exhibiting tumor cells with variable morphology and a higher degree of atypia is classified as pleomorphic subtype (H&E; 100×). (**b**) Observe the variability in the tumor cells nuclei, they are more pleomorphic than found in centrocytic/classic variant (H&E; 200×)

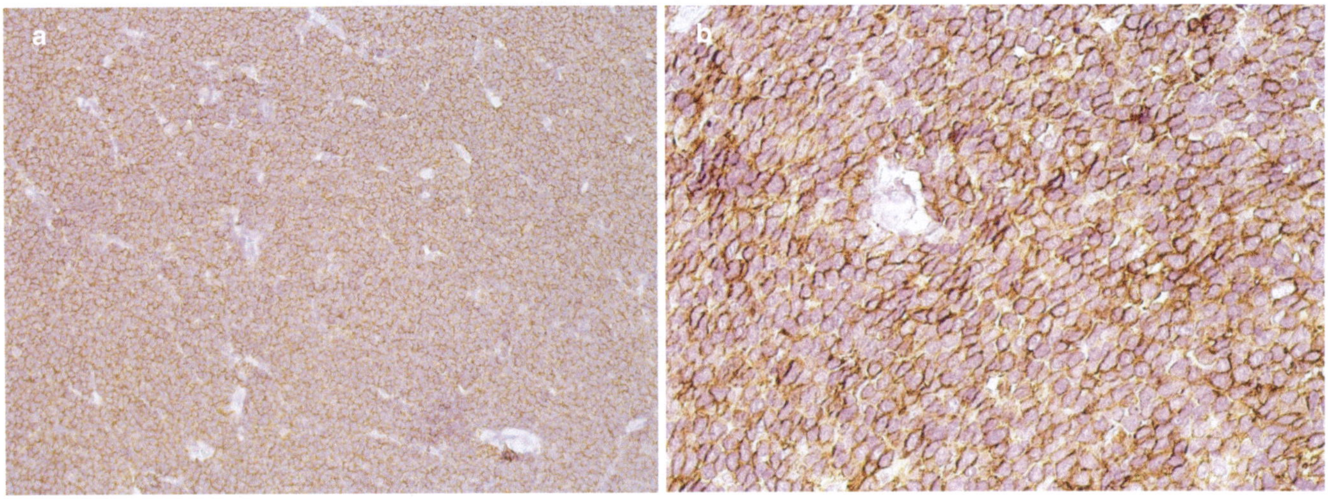

Fig. 38.6 Immunohistochemical features of mantle cell lymphoma. (**a**) Tumor cells are strongly and diffusely positive for CD20 (DAB; 100×), (**b**) Note the strong expression of CD20 in the membrane of tumor cells (DAB; 400×)

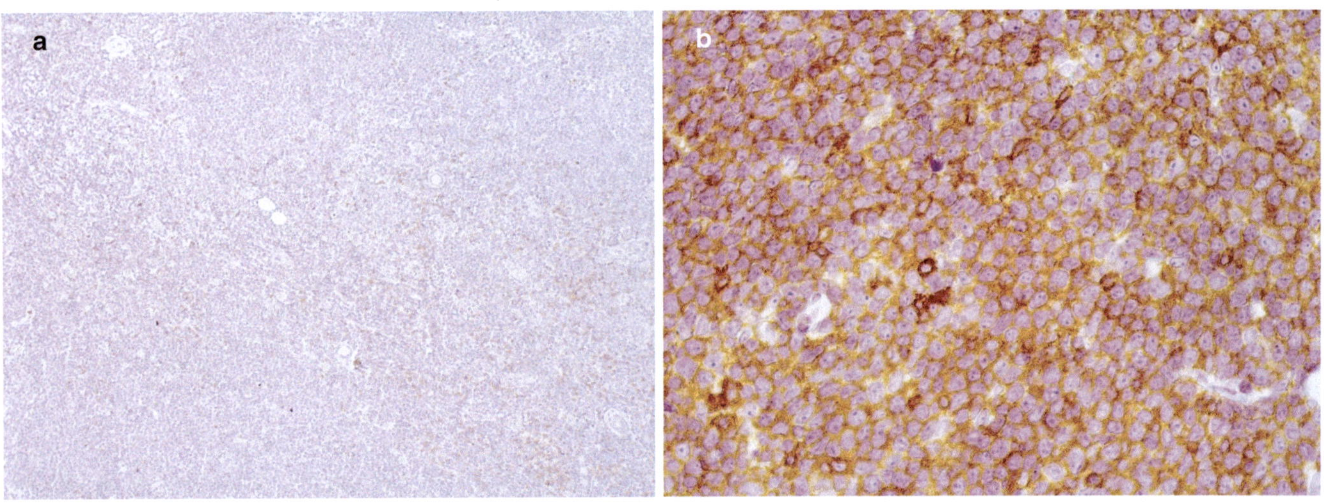

Fig. 38.7 Immunohistochemical features of mantle cell lymphoma. (**a**) Negative expression of CD3 in the tumor cells, with scattered positive cells representing reactive T lymphocytes (DAB; 50×). (**b**) Mantle cell lymphoma characteristically demonstrates the aberrant expression of CD5 protein. Note the diffuse expression in the membrane of the neoplastic cells (DAB; 400×)

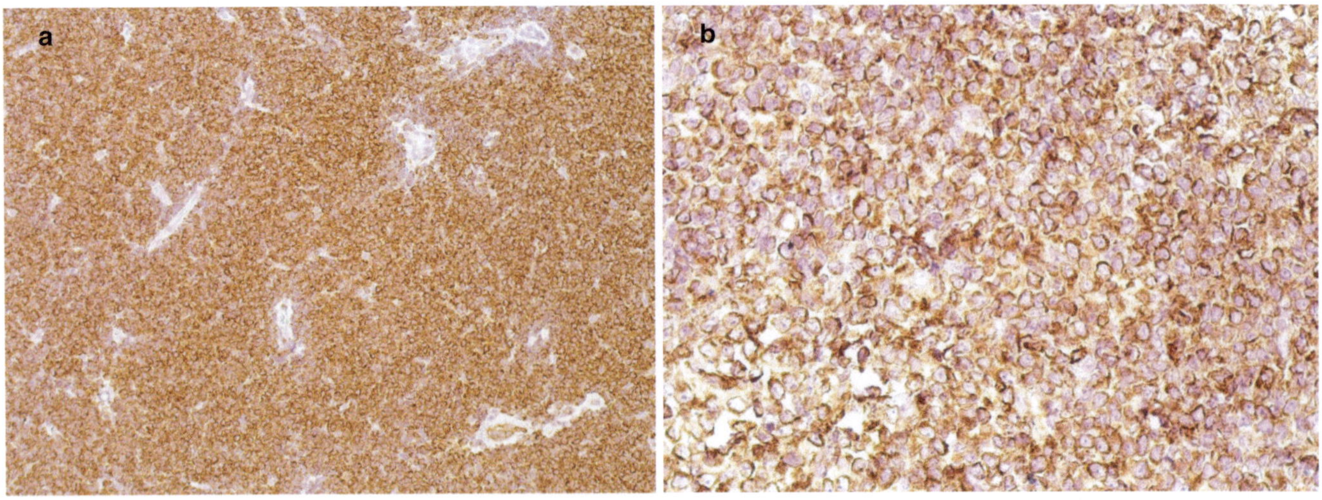

Fig. 38.8 Immunohistochemical features of mantle cell lymphoma. (**a**) Diffuse expression of BCL2 protein is a common finding in this neoplasm (DAB; 100×). (**b**) Observe the strong membranous expression pattern of BCL2 protein (DAB; 400×)

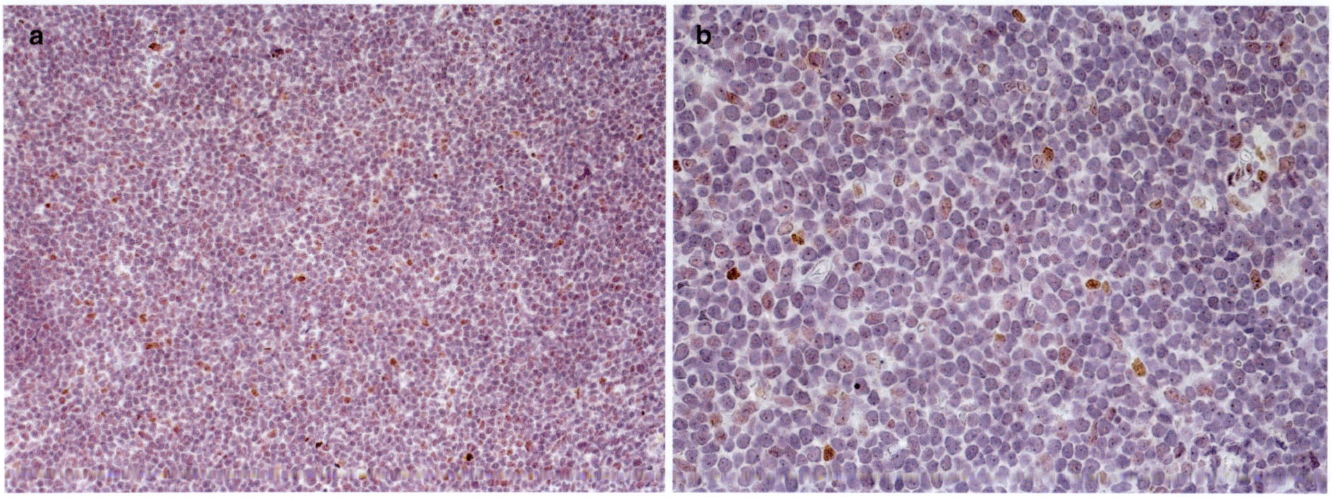

Fig. 38.9 Immunohistochemical features of mantle cell lymphoma. (**a**) Nuclear expression of p53 protein in tumor cells. A higher expression of this protein has been associated with a poorer prognosis for affected patients (DAB; 100×). (**b**) Note the nuclear expression pattern of p53 protein in some neoplastic cells (DAB; 400×)

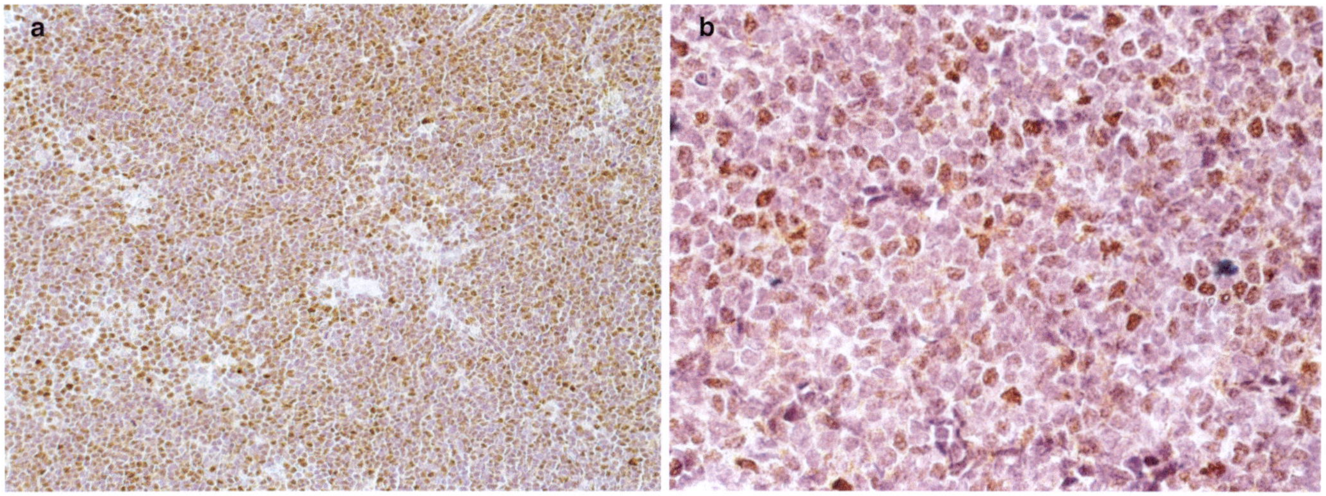

Fig. 38.10 Immunohistochemical features of mantle cell lymphoma. (**a**) Mantle cell lymphoma is typically positive for Cyclin D1 protein expression. The neoplasm exhibits a strong and diffuse expression of the protein (DAB; 100×). (**b**) Note the nuclear expression of Cyclin D1 protein in the majority of tumor cells and the different intensity in the protein expression among tumor cells (DAB; 400×)

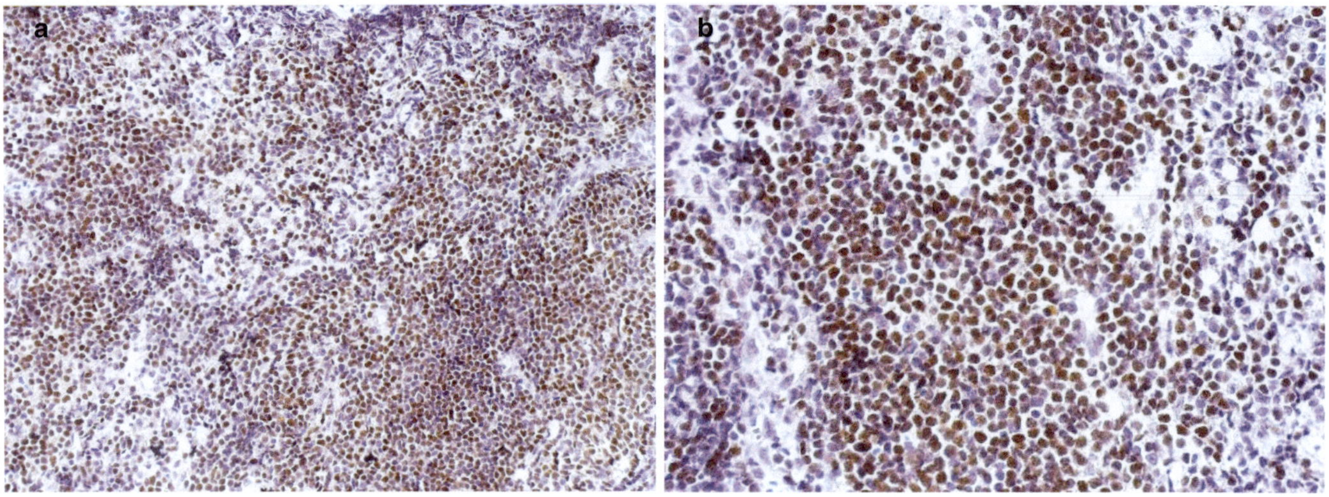

Fig. 38.11 Immunohistochemical features of mantle cell lymphoma. (**a**) The diffuse nuclear expression of SOX11 is frequently found in this neoplasm (DAB; 100×). (**b**) The nuclear expression of SOX11 protein is observed in this image. The presence of this protein is a very useful marker for Cyclin D1-negative mantle cell lymphomas (DAB; 400×)

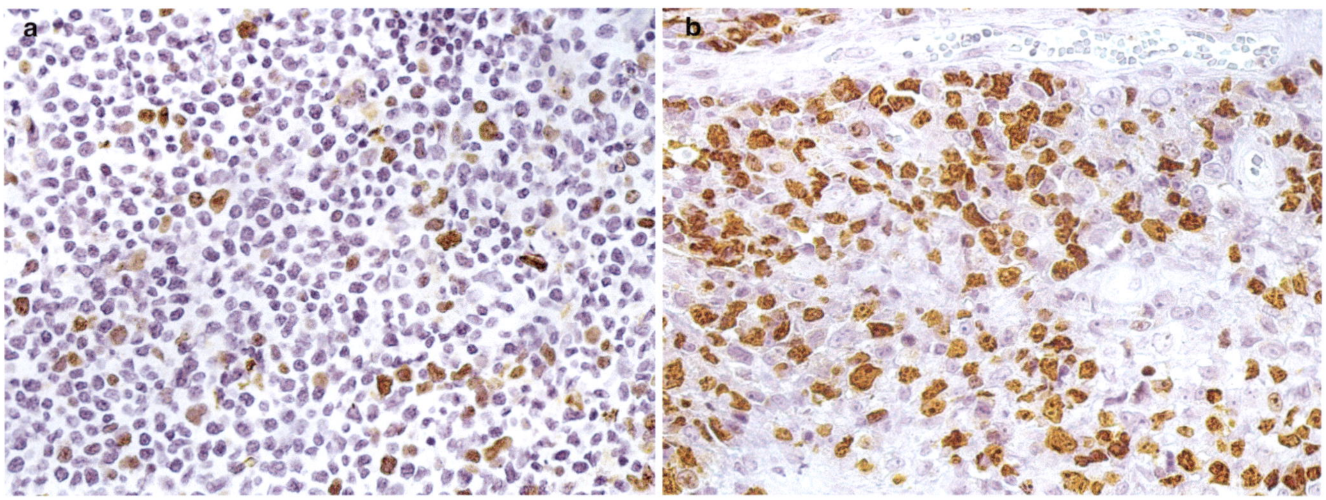

Fig. 38.12 Immunohistochemical features of mantle cell lymphoma. (**a**) The proliferative potential of mantle cell lymphoma varies. It is commonly associated with the microscopic pattern of the tumor, exhibiting a higher index in more pleomorphic subtypes. Observe in this image that Ki67 expression is lower than 30%, a cut-off value frequently associated with patients' prognosis (DAB; 400×). (**b**) An example of pleomorphic mantle cell lymphoma exhibiting a higher expression of Ki67 protein, higher than 30% and therefore, associated with a worse prognosis (DAB; 400×)

Sources

1. Rockacy J, Viozzi CF, Zent CS. Mantle cell lymphoma presenting as a slowly enlarging lesion of the floor of mouth in a healthy 72-year-old female: report of a case. J Oral Maxillofac Surg. 2007;65(2):333–7. https://doi.org/10.1016/j.joms.2005.06.024.
2. Guggisberg K, Jordan RC. Mantle cell lymphoma of the oral cavity: case series and comprehensive review of the literature. Oral Surg Oral Med Oral Pathol Oral Radiol Endod. 2010;109(1):98–104. https://doi.org/10.1016/j.tripleo.2009.08.010.
3. Eskelund CW, Dahl C, Hansen JW, Westman M, Kolstad A, Pedersen LB, et al. TP53 mutations identify younger mantle cell lymphoma patients who do not benefit from intensive chemoimmunotherapy. Blood. 2017;130(17):1903–10. https://doi.org/10.1182/blood-2017-04-779736.
4. Marcucci M, Marcucci G, Cordeiro MS, León JE, Araujo JP, de Oliveira JX, et al. Mantle cell lymphoma: involvement of nodal and extranodal sites in the head and neck, with multifocal oral lesions. Autops Case Rep. 2017;7(3):26–31. https://doi.org/10.4322/acr.2017.030.
5. Vergote V, Janssens A, André M, Bonnet C, Van Hende V, Van Den Neste E, et al. Results from the Belgian mantle cell lymphoma registry. Acta Clin Belg. 2017;72(3):172–8. https://doi.org/10.1080/17843286.2017.1293328.
6. Epperla N, Hamadani M, Fenske TS, Costa LJ. Incidence and survival trends in mantle cell lymphoma. Br J Haematol. 2018;181(5):703–6. https://doi.org/10.1111/bjh.14699.

7. Abukhiran I, Jasser J, Hoffman HT, Syrbu S. Mantle cell lymphoma involving major and minor salivary glands with parotid sparing. JAMA Otolaryngol Head Neck Surg. 2020;146(3):309–11. https://doi.org/10.1001/jamaoto.2019.4116.
8. Lukach L, Lehman H, Livoff A, Nahlieli O, Michaeli E, Allon I. Mantle cell lymphoma of the oral cavity: an uncommon site for an uncommon lesion, two new cases and literature review. Oral Oncol. 2020;103:104578. https://doi.org/10.1016/j.oraloncology.2020.104578.
9. Tashakori M, Kim DH, Kanagal-Shamanna R, Vega F, Miranda RN, Jain P, et al. Mantle cell lymphoma involving tonsils: a clinicopathologic study of 83 cases. Hum Pathol. 2021;118:60–8. https://doi.org/10.1016/j.humpath.2021.10.001.
10. Wagner VP, Rodrigues-Fernandes CI, Carvalho MVR, Dos Santos JN, Barra MB, Hunter KD, et al. Mantle cell lymphoma, malt lymphoma, small lymphocytic lymphoma, and follicular lymphoma of the oral cavity: an update. J Oral Pathol Med. 2021;50(6):622–30. https://doi.org/10.1111/jop.13214.
11. Breen CT, Chao J, Mehra S, Kohli N. Extranodal head and neck mantle cell lymphoma: characteristics, treatment, and survival. Ann Otol Rhinol Laryngol. 2022;131(4):412–9. https://doi.org/10.1177/00034894211025171.
12. Georgaki M, Theofilou VI, Pettas E, Piperi E, Stoufi E, Panayiotidis P, et al. Blastoid mantle cell lymphoma of the palate: report of a rare aggressive entity and review of the literature. Head Neck Pathol. 2022;16(2):631–42. https://doi.org/10.1007/s12105-021-01391-9.
13. Sander B, Campo E, Hsi ED. Chronic lymphocytic leukaemia/small lymphocytic lymphoma and mantle cell lymphoma: from early lesions to transformation. Virchows Arch. 2023 Jan;482(1):131–45. https://doi.org/10.1007/s00428-022-03460-y.
14. Carvalho MVR, Rodrigues-Fernandes CI, de Cáceres CVBL, Mesquita RA, Martins MD, Román Tager EMJ, et al. Mantle cell lymphoma involving the oral and maxillofacial region: a study of 20 cases. Oral Surg Oral Med Oral Pathol Oral Radiol. 2023;135(1):101–9. https://doi.org/10.1016/j.oooo.2022.08.018.
15. Zeng D, Fang Y, Fei Y, Liang R, Ye H, Liang Y, Sun X, et al. Treatment patterns and clinical outcomes of mantle cell lymphoma: a retrospective cohort study by CHOICE. Int J Cancer. 2023; https://doi.org/10.1002/ijc.34565.
16. Yang P, Cai QQ, Zhang W, Liu SZ, Liu H, Sun XH, et al. Real-world treatment and outcome patterns of patients with mantle cell lymphoma in China: a large, multicenter retrospective analysis. Cancer Med. 2023; https://doi.org/10.1002/cam4.6009.
17. Pahnke S, Abalo KD, Ekberg S, Albertsson-Lindblad A, Smedby KE, Jerkeman M, et al. Clinical characteristics and outcomes of 476 mantle cell lymphoma patients aged 80 years and older. Blood Cancer J. 2024;14(1):222. https://doi.org/10.1038/s41408-024-01204-6.
18. Muñoz J, Tsang M, Wang Y, Phillips T. Challenges of treating mantle cell lymphoma in older adults. Leuk Lymphoma. 2024:1–18. https://doi.org/10.1080/10428194.2024.2431563.
19. Barraclough A, Tang C, Lasica M, Smyth E, Cirillo M, Mutsando H, et al. Diagnosis and management of mantle cell lymphoma: a consensus practice statement from the Australasian Lymphoma Alliance. Intern Med J. 2024; https://doi.org/10.1111/imj.16561.

Burkitt Lymphoma

39

Chané Smit, Júlio Cesar Tanos de Lacerda, Javier Rendon Henao, Hélder Antônio Rebelo Pontes, and Felipe Paiva Fonseca

39.1 General Overview and Clinical Presentation

Burkitt lymphoma is an aggressive mature B-cell lymphoma. Although reports of possible examples of this malignancy had been published earlier at the beginning of the nineteenth century, it is accepted that this tumor was originally described as a more specific entity by the British surgeon Dr. Dennis Burkitt in 1958 as a round-cell sarcoma involving the jaws of African children in Uganda. It is currently defined by the World Health Organization classification of lymphoid tumors (WHO-HAEM5) as a monomorphic, medium-sized B-cell lymphoma with basophilic cytoplasm, multiple small nucleoli, a germinal-center B-cell phenotype, a high proliferation index, and an *IG::MYC* rearrangement. It is epidemiologically classified as endemic/African, sporadic/American or associated with immunosuppression. These subtypes demonstrate the same microscopic features but have different clinical presentations and different association rates with Epstein-Barr virus (EBV).

Burkitt lymphoma exhibits a male predominance and is reported to predominantly occur in young patients, ranging from less than a year to 19 years old, accounting for approximately 30 to 50% of all infantile lymphomas. Extranodal involvement is a frequent finding that usually affects the jaws, orbit bones, thyroid gland, nasal or oropharynx, ileocecal region, mediastinum, kidneys, ovaries, and breasts. Bone marrow infiltration may also occur and accounts for approximately 20% of the affected patients.

The *endemic* Burkitt lymphoma is typically diagnosed in the African continent, especially in the so-called "Lymphoma belt" region that includes countries like Papua New Guinea, Congo, Central African Republic, Zaire, and Cameroon. This region overlaps with endemic malaria infection, which is believed to interact with EBV and play some role in the etiology of the tumor. This variant more often affects children, and the mandible, maxilla and other facial bones are the most affected locations. Abdominal manifestation is also reported. There is a strong association with EBV infection that is present in virtually all cases. *Sporadic* Burkitt lymphoma occurs worldwide, but it is more commonly diagnosed in North America and Europe, and patients usually show abdominal or ileocecal tumors in children and young adults. In this variant, EBV is present in approximately 30% of the cases. In the variant *associated with immunosuppression*, more commonly HIV infection, the neoplasm more frequently affects the lymph nodes. Furthermore, the occurrence of leukemic presentation and bone marrow infiltration is more common than in the other variants, and the frequency of EBV is varied, ranging from 30 to 50% of the cases. The involvement of the central nervous system may occur in any of the epidemiological variants, and the characteristic rapid growth of the neoplasm due to the short doubling time of the tumor cells is an important clinical observation to support the diagnosis.

The etiology of Burkitt lymphoma is highly complex, and some cases have been strongly associated with chronic exposure to *Plasmodium falciparum* and EBV infection. Moreover, immunosuppression due to HIV infection and the prolonged course of post-transplant patients has been

C. Smit (✉)
Department of Oral and Maxillofacial Pathology, School of Dentistry, University of Pretoria, Pretoria, South Africa
e-mail: chane.smit@up.ac.za

J. C. T. de Lacerda
Department of Oral Medicine, Hospital Metropolitano Odilon Behrens (Odilon Behrens Metropolitan Hospital), Belo Horizonte, Brazil

J. R. Henao
Department of Hematopathology and Flow Cytometry, Ayudas Diagnósticas Sura Center, Cartagena, Colombia

H. A. R. Pontes
Service of Oral Pathology, João de Barros Barreto University Hospital, Federal University of Pará, Belém, Brazil

F. P. Fonseca
Department of Oral Surgery and Pathology, School of Dentistry, Universidade Federal de Minas Gerais, Belo Horizonte, Brazil

© The Author(s), under exclusive license to Springer Nature Switzerland AG 2025

F. P. Fonseca et al. (eds.), *Lymphoproliferative and Granulomatous Disorders of the Oral Cavity*,
https://doi.org/10.1007/978-3-031-98844-8_39

associated with an increased risk for developing this lymphoma. The WHO-HAEM5 guidelines now highlight the classification of Burkitt lymphoma according to EBV status, as either EBV-negative or EBV-positive cases, in addition to the classification based on epidemiological data, since this approach would better reflect the molecular characteristics of the tumor. The pathogenesis of this aggressive neoplasm has been better understood during the last decades, and Burkitt lymphoma is shown to carry a genetic hallmark characterized by chromosome translocation involving the *MYC* gene and one of the immunoglobulin genes. In approximately 85% of the cases, there is a t(8:14)/*IGH-MYC*, in 10% of the cases a t(8;22)(q24;q11) /*Ig-lambda* /*MYC* is found, and in approximately 5% of the cases, there is a t(2;8)(p12;q24) /*Ig-kappa*/*MYC* translocation.

In the oral cavity, Burkitt lymphoma commonly manifests as a painful swelling more frequently in the posterior region of the mandible. It often demonstrates a very rapid growth rate, usually extending to surrounding soft tissues of the palate, gingiva and buccal mucosa, with the presence of ulceration and areas of tissue necrosis. The occurrence of numb chin syndrome has been reported in a few cases. In many patients, the tumor manifests as simultaneous multiple lesions in both jaws, and radiographically, it presents as an ill-defined osteolytic image, which causes expansion and destruction of the cortical plates and alveolar bone, leading to tooth mobility and displacement. The so-called "floating tooth" radiographic appearance is frequently observed, especially when the alveolar bone is extensively destroyed.

Although Burkitt lymphoma is a highly aggressive neoplasm, it is considered a curable disease. Several combinations of immunochemotherapy, including the use of cyclophosphamide, prednisolone, and vincristine, with or without methotrexate and cytarabine, associated with the use of Rituximab, remain the primary choice of treatment. A bone marrow transplant is also recommended in some cases. Relapse and progression frequency vary, but the overall survival ranges from 70% to 90% after 5 years of follow-up with proper treatment access. The treatment outcomes differ significantly between children and adults; the latter present a worse outcome. The geographical distribution of the patients still holds a strong prognostic impact for Burkitt lymphoma, with patients living in developed countries presenting a much higher survival and excellent prognosis than those living in low-income/developing regions (Figs. 39.1, 39.2, 39.3, 39.4, 39.5, and 39.6).

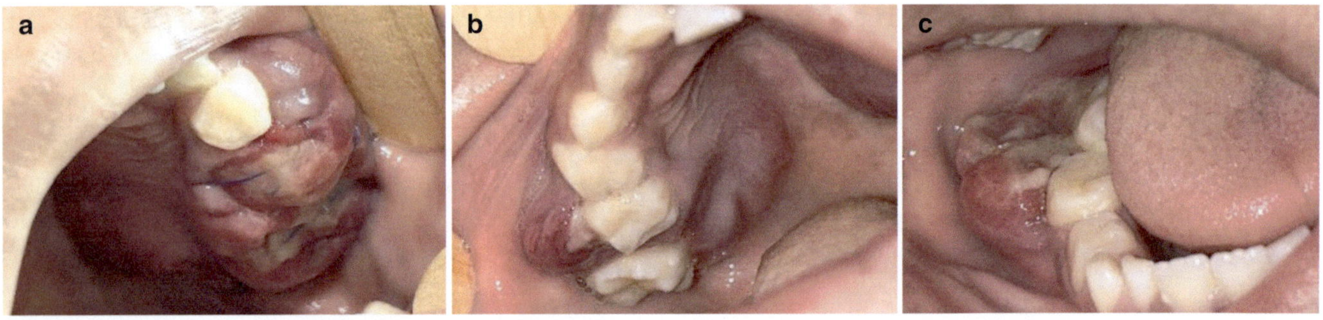

Fig. 39.1 Clinical presentation of Burkitt lymphoma affecting the oral cavity of an infant patient. (**a**) The neoplasm affected multiple regions simultaneously. Observe the lesion affecting the maxillary mucosa on the left side with an ulcerated surface and necrotic tissue. (**b**) The tumor also concurrently affected the right side of the maxilla, with expansion to the palate and the vestibular mucosa. (**c**) In the mandible, the tumor exhibited an ulcerated swelling, with areas of necrosis and displacement of adjacent teeth

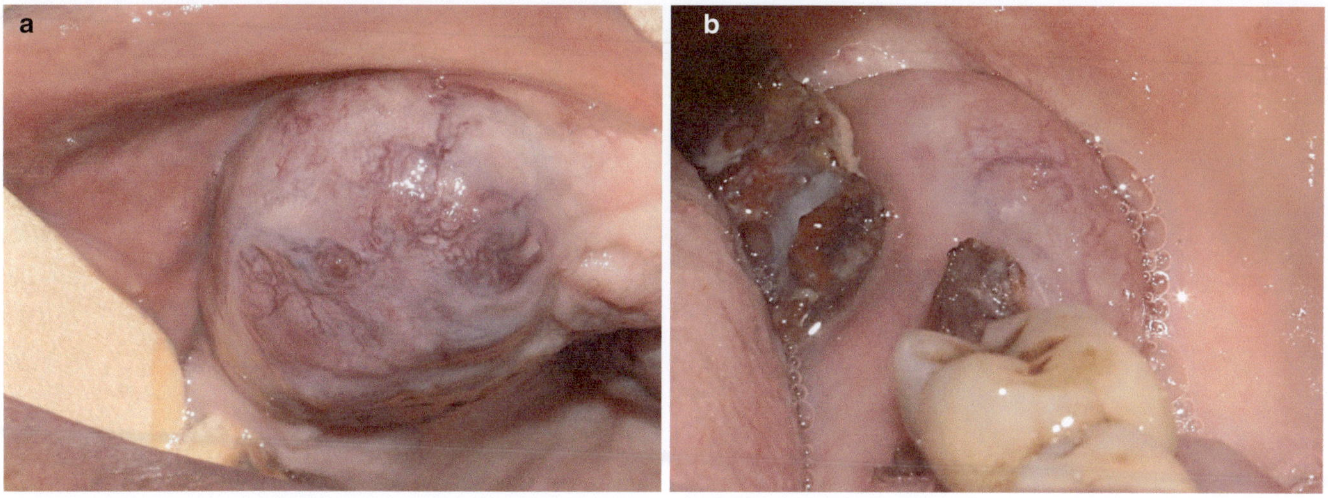

Fig. 39.2 Clinical presentation of Burkitt lymphoma affecting the oral cavity. (**a**) The patient had multiple lesions in the oral cavity. The maxilla exhibited an expansive tumor with purple-colored appearance and superficial telangiectasia. (**b**) The tumor also manifested in the left side of the mandible, causing an expansive growth around the second molar

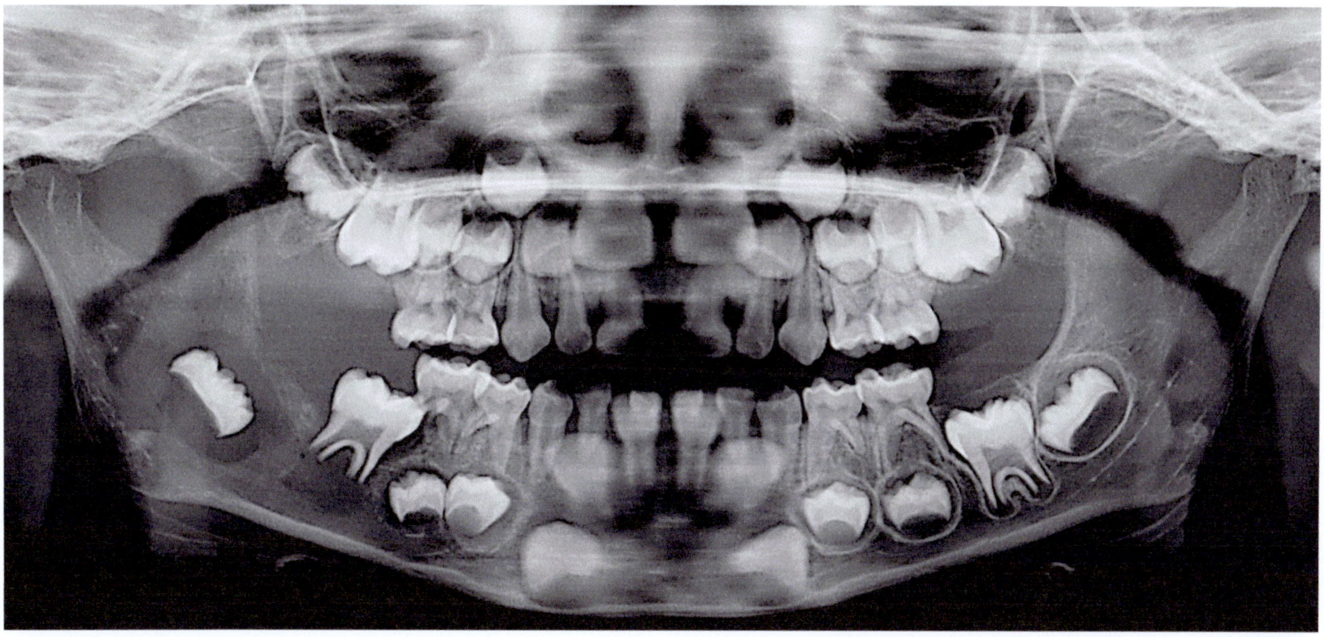

Fig. 39.3 Radiographic findings in a case of Burkitt lymphoma affecting a child. Observe the extensive radiolucent, poorly defined image affecting the posterior region of the mandible on the right side. There is a loss of cortication of the anterior ramus border, expansion of the follicular space around the second developing molar and loss of lamina dura around the first molar

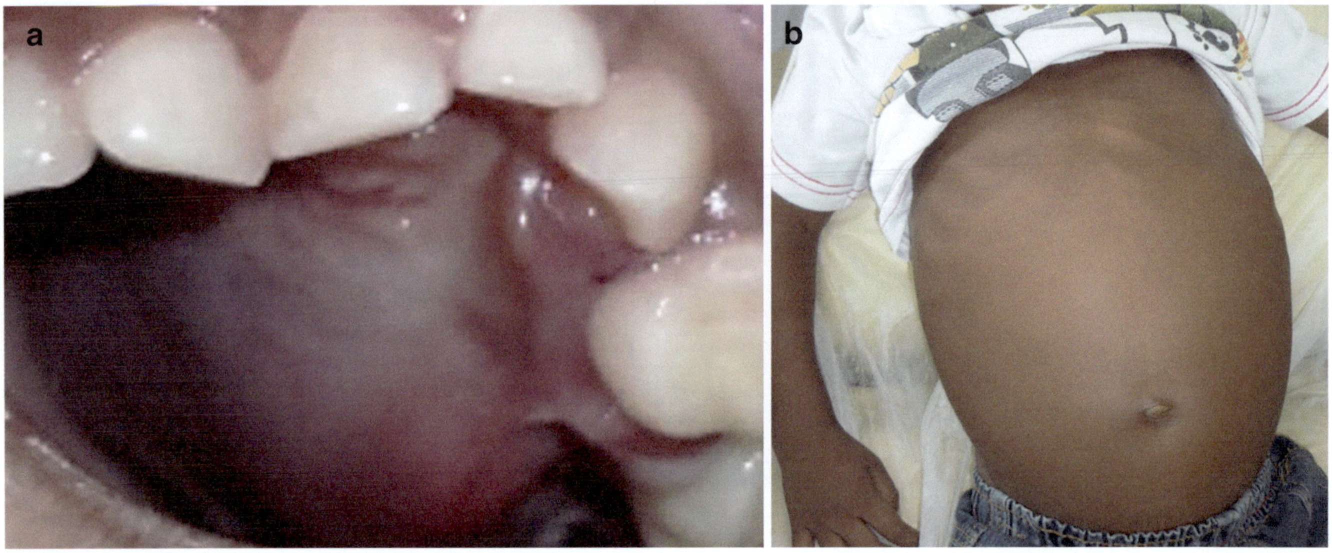

Fig. 39.4 Clinical presentation of Burkitt lymphoma affecting a pediatric patient. (**a**) Extensive swelling of the palate. (**b**) This patient also exhibited abdominal involvement by the neoplasm

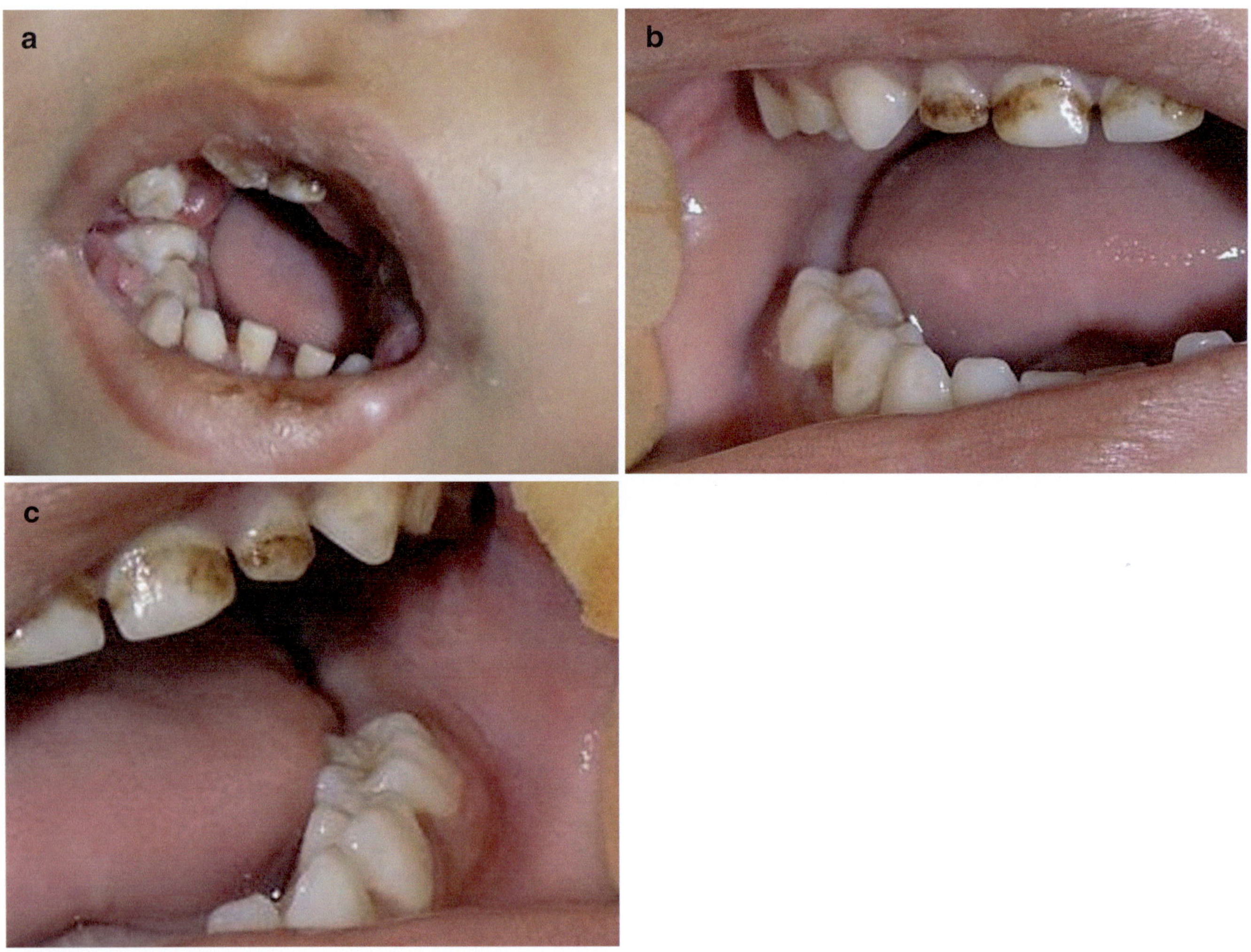

Fig. 39.5 Clinical presentation of Burkitt lymphoma affecting a pediatric patient. (**a**) The neoplasm simultaneously involved both maxilla and mandible bilaterally. The patient had a limited mouth opening. (**b**) Following chemotherapy, the neoplasm exhibited complete resolution as illustrated by these images of the right side and (**c**) the left side, demonstrating that despite its clinical aggressiveness, Burkitt lymphoma is a curable disease

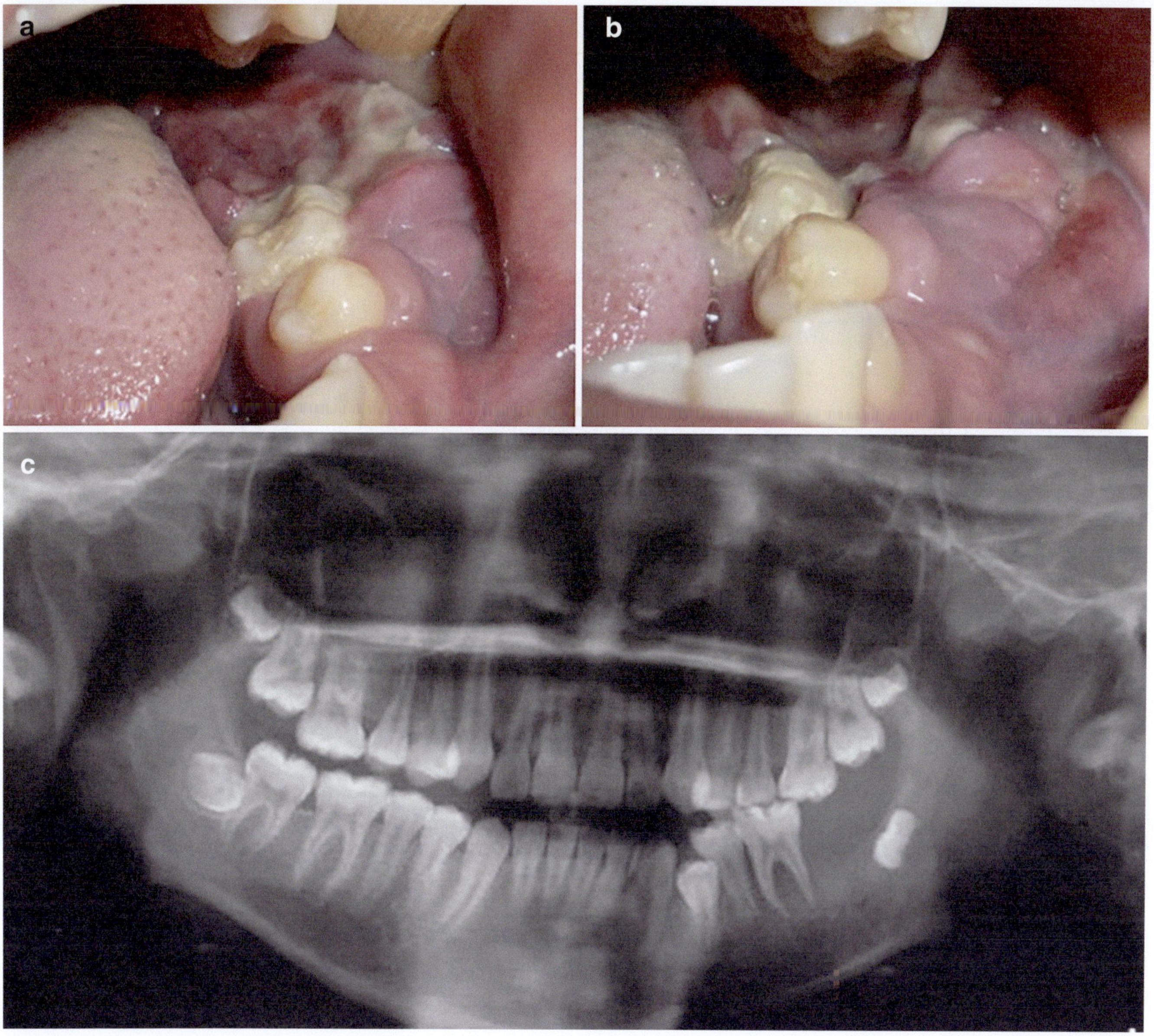

Fig. 39.6 Clinical presentation of Burkitt lymphoma affecting a young male patient. (**a**) Large painful swelling affecting the posterior region of the mandible, right side. (**b**) Note the first molar displacement and yellowish areas consistent with tissue necrosis. (**c**) Typical radiographic presentation of Burkitt lymphoma exhibiting alveolar bone destruction and the "floating tooth" appearance of the first lower left molar

39.2 Microscopic Findings

- The neoplasm characteristically demonstrates a diffuse growth pattern of monomorphic neoplastic cells, with little cytologic variability.
- Scant fibrous stroma.
- Presence of tingible body macrophages that give rise to the so-called "starry sky" or "water pot" microscopic pattern. This finding is a typical feature of Burkitt lymphoma, but it can also be observed in other lymphomas that also have high proliferative rates.
- Neoplastic cells are often organized very close to each other, leading to the "puzzle-like" or "squared-off" appearance.
- Predominance of intermediate-size neoplastic cells that exhibit hyperchromatic round nuclei and scant eosinophilic cytoplasm.
- Tumor cells are defined as predominantly intermediate in size because they are of a similar size to a macrophage nucleus.
- Multiple small nucleoli are usually observed, and can be more evident in some cases.
- Some degree of pleomorphism can be seen in some cases.
- The tingible body macrophages are typically clear cells and contain apoptotic debris inside the cytoplasm.
- Mitotic figures, apoptotic bodies and tissue necrosis are easily observed.
- Granulomatous reaction may be found in a few cases (Figs. 39.7, 39.8, 39.9, 39.10, 39.11, and 39.12).

39.3 Immunohistochemistry and/or Genetics

The tumor cells strongly and diffusely express mature B-cell markers like CD19, CD20, CD22, PAX5 and CD79a. Burkitt lymphoma is known to have a small number of reactive T lymphocytes, which is demonstrated by a few reactive cells staining for CD3. Due to the origin of tumor cells from the germinal center, CD10 and BCL6 are also strongly positive. BCL2 is negative or only focally positive, and any strong expression of BCL2 demands evaluation of a diffuse large B-cell lymphoma/high-grade B-cell lymphoma with dual rearrangements. The strong and diffuse expression of MYC protein in the nuclei of tumor cells (> 80%) is also common, and negative cases should be investigated for large B-cell lymphoma with mutation in 11q gain/loss aberration, especially in the presence of tingible body macrophages containing more than 10 apoptotic bodies/debris in their cytoplasm. The very high proliferative index demonstrated by Ki67 expression is typical of Burkitt lymphoma, approaching approximately 99% to 100% of positivity. It is important to differentiate Burkitt lymphoma from acute lymphoblastic lymphoma/leukemia, which also frequently affects pediatric patients and is microscopically similar; therefore, TdT negativity and CD20 strong positivity support the diagnosis of Burkitt lymphoma. The blastoid variant of mantle cell lymphoma must also be ruled out, and the lack of Cyclin D1 and SOX11 proteins contributes to a diagnosis of Burkitt lymphoma. The genetic hallmark of Burkitt lymphoma is the translocation involving *IG* and *MYC* genes, but other molec-

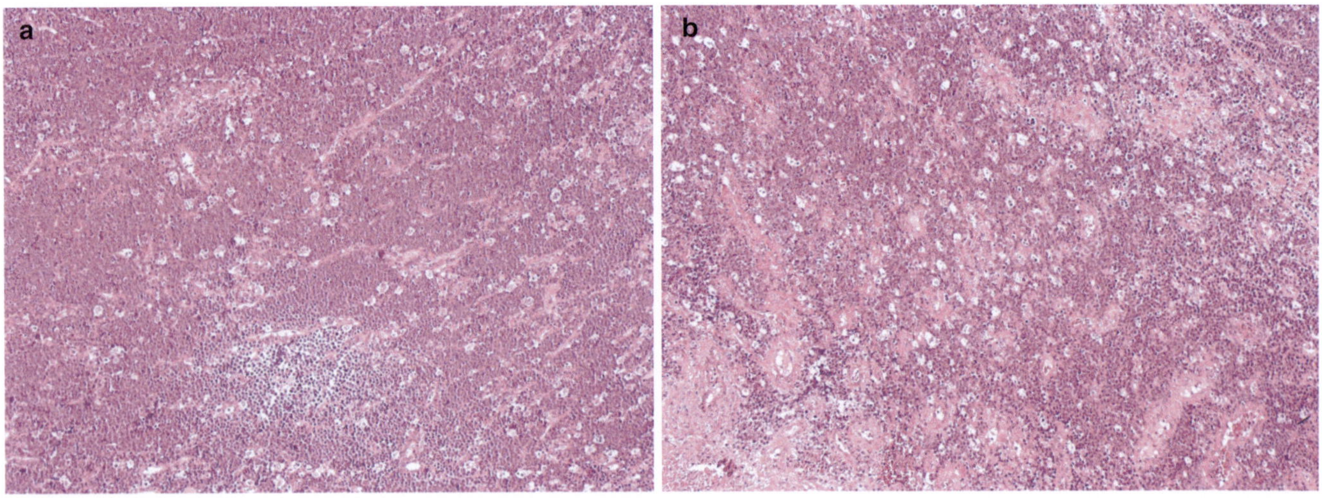

Fig. 39.7 Histopathologic features of Burkitt lymphoma. (**a**) Diffuse proliferation of tumor cells with the presence of a tingible body macrophage (H&E; 100×). (**b**) Observe the monophormous appearance of tumor cells with the characteristic "starry-sky" or "water pot" microscopic aspect (H&E; 100×)

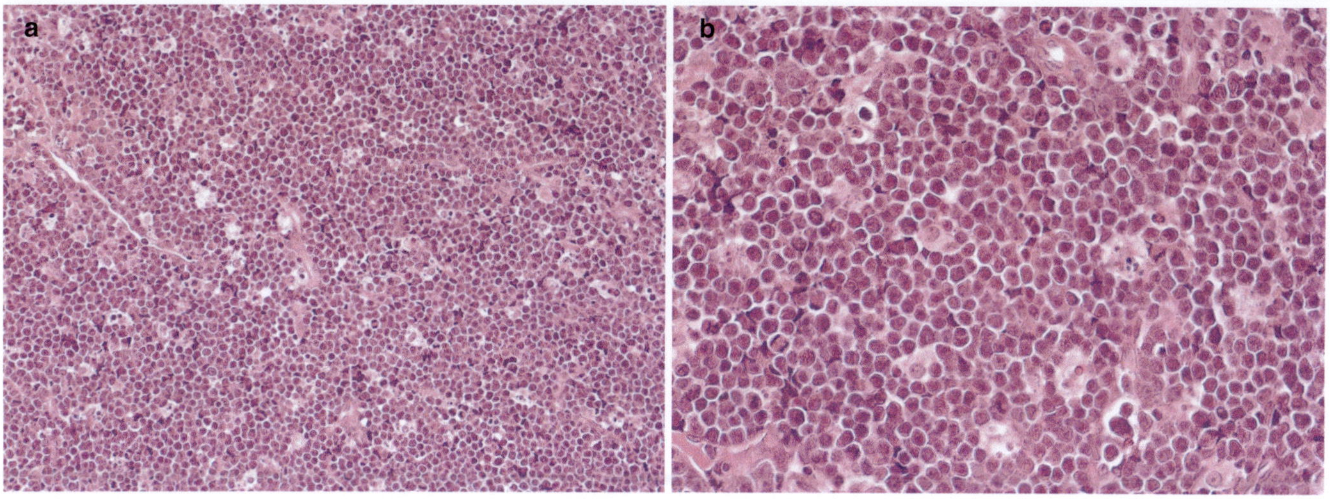

Fig. 39.8 Histopathologic features of Burkitt lymphoma. (**a**) Diffuse proliferation of tumor cells with the presence of a starry-sky pattern (H&E; 100×). (**b**) Neoplastic cells exhibited a predominantly monomorphic appearance. Tingible body macrophages presented a clear cytoplasm and were responsible for the starry-sky pattern (H&E; 200×)

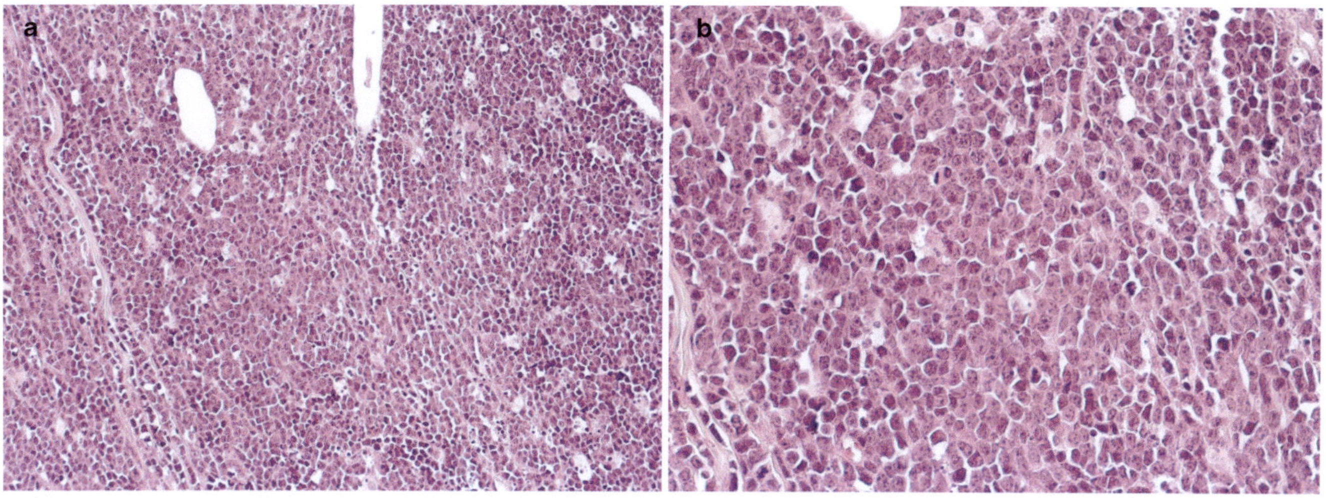

Fig. 39.9 Histopathologic features of Burkitt lymphoma. (**a**) Tumor cells are intermediate in size, exhibit round nuclei with inconspicuous nucleoli and scant basophilic cytoplasm (H&E; 100×). (**b**) Note that tumor cells are very close to each other, leading to a puzzle-like growth pattern (H&E; 200×)

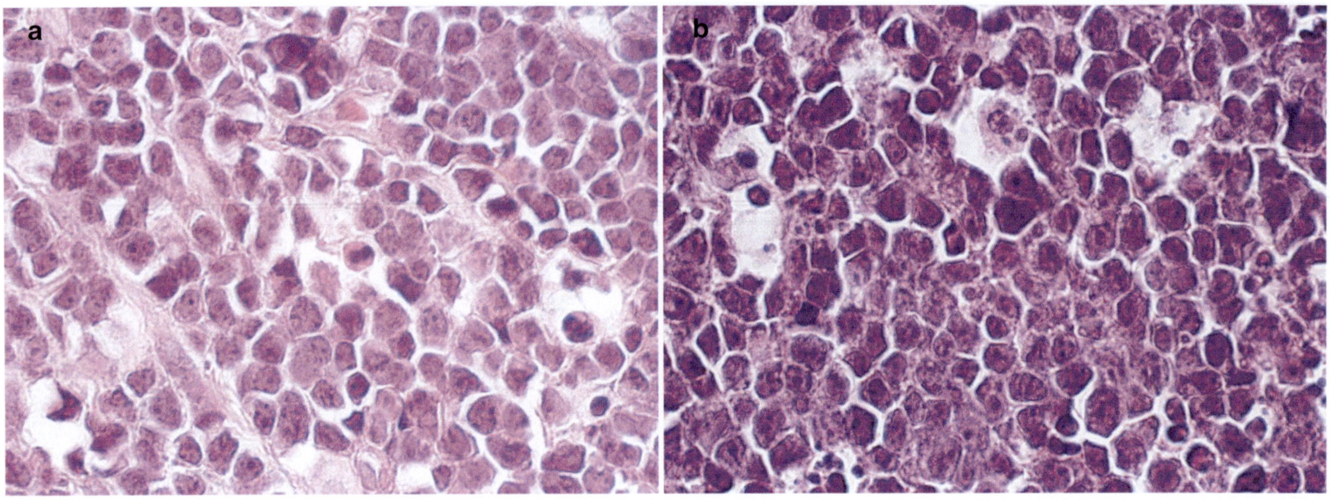

Fig. 39.10 Histopathologic features of Burkitt lymphoma. (**a**) Tumor cells are intermediate in size and exhibit round nuclei with multiple small nucleoli and scant basophilic cytoplasm (H&E; 400×). (**b**) Comparing the size of the nucleus of the macrophage and the size of the neoplastic cells, it is possible to observe a similar size, exemplifying an intermediate cell size lymphoma. Observe the presence of apoptotic bodies/debris in the cytoplasm of the tingible body macrophages (H&E; 400×)

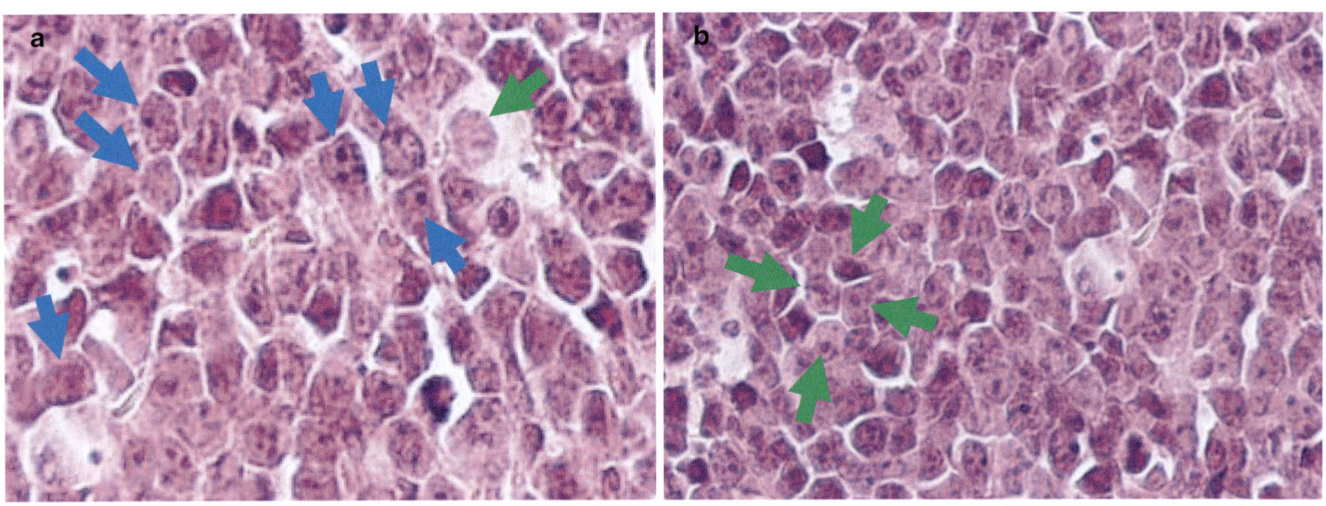

Fig. 39.11 Histopathologic features of Burkitt lymphoma. (**a**) Diffuse proliferation of neoplastic cells. Observe that the nuclear size of macrophages (green arrow) and the neoplastic cells (blue arrows) is very similar, leading to the classification of Burkitt lymphoma as an intermediate cell size lymphoma (H&E; 400×). (**b**) The tumor cells are very near to each other and the morphology of the cytoplasm of the cells seems to fit the neighboring cells, leading to the puzzle-like growth pattern of Burkitt lymphoma, as illustrated by the four cells indicated by green arrows (H&E; 400×)

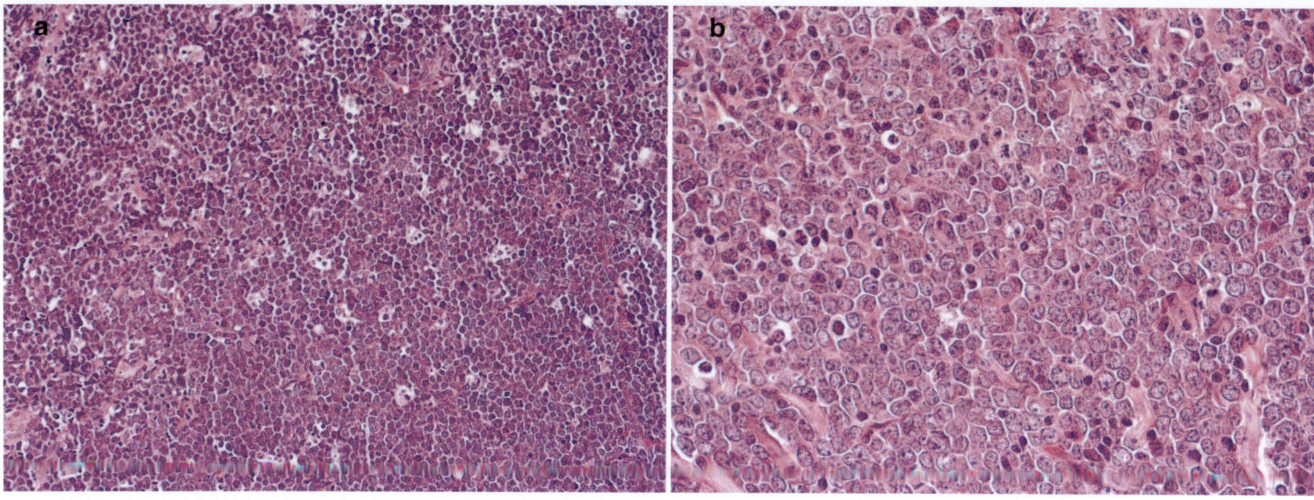

Fig. 39.12 Histopathologic features of Burkitt lymphoma. (**a**) The neoplasm is characterized by medium-sized tumor cells, with a starry sky pattern (H&E; 200×). (**b**) Note the small nucleoli and the square-off growth pattern of tumor cells. Mitotic figures are common (H&E; 400×)

Table 39.1 Summary of the main immunohistochemical reactions used for Burkitt lymphoma diagnosis. The main results for EBV detection and molecular findings are also described

Antibody/probe	Most frequent results	Pattern	Objective
CD20	Positive	Membrane	To demonstrate the B-cell origin
CD79a	Positive	Membrane	To demonstrate the B-cell origin
CD3	Negative	Membrane	To exclude a T-cell origin
CD10	Positive	Membrane	To demonstrate the germinal center origin of tumor cells
BCL2	Negative or only focally positive	Cytoplasm	To investigate a possible high-grade B-cell lymphoma
BCL6	Positive	Nucleus	To demonstrate the germinal center origin of tumor cells
MYC	Positive	Nucleus	Associated with the pathogenesis of the tumor
TdT	Negative	Nucleus	To exclude the diagnosis of lymphoblastic leukemia/lymphoma
Cyclin D1	Negative	Nucleus	To exclude the diagnosis of mantle cell lymphoma
SOX11	Variable[d]	Nucleus	To exclude the diagnosis of mantle cell lymphoma
Ki67	~99–100%	Nucleus	It illustrates the high proliferative potential of the tumor
EBER[a]	Variable positivity[c]	Nucleus	To demonstrate the presence of EBV
MYC[b]	Positive	–	Tumor biological and molecular characterization

[a]Investigated by in situ hybridization
[b]Investigated by fluorescent in situ hybridization or PCR
[c]The frequency of EBV positivity depends on the epidemiological variant of the tumor
[d]The expression of SOX11 is observed in EBV-negative Burkitt lymphomas

ular events have already been described in a varied frequency, including alterations in *TP53*, *TCF3, ID3* and the *PI3K* pathway, with molecular differences being observed between EBV-negative and EBV-positive Burkitt lymphomas, therefore, reinforcing the etiopathogenic role of this virus. (Table 39.1; Figs. 39.13, 39.14, 39.15, and 39.16).

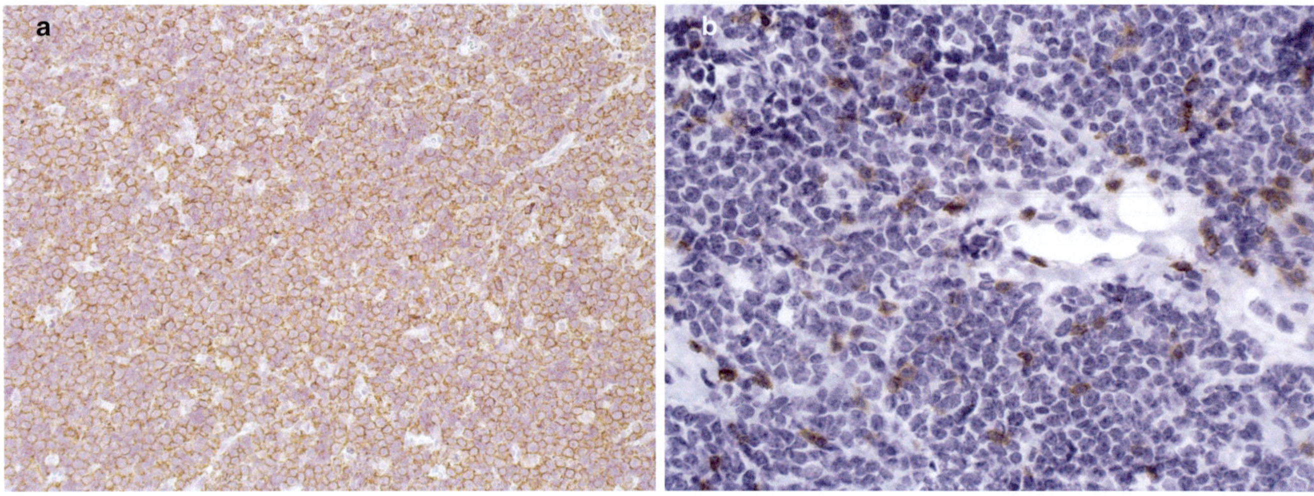

Fig. 39.13 Immunohistochemical features of Burkitt lymphoma. (**a**) Burkitt lymphoma is a mature B-cell neoplasm and exhibits a strong and diffuse expression for CD20 (DAB; 100×). (**b**) There is a small number of reactive T lymphocytes evidenced by CD3 staining (DAB; 200×)

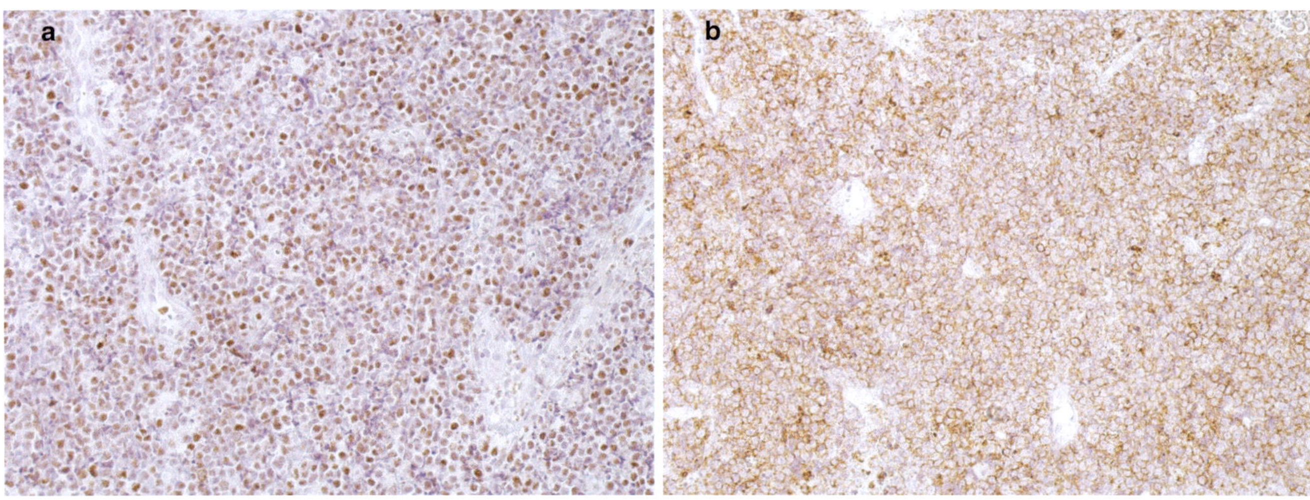

Fig. 39.14 Immunohistochemical features of Burkitt lymphoma. (**a**) Germinal center origin of the neoplastic cells of Burkitt lymphoma is demonstrated by a strong and diffuse nuclear expression of Bcl6 (DAB; 100×) and (**b**) membrane expression of CD10 (DAB; 100×)

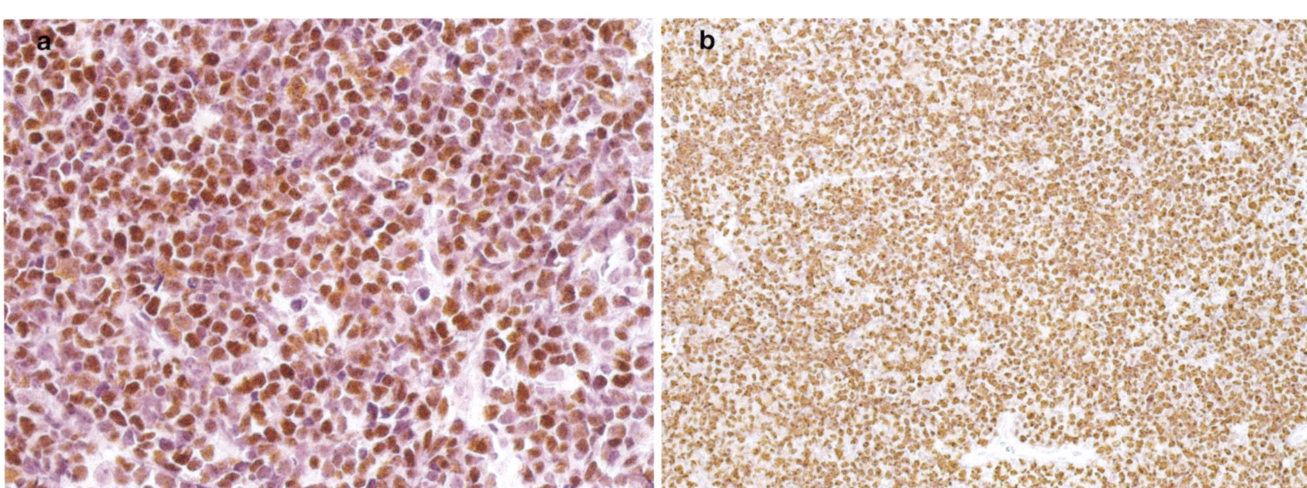

Fig. 39.15 Immunohistochemical features of Burkitt lymphoma. (**a**) Tumor cells are characteristically positive for the nuclear expression of c-Myc (DAB; 200×). (**b**) The very high proliferative index of Burkitt lymphoma is illustrated by the expression of Ki67 that achieves approximately 99% of positivity (DAB; 100×)

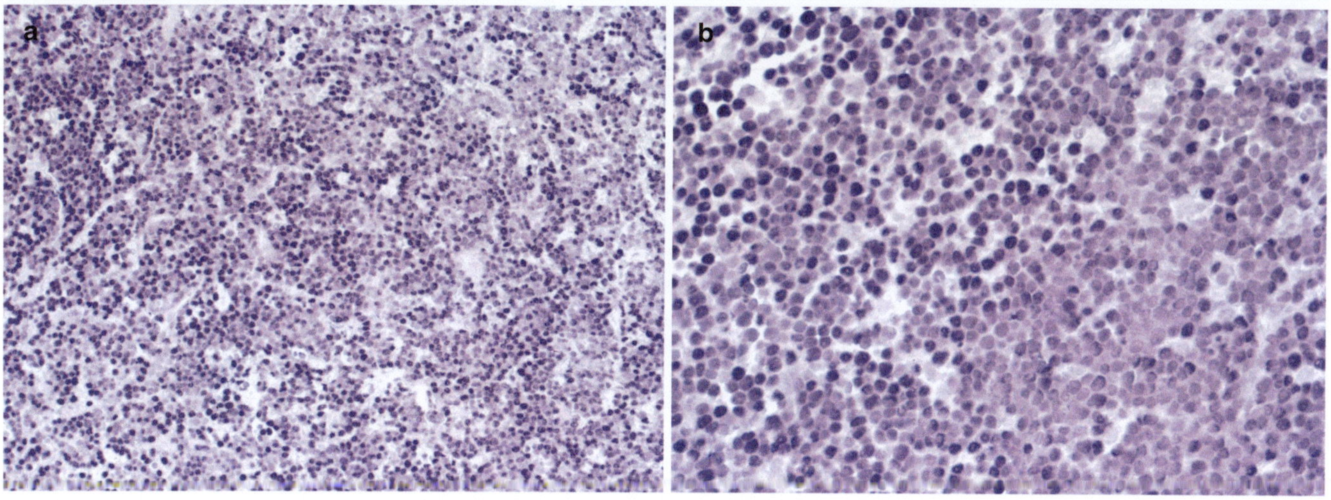

Fig. 39.16 Investigation of EBV-encoded small RNA (EBER) by in situ hybridization in Burkitt lymphoma. (**a**) Tumor cells are diffusely positive for EBV (EBER; 100×). (**b**) The presence of the virus is shown by the dark blue nuclear staining obtained during chromogenic in situ hybridization reaction (EBER; 200×)

Sources

1. Burkitt D. A sarcoma involving the jaws in African children. Br J Surg. 1958;46(197):218–23.
2. Queiroga EM, Gualco G, Weiss LM, et al. Burkitt lymphoma in Brazil is characterized by geographically distinct clinicopathologic features. Am J Clin Pathol. 2008;130(6):946–56.
3. Chene A, Donati D, Orem J, Mbidde ER, Kironde F, Wahlgren M, et al. Endemic Burkitt's lymphoma as a polymicrobial disease: new insights on the interaction between Plasmodium falciparum and Epstein-Barr virus. Semin Cancer Biol. 2009;19(6):411–20. https://doi.org/10.1016/j.semcancer.2009.10.002.
4. Rebelo-Pontes HA, Abreu MC, Guimarães DM, et al. Burkitt's lymphoma of the jaws in the Amazon region of Brazil. Med Oral Patol Oral Cir Bucal. 2014;19(1):e32–8.
5. Grande BM, Gerhard DS, Jiang A, Griner NB, Abramson JS, Alexander TB, et al. Genome-wide discovery of somatic coding and noncoding mutations in pediatric endemic and sporadic Burkitt lymphoma. Blood. 2019;133(12):1313–24. https://doi.org/10.1182/blood-2018-09-871418.
6. Rodrigues-Fernandes CI, Pérez-de-Oliveira ME, Aristizabal Arboleda LP, et al. Clinicopathological analysis of oral Burkitt's lymphoma in pediatric patients: a systematic review. Int J Pediatr Otorhinolaryngol. 2020;134:110033.
7. Benites BM, Miranda-Silva W, Rocha AC, Passos UL, Fonseca FP, da Silva CAR, et al. Late recurrence of Burkitt's lymphoma in the jaw: numb chin syndrome as the only symptom. Autops Case Rep. 2020;11:e2020218. https://doi.org/10.4322/acr.2020.218.
8. Arboleda LPA, Rodrigues-Fernandes CI, Mariz BALA, de Andrade BAB, Abrahão AC, Agostini M, et al. Burkitt lymphoma of the head and neck: an international collaborative study. J Oral Pathol Med. 2021;50(6):572–86. https://doi.org/10.1111/jop.13209.
9. Evens AM, Danilov A, Jagadeesh D, Sperling A, Kim SH, Vaca R, et al. Burkitt lymphoma in the modern era: real-world outcomes and prognostication across 30 US cancer centers. Blood. 2021;137(3):374–86. https://doi.org/10.1182/blood.2020006926.
10. Richter J, John K, Staiger AM, Rosenwald A, Kurz K, Michgehl U, et al. Epstein-Barr virus status of sporadic Burkitt lymphoma is associated with patient age and mutational features. Br J Haematol. 2022;196(3):681–9. https://doi.org/10.1111/bjh.17874.
11. Thomas N, Dreval K, Gerhard DS, Hilton LK, Abramson JS, Ambinder RF, et al. Genetic subgroups inform on pathobiology in adult and pediatric Burkitt lymphoma. Blood. 2023;141(8):904–16. https://doi.org/10.1182/blood.2022016534.
12. Fang H, Wang W, Medeiros LJ. Burkitt lymphoma. Hum Pathol. 2024:105703. https://doi.org/10.1016/j.humpath.2024.105703.
13. Solares S, León J, García-Gutiérrez L. The functional interaction between Epstein-Barr virus and MYC in the pathogenesis of Burkitt lymphoma. Cancers (Basel). 2024;16(24):4212. https://doi.org/10.3390/cancers16244212.
14. Choi JK, Quintanilla-Martinez L. Pediatric lymphomas: overview and diagnostic challenges. Virchows Arch. 2024; https://doi.org/10.1007/s00428-024-03980-9.
15. Chang J, Liang Y, Gao Y, Wu M, Lv F, Liu H, et al. High-grade B-cell lymphoma with 11q aberration in the HIV setting: a clinicopathological study of 10 cases and literature review. Infect Agent Cancer. 2024;19:42. https://doi.org/10.1186/s13027-024-00604-4.
16. Sureda-Gómez M, Iaccarino I, De Bolòs A, Meyer M, Balsas P, Richter J, Rodríguez ML, et al. SOX11 expression is restricted to EBV-negative Burkitt lymphoma and is associated with molecular genetic features. Blood. 2024;144(2):187–200. https://doi.org/10.1182/blood.2023023242.
17. Silva Filho NJD, Cardoso DM, Kayahara GM, Xavier-Júnior JCC, Cortopassi GM, Fonseca FP, et al. Primary manifestation of HIV-related Burkitt lymphoma in the oral and maxillofacial regions. J Am Dent Assoc. 2024;155(4):344–8. https://doi.org/10.1016/j.adaj.2023.11.012.
18. López C, Burkhardt B, Chan JKC, Leoncini L, Mbulaiteye SM, Ogwang MD, et al. Burkitt lymphoma. Nat Rev Dis Primers. 2022;8:78. https://doi.org/10.1038/s41572-022-00404-3.
19. Zhang DD, Medeiros CG, Liang M, Medeiros LJ. Origin of the terms 'water pot' and 'starry sky' in Burkitt lymphoma. Pathology. 2024;56(1):118–20. https://doi.org/10.1016/j.pathol.2023.06.003.

Diffuse Large B-Cell Lymphoma (Not Otherwise Specified)

40

Vitor Bonetti Valente, Javier Rendon Henao, and Felipe Paiva Fonseca

40.1 General Overview and Clinical Presentation

The World Health Organization classification of tumors of hematopoietic and lymphoid tissues recognizes a list of different lymphomas comprised of mature large B cells, most of them carrying morphological, immunophenotypic and genetic features that lead to specific diagnoses. However, many cases cannot be further classified and are, therefore, diagnosed as diffuse large B-cell lymphoma, not otherwise specified (DLBCL NOS). This entity is defined as a mature B-cell neoplasm composed of medium to large neoplastic cells that exhibit a diffuse growth pattern and it represents a diagnosis made by exclusion since other more specific large B-cell lymphomas must be ruled out by clinical, histologic, immunophenotypic and molecular analyses before a definitive DLBCL NOS diagnosis can be made, consequently, it represents a highly heterogeneous group of diseases.

DLBCL NOS is considered the most common non-Hodgkin lymphoma subtype and the most predominant in the oral and maxillofacial region too. It more commonly affects older males in their sixth to seventh decades of life and the lymph nodes are the most affected structures, although up to 40% of the cases arise in extranodal sites, especially in the gastrointestinal tract and the head and neck region. DLBCL NOS often manifests as rapidly growing swellings, usually asymptomatic, and B symptoms may be present. The involvement of the central nervous system is uncommon, but bone marrow involvement may occur in approximately 30% of the cases. The etiology of this tumor is poorly understood, but immunosuppression is an important risk factor for DLBCL onset (classified separately), and this neoplasm may develop secondary to a previous primary low-grade lymphoma. Genetic alterations in many different genes like *MYC*, *BCL2* and *BCL6*, have been identified as important events for DLBCL NOS pathogenesis and based on the molecular characteristics of this tumor more often observed using gene expression profiles, different molecular subtypes have been proposed; however, their importance for prognostic determination and future precision medicine approaches are still being validated and their reproducibility worldwide is very limited due to the difficult access to necessary facilities and its associated high costs.

In the oral cavity, the gingiva and the palate are the most affected locations, although virtually any site can be involved. The lesion has a very heterogeneous clinical presentation and can have a benign-looking appearance in rare cases, with a non-ulcerated, smooth, normal-colored aspect. However, oral DLBCL NOS more commonly manifests as an aggressive, rapidly growing neoplasm that may be asymptomatic or painful. Tumors are usually ulcerated and most have areas of tissue necrosis. Multiple simultaneous lesions may occur and adjacent teeth may be displaced or present different degrees of mobility. The tumor can affect both immunosuppressed and immunocompetent patients.

The neoplasm can extend towards the surrounding gnathic bones, or it may arise primarily from the bone tissues. Radiographically, DLBCL NOS exhibits irregular, ill-defined radiolucent images that infiltrate surrounding structures and that may extend to the maxillary sinus. The occurrence of periosteal reactions can be found, but is uncommon, while the tumor cells may also infiltrate the periodontal tissue, causing periodontal space widening. A diagnosis of oral DLBCL NOS must prompt clinicians to

V. B. Valente (✉)
Oral Oncology Center and Department of Diagnosis and Surgery, São Paulo State University (Unesp), School of Dentistry, Araçatuba, São Paulo, Brazil
e-mail: vitor.bonetti@unesp.br

J. R. Henao
Department of Hematopathology and Flow Cytometry, Ayudas Diagnósticas Sura Center, Cartagena, Colombia

F. P. Fonseca
Department of Oral Surgery and Pathology, School of Dentistry, Universidade Federal de Minas Gerais, Belo Horizonte, Brazil

© The Author(s), under exclusive license to Springer Nature Switzerland AG 2025

F. P. Fonseca et al. (eds.), *Lymphoproliferative and Granulomatous Disorders of the Oral Cavity*,
https://doi.org/10.1007/978-3-031-98844-8_40

recommend a systemic evaluation of the patient to investigate if the tumor represents a disseminated disease.

If the search for EBV, using either in situ hybridization or LMP-1 immunohistochemical expression results positive, the tumor should be reclassified and reported as diffuse large B-cell lymphoma EBV positive not otherwise specified (DLBCL EBV+ NOS), which is frequently associated with a poorer prognosis. Moreover, the presence of translocations in *MYC* and *BCL2* also demands reclassification of the disease to a high-grade B-cell lymphoma (HGBL), with double rearrangements. The presence of *BCL6* and *MYC* rearrangements is considered molecularly heterogeneous. In the latest World Health Organization classification of hematolymphoid tumors, it has been recommended that HGBL double rearrangements be grouped together with DLBCL.

DLBCL NOS is an aggressive neoplasm with an overall survival rate of approximately 65%, but different factors may impact patients' prognosis, including disease stage, patients' age, the international prognostic index, and bone marrow involvement, among several others. CHOP regimen that included the use of cyclophosphamide, doxorubicin, vincristine and prednisone was the standard of care in the 1990s, but the development and introduction of rituximab, a chimeric type 1 monoclonal antibody against CD20 that led to the R-CHOP scheme, improved the therapeutic management of these patients and increased their survival rate. However, tumor relapse and progression still occur in a variable number of cases (Table 40.1; Fig. 40.1).

Observe that the current classification of hematolymphoid tumors proposed by the World Health Organization (WHO-HAEME5) recognizes 18 different types of large B-cell lymphomas, 17 of them with specific clinicopathological, immunophenotypic and/or genetic features, which should be excluded before a diagnosis of diffuse large B-cell lymphoma NOS can be made. Moreover, other small/medium-sized cell lymphomas like mantle cell lymphoma can also have variants represented by large B-cell proliferations and should also be excluded during diagnostic work-up. However, considering the current epidemiological data, plasmablastic lymphoma and DLBCL NOS represent the two most frequent entities of this group of large B-cell lymphomas diagnosed in the oral cavity and gnathic bones, although the limited access to molecular tests to investigate the occurrence of genetic events may impair a better understanding on the incidence in the oral cavity of large B-cell lymphomas whose diagnoses depend on the identification of genetic abnormalities.

Table 40.1 Current variants of large B-cell lymphomas recognized by the World Health Organization Classification of hematolymphoid tumors

1	Diffuse large B-cell lymphoma, not otherwise specified (DLBCL, NOS)
2	T-cell/histiocyte-rich large B-cell lymphoma
3	Diffuse large B-cell lymphoma/high-grade B-cell lymphoma with *MYC* and *BCL2* rearrangements
4	ALK-positive large B-cell lymphoma
5	Large B-cell lymphoma with *IRF4* rearrangement
6	High-grade B-cell lymphoma with 11q aberration
7	Lymphomatoid granulomatosis
8	EBV-positive diffuse large B-cell lymphoma
9	Diffuse large B-cell lymphoma associated with chronic inflammation
10	Fibrin-associated large B-cell lymphoma
11	Fluid overload-associated large B-cell lymphoma
12	Plasmablastic lymphoma
13	Primary large B-cell lymphoma of immune-privileged sites
14	Primary cutaneous diffuse large B-cell lymphoma, leg type
15	Intravascular large B-cell lymphoma
16	Primary mediastinal large B-cell lymphoma
17	Mediastinal grey zone lymphoma
18	High-grade B-cell lymphoma NOS

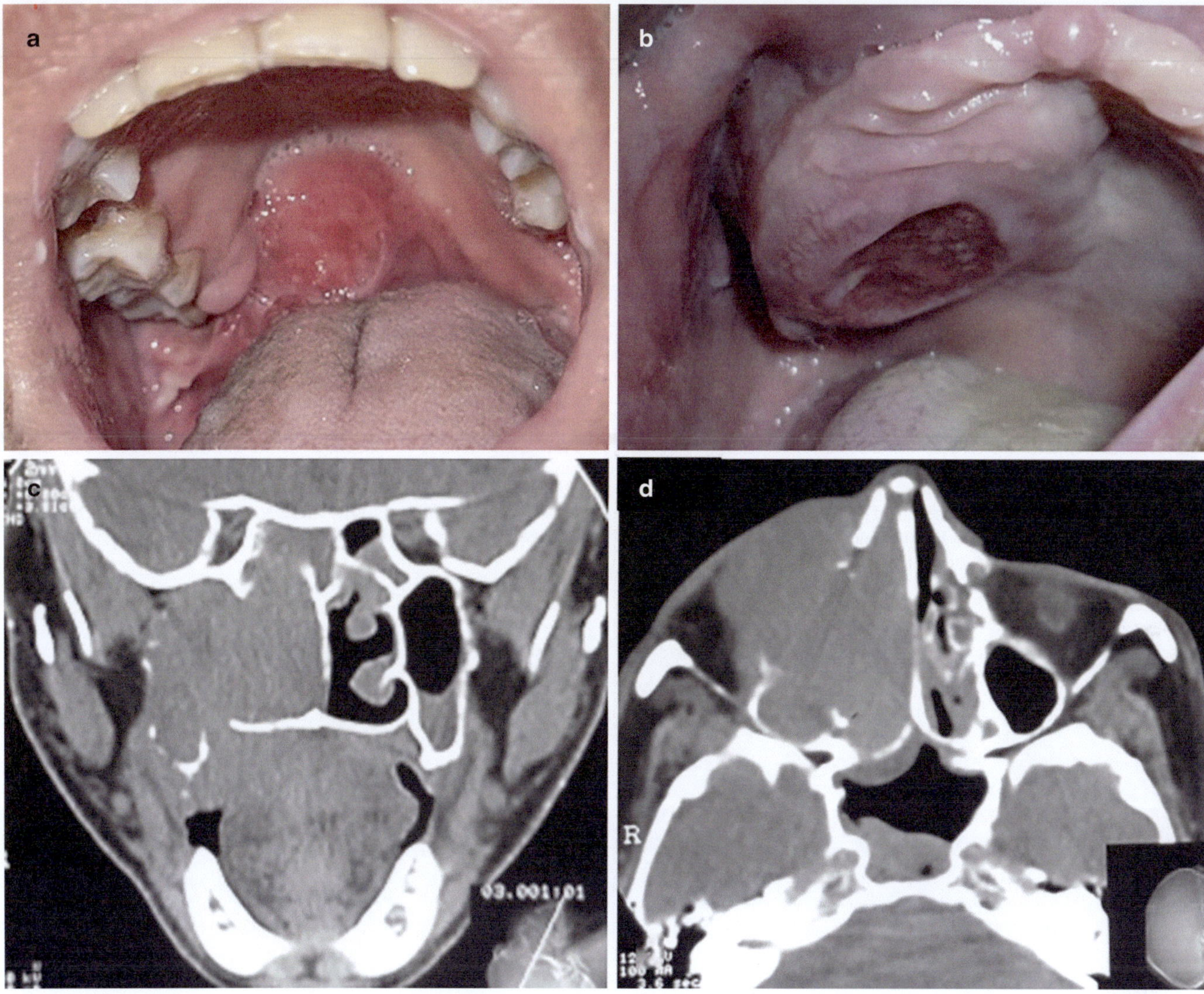

Fig. 40.1 Clinical presentation of DLBCL NOS affecting the oral cavity. (**a**) A 53-years-old male patient affected by an ulcerated tumor in the palate. (**b**) A 57-years-old male patient affected by DLBCL NOS with two months of duration exhibiting an ulcerated swelling of the hard palate. (**c**) The coronal section of computed tomography exam reveals the involvement of the maxillary sinus and other surrounding structures, while the (**d**) axial section illustrates the vestibular expansion of the tumor with cortical bone destruction

40.2 Microscopic Findings

- The tumor typically exhibits a diffuse growth pattern of the neoplastic cells.
- Some cases can exhibit tingible body macrophages and the starry sky pattern.
- A fibrous stroma can be present, but most cases have a scarce or no stroma.
- The neoplastic cells frequently invade the surrounding normal tissues.
- Areas of necrosis can be frequently observed, and geographic necrosis is more frequent in DLBCL EBV+ NOS.
- There is a predominance of medium to large neoplastic cells that exhibit a large round nucleus containing one central nucleolus (consistent with immunoblasts) or three or more peripherally located nucleoli (consistent with centroblasts).
- Smaller neoplastic cells (consistent with centrocytes) are also present, but in a lower number.
- Many of the small cells are reactive T lymphocytes and express CD3 protein.
- The cytoplasm of the tumor cells is usually scarce.
- Typical and atypical mitotic figures are frequent.
- Some cases exhibit an increased number of pleomorphic cells.
- Rare cases may demonstrate areas containing clear cells, spindle cells and signet ring-like cells.
- HGBL may have the same microscopic features of DLBCL NOS, but it may also have a blastoid appearance with medium-sized cells with darker nuclei and less prominent nucleoli, often resembling Burkitt lymphoma or lymphoblastic lymphoma (Figs. 40.2, 40.3, and 40.4).

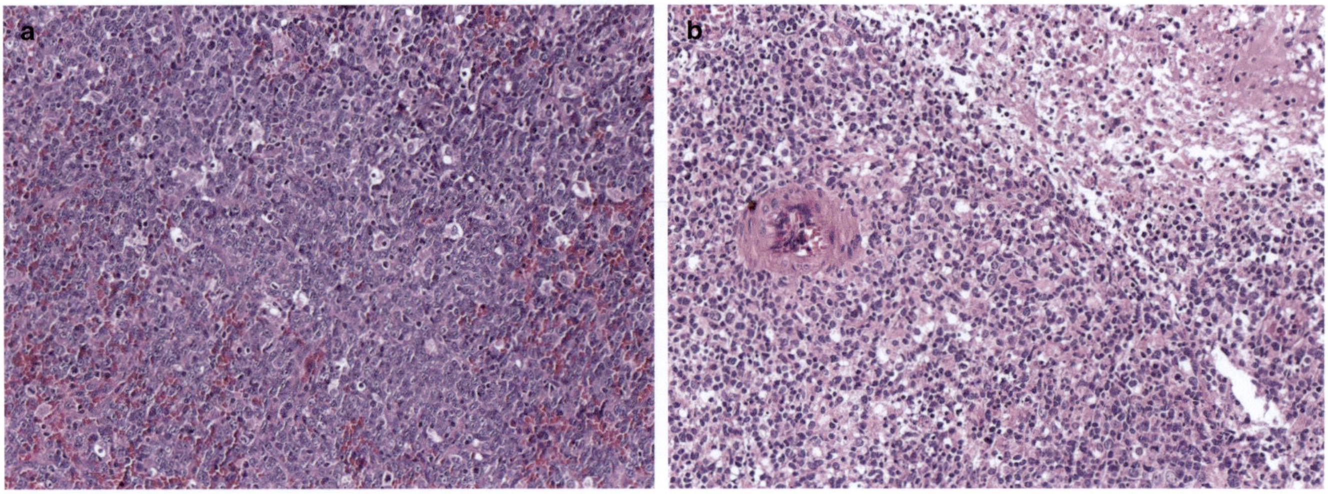

Fig. 40.2 Histopathological features of DLBCL NOS. (**a**) The neoplastic cells proliferate in a diffuse, sheet-like growth pattern. In some cases, it is possible to observe the presence of tingible body macrophages and the starry sky pattern (H&E; 100×). (**b**) Areas of tissue necrosis are common due to the high grade of the neoplasm. The necrotic region is located in the more eosinophilic region of the upper right area of the image (H&E; 200×)

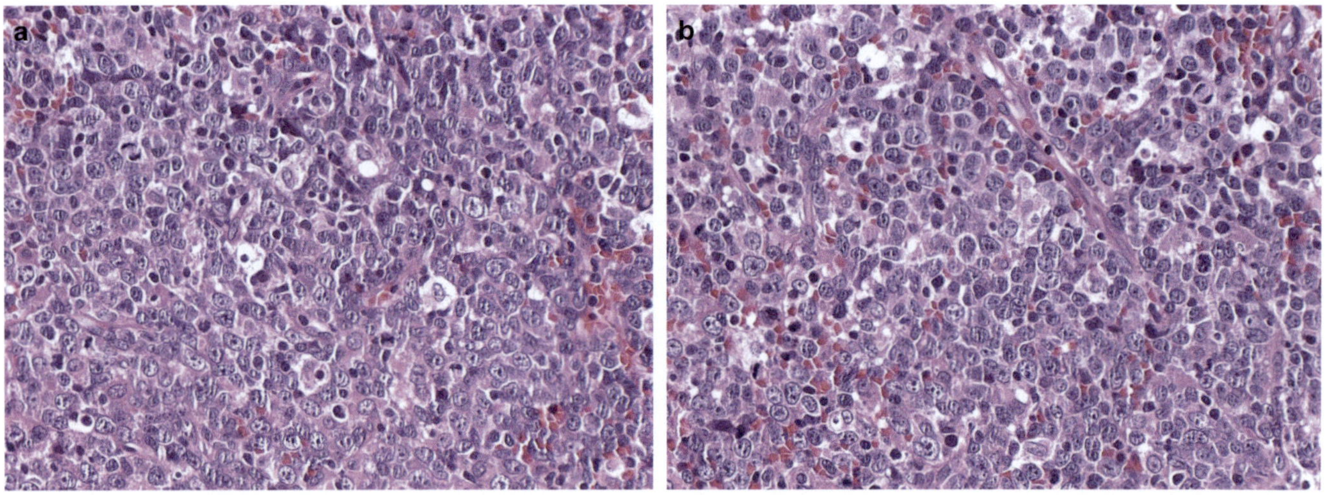

Fig. 40.3 Histopathological features of DLBCL NOS. (**a**) Under higher-power magnification it is possible to determine the cell size by comparing the nuclei of the macrophages and the neoplastic cells. Immunoblasts are large cells characterized by the presence of a prominent centrally located nucleolus, while centroblasts are large cells with three or more nucleoli distributed in the nucleus (H&E; 200×). (**b**) In the absence of a macrophage to be used as a reference to determine the tumor cell size, it is possible to use a normal endothelial cell. Large tumor cells will be approximately two-fold larger than endothelial cells (H&E; 200×)

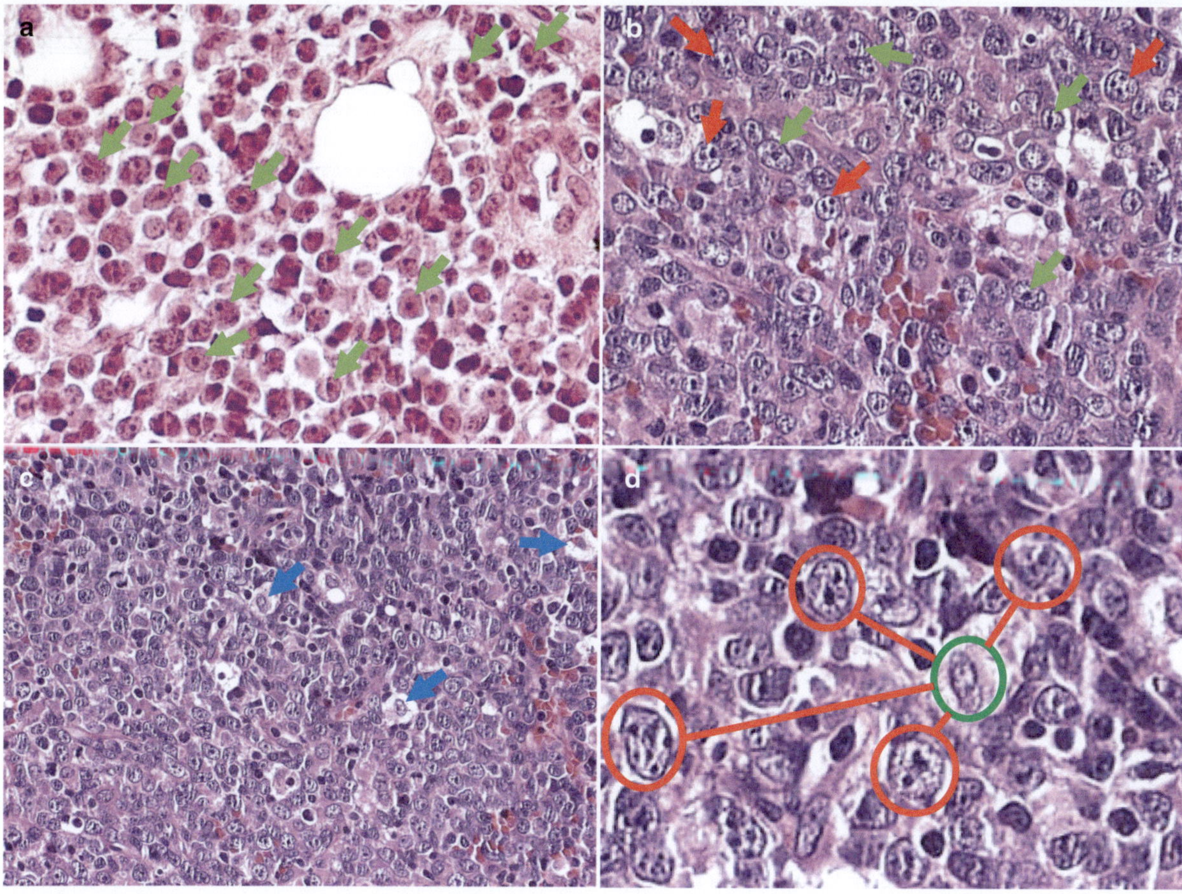

Fig. 40.4 Microscopic features of diffuse large B-cell lymphoma not otherwise specified (DLBCL NOS) affecting the oral mucosa. (**a**) Diffuse proliferation of large neoplastic B cells predominantly showing a single centrally located nucleolus consistent with immunoblasts (green arrows). (**b**) Another example of DLBCL NOS affecting the palate showing the same diffuse growth pattern of the previous case, but now containing tumor cells with one centrally located nucleolus representing immunoblasts (green arrows), and some tumor cells with three or more nucleoli representing centroblasts (red arrows). (**c**) Note the presence of tingible body macrophages with their clear cytoplasm (blue arrows) that impart the starry sky microscopic pattern. (**d**) Using the nucleus of one tingible body macrophage (green balloon) as a histologic reference to determine the cell size of the neoplastic cells that predominate in this tumor, it is possible to observe that the nuclei of tumor cells (red balloons) are larger than the nucleus size of the macrophage

40.3 Immunohistochemistry and/or Genetics

Considering that the diagnosis of DLBCL NOS is made by excluding other more specific large B-cell lymphomas, the immunohistochemical panel recommended for the diagnosis of this entity may vary and will depend on the list of the main microscopic differential diagnoses considered for each case. The mature B-cell nature of the tumor is shown by the expression of CD20, CD22, PAX5 and/or CD79a, while CD3 is negative and stain reactive T lymphocytes.

The use of gene expression profile (GEP) assay identified two main biological groups of DLBCL according to their cell of origin (COO) termed germinal center B-cell type (GCB) and activated B-cell type (ABC), whose importance was still recognized in the International Consensus Classification (ICC) group position paper and the World Health Organization classification (WHO-HAEME5). The GCB type is more common and is associated with a more favorable prognosis. More recently, a series of publications has used genomics to subclassify DLBCL cases according to their gene expression (LymphGen, Haematological Malignancy Research Network and Harvard, for instance).

However, the use of large-scale genetic approaches is difficult to reproduce in diagnostic laboratories and as an attempt to find immunohistochemical markers that could carry prognostic significance, a series of algorithms based on immunophenotype have been proposed. In 2004, Hans et al. suggested the use of the combination of CD10, BCL6 and MUM1 antibodies by immunohistochemistry as an attempt to reproduce GEP studies, considering for a positive result a staining pattern >30% in neoplastic cells for each marker, classifying DLBCL cases as GCB type and non-GCB type. However, only a small concordance between Hans' algorithm and the GEP assay was observed, ranging from 72% to 86% in available studies. Moreover, an unclassifiable group of cases was still present and the prognostic reproducibility of this algorithm is usually considered limited, although its use remains recommended by the WHO-HAEM5 classification. Many cases express BCL2 (>50% of the neoplastic cells) and MYC (> 40% of the neoplastic cells) proteins.

Other frequent B-cell neoplasms that may have similar microscopic features should be ruled out: Cyclin D1 and SOX11 should be investigated to exclude mantle cell lymphoma, CD138 to exclude plasmablastic lymphoma, and CD21/CD23 to contribute to identifying follicular dendritic cell meshwork that could lead to a high-grade follicular lymphoma diagnosis. The occurrence of a high-grade transformation in a previous low-grade lymphoma must be investigated morphologically and immunohistochemically. MALT lymphoma does not have a specific marker and should be considered from a histological basis, while chronic lymphocytic leukemia/small lymphocytic lymphoma (Richter transformation) should be evaluated using the expression of CD5 and CD23 combined with morphological evaluation, given that a small subset of DLBCL NOS may also express both markers.

The presence of EBV must be investigated to exclude a DLBCL EBV+ NOS, and the presence of mutations in *MYC* and *BCL2* should be evaluated to investigate a HGBL with dual rearrangements. The presence of BCL6 rearrangement should also be reported (Table 40.2; Figs. 40.5, 40.6, 40.7, 40.8, 40.9, 40.10, 40.11, 40.12, and 40.13).

Table 40.2 Summary of the main immunohistochemical reactions used for DLBCL NOS diagnosis

Antibody/probe	Most frequent results	Pattern	Objective
CD20	Positive	Membrane	To demonstrate the B-cell nature of the tumor
PAX5	Positive	Nucleus	To demonstrate the B-cell nature of the tumor
CD79a	Positive	Membrane	To demonstrate the B-cell nature of the tumor
CD3	Negative	Membrane	To exclude a T-cell nature of the tumor
CD138	Negative	Membrane	To exclude a plasmablastic lymphoma
Cyclin D1	Negative	Nucleus	To exclude a mantle cell lymphoma
CD5	Positive or negative	Membrane	To investigate the possible presence of CLL/SLL
CD23	Positive or negative	Membrane	To investigate the possible presence of CLL/SLL
CD21	Negative	Membrane	To investigate a possible follicular lymphoma, identifying follicular dendritic cells meshwork
CD30	Positive and Negative	Membrane	Prognostic and therapeutic determination. More commonly expressed in EBV-positive cases
MUM1	Positive or negative	Nucleus	To classify the tumor according to Hans algorithm
CD10	Positive or negative	Membrane	To classify the tumor according to Hans algorithm
BCL6	Positive or negative	Nucleus	To classify the tumor according to Hans algorithm
BCL2	Positive	Cytoplasm	Frequently expressed in DLBCL NOS (correlate with *BCL2* translocation)
MYC	Positive	Nucleus	Frequently expressed in DLBCL NOS (correlate with *MYC* translocation)
Ki67	~40–70%	Nucleus	To determine the proliferative index
EBER[a]	Positive in a subset of the cases	Nucleus	To demonstrate the presence of EBV
MYC[b]	Positive in a subset of the cases	–	To investigate a possible HGBL double rearrangements
BCL2[b]	Positive in a subset of the cases	–	To investigate a possible HGBL double rearrangements
BCL6[b]	Positive in a subset of the cases	–	To characterize the molecular basis of DLBCL

The main results for EBV detection and molecular findings are also described

EBV Epstein-Barr virus, *HGBL* High-grade B-cell lymphoma, *CLLS/SLL* Chronic lymphocytic leukemia/Small lymphocytic lymphoma

[a]Investigated by in situ hybridization

[b]Investigated by fluorescent in situ hybridization

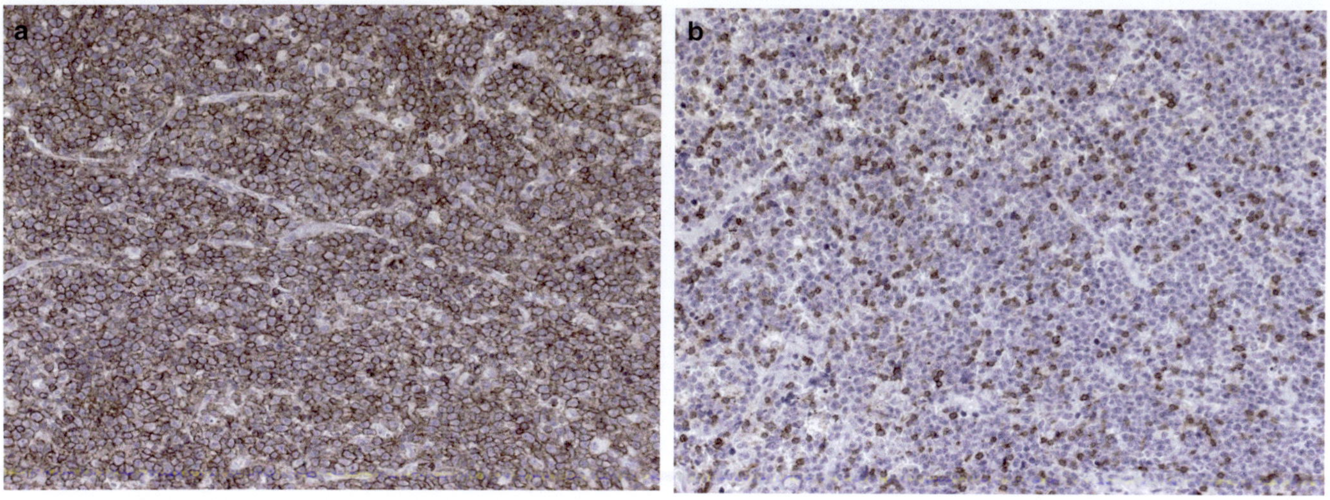

Fig. 40.5 Immunohistochemical features of DLBCL NOS. (**a**) Tumor cells show a strong and diffuse membrane positivity to CD20 (DAB; 100×). (**b**) Only reactive T lymphocytes express CD3 (DAB; 100×)

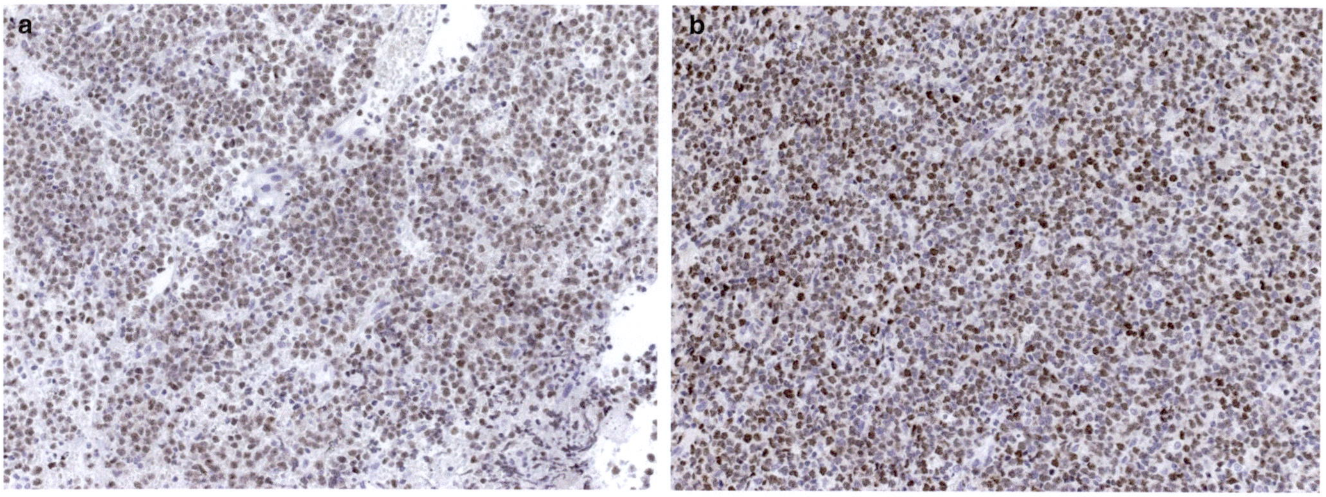

Fig. 40.6 Immunohistochemical features of DLBCL NOS. (**a**) The mature B-cell phenotype of DLBCL NOS can be demonstrated by PAX5 nuclear expression (DAB; 100×). (**b**) MUM1 can be expressed in many cases, and its presence indicates that this case is classified as non-germinal center type DLBCL NOS according to Hans' algorithm, which is determined also together with the evaluation of BCL6 and CD10 proteins (DAB; 100×)

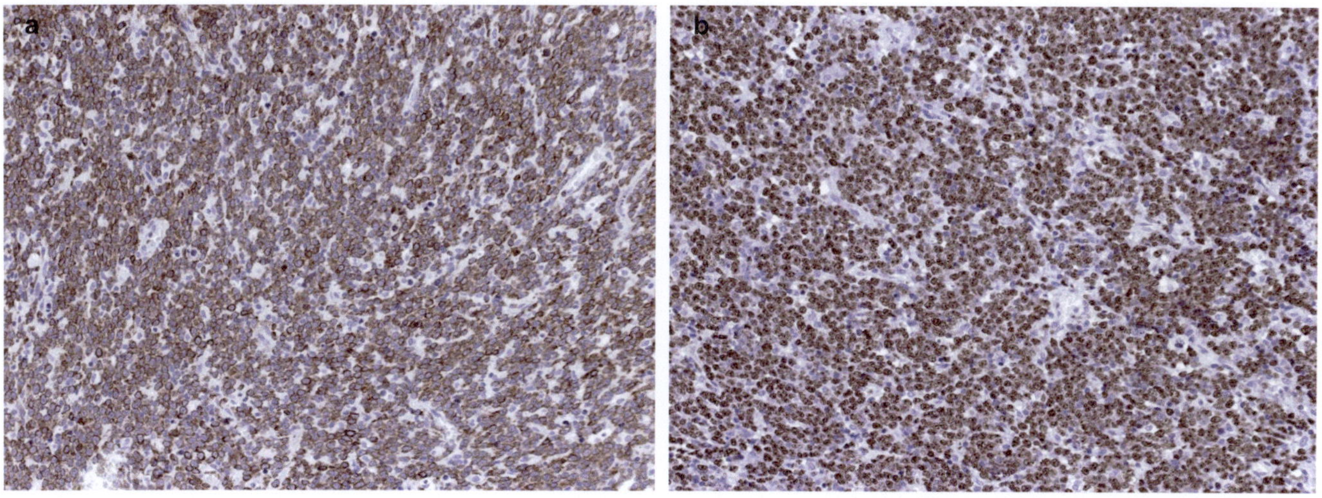

Fig. 40.7 Immunohistochemical features of DLBCL NOS. (**a**) Tumor cells exhibit cytoplasmic expression of BCL2 (DAB; 100×). (**b**) Proliferative index measured by Ki67 may vary, but it is usually high, possibly achieving 90% of positivity in some cases (DAB; 100×)

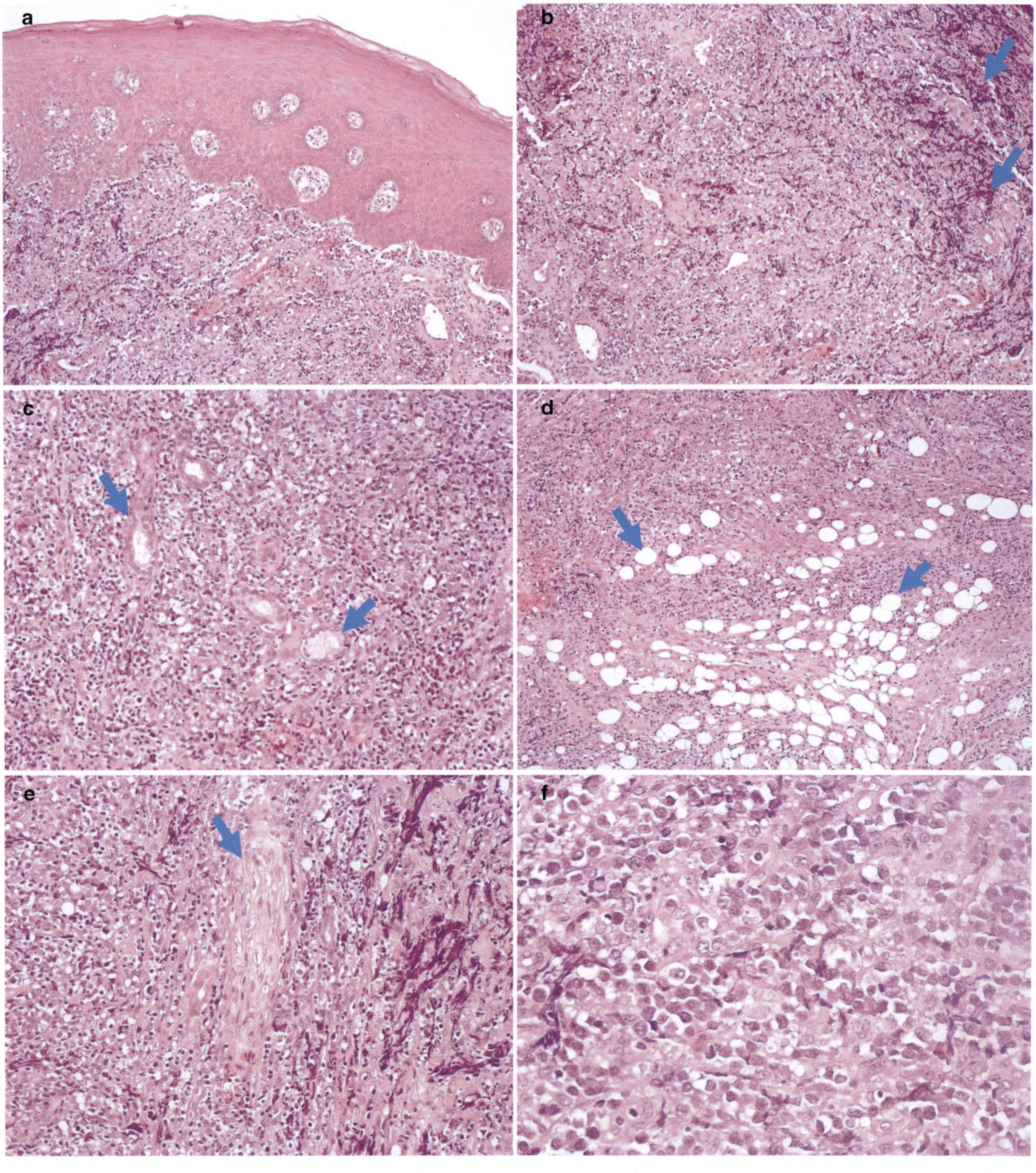

Fig. 40.8 Histopathological features of DLBCL NOS affecting the palate of a male patient. (**a**) Overlying squamous epithelium and a diffuse proliferation of tumor cells in the lamina propria (H&E; 100×). (**b**) The neoplastic cells are diffusely distributed in the lamina propria. Histological artifacts are very commonly observed in lymphoid neoplasms and can be seen in the right side of this image (blue arrows), where the morphological features of the tumor are lost (H&E; 100×). (**c**) Tumor cells infiltrate salivary gland ducts and acini (blue arrows) (H&E; 100×), (**d**) mature adipocytes (blue arrows) (H&E; 100×), (**e**) and nerve bundles (blue arrow) (H&E; 100×). (**f**) Note the large size of the tumor cells with prominent nucleoli (H&E; 200×)

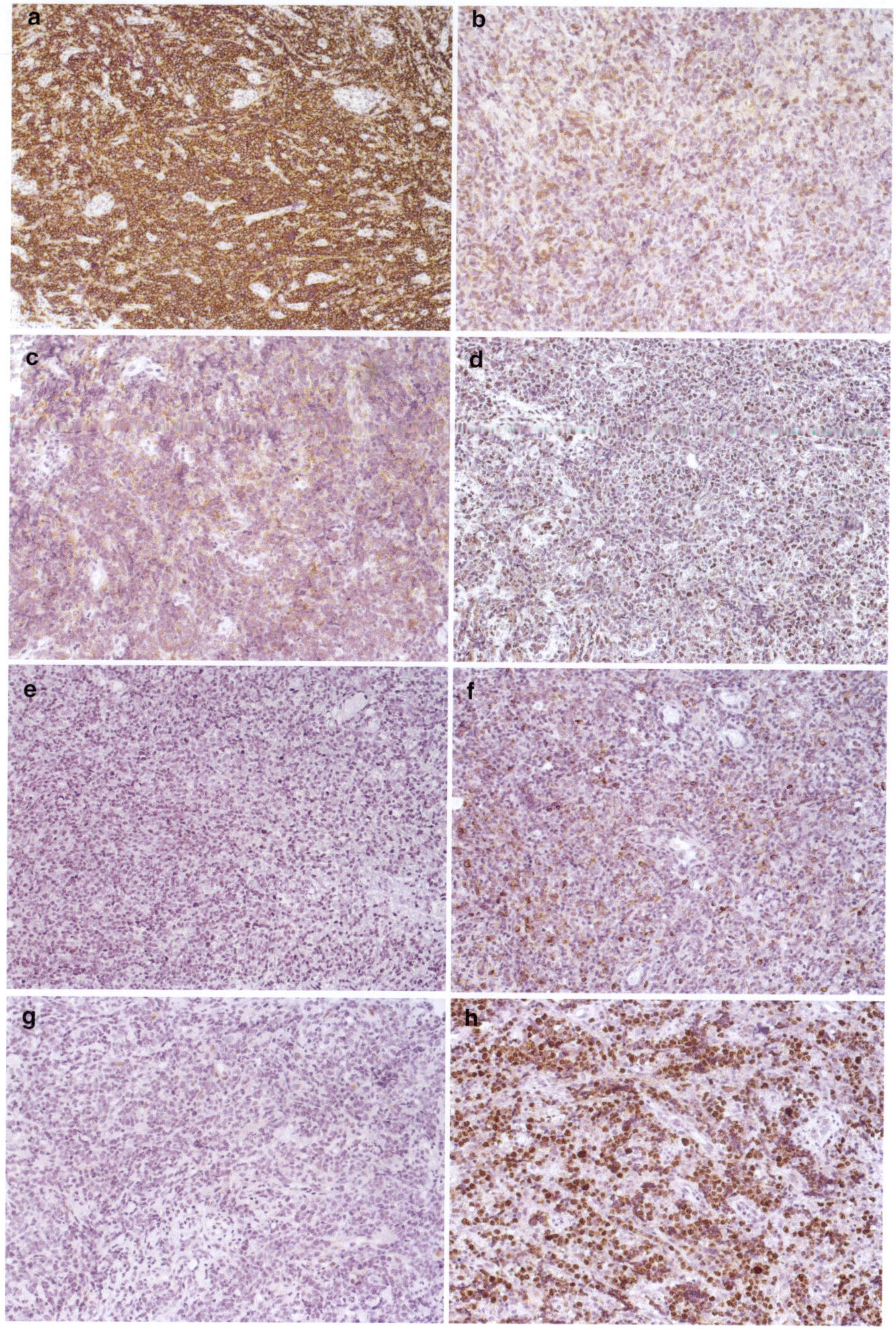

Fig. 40.9 Immunohistochemical features of DLBCL NOS affecting the palate of a male patient (same patient as in Fig. 40.8). (**a**) Tumor cells demonstrate a strong and diffuse membrane positivity to CD20 (DAB; 100×). (**b**) Negative result for CD3. Reactive T lymphocytes express the protein (DAB; 100×). (**c**) Diffuse positivity to CD10 (DAB; 100×), and (**d**) BCL6 (DAB; 100×), and (**e**) negative result for MUM1 (DAB; 100×), denoting a germinal center B-cell (GCB) DLBCL NOS subtype. (**f**) Expression of BCL2 protein (DAB; 100×). (**g**) Negative result for Cyclin D1 helps to exclude the diagnosis of mantle cell lymphoma (DAB; 100×). (**h**) High proliferative index measured by Ki67 expression (DAB; 100×)

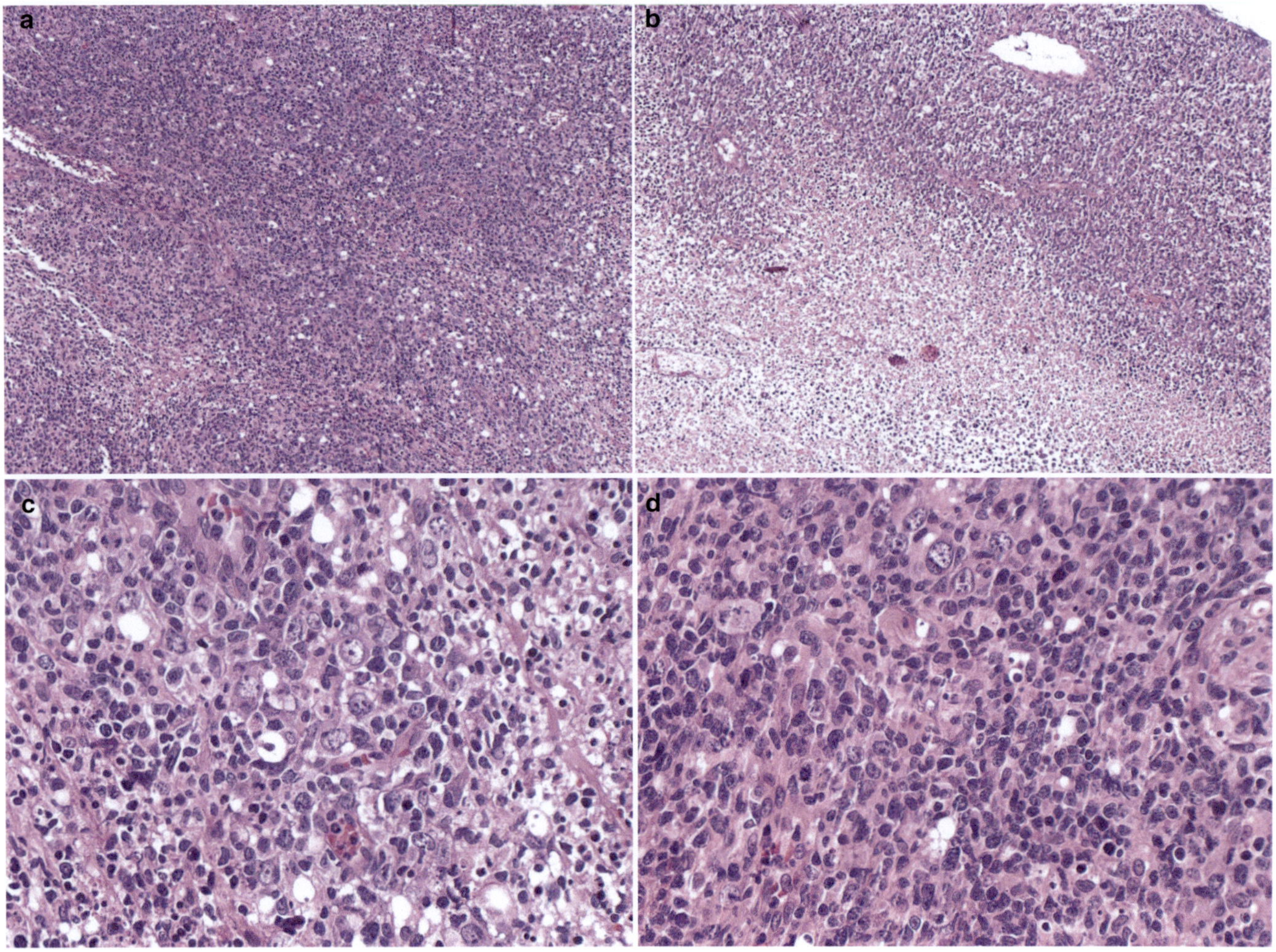

Fig. 40.10 Histopathological features of DLBCL, EBV positive, NOS. (**a**) Tumor cells exhibit a diffuse growth pattern (H&E; 50×). (**b**) Extensive areas of geographic necrosis is a common finding (H&E; 50×). (**c**) The neoplasm is predominantly composed of large cells containing one centrally located nucleolus (immunoblasts) or multiple nucleoli (centroblasts) (DAB; 200×). (**d**) Atypical mitotic figures and a high grade of pleomorphism are frequently observed (H&E; 200×)

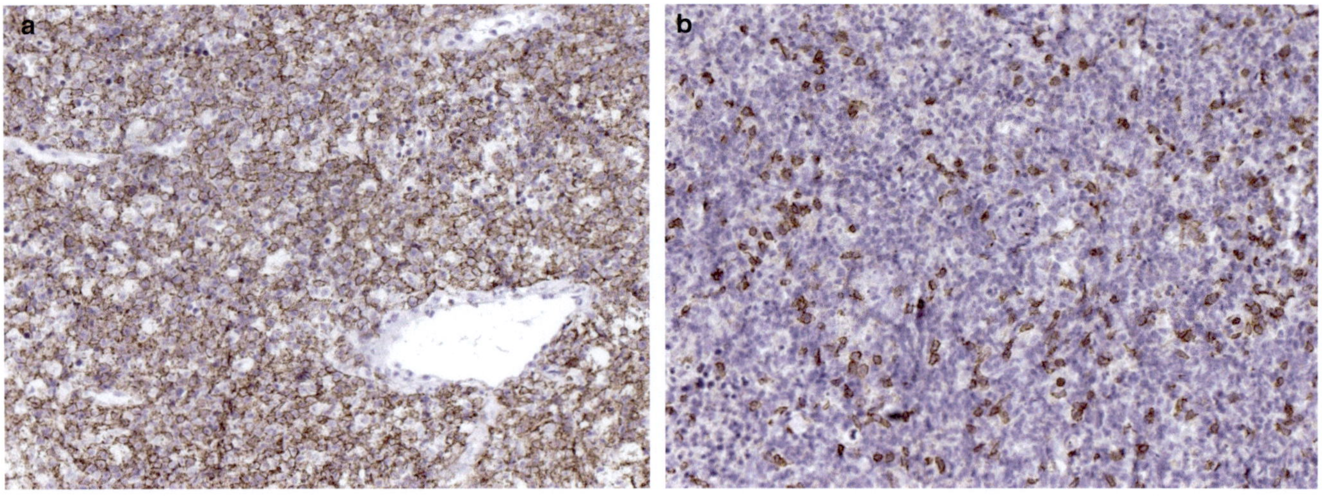

Fig. 40.11 Immunohistochemical features of DLBCL, EBV positive, NOS. (**a**) Tumor cells show a strong and diffuse membrane positivity to CD20 (DAB; 100×). (**b**) Only reactive T lymphocytes express CD3 (DAB; 100×)

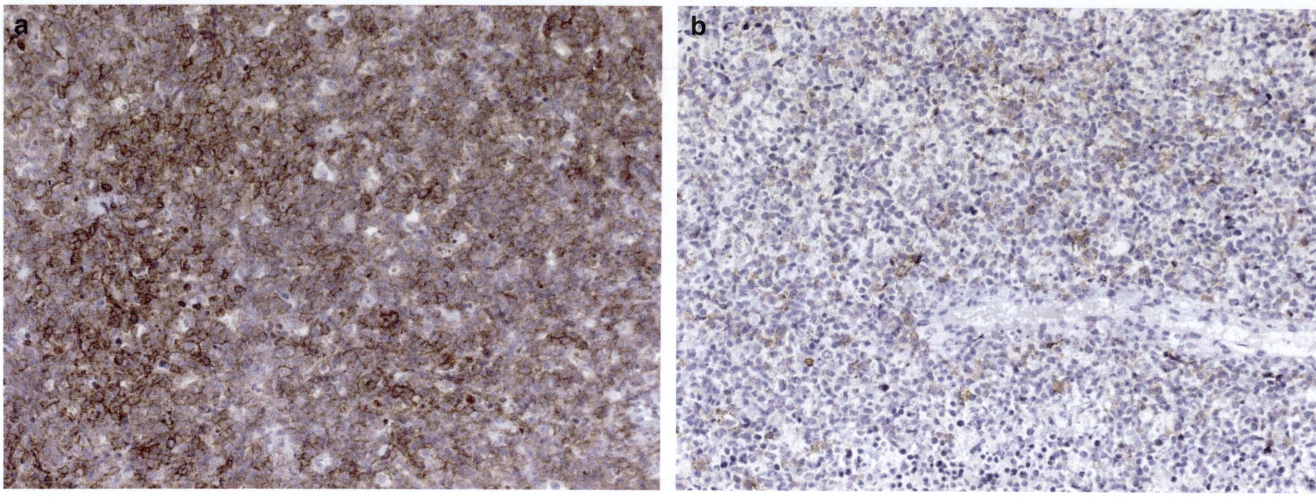

Fig. 40.12 Immunohistochemical features of DLBCL, EBV positive, NOS. (**a**) Strong expression of CD10 can be found in some cases, and it is investigated together with BCL6 and MUM1 markers to determine if the case is subclassified as germinal center DLBCL or non-germinal center DLBCL according to Hans' algorithm (DAB; 100×). (**b**) CD30 can be expressed by approximately 10% of DLBCL NOS cases, and it is more commonly found in EBV-positive cases (DAB; 100×)

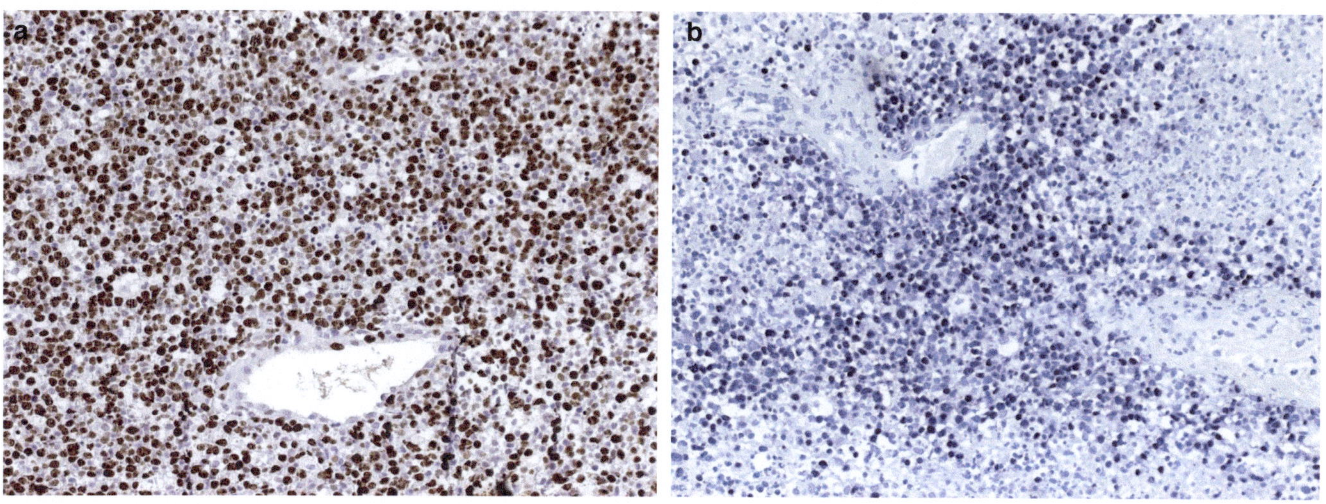

Fig. 40.13 Immunohistochemical features of DLBCL NOS. (**a**) Proliferative index measured by Ki67 is usually very high, achieving 90% of positivity in some cases (DAB; 100×). (**b**) The presence of EBV virus is demonstrated by in situ hybridization (EBER; 100×)

Sources

1. Alizadeh AA, Eisen MB, Davis RE, Ma C, Lossos IS, Rosenwald A, et al. Distinct types of diffuse large B-cell lymphoma identified by gene expression profiling. Nature. 2000;403(6769):503–11. https://doi.org/10.1038/35000501.
2. Hans CP, Weisenburger DD, Greiner TC, Gascoyne RD, Delabie J, Ott G, et al. Confirmation of the molecular classification of diffuse large B-cell lymphoma by immunohistochemistry using a tissue microarray. Blood. 2004;103(1):275–82. https://doi.org/10.1182/blood-2003-05-1545.
3. Chapuy B, Stewart C, Dunford AJ, Kim J, Kamburov A, Redd RA, et al. Molecular subtypes of diffuse large B cell lymphoma are associated with distinct pathogenic mechanisms and outcomes. Nat Med. 2018;24(5):679–90. https://doi.org/10.1038/s41591-018-0016-8.
4. Pasqualucci L, Dalla-Favera R. Genetics of diffuse large B-cell lymphoma. Blood. 2018;131(21):2307–19. https://doi.org/10.1182/blood-2017-11-764332.
5. Schmitz R, Wright GW, Huang DW, Johnson CA, Phelan JD, Wang JQ, et al. Genetics and pathogenesis of diffuse large B-cell lymphoma. N Engl J Med. 2018;378(15):1396–407. https://doi.org/10.1056/NEJMoa1801445.
6. Wright GW, Huang DW, Phelan JD, Coulibaly ZA, Roulland S, Young RM, et al. A probabilistic classification tool for genetic subtypes of diffuse large B cell lymphoma with therapeutic implications. Cancer Cell. 2020;37(4):551–568.e14. https://doi.org/10.1016/j.ccell.2020.03.015.
7. Rodrigues-Fernandes CI, de Souza LL, Santos-Costa SFD, Pontes HAR, et al. Clinicopathological analysis of oral diffuse large B-cell lymphoma, NOS: a systematic review. J Oral Pathol Med. 2019;48(3):185–91. https://doi.org/10.1111/jop.12802.

8. Costa SFDS, Silva AMB, Amaral-Silva GK, Pontes HAR, Pontes FSC, Fonseca FP, et al. Epstein-Barr virus-positive diffuse large B-cell lymphoma, not otherwise specified, in the Oral cavity. J Craniofac Surg. 2019;30(3):e259–62. https://doi.org/10.1097/SCS.0000000000005302.
9. de Arruda JAA, Schuch LF, Conte Neto N, de Souza LL, Rodrigues-Fernandes CI, Abreu LG, et al. Oral and oropharyngeal lymphomas: a multi-institutional collaborative study. J Oral Pathol Med. 2021;50(6):603–12. https://doi.org/10.1111/jop.13211.
10. Candelaria M, Dueñas-Gonzalez A. Rituximab in combination with cyclophosphamide, doxorubicin, vincristine, and prednisone (R-CHOP) in diffuse large B-cell lymphoma. Ther Adv Hematol. 2021;12:2040620721989579. https://doi.org/10.1177/2040620721989579.
11. Rodrigues-Fernandes CI, Junior AG, Soares CD, Morais TML, do Amaral-Silva GK, MGF d C, et al. Oral and oropharyngeal diffuse large B-cell lymphoma and high-grade B-cell lymphoma: a clinicopathologic and prognostic study of 69 cases. Oral Surg Oral Med Oral Pathol Oral Radiol. 2021;131(4):452–462.e4. https://doi.org/10.1016/j.oooo.2020.11.005.
12. Rodrigues-Fernandes CI, Abreu LG, Radhakrishnan R, Perez DEDC, Amaral-Silva GK, Gondak RO, et al. Prognostic significance of CD30 expression in diffuse large B-cell lymphoma: a systematic review with meta-analysis. J Oral Pathol Med. 2021;50(6):587–93. https://doi.org/10.1111/jop.13208.
13. Runge HFP, Lacy S, Barrans S, Beer PA, Painter D, Smith A, et al. Application of the LymphGen classification tool to 928 clinically and genetically-characterised cases of diffuse large B cell lymphoma (DLBCL). Br J Haematol. 2021;192(1):216–20. https://doi.org/10.1111/bjh.17132.
14. Morais-Perdigão AL, Rodrigues-Fernandes CI, Araújo GR, Soares CD, de Andrade BAB, Martins MD, et al. CD30 expression in oral and oropharyngeal diffuse large B cell lymphoma, not otherwise specified. Head Neck Pathol. 2022;16(2):476–85. https://doi.org/10.1007/s12105-021-01387-5.
15. Song JY, Dirnhofer S, Piris MA, Quintanilla-Martínez L, Pileri S, Campo E. Diffuse large B-cell lymphomas, not otherwise specified, and emerging entities. Virchows Arch. 2023;482(1):179–92. https://doi.org/10.1007/s00428-022-03466-6.

Plasmablastic Lymphoma

41

Willie F. P. van Heerden,
Guilherme Rossi Assis de Mendonça,
Ana Carolina Prado Ribeiro, Márcio Ajudarte Lopes,
and Felipe Paiva Fonseca

41.1 General Overview and Clinical Presentation

Plasmablastic lymphoma is a high-grade B-cell lymphoma described in 1997 by Delecluse et al. that more commonly affects the oral cavity of immunosuppressed patients, but it is considered very uncommon, representing no more than 1% of all cases of large B-cell lymphomas. It is defined as an aggressive lymphoid neoplasm comprising a diffuse proliferation of immunoblasts and plasmablasts that are typically negative or only focally positive for mature B-cell markers like CD20 and PAX5, carrying a plasma cell immunophenotype. Although the etiology of plasmablastic lymphoma remains poorly understood, EBV is present in approximately 70% of the cases especially in the setting of immunosuppression, and is believed to play an important role in the development of this neoplasm, with the presence of EBV being associated with a different molecular landscape than cases negative for this virus, illustrating the pathogenic importance of this microorganism. Moreover, chromosomal translocations involving the *MYC* gene and immunoglobulin group genes are found in approximately 50–60% of the cases, and these genetic abnormalities are also implicated in the pathogenesis of plasmablastic lymphoma. More recently, mutations in other important members of the *JAK/STAT*, *MAPK/ERK* and *NOTCH* families of genes, as well as in *TP53*, have been described.

Adult males are more affected than females, usually in their fourth to sixth decades of life. Following the oral cavity, the gastrointestinal tract and the skin are the most affected locations. The bone and soft tissues, as well as the lymph nodes, can also be affected by plasmablastic lymphoma. The neoplasm usually presents as rapidly growing tumors, with ulcerated regions and areas of tissue necrosis. The mucosa of the upper gingiva/alveolar ridge and the palate are the most affected locations in the oral cavity and in some cases the gingival growth may be misinterpreted as a reactive hyperplastic condition like pyogenic granuloma. Plasmablastic lymphomas are most often diagnosed in advanced Ann-Arbor stages, but B-symptoms are usually not reported by patients.

This lymphoma is more often diagnosed in HIV-positive patients, accounting for approximately 2.6–3% of all lymphomas diagnosed in this population, and it is considered an AIDS-defining disease. Most of the patients present a CD4+ T-cell count below 200 cells/ml^3 and a highly variable viral load. However, immunosuppressed patients due to other reasons like oncological treatment, organ transplantation, autoimmune disease and aging immunosenescence may also develop the neoplasm; moreover, immunocompetent patients may also be rarely affected.

Although plasmablastic lymphoma most often manifests in the soft tissue, it may also be associated with some destruction of the surrounding bone, more frequently like an infiltrative process rather than a primary intra-osseous tumor causing

W. F. P. van Heerden (✉)
Department of Oral and Maxillofacial Pathology, School of Dentistry University of Pretoria, Pretoria, South Africa

PathCare Vermaak Histopathology Laboratory, Pretoria, South Africa
e-mail: willie.vanheerden@up.ac.za

G. R. A. de Mendonça
Department of Pathology, School of Medical Sciences, University of Campinas, Campinas, Brazil

A. C. P. Ribeiro
Dental Oncology Service, São Paulo State Cancer Institute (ICESP-FMUSP), São Paulo, Brazil

M. A. Lopes
Department of Oral Diagnosis (Semiology), Piracicaba Dental School, University of Campinas (UNICAMP), Piracicaba, Brazil
e-mail: malopes@fop.unicamp.br

F. P. Fonseca
Department of Oral Surgery and Pathology, School of Dentistry, Universidade Federal de Minas Gerais, Belo Horizonte, Brazil

© The Author(s), under exclusive license to Springer Nature Switzerland AG 2025
F. P. Fonseca et al. (eds.), *Lymphoproliferative and Granulomatous Disorders of the Oral Cavity*,
https://doi.org/10.1007/978-3-031-98844-8_41

cortical bone expansion. Therefore, in these cases and also because of the histological features and the plasmacytic immunophenotype of the tumor, the distinction between plasmablastic lymphoma and plasmacytoma/multiple myeloma may be very difficult, and full clinical and laboratorial data need to be investigated. In this setting, the presence of paraproteinemia and combination of CRAB criteria (hypercalcemia, renal dysfunction, anemia and bone lesions) favors a plasmacytoma/multiple myeloma, whereas demonstration of EBV in tumor cells favors plasmablastic lymphoma. In addition, other lymphomas demonstrating a plasmablastic morphology like anaplastic large cell lymphoma, ALK+ large B-cell lymphoma and primary effusion lymphoma (solid variant) should also be ruled out by investigating the expression of CD30 and T-cell markers, the expression of ALK protein, and the presence of HHV8 infection, respectively.

There is currently no gold standard chemotherapeutic approach for patients affected by plasmablastic lymphoma, and different regimens have been used. Bone marrow transplant and adjuvant radiotherapy have also been applied. Although plasmablastic lymphoma is usually negative for CD20, the use of Rituximab has been reported in some studies. The prognosis of the affected patients is very poor, and survival achieves a median of only 6–7 months in some studies and an estimated 5-year overall survival of 36% (95% CI, 30–42%). The importance of HIV and EBV infections for patients' prognosis remains debatable. Some reports describing total remission of the neoplasm after initiation of HAART therapy in HIV immunosuppressed patients have been published, but the neoplasm often recurs and patients' survival remains short (Figs. 41.1, 41.2, and 41.3).

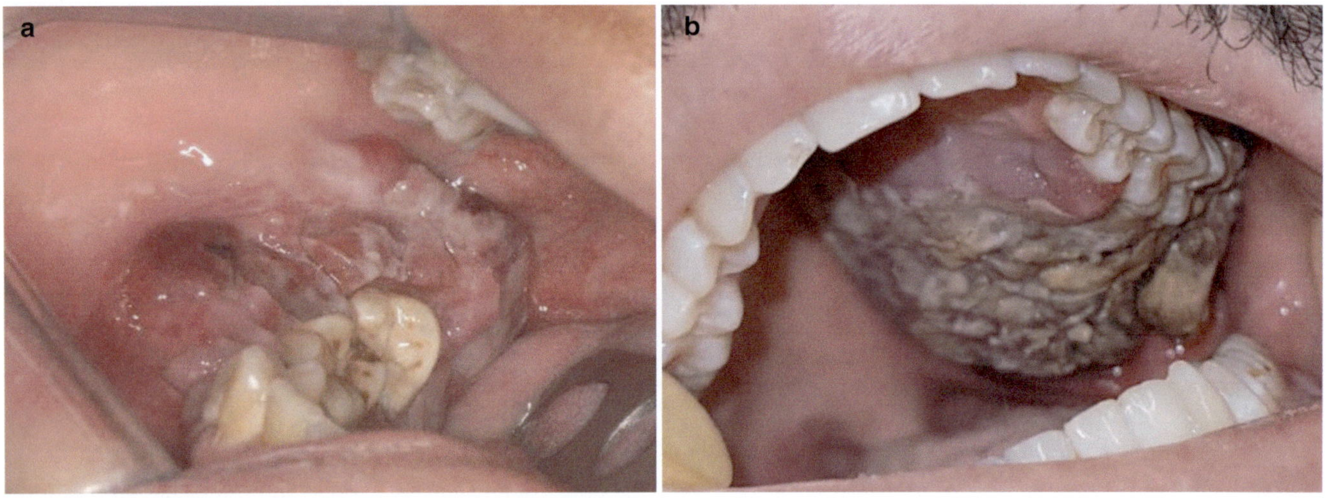

Fig. 41.1 Clinical presentation of plasmablastic lymphoma. (**a**) Ulcerated tumor affecting the lower gingiva of a 23-year-old, HIV-positive, male patient. (**b**) Aggressive neoplasm with extensive areas of tissue necrosis affecting the palate and the upper gingiva of a 32-year-old, HIV-positive, male patient. (Courtesy image: Dr. Juliana Diogo de Almeida Sampaio)

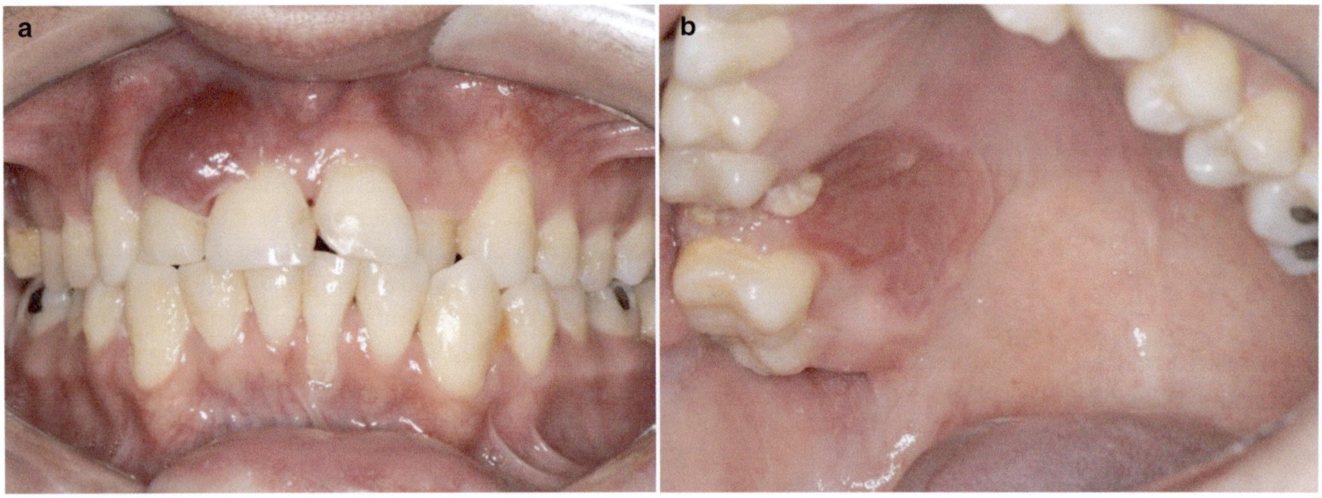

Fig. 41.2 Clinical presentation of plasmablastic lymphoma. (**a**) Asymptomatic, reddish nodule affecting the upper gingiva of a 23-year-old, HIV-positive, male patient. (**b**) The patient also presented a large ulcer in the hard palate

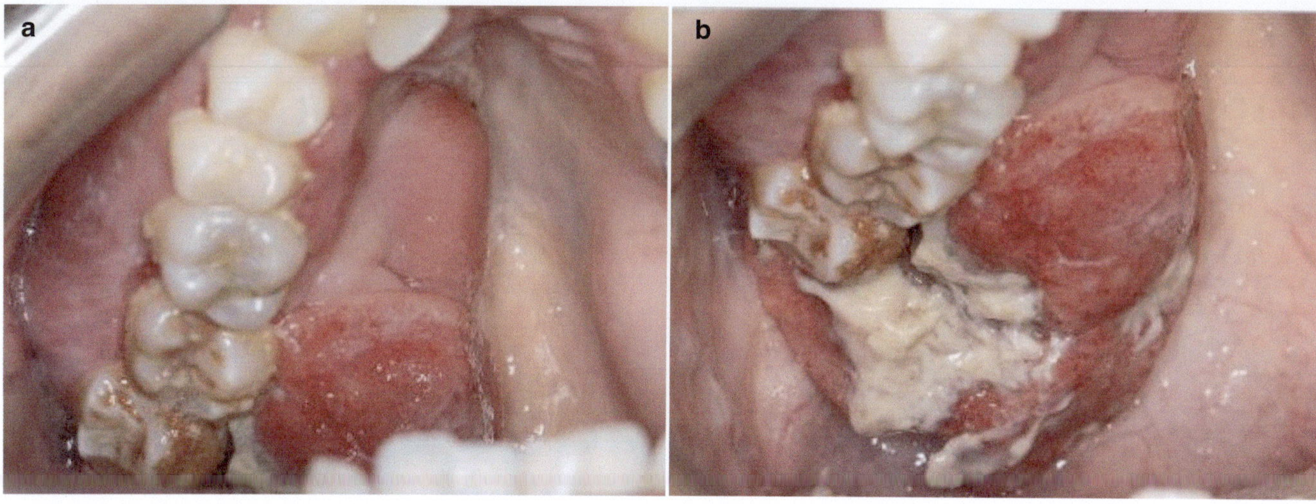

Fig. 41.3 Clinical presentation of plasmablastic lymphoma. (**a**) Painful, tumoral lesion affecting the vestibular mucosa, upper right gingiva and the palate of a 38-year-old male patient. (**b**) Note the extensive necrotic regions present in the neoplasm after a few days of follow-up. This clinical presentation is consistent with the highly aggressive biological nature of the disease and its microscopic features, characterized by a high proliferative rate

41.2 Microscopic Findings

- The neoplasm usually demonstrates a diffuse growth pattern of tumor cells.
- There usually is a scant vascularized and fibrous stroma.
- The presence of tingible body macrophages that give rise to the so-called "starry sky" microscopic pattern is commonly observed.
- Neoplastic cells are frequently distributed very close to each other, occasionally resulting in an epithelioid-like arrangement.
- The neoplasm is predominantly comprised of large neoplastic cells that exhibit a displaced nucleus to the periphery and an abundant basophilic to eosinophilic cytoplasm resembling large plasma cells called plasmablasts.
- Plasmablasts usually exhibit dispersed chromatin and one central nucleolus (resembling an immunoblast) or three or more peripherally located nucleoli (resembling centroblasts).
- Numerous typical and atypical mitotic figures are present.
- Some cases exhibit an increased number of smaller neoplastic cells more similar to normal plasma cells, being described as plasmacytic differentiation.
- Pleomorphic cells can also be seen.
- Necrotic regions are common (Figs. 41.4, 41.5, 41.6, 41.7, and 41.8).

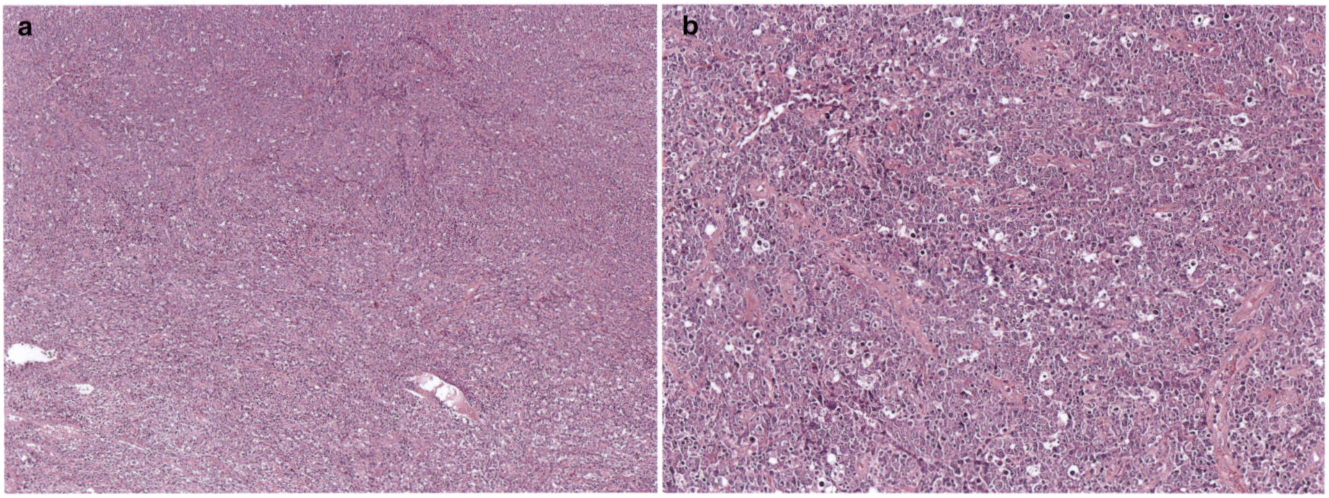

Fig. 41.4 Histopathologic features of plasmablastic lymphoma. (**a**) Diffuse proliferation of tumor cells and presence of the starry sky appearance (H&E; 25×). (**b**) The presence of clear tingible body macrophages gives rise to the starry sky pattern, indicative of a high proliferative index (H&E; 50×)

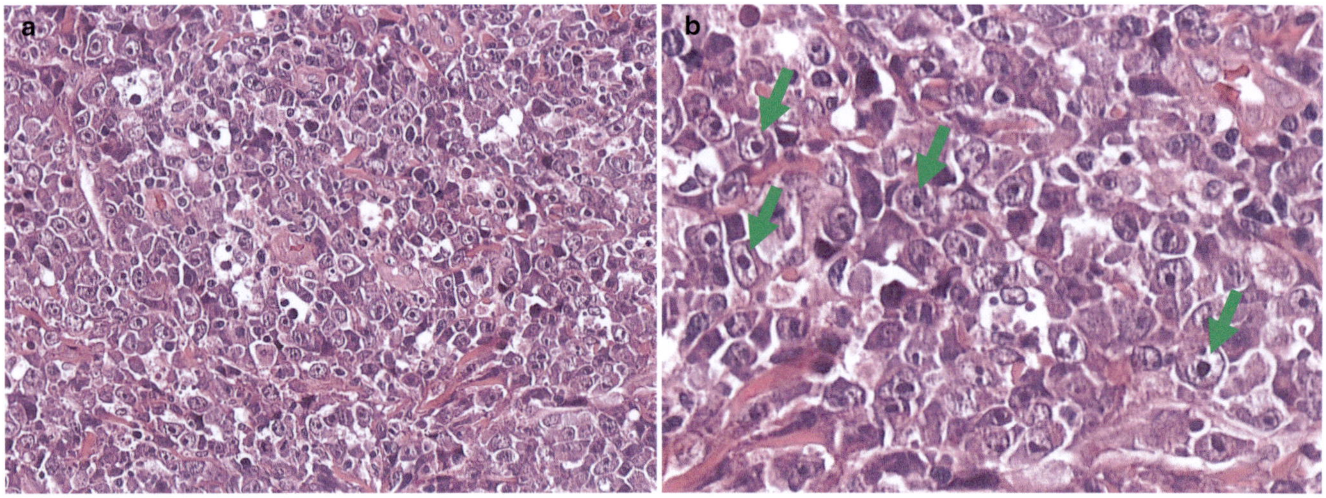

Fig. 41.5 Histopathologic features of plasmablastic lymphoma. (**a**) Tumor cells are large with loose chromatin that allows the observation of one or more prominent nucleoli in the center or in the periphery of the nuclei. Cytoplasm is ample and eosinophilic. Stroma is scarce and fibrotic (H&E; 100×). (**b**) The large neoplastic cells contain a prominent centrally-located nucleolus resembling immunoblasts or multiple peripherally located nucleoli resembling centroblasts (green arrows). The nucleus of these large neoplastic cells is frequently displaced to the periphery, consistent with plasmablasts. Some smaller neoplastic cells more similar to normal plasma cells are also present and in some cases they predominate, when the terminology plasmacytic differentiation is often used (H&E; 200×)

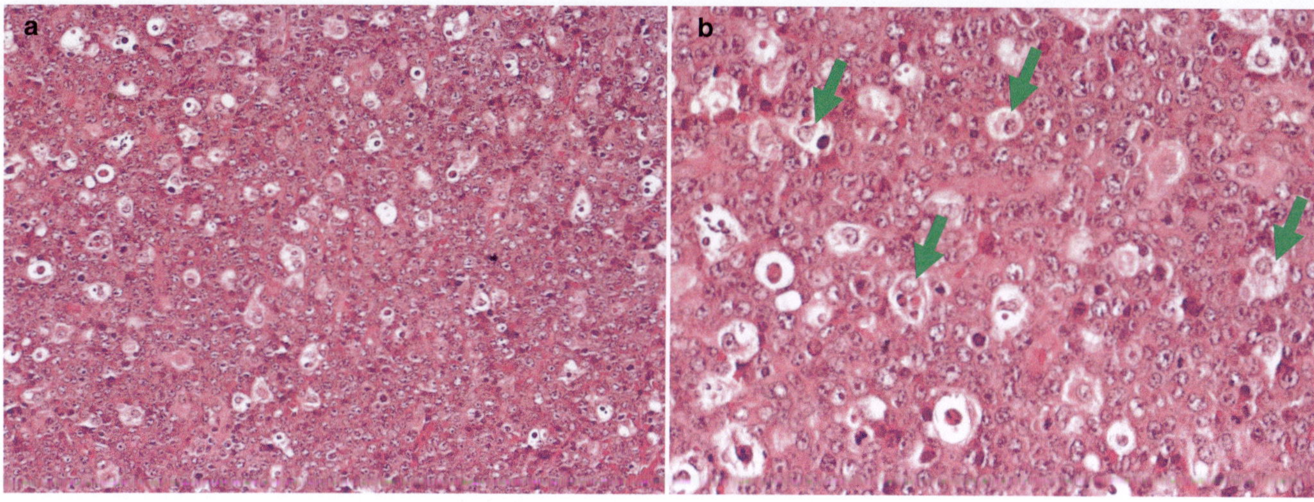

Fig. 41.6 Histopathologic features of plasmablastic lymphoma. (**a**) Observe the typical starry-sky microscopic pattern that can be observed in the majority of the cases due to the presence of tingible body macrophages (H&E;100X). (**b**) Tumor cells exhibit a very cohesive, sheet-like distribution, leading to a syncytial growth pattern that may give rise to an epithelioid aspect. Observe the presence of the tingible body macrophages (green arrows) with their characteristic clear cytoplasms, very often containing apoptotic debris (H&E;200X)

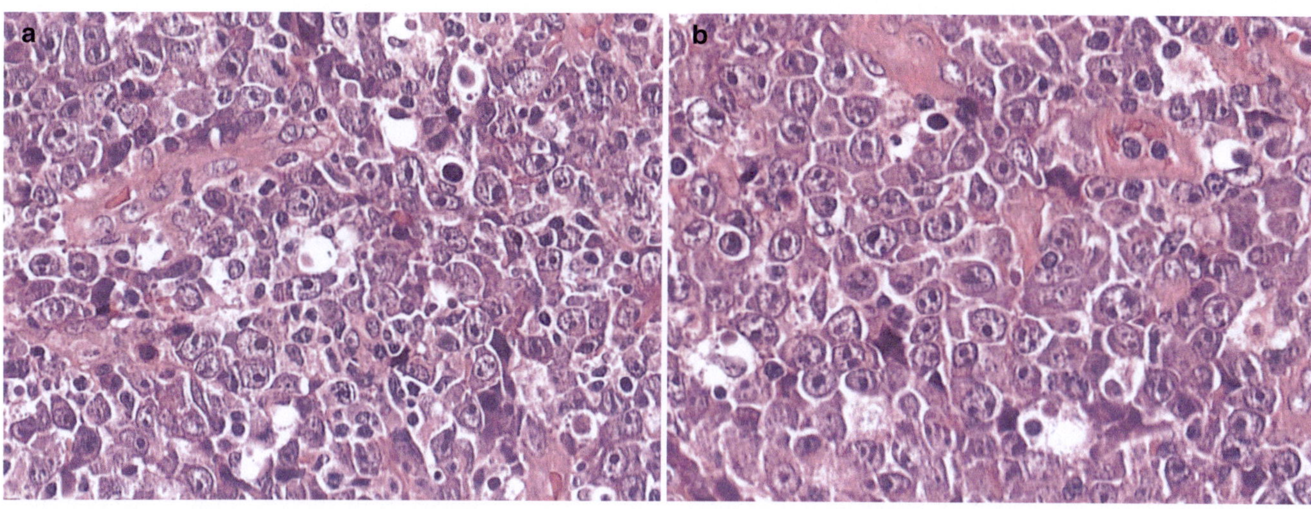

Fig. 41.7 Histopathologic features of plasmablastic lymphoma. (**a**) Observe the presence of centroblasts, immunoblasts and plasmablasts. Some tingible body macrophages phagocytizing apoptotic bodies and debris can also be seen (H&E; 200×). (**b**) Tumor cells have one or more prominent nucleoli. Plasmablasts exhibit the same nuclear features, but the nucleus is displaced, resembling plasma cells. The cytoplasm may show a clearer region near the nuclear membrane, which is reminiscent of the Hof region of plasma cells that corresponds to the negative image of the Golgi complex (H&E; 200×)

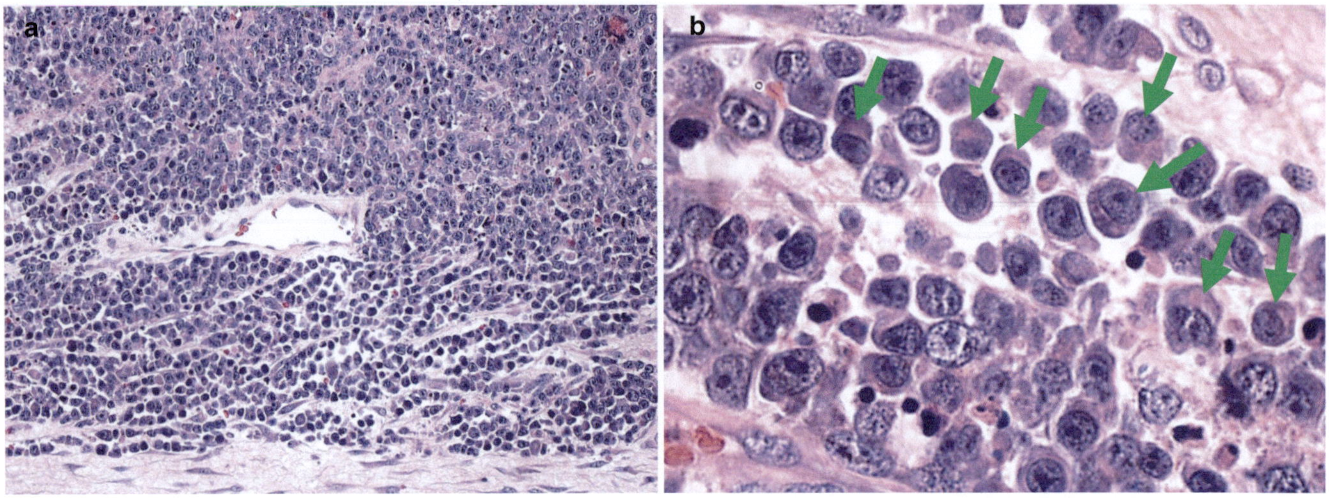

Fig. 41.8 Histopathologic features of plasmablastic lymphoma. (**a**) The upper part of the image shows a plasmablastic differentiation with predominantly large neoplastic cells with prominent central nucleolus, while the lower part of the image illustrates a plasmacytic differentiation with predominance of intermediary-sized cells (H&E; 100×). (**b**) Under high magnification it is possible to observe the plasmablastic cells with their prominent nucleoli (green arrows) and smaller plasmacytic cells (H&E; 400×)

41.3 Immunohistochemistry and/or Genetics

The main immunohistochemical markers used to diagnose plasmablastic lymphoma are those that demonstrate plasma cell differentiation. It is also important to demonstrate the lack of CD20 expression. Although very rare, ALK+ large B-cell lymphoma and extracavitary primary effusion lymphoma affecting the oral cavity should be considered as differential diagnoses when dealing with lymphomas demonstrating plasmablastic differentiation, and therefore, they will demand the investigation of ALK and HHV8, especially in those cases that do not demonstrate the typical immunohistochemical presentation or those negative for EBV. Anaplastic large cell lymphoma is another morphologically important differential diagnosis, also because plasmablastic lymphoma may express CD30 in up to 30% of the cases. However, the expression of CD30 in a diffuse and strong membranous staining with perinuclear dot-like pattern favors an anaplastic large cell lymphoma, while the expression of plasma cell markers and the presence of EBV are more consistent with a plasmablastic lymphoma.

It is important to investigate the presence of EBV by in situ hybridization (EBER) because most cases of plasmablastic lymphoma are associated with this virus, usually with a latency I program (EBER+, LMP1−, EBNA 2/3−), but occasionally with a latency II pattern (EBER+, LMP1+, EBNA 2/3−) and rarely latency type III (EBER+, LMP1+, EBNA 2/3+) in patients with a more severe immunosuppression. Of note, plasmacytoma/multiple myeloma, one of the main differential diagnoses, is more commonly negative for this virus. The proliferative index measured by K67 expression is usually very high in plasmablastic lymphoma, achieving up to 90% of positivity, which is usually much higher than the proliferative potential observed in plasmacytoma/multiple myeloma.

The molecular landscape of plasmablastic lymphoma is now better described with the presence of chromosome translocation involving *MYC* and immunoglobulin genes, alterations in members of the *JAK/STAT*, *MAPK/ERK* and *NOTCH* pathways, mutations in the *TP53* gene and somatic mutations in the *PRDM1* gene representing the most frequent genetic events described in this neoplasm (Table 41.1; Figs. 41.9, 41.10, 41.11, 41.12, 41.13, 41.14, 41.15, 41.16, and 41.17).

Table 41.1 Summary of the main immunohistochemical reactions used for plasmablastic lymphoma diagnosis

Antibody/probe	Most frequent results	Pattern	Objective
CD20	Negative or focally positive	Membrane	To exclude a DLBCL NOS
CD3	Negative	Membrane	To exclude the T-cell nature of the tumor
MUM1	Positive	Nucleus	To demonstrate the plasmablastic differentiation
Plasma cell	Positive	Cytoplasm	To demonstrate the plasmablastic differentiation
EMA	Positive	Membrane	To demonstrate the plasmablastic differentiation
CD138	Positive	Membrane	To demonstrate the plasmablastic differentiation
MYC	Positive	Nucleus	Tumor biological and molecular characterization
Ki67	~90%	Nucleus	To demonstrate the proliferative index of the tumor
ALK	Negative	Variable	To exclude an ALK+ LBCL
HHV8	Negative	Nucleus	To exclude an extracavitary PEL
EBER[a]	Positive in ~70% of the cases	Nucleus	To demonstrate the presence of EBV
MYC[b]	Positive in ~50% of the cases	–	Tumor biological and molecular characterization
JAK/STAT[b]	Positive in some cases	–	Tumor biological and molecular characterization
MAPK/ERK[b]	Positive in some cases	–	Tumor biological and molecular characterization
NOTCH[b]	Positive in some cases	–	Tumor biological and molecular characterization
TP53[b]	Positive in some cases	–	Tumor biological and molecular characterization
PRDM1[b]	Positive in some cases	–	Tumor biological and molecular characterization

The main results for EBV detection and molecular findings are also described

DLBCL NOS Diffuse large B-cell lymphoma not otherwise specified, *LBCL* Large B-cell lymphoma, *PEL* primary effusion lymphoma

[a]Investigated by in situ hybridization

[b]Investigated by fluorescent in situ hybridization or PCR

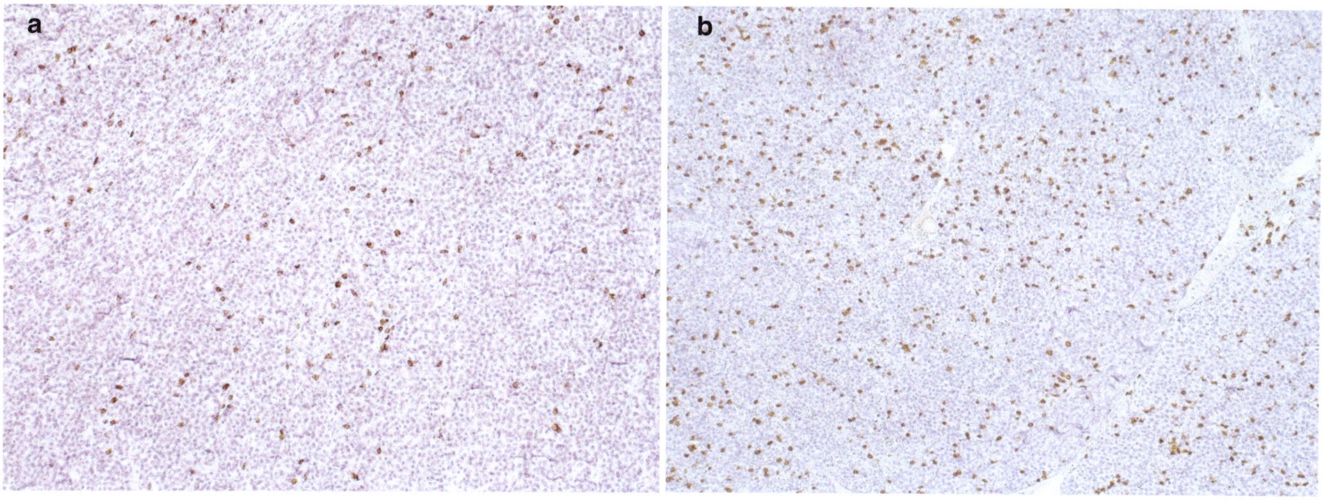

Fig. 41.9 Immunohistochemical features of Plasmablastic lymphoma. (**a**) Tumor cells are negative for mature B-cell markers like CD20 or are only focally positive. Observe the positivity only in reactive B lymphocytes (DAB; 100×). (**b**) The T-cell marker CD3 is also negative. Observe the positivity only in reactive T lymphocytes (DAB; 100×)

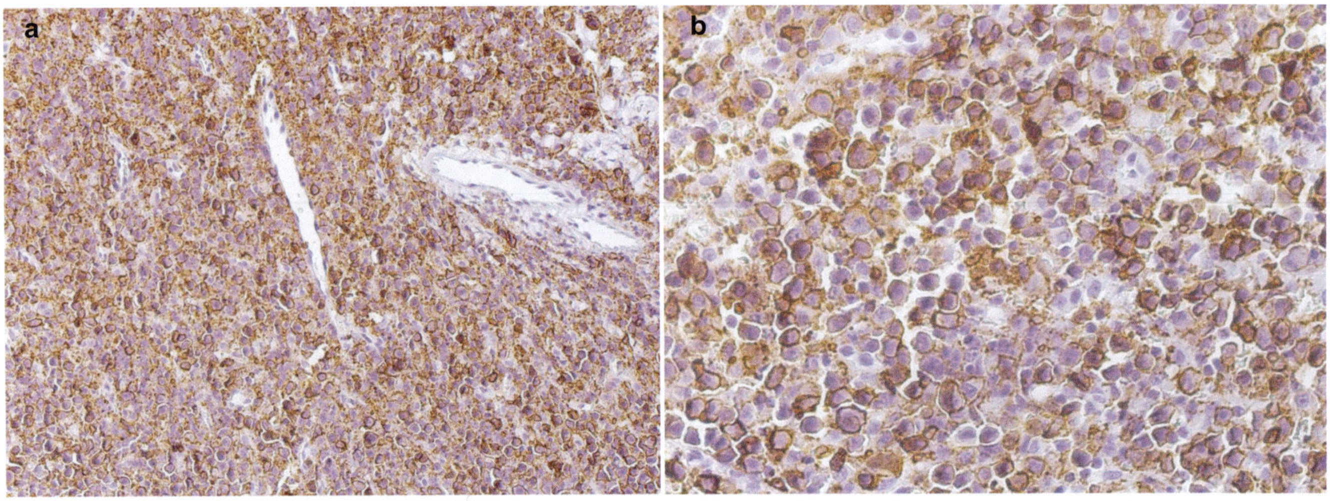

Fig. 41.10 Immunohistochemical features of Plasmablastic lymphoma. (**a**) Tumor cells are strongly and diffusely positive for CD138 in most cases (DAB; 100×). (**b**) Note the membranous staining pattern of CD138 in the plasmablastic lymphoma cells (DAB; 400×)

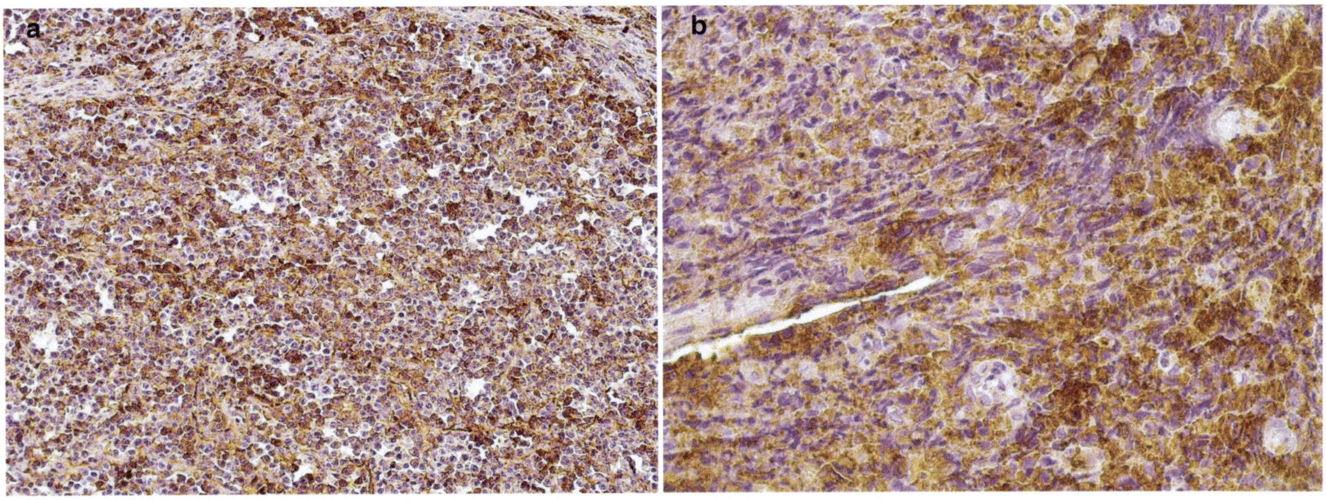

Fig. 41.11 Immunohistochemical features of Plasmablastic lymphoma. (**a**) Diffuse and cytoplasmic expression of plasma cell antibody (clone VS38c) (DAB; 100×). (**b**) Observe the cytoplasmic expression of the protein in tumor cells. It also demonstrates the plasmacytic immunophenotype of the tumor (DAB; 400×)

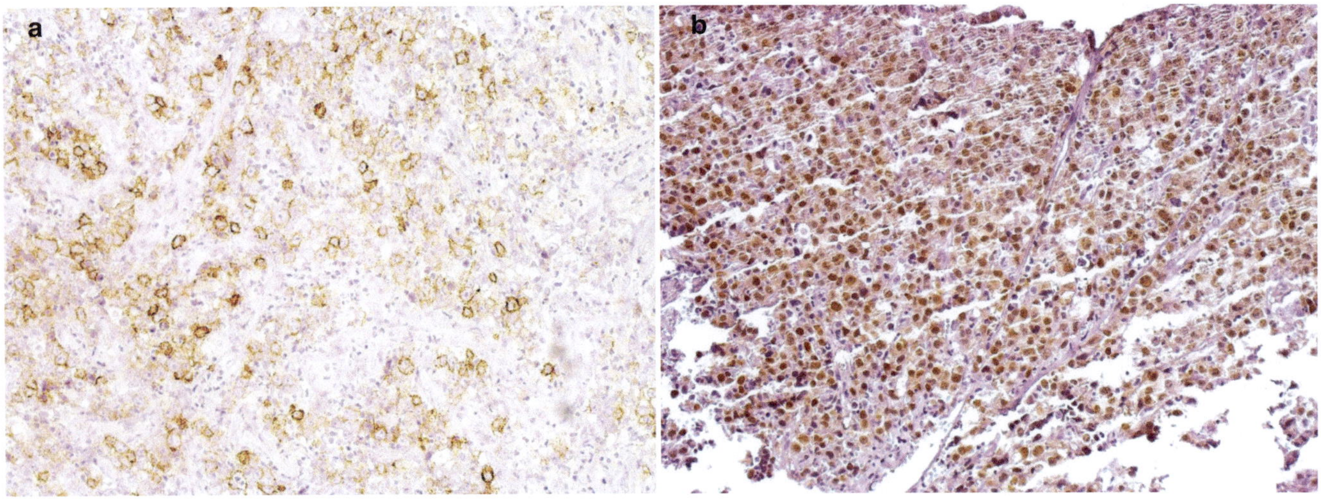

Fig. 41.12 Immunohistochemical features of Plasmablastic lymphoma. (**a**) The expression of EMA (DAB; 100×), and (**b**) MUM1 are also consistent with the plasmacytic differentiation of tumor cells (DAB; 100×)

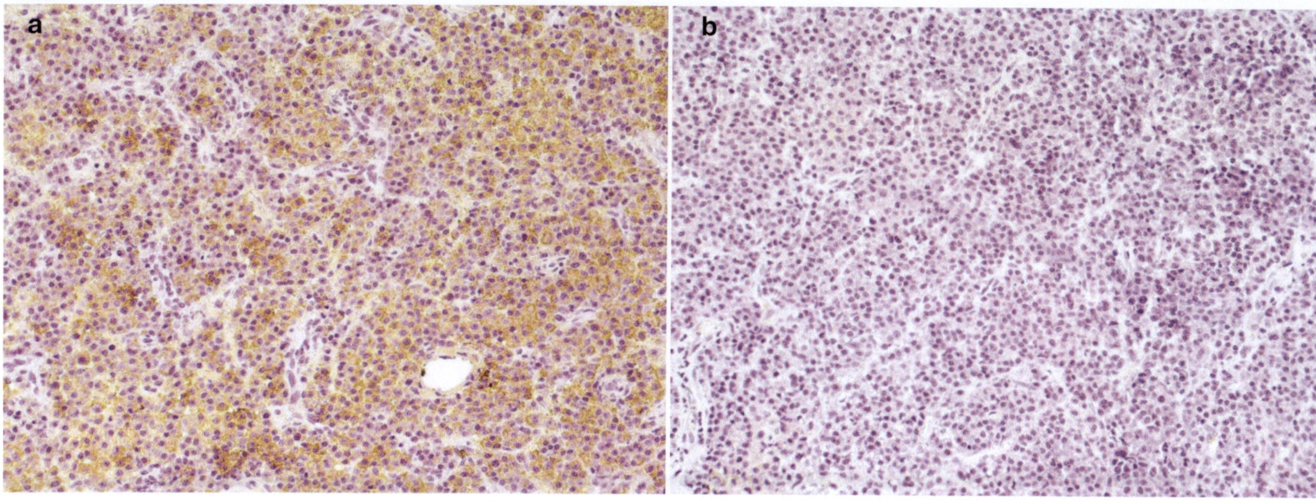

Fig. 41.13 Immunohistochemical features of Plasmablastic lymphoma. (**a**) Monoclonality of tumor cells is demonstrated by diffuse expression of immunoglobulin light chain Kappa (DAB; 200×), and (**b**) negativity to the immunoglobulin light chain Lambda (DAB; 200×)

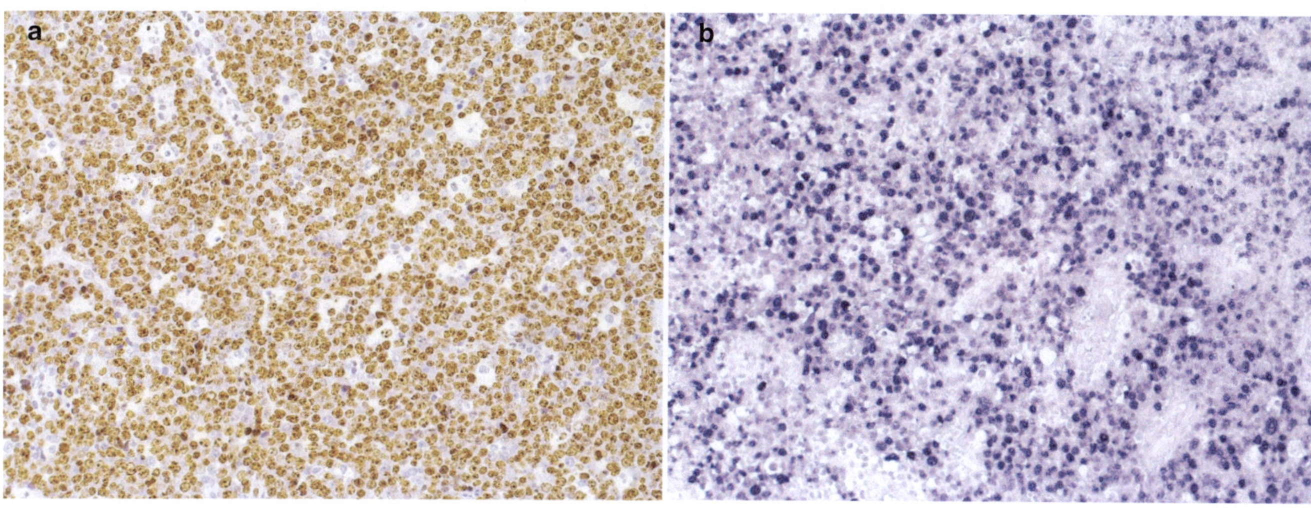

Fig. 41.14 Immunohistochemical features of Plasmablastic lymphoma. (**a**) The proliferative potential of plasmablastic lymphoma is very high, achieving up to 95% in some cases. Observe almost all cells expressing the Ki67 protein (DAB; 100×). (**b**) The presence of EBV is demonstrated using in situ hybridization. Observe the dark blue color in the nuclei of tumor cells (EBER; 100×)

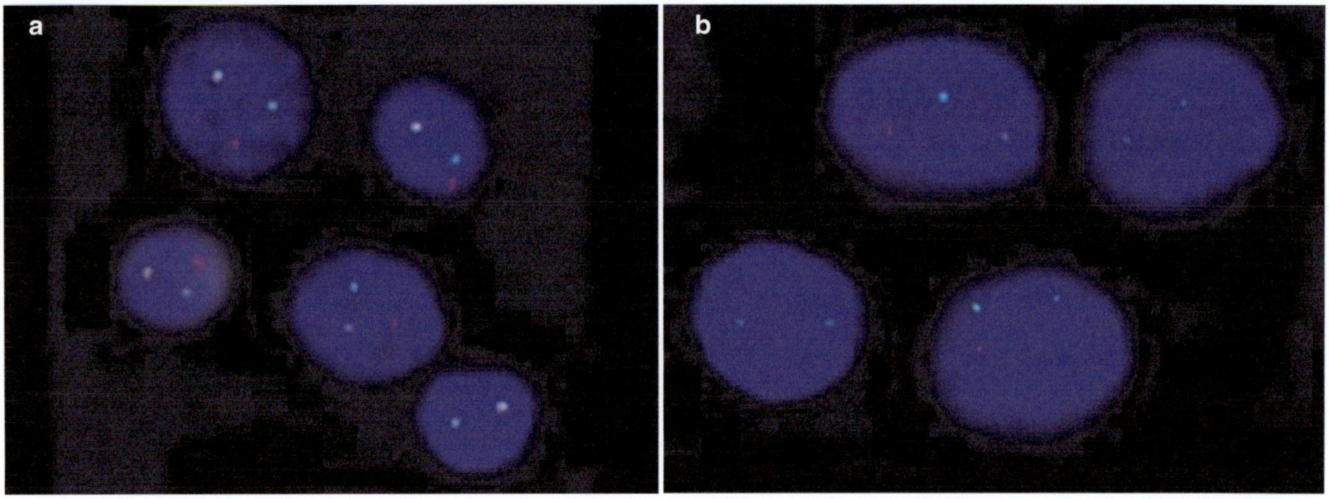

Fig. 41.15 Genetic features of plasmablastic lymphoma. Approximately 50% of the cases carry *MYC* translocation. (**a**) Observe the separated red and green signals illustrating the mutation by using a break-apart probe (FISH; 1000×). (**b**) Another example of *MYC* break-apart probe that illustrates the separation of green and red signals, denoting the occurrence of *MYC* translocation (FISH; 1000×)

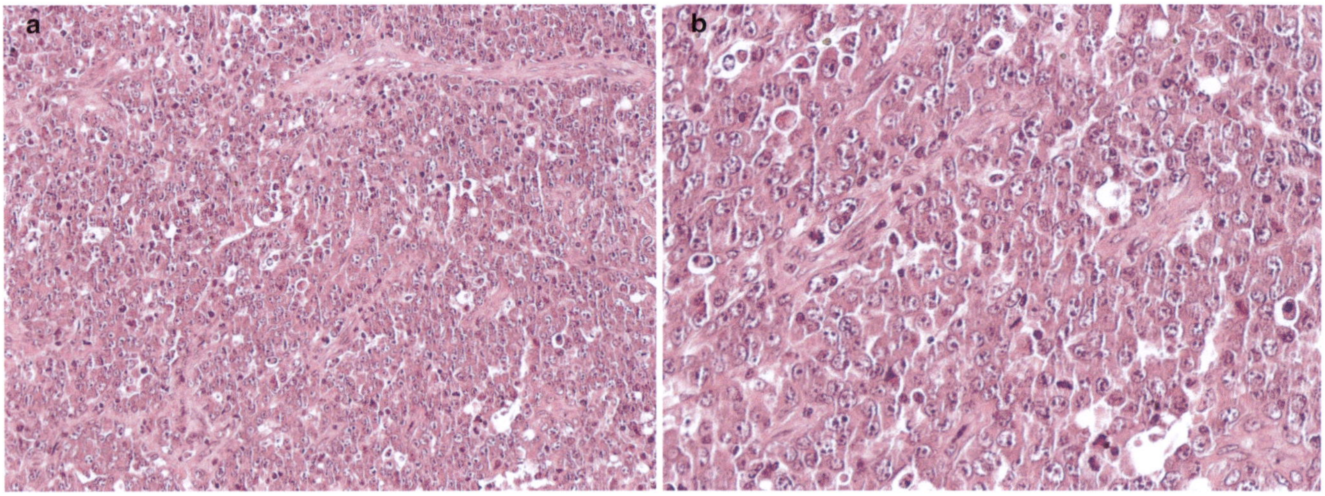

Fig. 41.16 Microscopic features of a primary effusion lymphoma. (**a**) The starry sky pattern is also present in this entity that exhibits a diffuse growth pattern of tumor cells (H&E; 100×). (**b**) The neoplastic cells also demonstrate an immunoblastic or plasmablastic appearance, strongly resembling plasmablastic lymphoma (H&E; 200×)

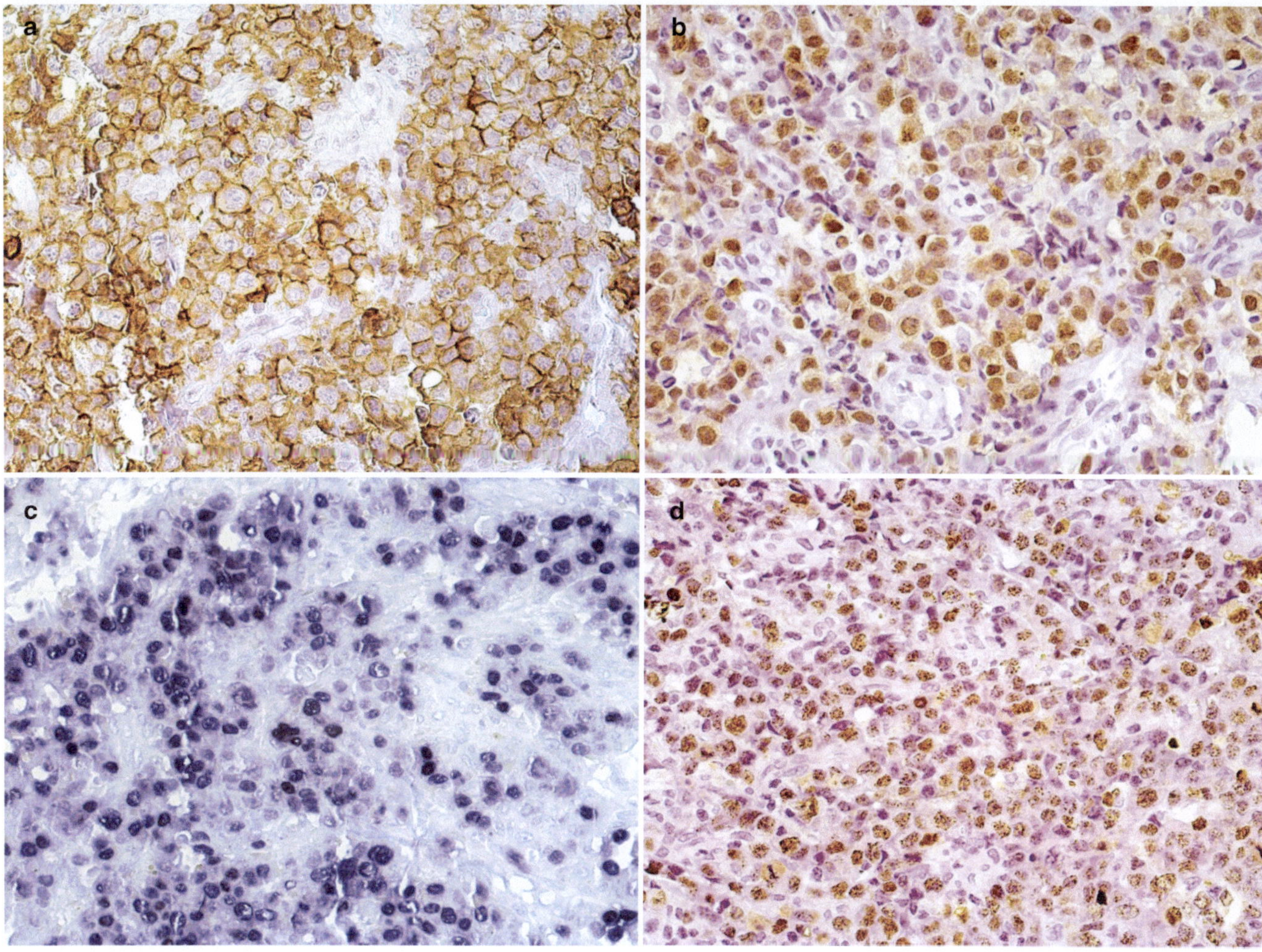

Fig. 41.17 Immunohistochemical features of primary effusion lymphoma and association with EBV and HHV8 infection. This is an important differential diagnosis for plasmablastic lymphomas. (**a**) diffusely positive for markers of plasmacytic differentiation like CD138 (DAB; 200×), and (**b**) MUM1 (DAB; 200×). (**c**) EBV is present in most of the cases and is demonstrated by in situ hybridization (EBER; 200×). (**d**) The presence of HHV8 in tumor cells is mandatory to confirm the diagnosis and very useful to differentiate this entity from plasmablastic lymphoma. Observe the nuclear positivity using LANA1 antibody (DAB; 200×)

Sources

1. Vega F, Chang CC, Medeiros LJ, et al. Plasmablastic lymphomas and plasmablastic plasma cell myelomas have nearly identical immunophenotypic profiles. Mod Pathol. 2005;18:806–15.
2. Valera A, Balagué O, Colomo L, et al. IG/MYC rearrangements are the main cytogenetic alteration in plasmablastic lymphomas. Am J Surg Pathol. 2010;34:1686–94.
3. Loghavi S, Alayed K, Aladily TN, et al. Stage, age, and EBV status impact outcomes of plasmablastic lymphoma patients: a clinicopathologic analysis of 61 patients. J Hematol Oncol. 2015;8:65–76.
4. Tchernonog E, Faurie P, Coppo P, et al. Clinical characteristics and prognostic factors of plasmablastic lymphoma patients: analysis of 135 patients from the LYSA group. Ann Oncol. 2017;28:843–8.
5. Rodrigues-Fernandes CI, de Souza LL, Santos-Costa SFD, Silva AMB, Pontes HAR, Lopes MA, de Almeida OP, Brennan PA, Fonseca FP. Clinicopathological analysis of oral plasmablastic lymphoma: a systematic review. J Oral Pathol Med. 2018;47(10):915–22. https://doi.org/10.1111/jop.12753.
6. Liu Z, Filip I, Gomez K, Engelbrecht D, Meer S, Lalloo PN, et al. Genomic characterization of HIV-associated plasmablastic lymphoma identifies pervasive mutations in the JAK-STAT pathway. Blood Cancer Discov. 2020;1(1):112–25. https://doi.org/10.1158/2643-3230.BCD-20-0051.
7. Ramis-Zaldivar JE, Gonzalez-Farre B, Nicolae A, Pack S, Clot G, Nadeu F, et al. MAPK and JAK-STAT pathways dysregulation in plasmablastic lymphoma. Haematologica. 2021;106(10):2682–93. https://doi.org/10.3324/haematol.2020.271957.
8. Fonseca FP, Robinson L, van Heerden MB, van Heerden WFP. Oral plasmablastic lymphoma: a clinicopathological study of 113 cases. J Oral Pathol Med. 2021;50(6):594–602. https://doi.org/10.1111/jop.13210.
9. Nel C, Robinson L, Ker-Fox J, van Heerden WFP. Radiological features of oral and maxillofacial plasmablastic lymphomas. Oral Radiol. 2022;38(4):610–7. https://doi.org/10.1007/s11282-022-00598-y.
10. Dotlic S, Gibson SE, Hartmann S, Hsi ED, Klimkowska M, Rodriguez-Pinilla SM, et al. Lymphomas with plasmablastic features: a report of the lymphoma workshop of the 20th meeting of the European Association for Haematopathology.

Virchows Arch. 2023;483(5):591–609. https://doi.org/10.1007/s00428-023-03585-8.

11. Gomes NR, Lima LA, Morais-Perdigão AL, de Caceres CVBL, Sant'Ana MSP, Pontes HAR, et al. Radiological aspects of lymphomas and leukaemias affecting the jaws: a systematic review. J Oral Pathol Med. 2023;52(4):315–23. https://doi.org/10.1111/jop.13422.
12. Ramirez-Gamero A, Martínez-Cordero H, Beltrán BE, Florindez J, Malpica L, Castillo JJ. Plasmablastic lymphoma: 2024 update on diagnosis, risk stratification, and management. Am J Hematol. 2024;99(8):1586–94. https://doi.org/10.1002/ajh.27376.
13. Hansen AR, Vardell VA, Fitzgerald LA. Epidemiologic characteristics, treatment patterns, and survival analysis of plasmablastic lymphoma in the United States: a SEER and NCDB analysis. Clin Lymphoma Myeloma Leuk. 2024;24(4):e152–e160.e3. https://doi.org/10.1016/j.clml.2023.12.014.
14. Chen BJ, Hsieh TH, Yuan CT, Wang RC, Yang CF, Chuang WY, et al. Clinicopathological and genetic landscape of plasmablastic lymphoma in Taiwan. Pathol Res Pract. 2024;253:155059. https://doi.org/10.1016/j.prp.2023.155059.
15. Di Ciaccio PR, Polizzotto MN, Cwynarski K, et al. The influence of immunodeficiency, disease features, and patient characteristics on survival in plasmablastic lymphoma. Blood. 2024;143(2):152–65. https://doi.org/10.1182/blood.2023021348.

Plasmacytoma and Multiple Myeloma

42

Ricardo Alves Mesquita, Chané Smit, Nathalia Rodrigues Gomes, Mauricio Augusto Aquino de Castro, and Felipe Paiva Fonseca

42.1 General Overview and Clinical Presentation

Plasmacytoma and multiple myeloma represent malignant proliferations originating from plasma cells, which are post-germinal center, class-switched, terminally differentiated B-cells that secrete monoclonal immunoglobulins called M-proteins or paraproteins. The International Agency for Research on Cancer (IARC) estimated for 2018 a total of 160,000 new cases worldwide, and 106,000 deaths, accounting for approximately 10% of all malignant hematolymphoid tumors, therefore, representing the second most common intra-osseous malignancy after osteosarcomas. Although extramedullary plasmacytoma is well known, this presentation is unusual and should be carefully differentiated from other malignant hematolymphoid tumors that may also contain a large number of plasma cells like marginal zone lymphoma of the mucosa-associated lymphoid tissue (MALT lymphoma).

Plasmacytoma and multiple myeloma are conditions that commonly affect the bones, typically those with active hematopoiesis like the spine, followed by the pelvis, skull, ribs, vertebrae and long bones. The axial skeleton is more affected than the appendicular, while the gnathic bones are affected in up to 30% of cases. Males are more affected and patients are usually in their sixth to seventh decades of life. Plasmacytoma manifests as a solitary lesion in the bone (solitary plasmacytoma of bone) or in an extramedullary site (extramedullary plasmacytoma), whereas multiple myeloma is characterized by a group of different clinical, radiological and laboratorial manifestations that include multiple bone lesions, anemia, hypocalcemia, renal impairment (CRAB features), monoclonal protein (M-protein) deposition and Bence-Jones proteinuria. It is estimated that approximately 50% of plasmacytomas will evolve to multiple myeloma during patients' follow-up. Immunosuppressed patients may also develop plasmacytoma/multiple myeloma, but a higher incidence in this group of patients is not observed, in contrast to plasmablastic lymphoma.

In the jaws, plasmacytoma presents with a solitary bone lesion, while multiple myeloma shows multiple radiolucent, ill-defined lesions on panoramic radiography, more commonly seen in the posterior region of the mandible. Both maxilla and mandible can be simultaneously affected in some cases. The so-called "punch out" radiographic feature is common and can also be appreciated on cone-beam computed tomography. Periosteal reactions can be variably identified, either as "sun-burst aspect" or as "Codman triangle." Large areas of bone destruction can be seen in advanced cases, leading to tooth displacement or mobility. In cases of multiple myeloma, lateral cephalogram can have a 'pepper-pot' skull appearance due to the multiple punched-out lesions affecting the calvarium. Intra-oral manifestations result from cortical bone destruction and may be painful or asymptomatic. The lesions present as non-ulcerated growths or may reveal extensive regions of tissue necrosis or ulcerations. Numb chin syndrome is uncommon, but has been described in some patients affected by plasmacytoma and multiple myeloma. Bone fractures may occur in more advanced diseases.

In some cases, the occurrence of amyloid deposition in oral and maxillofacial structures can be found, and the diagnosis of oral amyloidosis in patients affected by plasmacytoma and multiple myeloma is well described. Oral amyloidosis more commonly manifests as diffuse and asymptomatic enlargement of the tongue, which may present a range from normal to a yellowish-colored mucosa.

R. A. Mesquita (✉) · N. R. Gomes · M. A. A. de Castro · F. P. Fonseca
Department of Oral Surgery and Pathology, School of Dentistry, Universidade Federal de Minas Gerais, Belo Horizonte, Brazil
e-mail: ramesquita@ufmg.br

C. Smit
Department of Oral and Maxillofacial Pathology, School of Dentistry University of Pretoria, Pretoria, South Africa
e-mail: chane.smit@up.ac.za

© The Author(s), under exclusive license to Springer Nature Switzerland AG 2025
F. P. Fonseca et al. (eds.), *Lymphoproliferative and Granulomatous Disorders of the Oral Cavity*,
https://doi.org/10.1007/978-3-031-98844-8_42

Macroglossia often presents with indented lateral borders due to pressure from the adjacent teeth. Other sites like the buccal mucosa, palate and lips may also be affected as asymptomatic nodules or tumors, and the presence of ulceration may be found. The amyloid deposits can also be observed in other organs like the kidneys, liver and heart, potentially resulting in severe organ damage.

Extramedullary plasmacytoma presents with a more favorable prognosis. Solitary plasmacytoma of the bone has been treated by surgery, radiation and/or systemic therapy, with a variable recurrence rate and prognosis. Progression to multiple myeloma may occur, and the risk depends on some parameters like tumor size, bone marrow involvement and patient's age. Multiple myeloma is considered an incurable disease in most instances, despite the important improvements in the current treatment modalities, which have significantly improved survival rates. Therapeutic schemes range from different chemotherapy approaches associated with the use of anti-resorptive drugs, to target immunotherapy to bone marrow transplantation.

During the last decades, the prognosis of patients affected by multiple myeloma has improved, but it may still range from as low as 6 months for widespread aggressive variants to over 10 years for the smoldering subtype of multiple myeloma, with a mean 5-year survival rate of 55.6%. Different clinical and biochemical parameters, including the International Staging System, clinical stage and Eastern Cooperative Oncology Group scale, microscopic features and genetic findings, among others, are considered important prognostic determinants (Figs. 42.1, 42.2, 42.3, 42.4, 42.5, and 42.6).

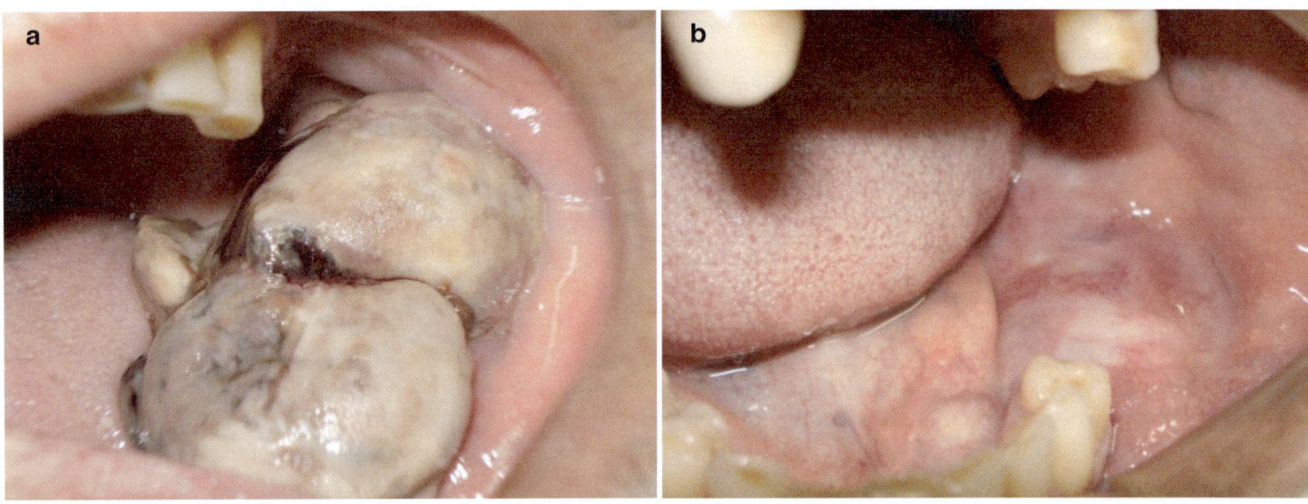

Fig. 42.1 Clinical presentation of multiple myeloma affecting the oral cavity. (**a**) An aggressive tumor affecting the mandible with extensive areas of necrosis. The patients also had osteolytic lesions in other bones. (**b**) A non-ulcerated expansion of the mandible left side. The patient also had lesions in the ribs and skull

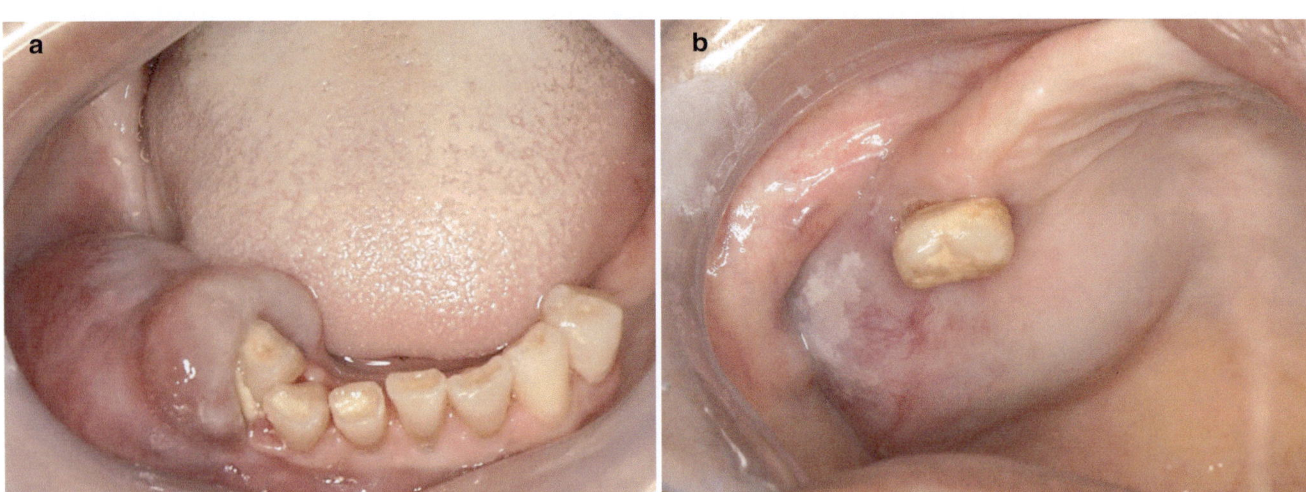

Fig. 42.2 Clinical presentation of multiple myeloma affecting the oral cavity. (**a**) A male patient was affected by multiple bone lesions that caused a large tumor growth in the mandible. The lesion was asymptomatic. (**b**) The same patient also had a lesion in the maxillary bone that caused an expansive growth in the upper alveolar ridge and hard palate

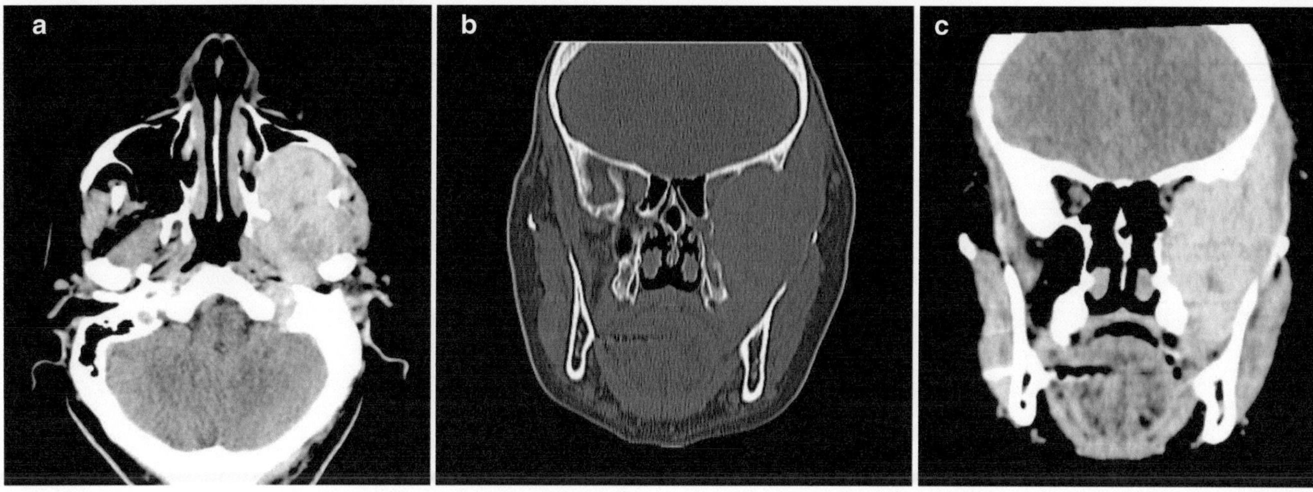

Fig. 42.3 Computed tomography features of solitary plasmacytoma of bone affecting the maxilla. (**a**) Axial section showing the hypodense image of an extensive, destructive and infiltrative neoplasm in the maxilla of the left side. The tumor infiltrates the maxillary sinus. (**b**) Coronal section showing the infiltrative growth of the neoplasm toward the temporal bone and base of the skull. (**c**) Coronal section showing that the orbital cavity was already infiltrated by neoplastic cells

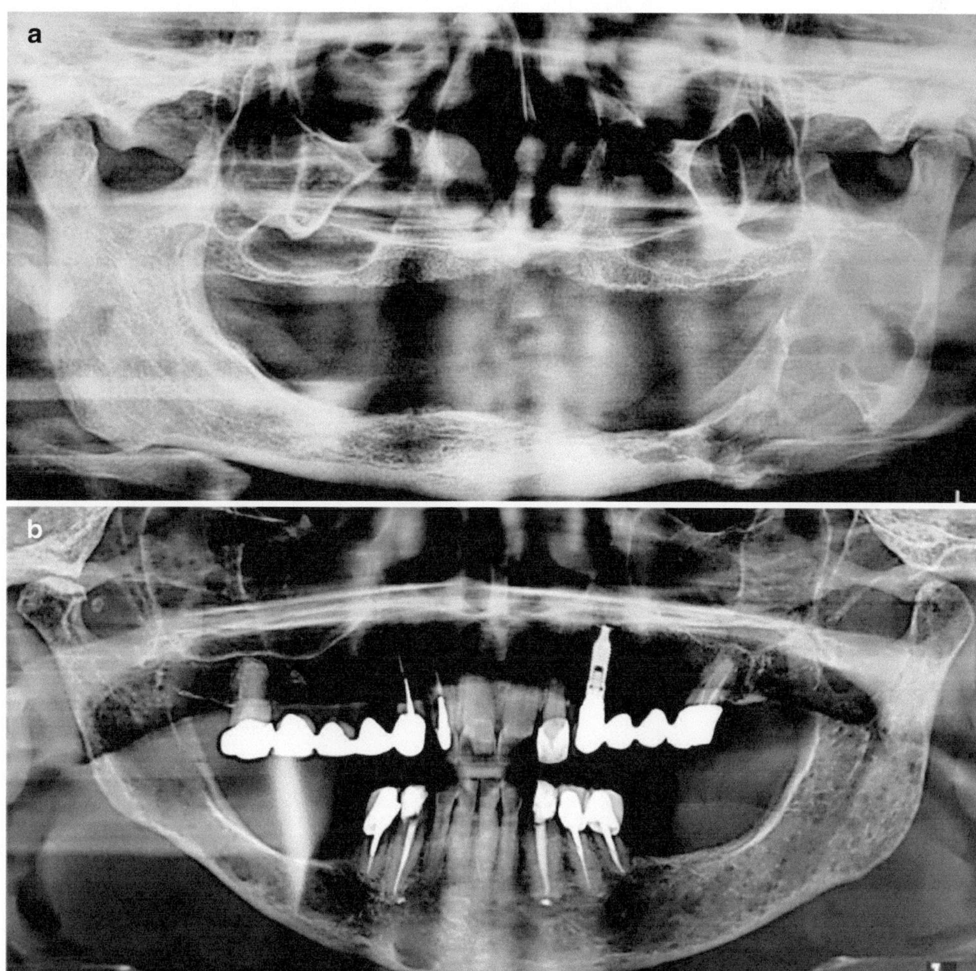

Fig. 42.4 Radiographic features of multiple myeloma affecting the gnathic bones. (**a**) Radiolucent lesion affecting the posterior region and ascending ramus of the mandible, left side. The image borders are irregular and ill-defined. (**b**) Multiple radiolucent lesions affecting the mandible and the maxilla bilaterally. In the mandible body, it is possible to observe the so-called "punched-out" aspect of the tumor. The posterior regions of the maxilla, the tuberosity region, exhibiting radiolucent lesions

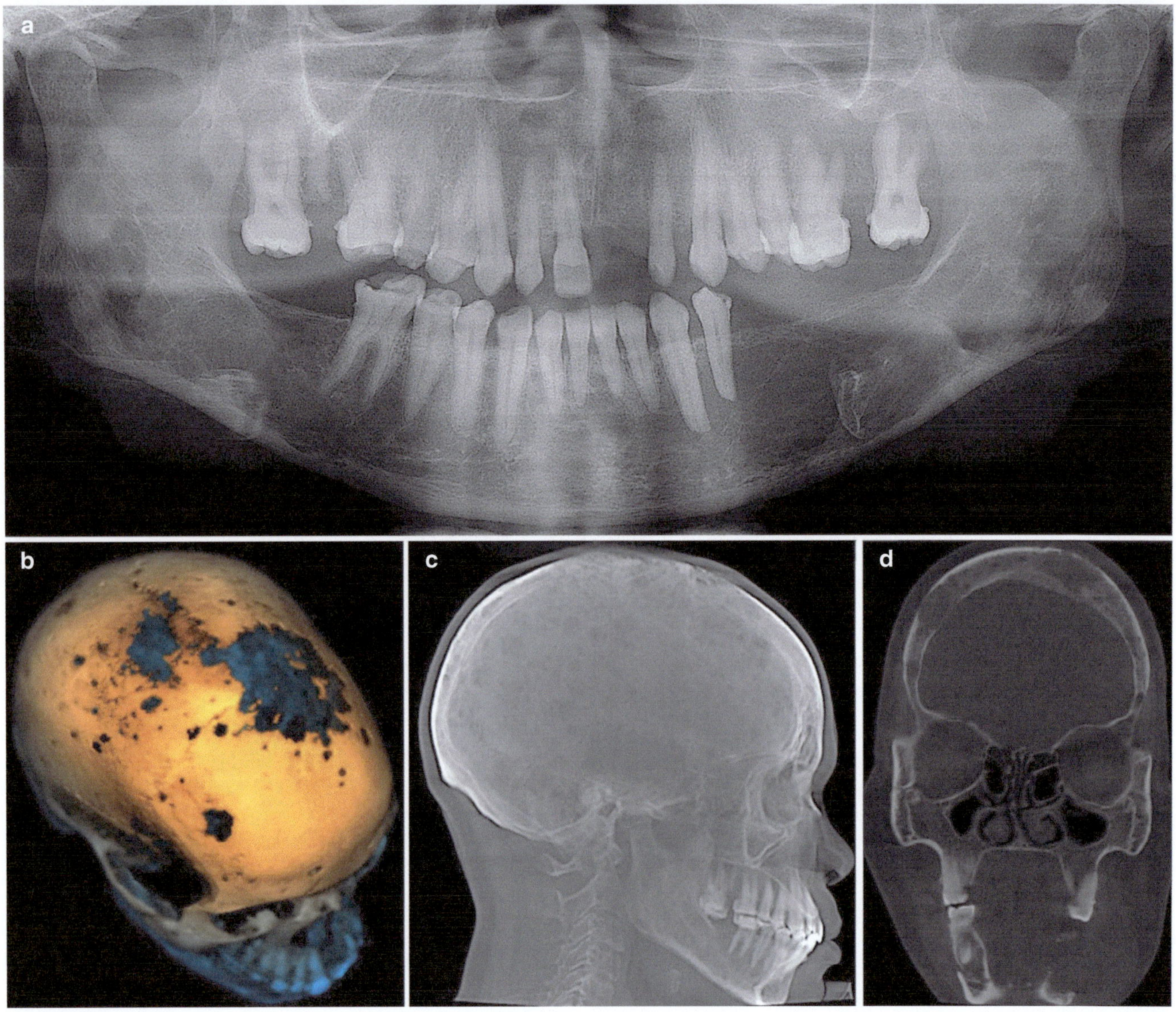

Fig. 42.5 Radiographic features of multiple myeloma affecting the gnathic bones. (**a**) Panoramic radiograph showing multiple ill-defined radiolucent lesions diffusely affecting the whole mandible. (**b**) Cone-beam computed tomography (CBCT) volumetric reconstruction of the skull bone showing the punched-out lesions. (**c**) Sagittal skull view demonstrating the characteristic pepper-pot skull radiographic appearance. (**d**) Coronal section of CBCT illustrating the presence of multiple ill-defined hypodense images affecting the skull, maxilla and mandible

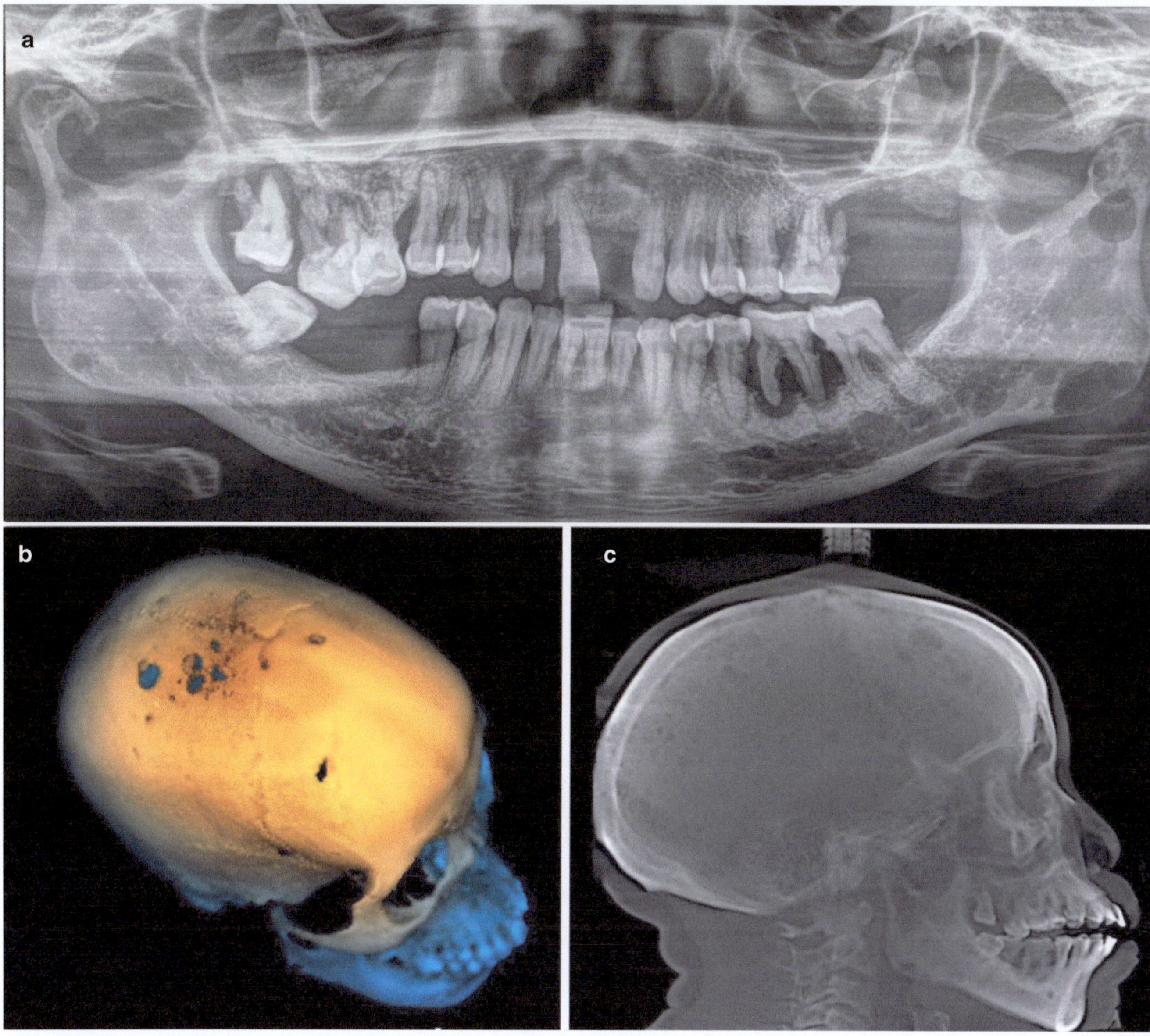

Fig. 42.6 Radiographic features of multiple myeloma affecting the gnathic bones. (**a**) Multiple irregular and ill-defined radiolucent images diffusely affecting the whole mandibular body. (**b**) CBCT volumetric reconstruction of the skull bone showing the osseous lesions. (**c**) Skull sagittal view demonstrating the characteristic punch-out radiographic aspect

42.2 Microscopic Findings

- Plasmacytoma and multiple myeloma cannot be differentiated based on microscopic or immunophenotypic findings, since they present similar histopathologic aspects.
- Tumor cells commonly exhibit a solid, diffuse growth pattern.
- Fibrous stroma is usually present, but scarce.
- Neoplastic plasma cells present different grades of pleomorphism and atypia.
- Neoplastic plasma cells may exhibit normal appearance in many cases or exhibit dysplastic features like nuclear hyperchromatism without the typical nucleoli located in the periphery of the nuclear membrane.
- Some cases may have plasmablasts (large cells with prominent central nucleolus) and should be differentiated from plasmablastic lymphomas.
- Highly pleomorphic cases with a high proliferative index may be seen and represent an anaplastic variant of the disease.
- Dutcher bodies and Russel bodies are frequently seen.
- Amyloid deposits present as pink, amorphous, waxy-looking material and are more commonly found around blood vessels.

- A characteristic cracking artefact is present in amyloid deposits.
- Amyloid deposits can be surrounded by multinucleated giant cells.
- Congo red stains amyloid as pink to red color under light microscopy, while polarized microscopy is used to confirm the presence of these deposits by demonstrating an apple-green birefringence.
- The oral cavity may also be affected by several other conditions like lipoid proteinosis, hyaline fibromatosis syndrome, ligneous gingivitis/periodontitis, lichen sclerosus, local scleroderma, and oral submucous fibrosis, that may microscopically resemble amyloidosis; however, microscopic and clinical correlation usually lead to correct diagnosis (Figs. 42.7, 42.8, 42.9, and 42.10).

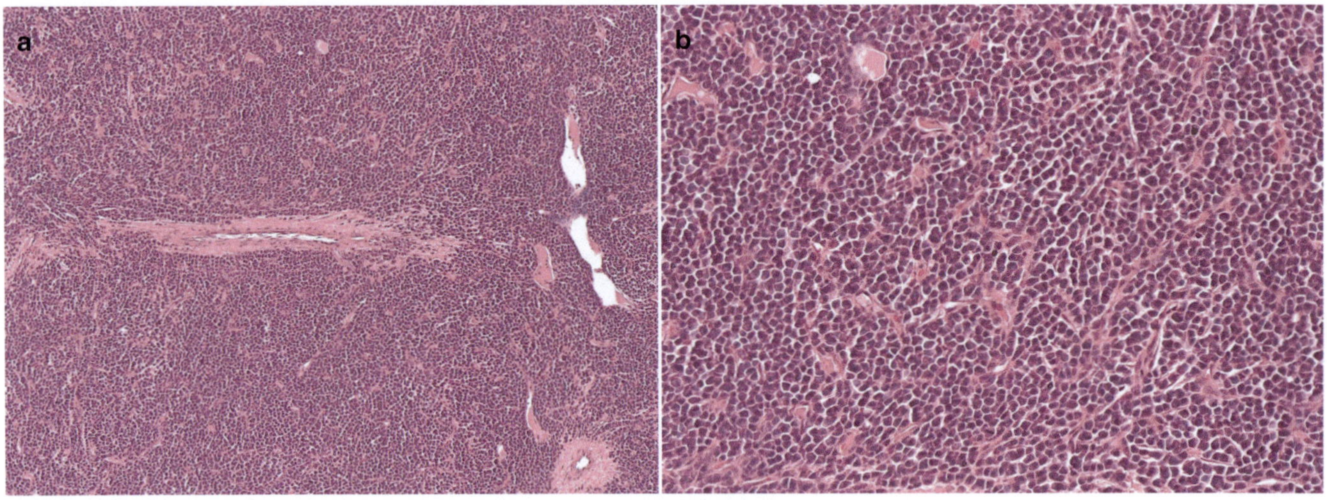

Fig. 42.7 Microscopic findings of plasmacytoma and multiple myeloma. (**a**) Diffuse proliferation of neoplastic cells (H&E; 25×). (**b**) Tumor cells exhibit plasma cell differentiation with a predominance of hyperchromatic nuclei and an eosinophilic cytoplasm (H&E; 100×)

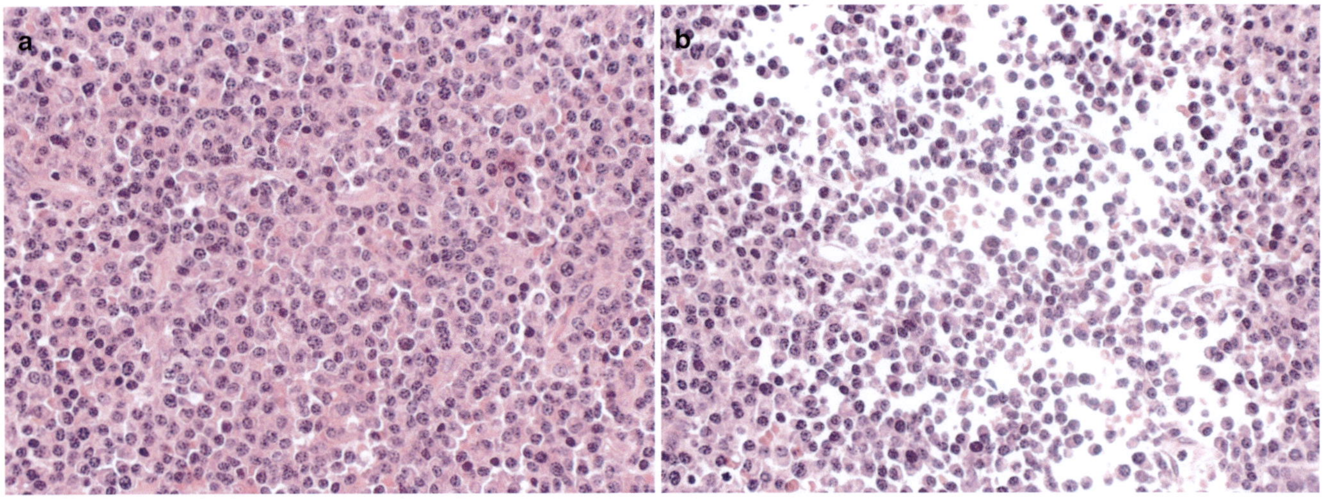

Fig. 42.8 Microscopic findings of plasmacytoma and multiple myeloma. (**a**) Diffuse proliferation of neoplastic plasma cells that show multiple, small nucleoli and an abundant eosinophilic cytoplasm, resembling normal plasmacytic differentiation. Some atypia can be found (H&E; 100×). (**b**) In areas where tumor cells are more loosely distributed, the plasma cell morphology can be more easily observed. Mitotic figures and nuclear pleomorphism can also be seen in this image (H&E; 100×)

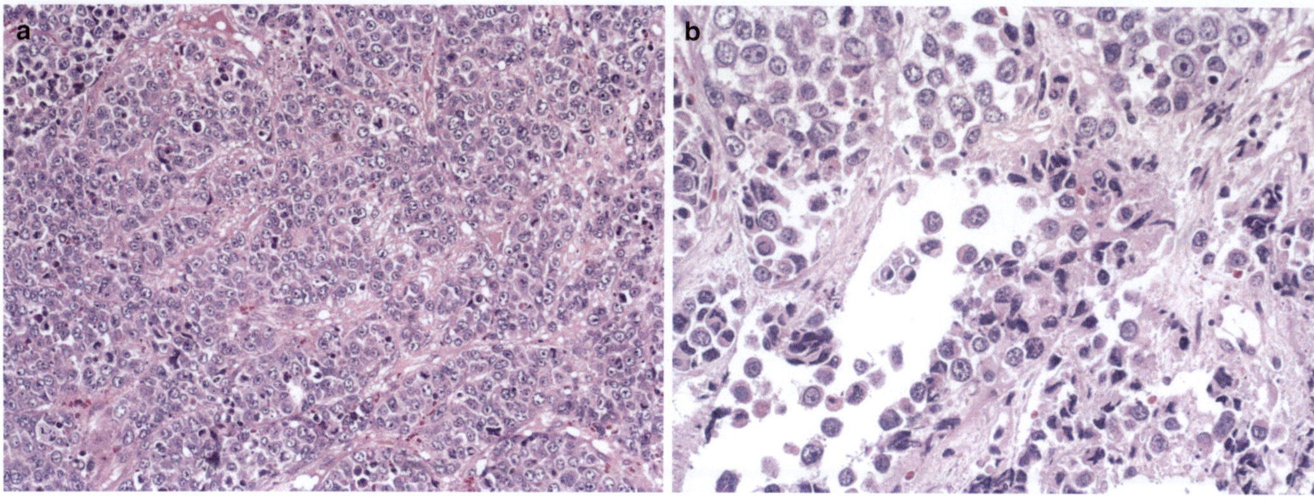

Fig. 42.9 Microscopic findings of plasmacytoma and multiple myeloma. (**a**) In some cases of plasmacytoma/multiple myeloma, tumor cells are larger and exhibit one or more prominent nucleoli resembling plasmablasts (H&E; 100×). (**b**) A higher degree of pleomorphism can be seen in these cases. Observe the larger neoplastic cells showing a displaced nucleus containing prominent nucleoli and an eosinophilic cytoplasm. This microscopic presentation is more difficult to be differentiated from plasmablastic lymphoma (H&E; 200×)

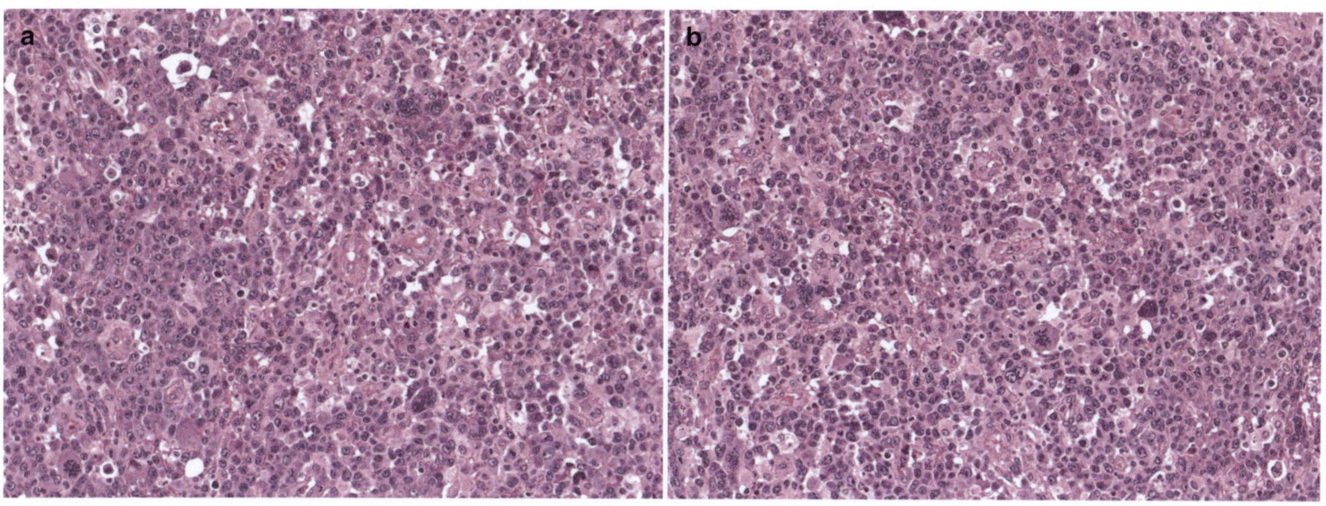

Fig. 42.10 Microscopic findings of plasmacytoma and multiple myeloma. (**a**) Plasmacytoma/multiple myeloma may exhibit a higher degree of cellular pleomorphism with the presence of anaplastic cells. Observe the very atypical mitotic figs. (H&E; 100×). (**b**) In addition to the tumor cells with the typical plasma cell differentiation, anaplastic cells exhibiting hyperchromatic and multilobated nuclei is observed (H&E; 100×)

42.3 Immunohistochemistry and/or Genetics

Immunohistochemistry demonstrates the plasmacytic origin of the neoplasm through positivity to CD38, CD138, plasma cell (VS38c), MUM1 and/or EMA. Mature B-cell markers like CD20 are negative, but CD79a can be focally positive. In addition, mature T-cell markers like CD3 are negative. Immunoglobulin light chain restriction is considered mandatory and is established by demonstrating kappa or lambda expression. Monoclonality for kappa is more frequently found than for lambda. The investigation of monoclonality by immunohistochemistry may be problematic in many cases due to important and frequent unspecific staining, which is improved using chromogenic in situ hybridization (CISH). The proliferative index varies, but it is usually lower than observed in plasmablastic lymphoma, ranging from 30% to 40% in most cases, except for the anaplastic variant that may achieve 90% of positivity. Expression of CD56 and cyclin D1 can be found in a minority of cases. Plasmacytoma and multiple myeloma are usually EBV-negative, but rare EBV-positive cases are described and may cause significant overlap with plasmablastic lymphoma. In the absence of full clinical, radiological and laboratorial data, some cases can be impossible to be differentiated from plasmablastic lymphoma. The mutational landscape of plasmacytoma and multiple myeloma is very complex and includes, in early phases of the pathogenesis, multiple trisomies and recurrent chromosomal translocations involving the *IGH* locus that result in overexpression of oncogenes, like *CCND1*, *CCND2*, *CCND3*, *NSD2* (*MMSET*, *WHSC1*), *MAF*, *MAFA*, and *MAFB*. Secondary events that occur later in the pathological process include activation of the *RAS/MAPK* and *NF-κB* pathways, the DNA repair pathway and the *MYC* gene (Table 42.1; Figs. 42.11, 42.12, 42.13, 42.14, 42.15, 42.16, 42.17, and 42.18).

Table 42.1 Summary of the main immunohistochemical reactions used for plasmacytoma and multiple myeloma diagnosis

Antibody/ probes	Most frequent results	Pattern	Objective
CD20	Negative	Membrane	To exclude other B-cell neoplasm
CD3	Negative	Membrane	To exclude a T-cell neoplasm
MUM1	Positive	Nucleus	To demonstrate the plasma cell phenotype of the neoplasm
Plasma cell (VS38c)	Positive	Cytoplasm	To demonstrate the plasma cell phenotype of the neoplasm
EMA	Positive	Membrane	To demonstrate the plasma cell phenotype of the neoplasm
CD138	Positive	Membrane	To demonstrate the plasma cell phenotype of the neoplasm
Kappa/lambda	Monoclonality (more frequently kappa)	Cytoplasm	To demonstrate the monoclonality of the neoplasm
Cyclin D1	Variably positive	Nucleus	Expressed in a varied number of cases
CD56	Variably positive	Membrane	Expressed in a varied number of cases
Ki67	~30–40% and ~90% in anaplastic variant	Nucleus	To demonstrate the proliferative potential of the neoplasm
EBER[a]	Usually negative, with rare positive cases	Nucleus	To investigate the presence of EBV
Gene hyperdiploidy[b]	Variable	–	To characterize the molecular features of the tumor
IGH translocations[b]	Variable	–	To characterize the molecular features of the tumor
RAS/MAPK activation[b]	Variable	–	To characterize the molecular features of the tumor
NF-kB pathway activation[b]	Variable	–	To characterize the molecular features of the tumor
DNA repair pathway[b]	Variable	–	To characterize the molecular features of the tumor
MYC activation[b]	Variable	–	To characterize the molecular features of the tumor

The analysis of EBV and the main molecular features is also described
[a]Investigated by in situ hybridization
[b]Investigated by fluorescent in situ hybridization or PCR

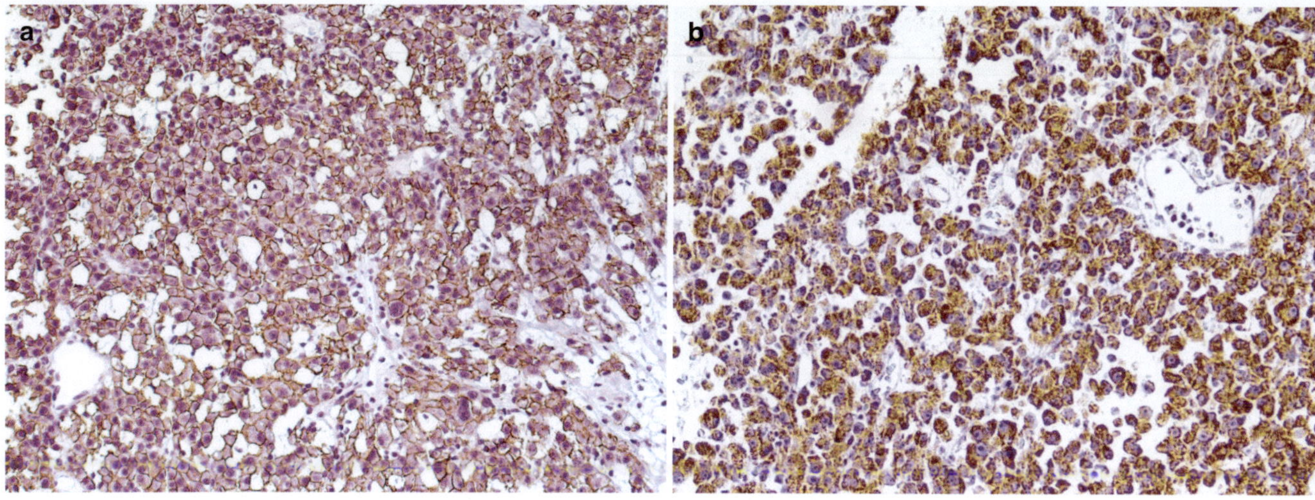

Fig. 42.11 Immunohistochemical findings of plasmacytoma and multiple myeloma. (**a**) Tumor cells in plasmacytoma/multiple myeloma exhibit diffuse membrane expression of CD138 (DAB; 100×). (**b**) The cytoplasmic expression of VS38c (plasma cell) antibody is also a common finding (DAB; 100×)

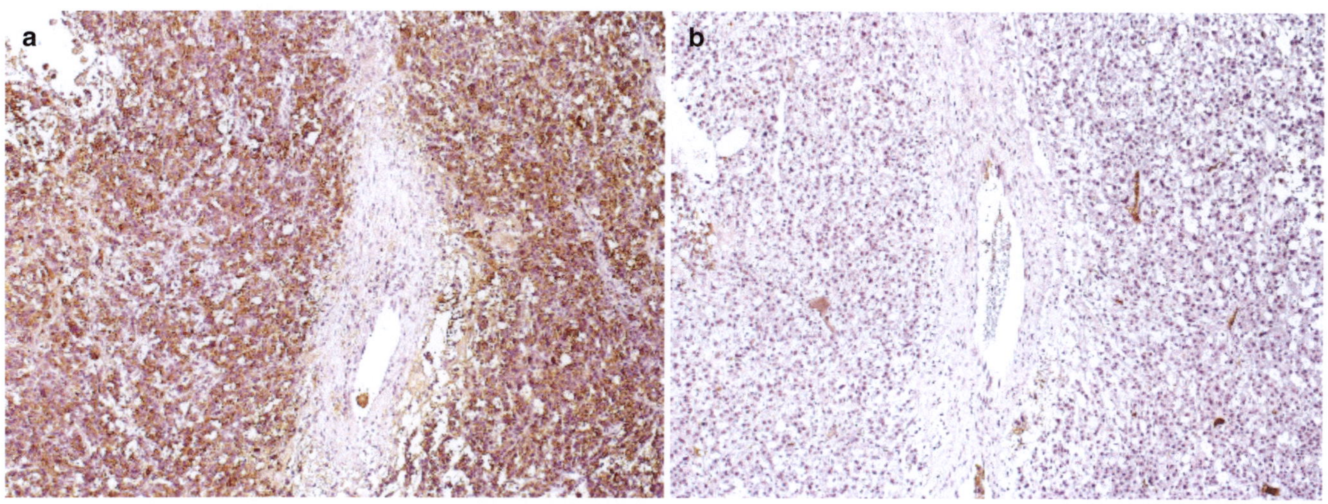

Fig. 42.12 Immunohistochemical reaction to demonstrate monoclonality of plasmacytoma and multiple myeloma cells. (**a**) In this case tumor cells were monoclonal to kappa light chain. Observe the strong and diffuse staining for kappa in the cytoplasm of the cell (DAB; 50×). (**b**) The reaction to lambda light chain proved negative and stained only scattered reactive plasma cells (DAB; 50×)

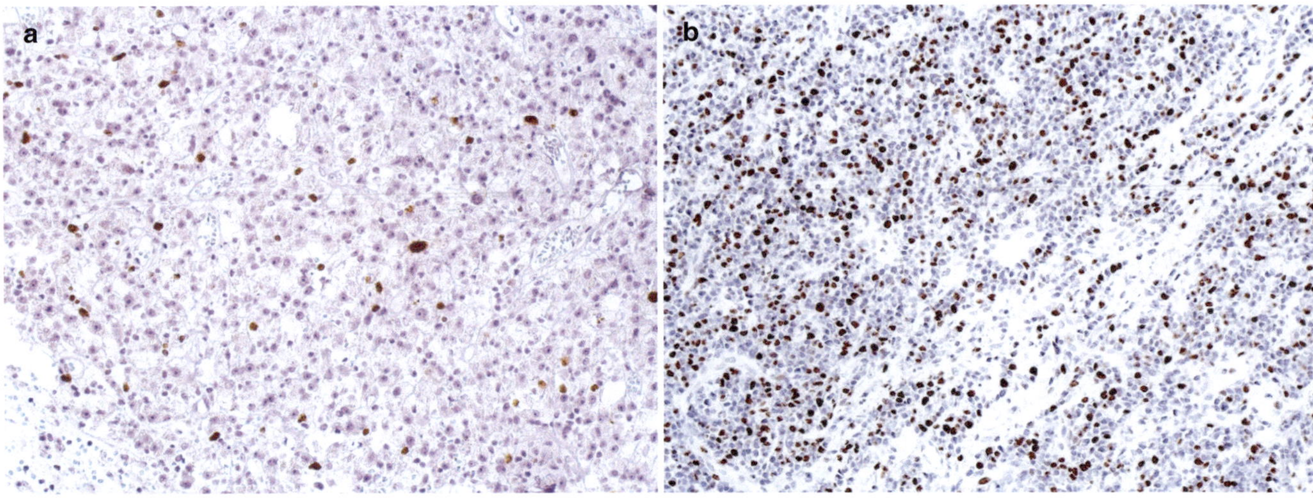

Fig. 42.13 Proliferative features of plasmacytoma and multiple myeloma demonstrated using Ki67 nuclear expression. (**a**) Tumor cells in plasmacytoma/multiple myeloma exhibit a variable proliferative potential. Although it can achieve up to 90% positivity in anaplastic variant, it is usually lower than the proliferative rate found in plasmablastic lymphoma. In this case, proliferation is low, with approximately 15% positivity (DAB; 100×). (**b**) Another example of plasmacytoma/multiple myeloma exhibiting a higher proliferative index, of approximately 50% in hotspot areas (DAB; 100×)

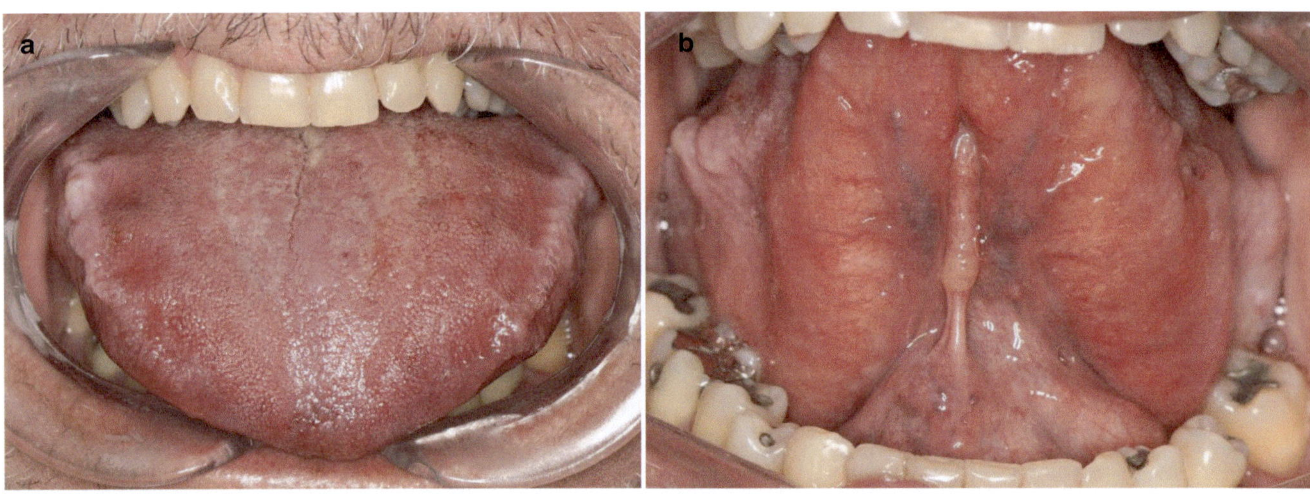

Fig. 42.14 Clinical presentation of oral amyloidosis. (**a**) The most common manifestation of oral amyloidosis is the enlarged tongue with indented lateral borders. Under palpation, the tongue is hard, and mobility may decrease significantly. (**b**) In the ventral portion of the tongue it is possible to observe the yellowish aspect of amyloidosis. This clinical finding is very suggestive of the diagnosis

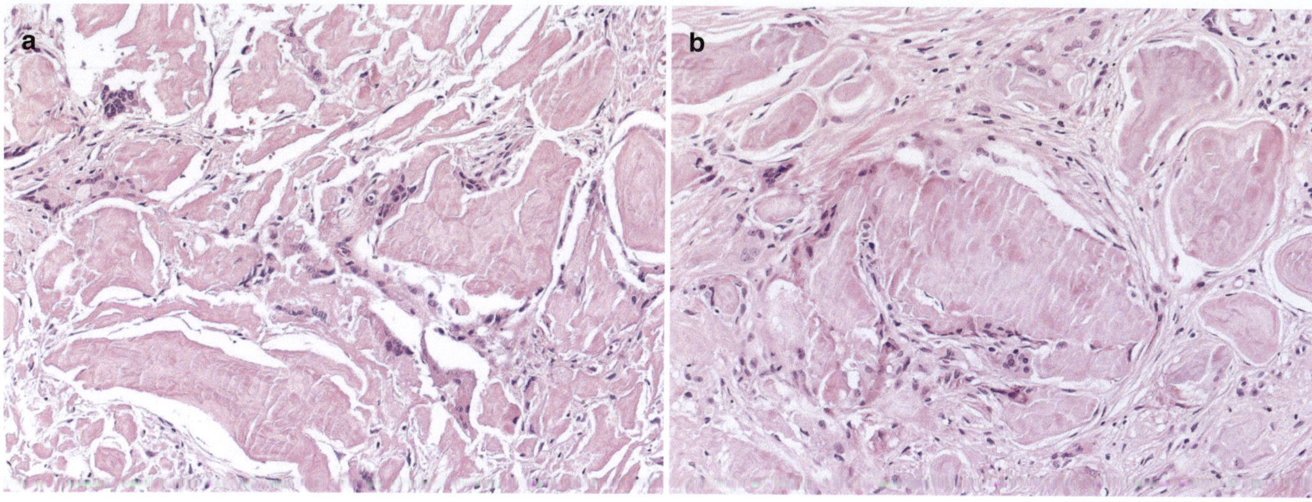

Fig. 42.15 Microscopic findings of amyloidosis affecting the tongue. (**a**) The amyloid deposits can be found as eosinophilic amorphous material diffusely or locally distributed in the connective tissue. In some cases, multinucleated giant cells are found surrounding the amyloid deposits (H&E; 100×). (**b**) The cracking artefact is usually observed in the amyloid deposits (H&E; 100×)

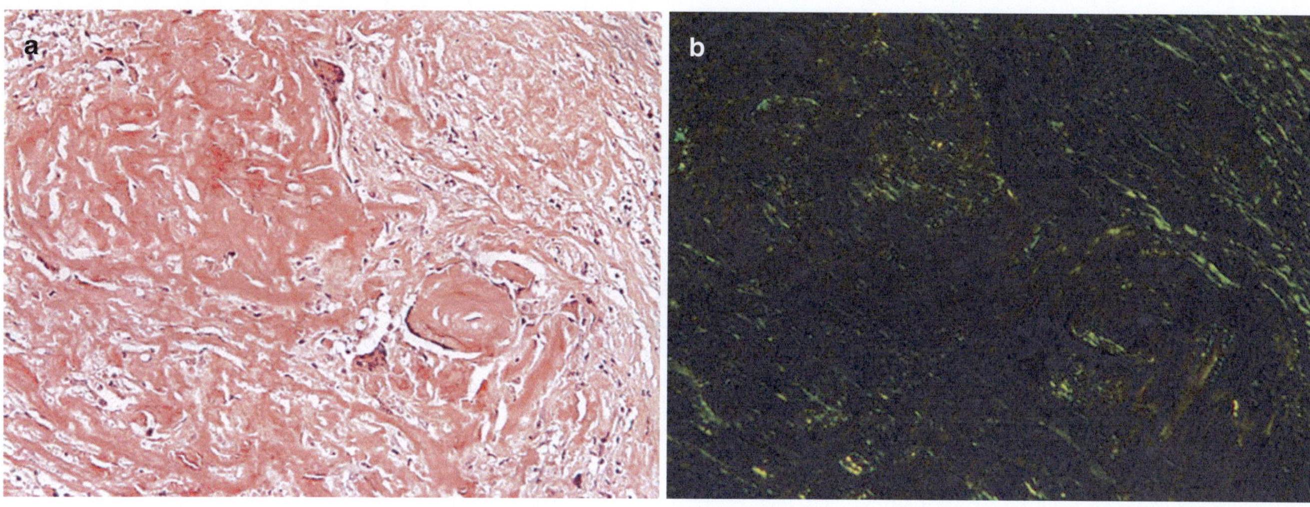

Fig. 42.16 Microscopic findings of amyloidosis affecting the tongue. (**a**) Congo red staining is used to confirm the amyloid nature of the amorphous deposits. Under conventional microscopy, a reddish staining of the amyloid is observed (Congo red; 100×). (**b**) Confirmation comes with polarized microscopy that shows the typical apple-green refringence (Polarized Congo Red; 100×)

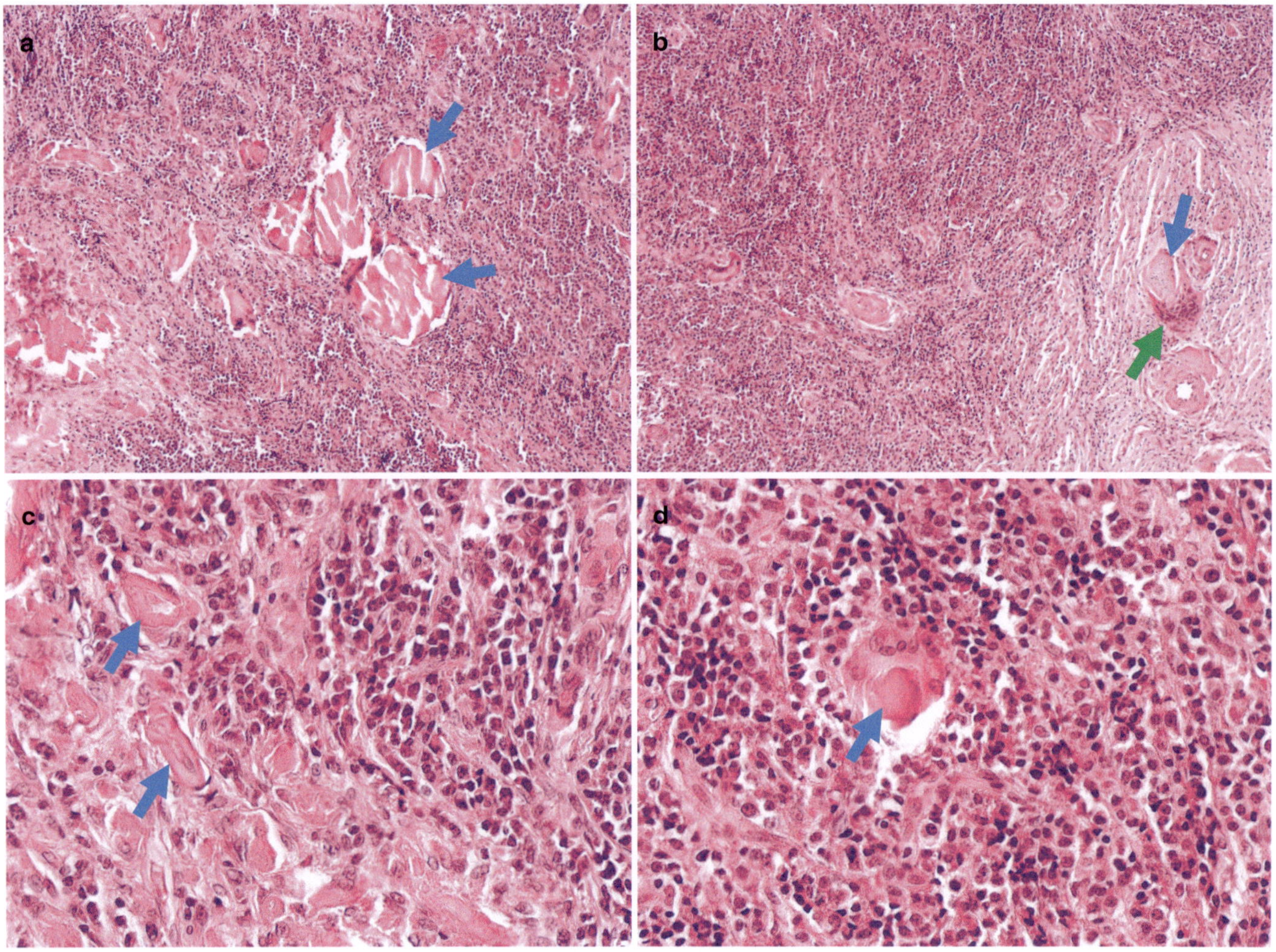

Fig. 42.17 Microscopic findings of multiple myeloma affecting the mandible and maxilla of a male patient. (**a**) Diffuse proliferation of neoplastic plasma cells with the presence of hyaline structures compatible with amyloid deposits (blue arrows) (H&E; 100×). (**b**) Some foreign body-type multinucleated giant cells (green arrow) were seen around amyloid deposits (blue arrow) (H&E; 100×). (**c**) Amyloid deposits were also found as small eosinophilic aggregates in the tumor (Blue arrows) (H&E; 200×). (**d**) Another example of multinucleated giant cell surrounding the amyloid deposit. Note the diffuse proliferation of the neoplastic plasma cells (H&E; 200×)

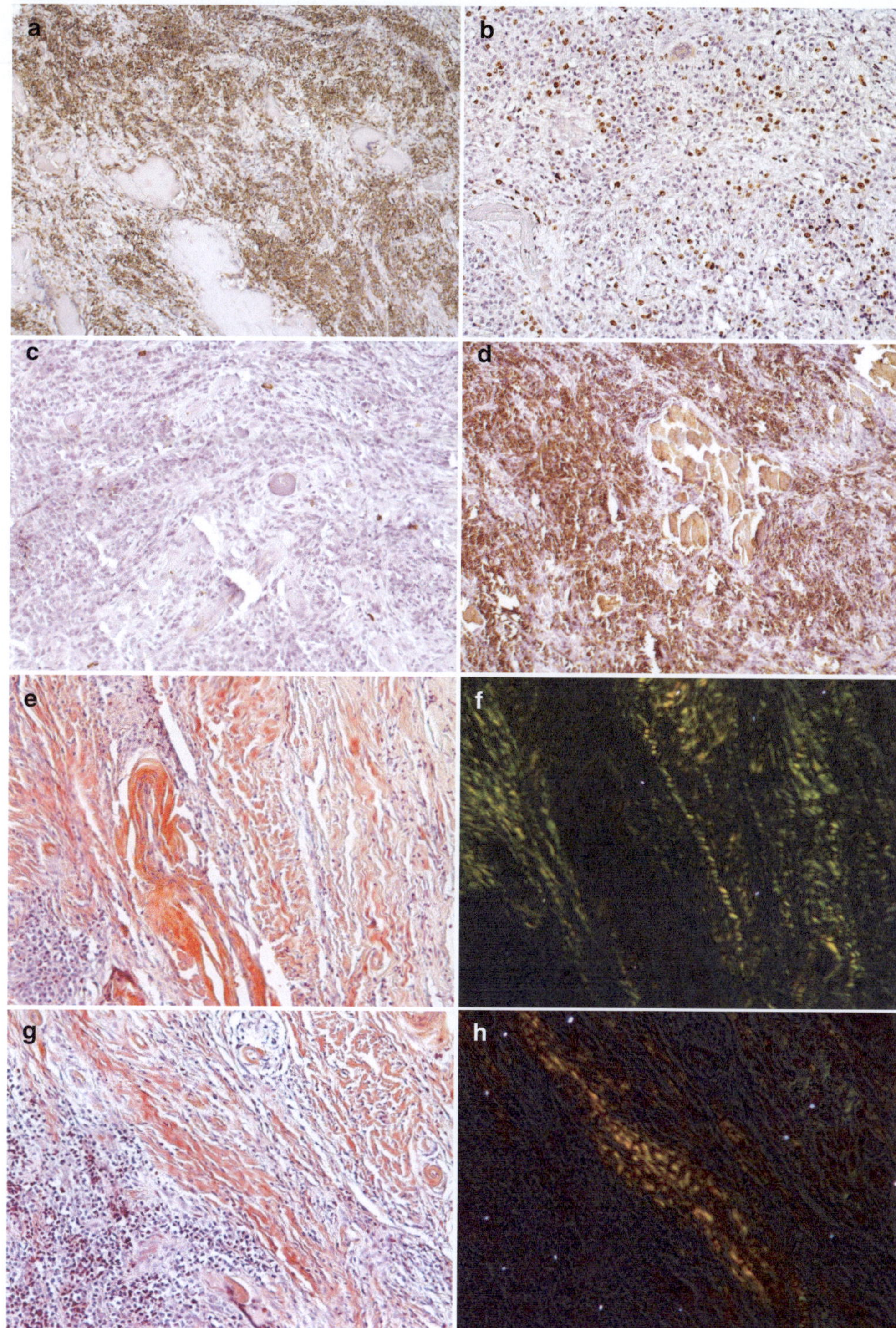

Fig. 42.18 Microscopic and immunohistochemical findings of multiple myeloma affecting the mandible and maxilla of a male patient. (**a**) Strong and diffuse cytoplasmic expression of plasma cell protein (clone VS38c) in the neoplastic cells (DAB; 100×). (**b**) Proliferative index achieving approximately 30% is lower than usually observed for plasmablastic lymphomas (DAB; 100×). (**c**) Monoclonality analysis demonstrated a negative result for kappa (DAB; 100×), and (**d**) positivity for lambda light chain (DAB; 100×). (**e**) Strong Congo red stain in the amyloid material (Congo red; 200×), (**f**) which is confirmed by polarized microscopy. Observe the apple green aspect under polarization (polarized Congo red; 200×). (**g**) Another example of Congo red staining the amyloid tissue deposited. Observe the tumor cells in the lower left region of the image (Congo red; 200×). (**h**) Amyloid nature of the material is confirmed under polarization (polarized Congo red; 200×)

Sources

1. Lae ME, Vencio EF, Inwards CY, Unni KK, Nascimento AG. Myeloma of the jaw bones: a clinicopathologic study of 33 cases. Head Neck. 2003;25(5):373–81.
2. Owotade F, Ugboko V, Ajike S, Salawu L, Amusa Y, Omole M. Head and neck manifestations of myeloma in Nigerians. Int J Oral Maxillofac Surg. 2005;34(7):761–5.
3. Gerry D, Lentsch EJ. Epidemiologic evidence of superior outcomes for extramedullary plasmacytoma of the head and neck. Otolaryngol Head Neck Surg. 2013;148(6):974–81. https://doi.org/10.1177/0194599813481334.
4. de Waal EG, Leene M, Veeger N, et al. Progression of a solitary plasmacytoma to multiple myeloma. A population-based registry of the northern Netherlands. Br J Haematol. 2016;175(4):661–7.
5. Faria KM, Ribeiro ACP, Brandão TB, et al. Radiographic patterns of multiple myeloma in the jawbones of patients treated with intravenous bisphosphonates. J Am Dent Assoc. 2018;149(5):382–91.
6. Faria KM, Brandão TB, Silva WG, et al. Panoramic and skull imaging may aid in the identification of multiple myeloma lesions. Med Oral Patol Oral Cir Bucal. 2018;23(1):e38–43.
7. Pontes FSC, De Souza LL, Fonseca FP, Pontes HAR. Mandibular lesion as the first sign of multiple myeloma in a young patient. J Oral Maxillofac Pathol. 2019;23(Suppl 1):94–6. https://doi.org/10.4103/jomfp.JOMFP_109_17.
8. Ludwig H, Novis Durie S, Meckl A, Hinke A, Durie B. Multiple myeloma incidence and mortality around the globe; interrelations between health access and quality, economic resources, and patient empowerment. Oncologist. 2020;25(9):e1406–13.
9. Rajkumar SV. Multiple myeloma: 2020 update on diagnosis, risk-stratification and management. Am J Hematol. 2020;95(5):548–67.
10. Rodrigues-Fernandes CI, de Cáceres CBL, Sant'Ana MSP, Soares CD, de Carvalho MGF, van Heerden WFP, et al. Oral lesions containing amyloid-like material. Oral Surg Oral Med Oral Pathol Oral Radiol. 2021;132(2):190–201. https://doi.org/10.1016/j.oooo.2021.01.016.
11. Souza LL, Cáceres CVBL, Vargas PA, Lopes MA, Santos-Silva AR, Silva WGD, et al. Plasmacytoma and plasma cell myeloma affecting the jaws: a multi-institutional collaborative study. J Oral Pathol Med. 2021;50(6):613–21. https://doi.org/10.1111/jop.13213.
12. Akyol R, Şirin Sarıbal G, Amuk M. Evaluation of mandibular bone changes in multiple myeloma patients on dental panoramic radiographs. Oral Radiol. 2022;38(4):575–85. https://doi.org/10.1007/s11282-022-00590-6.
13. Danskin Y, Alhajji D, Singh A, Rota A, Huryn JM, Estilo CL. Multiple myeloma masquerading as mandibular medication-related osteonecrosis of the jaw: a case report. Aust Dent J. 2022 Mar;67(1):94–9. https://doi.org/10.1111/adj.12882.
14. Felix FA, de Sena ACVP, de Arruda JAA, Tavares TS, Rocha AL, Rodrigues-Fernandes CI, et al. Fine-needle aspiration cytology for the diagnosis of plasma cell neoplasms in the head and neck region: a systematic analysis of the literature. Diagn Cytopathol. 2023;51(3):198–210. https://doi.org/10.1002/dc.25095.
15. Chuang PW, Chuang WY, Lee TJ, Chang PH, Chen YW, Fu CH. Outcome analysis of solitary extramedullary plasmacytoma in the head and neck: a clinical perspective. Head Neck. 2024;47:983–9. https://doi.org/10.1002/hed.27998.
16. Ganzel C, Trestman S, Levi S, Gatt ME, Lavi N, Vaxman I, et al. Clinical features, therapy patterns, outcomes and prognostic factors of solitary plasmacytomas: a report of the Israeli Myeloma Study Group. Leuk Lymphoma. 2022;63(14):3448–55. https://doi.org/10.1080/10428194.2022.2118535.

Part VII

Mature NK/T Cell Lymphomas

Extranodal NK/T-Cell Lymphoma

43

Silvia Ferreira de Sousa,
Cinthia Veronica Bardalez Lopez de Caceres,
Guilherme Rossi Assis de Mendonça,
and Felipe Paiva Fonseca

43.1 General Overview and Clinical Presentation

Extranodal NK/T-cell lymphoma is an aggressive lymphoma that typically affects the nasal cavity and upper aerodigestive structures and, less commonly, extranasal sites such as skin, soft tissue, testes and the gastrointestinal tract. A primary nodal EBV-positive T and NK cell lymphoma has been recognized, but the involvement of the superior respiratory tract must be ruled out to confirm the diagnosis of this recently described entity. Extranodal NK/T-cell lymphoma represents the most common T-cell lymphoma subtype in some regions of the world, especially in Asia and in some regions of Central and South America, accounting for approximately 10% of all non-Hodgkin lymphomas in these regions. The diagnosis of this lymphoma can be very challenging, especially in nonendemic regions and in children, given the clinical similarities to other infectious or inflammatory processes that may also cause destruction of the midline tissues and palate perforation like cocaine abuse, leishmaniasis, tertiary syphilis, granulomatosis with polyangiitis, mucormycosis and rhinoscleroma.

This entity had already been described since the nineteenth century as ulcerative necrotizing and destructive lesions of unknown nature, affecting the midface, the nose and/or the upper airways with fatal outcome. Of note, one of its former terminologies, midline lethal granuloma, appropriately illustrated the most common clinical manifestation of the disease and its highly aggressive behavior, typically associated with a dismal outcome. The etiology of the tumor is not completely understood, but EBV infection is believed to play an important role in this process since viral RNA is detected in virtually all cases. Rare examples of EBV-negative tumors are rarely described, but these reports should be taken with caution since a false negative result for EBER detection may occur, for example, because of the lack of viable neoplastic cells given the extensive necrotic tissues. These cases would rather be better diagnosed as peripheral T-cell lymphoma not otherwise specified. More recently, the genetic basis of extranodal NK/T-cell lymphoma has been more detailed described, and it was shown that a diverse number of genetic mutations seem to be involved in its pathogenesis, including the chromosomal deletion of 6q21–25 region, alterations in members of the *JAK/STAT* pathway, epigenetic regulators, tumor suppressor genes, RNA helicase and *PD-1/PD-L1* pathway. Several other genes and pathways have been described to be altered in this aggressive lymphoma, illustrating its complex genetic landscape.

Adults with a median age of 46–60 years are the most affected group, although children can also be affected, especially in countries like China, Japan and Guatemala. Males seem to be more affected, but some studies have found a female predominance. This lymphoma can be sub-classified according to the anatomical involvement as nasal or non-nasal extranodal NK/T-cell lymphoma. The patients are more often diagnosed with the nasal presentation, which usually exhibits nasal obstruction, with discharge or epistaxis, followed by edema and ulceration. The occurrence of a diffuse edema of the lower eyelid is a frequent manifestation. The highly aggressive clinical evolution of the disease commonly leads to a necrotic destruction of nasal skin and mucosa, nasal septum, paranasal sinuses and nasopharynx, frequently perforating the central part of the palate, and leading to an oroantral communication. The occurrence of lesions in the upper alveolar ridge and/or gingiva may resemble aggressive periodontal disease and it may cause misdiag-

S. F. de Sousa (✉) · C. V. B. L. de Caceres · F. P. Fonseca
Department of Oral Surgery and Pathology, School of Dentistry, Universidade Federal de Minas Gerais, Belo Horizonte, Brazil
e-mail: silviafsousa@ufmg.br

G. R. A. de Mendonça
Department of Pathology, School of Medical Sciences, University of Campinas, Campinas, Brazil

© The Author(s), under exclusive license to Springer Nature Switzerland AG 2025

F. P. Fonseca et al. (eds.), *Lymphoproliferative and Granulomatous Disorders of the Oral Cavity*,
https://doi.org/10.1007/978-3-031-98844-8_43

noses. The non-nasal presentation of the tumor is more often diagnosed in the skin, gastrointestinal tract and testis, accounting for approximately 20% of all cases.

The presence of extensive areas of necrotic tissue in extranodal NK/T-cell lymphoma may hamper the acquisition of adequate tissue for microscopic evaluation, often demanding multiple biopsies. This necrosis is believed to be a consequence of the angioinvasion and angiodestruction caused by tumor cells, which also produce chemical mediators that contribute to this clinical manifestation. Most of the cases are diagnosed in stages I and II, but disseminated and more advanced stage disease can also be found. The frequency of B-symptoms varies from 3% to 57% of the patients, while bone marrow involvement is considered uncommon.

The prognosis of patients affected by extranodal NK/T--cell lymphoma is poor, but has improved significantly with the use of new chemotherapeutic schemes. Radiotherapy alone can be used for localized diseases, while its combination with chemotherapy is recommended for more advanced manifestations. The effectiveness of chemotherapy improved with the use of non-anthracycline-containing regimens based on platinum or L-asparaginase, such as DeVIC (dexamethasone, etoposide, ifosfamide, and carboplatin), DICE (dexamethasone, ifosfamide, cisplatin, etoposide), GDP (gemcitabine, dexamethasone, and cisplatin), VIPD (etoposide, ifosfamide, cisplatin, and dexamethasone), LVP (L-asparaginase, vincristine, and prednisolone), GELOX (gemcitabine, L-asparaginase, and oxaliplatin), SMILE (dexamethasone, methotrexate, ifosfamide, L-asparaginase, and etoposide) and AspaMetDex (L-asparaginase, methotrexate, and dexamethasone). Hematopoietic stem cell transplantation has also been described in some studies.

Despite improvements in the therapeutic modalities, relapses are common and current survival rates remain low, achieving approximately 50%. Different factors may impact survival, such as age >60 years, advanced stage (III/IV) disease, lymph node involvement, presence of B-symptoms and circulating EBV DNA (Figs. 43.1, 43.2, and 43.3).

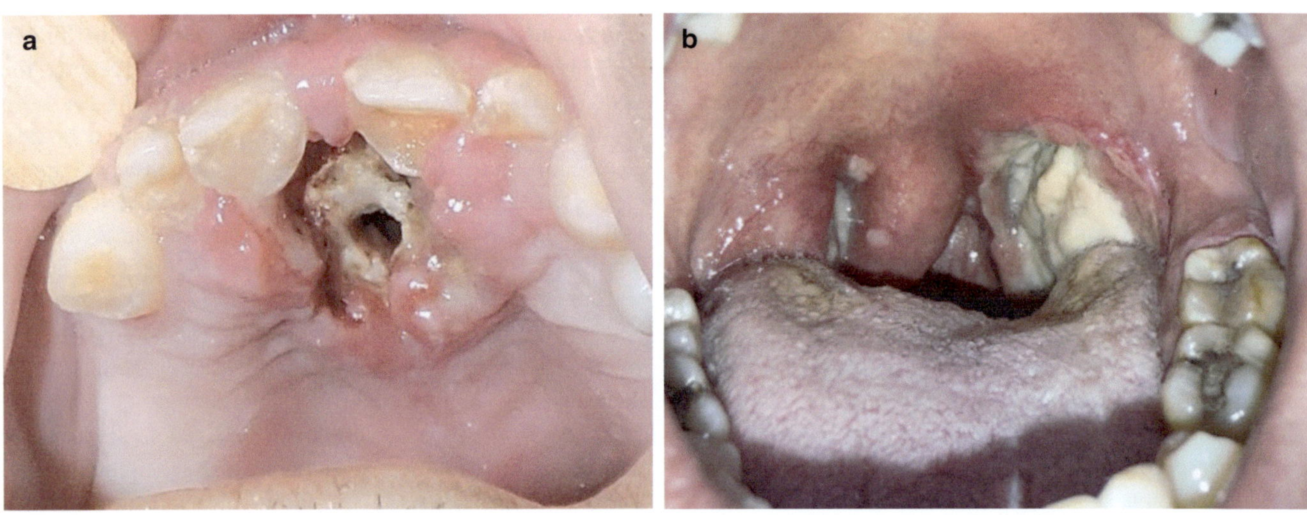

Fig. 43.1 Clinical manifestations of extranodal NK/T-cell lymphoma affecting the oral cavity. (**a**) The most common clinical presentation of the disease manifesting as a palate perforation associated with extensive areas of tissue necrosis. (**b**) The neoplasm may manifest as an aggressive ulcer in the soft palate covered by a yellowish necrotic tissue, which makes the biopsy procedure difficult. Microscopically, the lack of a satisfactory number of neoplastic cells may hamper the correct interpretation and delay the diagnosis

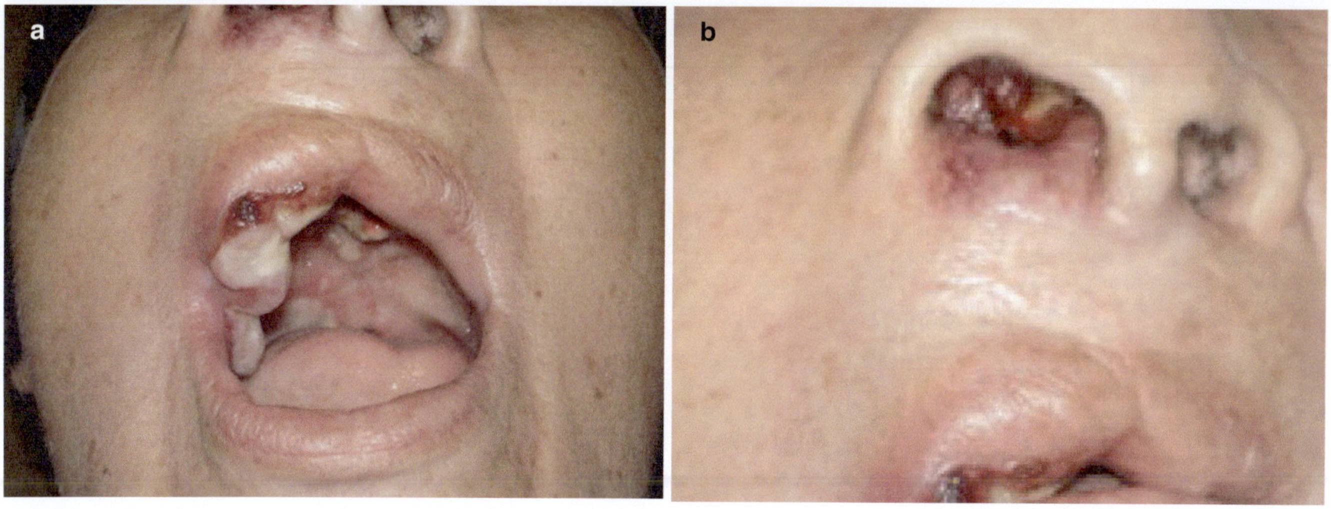

Fig. 43.2 Clinical manifestation of extranodal NK/T-cell lymphoma affecting the oral cavity. (**a**) A female patient showing the neoplasm extending towards the oral cavity through palatine perforation and further affecting the surrounding soft tissues of the mouth and the upper lip. (**b**) Note the destruction of nasal tissue by the tumor cells. It is possible to observe the elevation of the right nasal wing

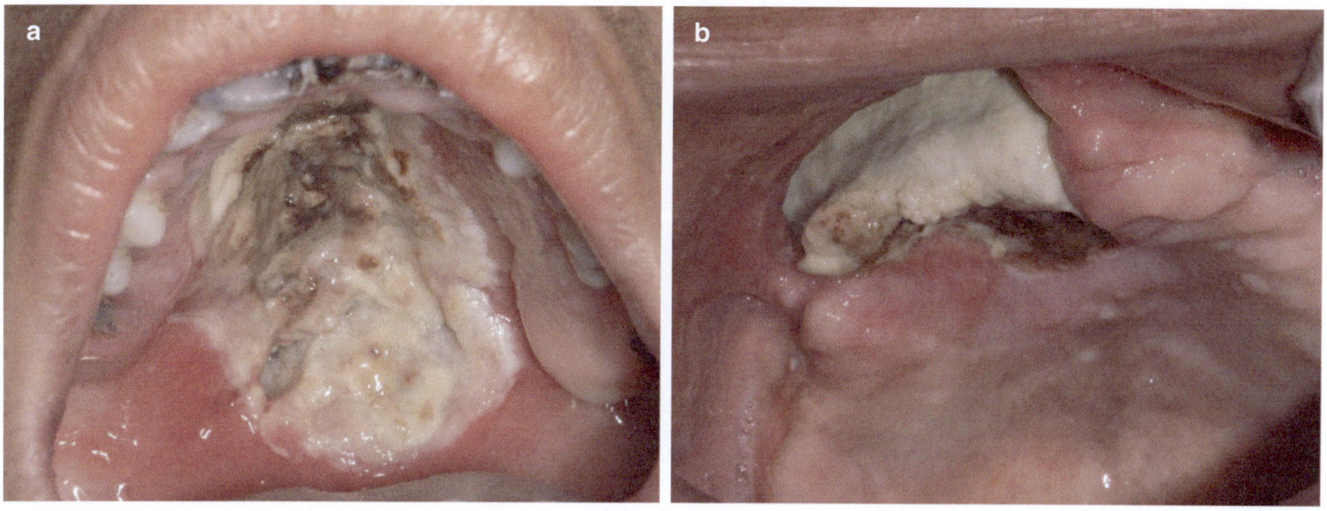

Fig. 43.3 Clinical manifestation of extranodal NK/T-cell lymphoma affecting the oral cavity. (**a**) A patient showing the typical destruction of the central region of the palate with extensive areas of necrosis. (**b**) A male patient affected by extranodal NK/T-cell lymphoma exhibiting a large ulcerated and necrotic area in the oral cavity. Observe the occurrence of bone necrosis associated with neoplastic infiltration

43.2 Microscopic Findings

- The tumor typically exhibits a diffuse growth pattern in an edematous, necrotic and loosely arranged fibrous stroma.
- The presence of extensive areas of necrosis is common and may make the diagnosis difficult.
- Blood vessels surrounded by neoplastic cells are frequently observed (angiocentricity).
- Perivascular hyaline necrosis (fibrinoid changes in the blood vessel wall) is a common finding.
- Neoplastic cells exhibit a highly variable size and morphology, being composed of atypical cells ranging from small to medium to large.

- Characteristically, a large number of reactive inflammatory cells, including plasma cells, neutrophils, eosinophils and macrophages are present, which sometimes may make the correct diagnosis difficult.
- Numerous typical and atypical mitotic figures are found.
- Karyorrhexis and apoptotic bodies are commonly present.
- Angioinvasion and angiodestruction are common findings and are characterized by the presence of tumor cells disposed around small and/or large blood vessels, infiltrating and destroying their vascular walls.
- The occurrence of pseudoepitheliomatous hyperplasia demands the exclusion of an oral squamous cell carcinoma (Figs. 43.4, 43.5, 43.6, and 43.7).

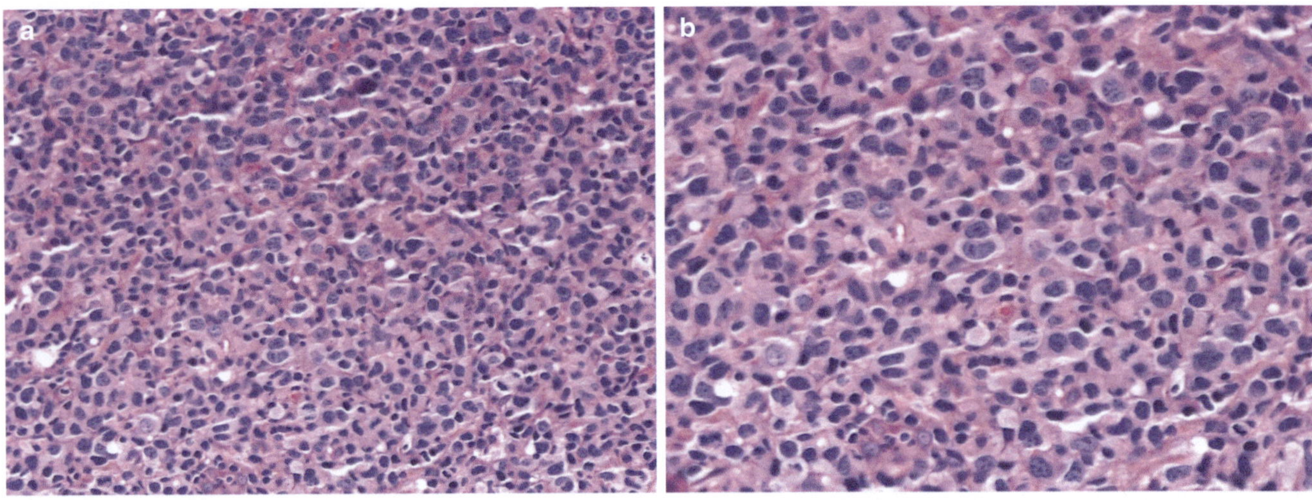

Fig. 43.4 Microscopic features of extranodal NK/T-cell lymphoma. (**a**) Tumor cells exhibit a diffuse proliferation pattern (H&E; 200×). (**b**) The neoplastic cells are typically polymorphic, ranging from large cells to small cells. Mitotic figures are often easily found (H&E; 200×)

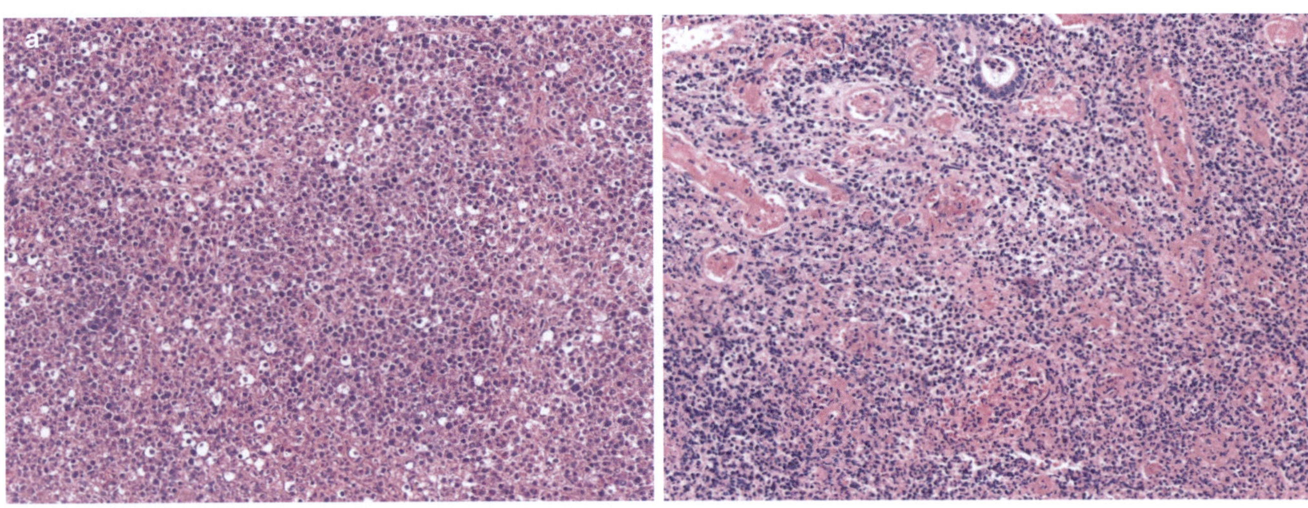

Fig. 43.5 Microscopic features of extranodal NK/T-cell lymphoma. (**a**) The presence of macrophages (the clear cells in this image) is commonly observed and may focally resemble the starry-sky pattern in this neoplasm (H&E; 100×). (**b**) The presence of reactive inflammatory cells like neutrophils and plasma cells is another very common microscopic characteristic of extranodal NK/T-cell lymphoma and it may make the correct diagnosis difficult. Observe the mixture of neoplastic cells and reactive cells surrounding blood vessels and normal glandular structures (H&E; 100×)

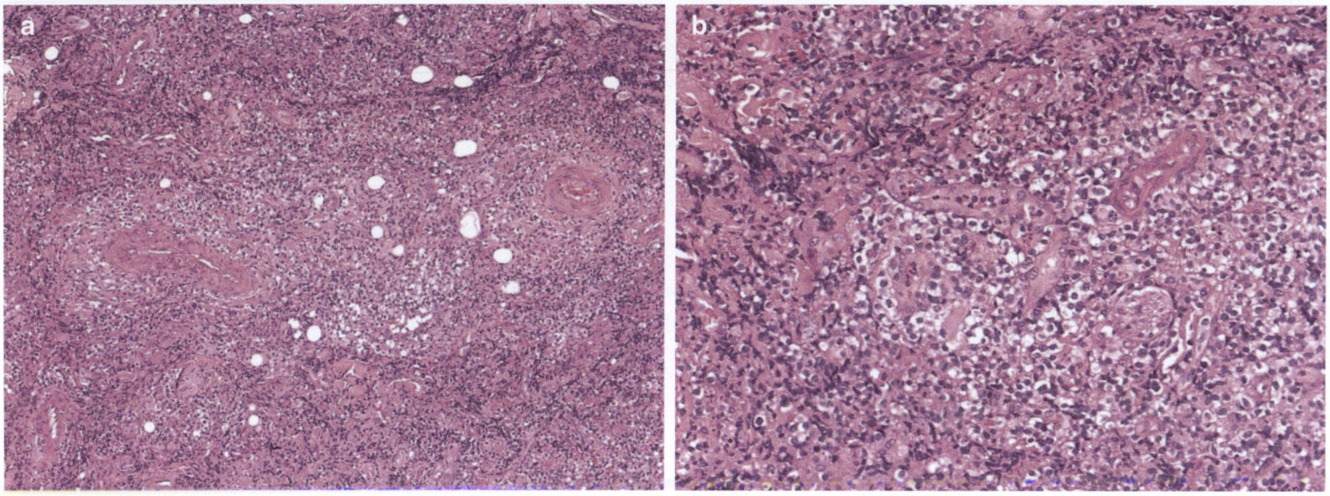

Fig. 43.6 Microscopic features of extranodal NK/T-cell lymphoma. (**a**) Angiocentric growth pattern is a hallmark of extranodal NK/T-cell lymphoma. Observe the presence of large blood vessels being surrounded and infiltrated by tumor cells (H&E; 100×). (**b**) The angiocentric potential of tumor cells also occurs related to smaller vessels and is shown in this image, where neoplastic cells invade the walls of blood vessels (H&E; 100×)

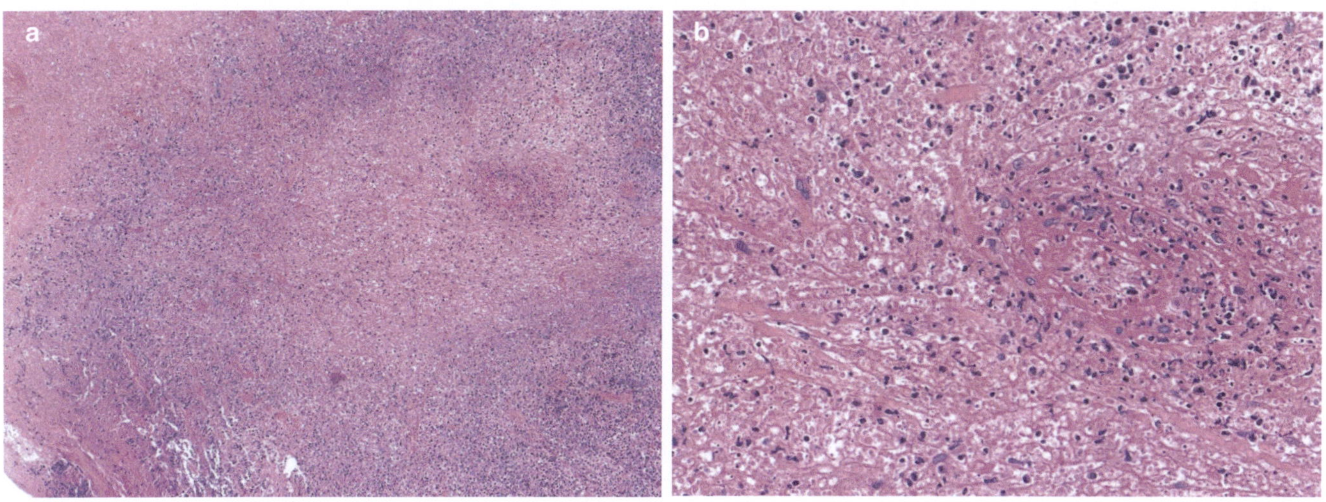

Fig. 43.7 Microscopic features of extranodal NK/T-cell lymphoma. (**a**) Given the angiocentricity and angiodestruction of the tumor cells, extensive areas of necrosis are common in the biopsied tissue, which may hamper the correct diagnosis due to a lack of viable cells to run immunohistochemical analysis and detection of EBV (H&E; 50×). (**b**) Observe in this image the presence of fibrinoid necrosis around the blood vessel and the necrotic stroma of the lesion (H&E; 100×)

43.3 Immunohistochemistry and/or Genetics

Extranodal NK/T-cell lymphoma has a cytotoxic phenotype, and the immunohistochemical reactions aim to demonstrate its NK and T-cell origin with positivity to CD2, CD3ε, CD45RO, granzyme B, perforin and TIA-1. Approximately 85% of the cases exhibit CD56 positivity. The expression of CD30 is observed in 55% of the cases, but it usually does not exhibit the characteristic strong and diffuse, perinuclear Golgi-like staining pattern observed in anaplastic large B-cell lymphomas. The neoplasm is usually negative for CD4, CD8, and CD57. CD20, CD68 and CD138 are also negative, but illustrate the reactive background of the tumor that contains B lymphocytes, macrophages and plasma cells, respectively. The angiocentricity of the neoplasm can be highlighted by immunohistochemical stains. In addition, the presence of EBV demonstrated by in situ hybridization is considered mandatory for the diagnosis. The genetic landscape is complex, but alterations in the *JAK/STAT* pathway and chromosomal deletion of 6q21–25 region are considered the most frequent molecular events (Table 43.1; Figs. 43.8, 43.9, 43.10, 43.11, 43.12, and 43.13).

Table 43.1 Summary of the main immunohistochemical reactions used for extranodal NK/T-cell lymphoma diagnosis

Antibody/probe	Most frequent results	Pattern	Objective
CD20	Negative	Membrane	To rule out a B-cell lymphoma
CD2	Positive	Membrane	To demonstrate the NK/T-cell nature of the neoplasm
CD3/CD3ε	Positive	Membrane/cytoplasm	To demonstrate the NK/T-cell nature of the neoplasm
CD45RO	Positive	Membrane	To demonstrate the NK/T-cell nature of the neoplasm
CD56	Positive	Membrane	To demonstrate the NK/T-cell nature of the neoplasm
CD43	Positive	Membrane	To demonstrate the NK/T-cell nature of the neoplasm
CD30	Positive	Membrane	This marker is positive in ~55% of the cases
Granzyme B	Positive	Granules in the cytoplasm	To demonstrate the cytotoxic phenotype
TIA-1	Positive	Granules in the cytoplasm	To demonstrate the cytotoxic phenotype
Perforin	Positive	Granules in the cytoplasm	To demonstrate the cytotoxic phenotype
Ki67	~60–70%	Nucleus	To demonstrate the proliferative index of the neoplasm
EBER[a]	Positive	Nucleus	To demonstrate the presence of EBV
JAK/STAT[b]	Variable	–	To genetically characterize the disease
Deletion of 6q21–25[b]	Variable	–	To genetically characterize the disease

The main results for EBV detection and molecular findings are also described
[a]Investigated by in situ hybridization
[b]Investigated by fluorescent in situ hybridization or PCR

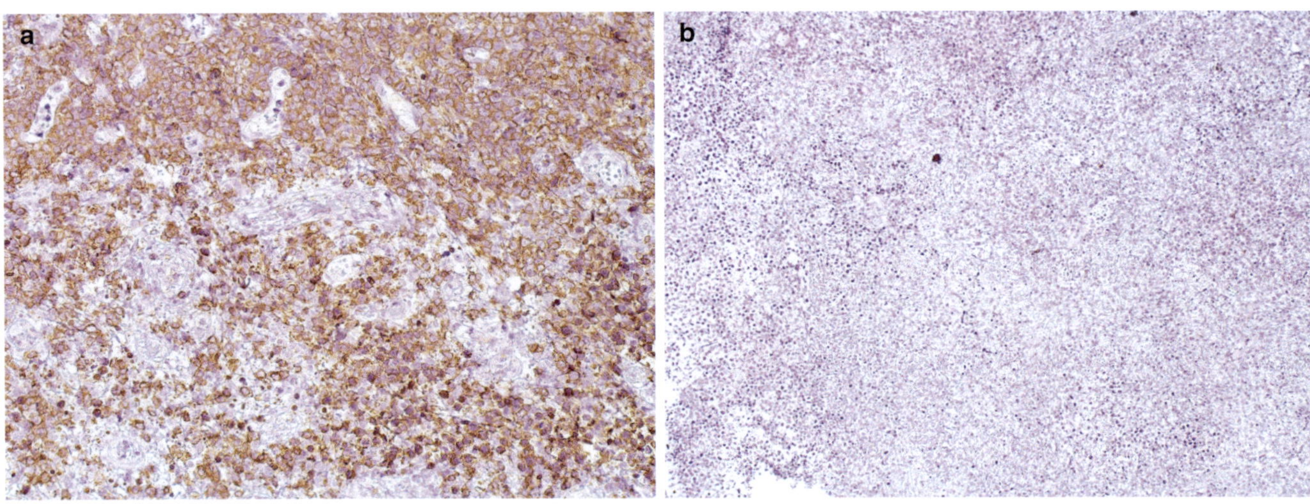

Fig. 43.8 Immunohistochemical features of extranodal NK/T-cell lymphoma. (**a**) The T-cell marker CD3 is strongly and diffusely expressed by tumor cells (DAB; 100×). (**b**) The mature B-cell marker CD20 is negative in tumor cells (DAB; 100×)

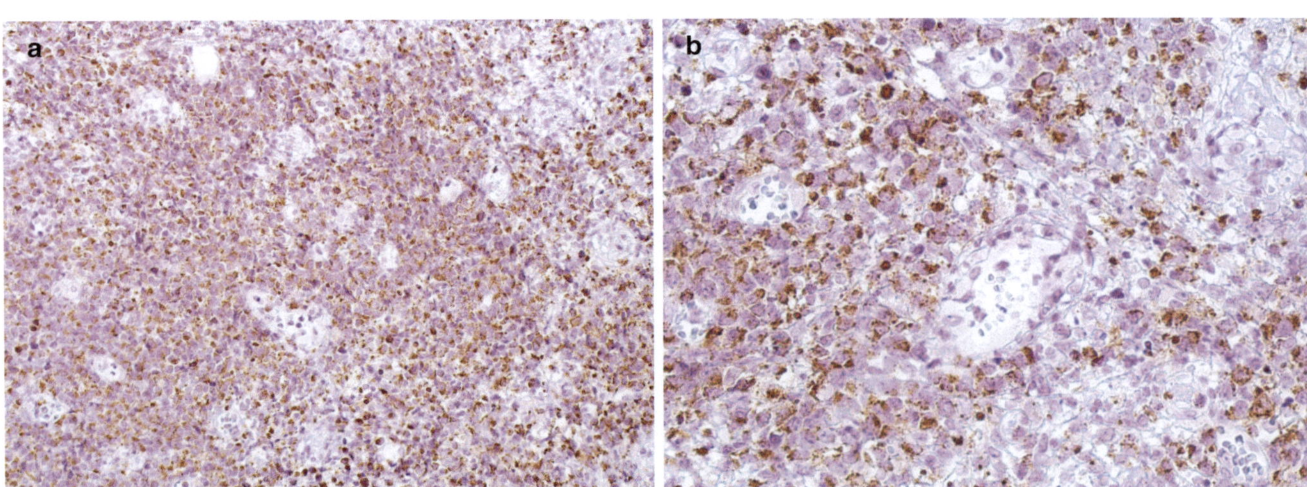

Fig. 43.9 Immunohistochemical features of extranodal NK/T-cell lymphoma. (**a**) Cytotoxic granules are usually present in the tumor cells. Granzyme B shows a granular staining pattern in the cytoplasm of the neoplastic cells (DAB; 100×). (**b**) In some cases, it is possible to observe the perivascular distribution of the tumor cells using some antibodies, like Granzyme B in this image (DAB; 200×)

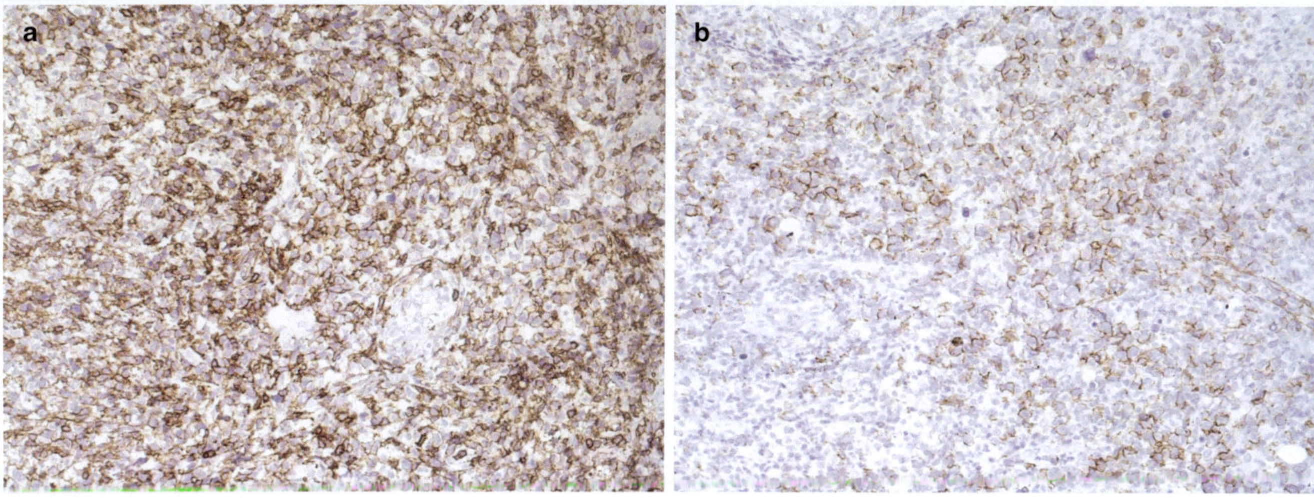

Fig. 43.10 Immunohistochemical features of extranodal NK/T-cell lymphoma. (**a**) The expression of CD43 is common in extranodal NK/T-cell marker, but due to its low specificity, demonstration of the T and NK cell markers is mandatory for the diagnosis (DAB; 100×). (**b**) The NK-cell marker CD56 is present in the majority of the cases. Observe the membrane staining pattern in this image (DAB; 100×)

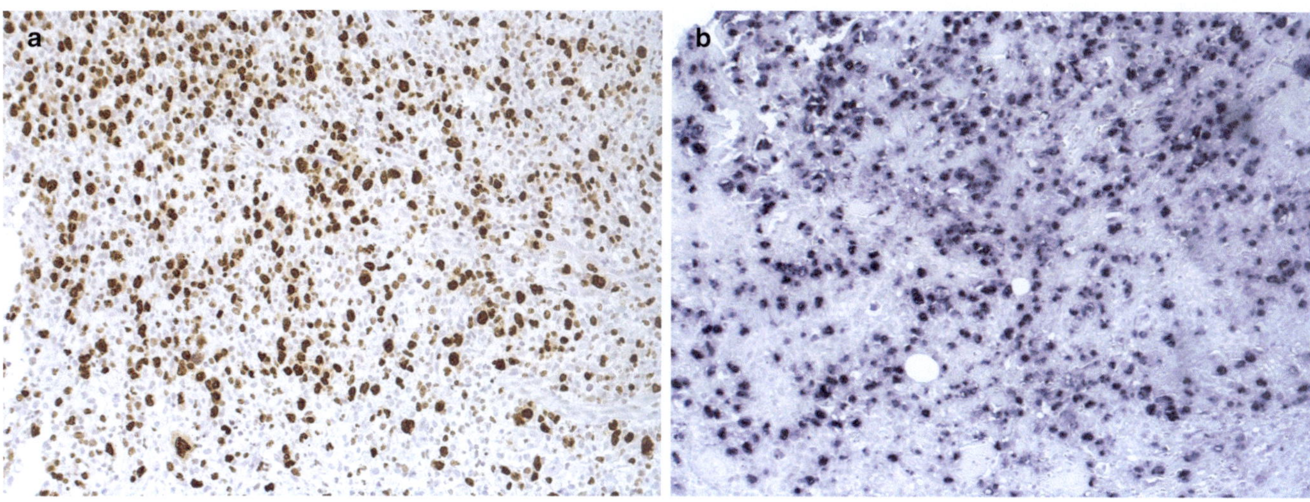

Fig. 43.11 Immunohistochemical features of extranodal NK/T-cell lymphoma. (**a**) Proliferative index measured by Ki67 is variable, but usually high, approaching 70% or more in some cases (DAB; 100×). (**b**) The presence of EBV demonstrated by in situ hybridization is mandatory for the correct diagnosis (EBER; 100×)

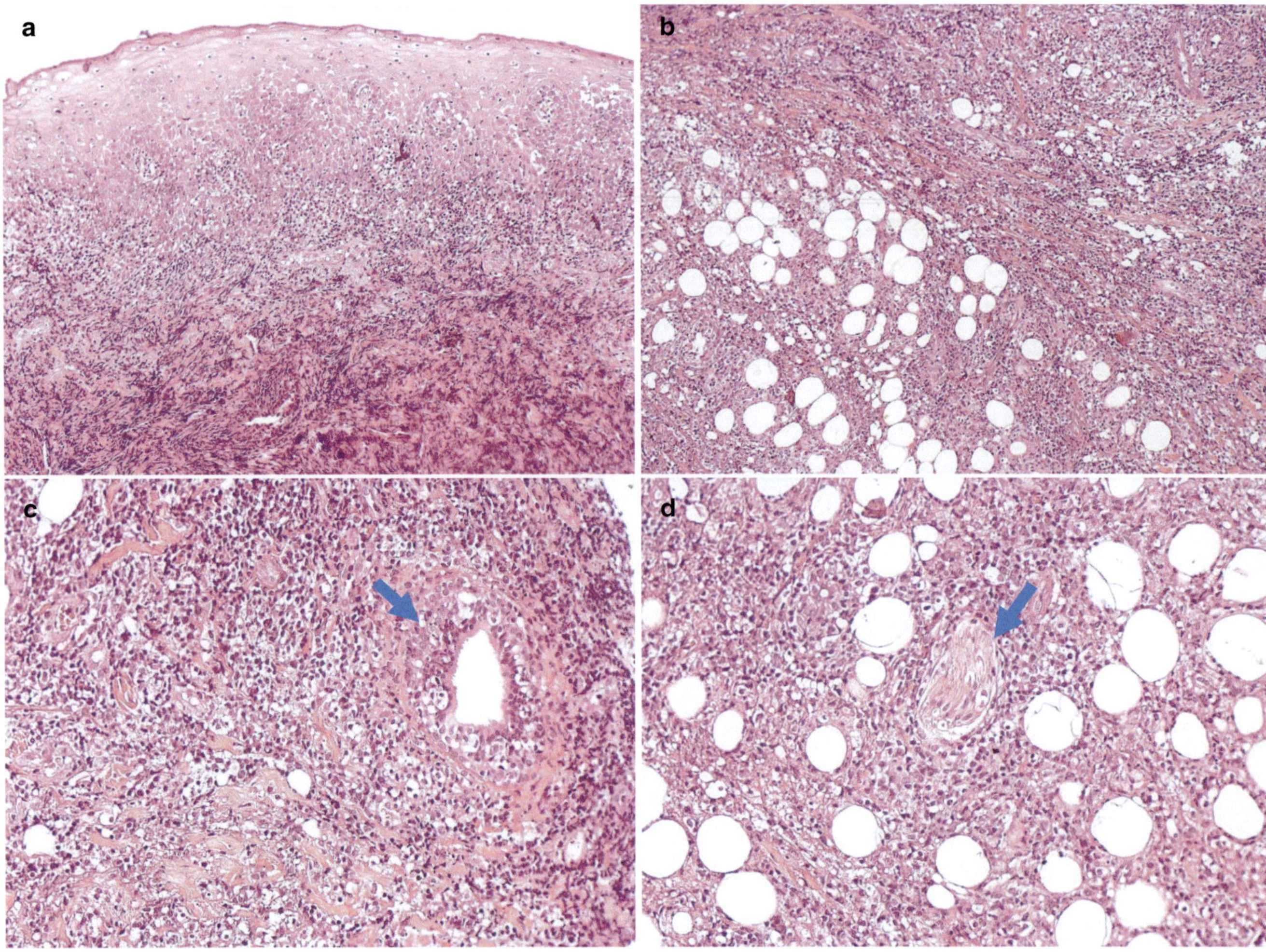

Fig. 43.12 Microscopic features of extranodal NK/T-cell lymphoma affecting the palate of a female patient. (**a**) Overlying squamous epithelium with a diffuse infiltration of neoplastic cells in the lamina propria (H&E; 100×). (**b**) Tumor cells proliferate diffusely and infiltrate the mature adipocytes (H&E; 100×). (**c**) Observe the angiocentric distribution of tumor cells (H&E; 200×). (**d**) Perineural distribution is also identified (blue arrow) (H&E; 200×)

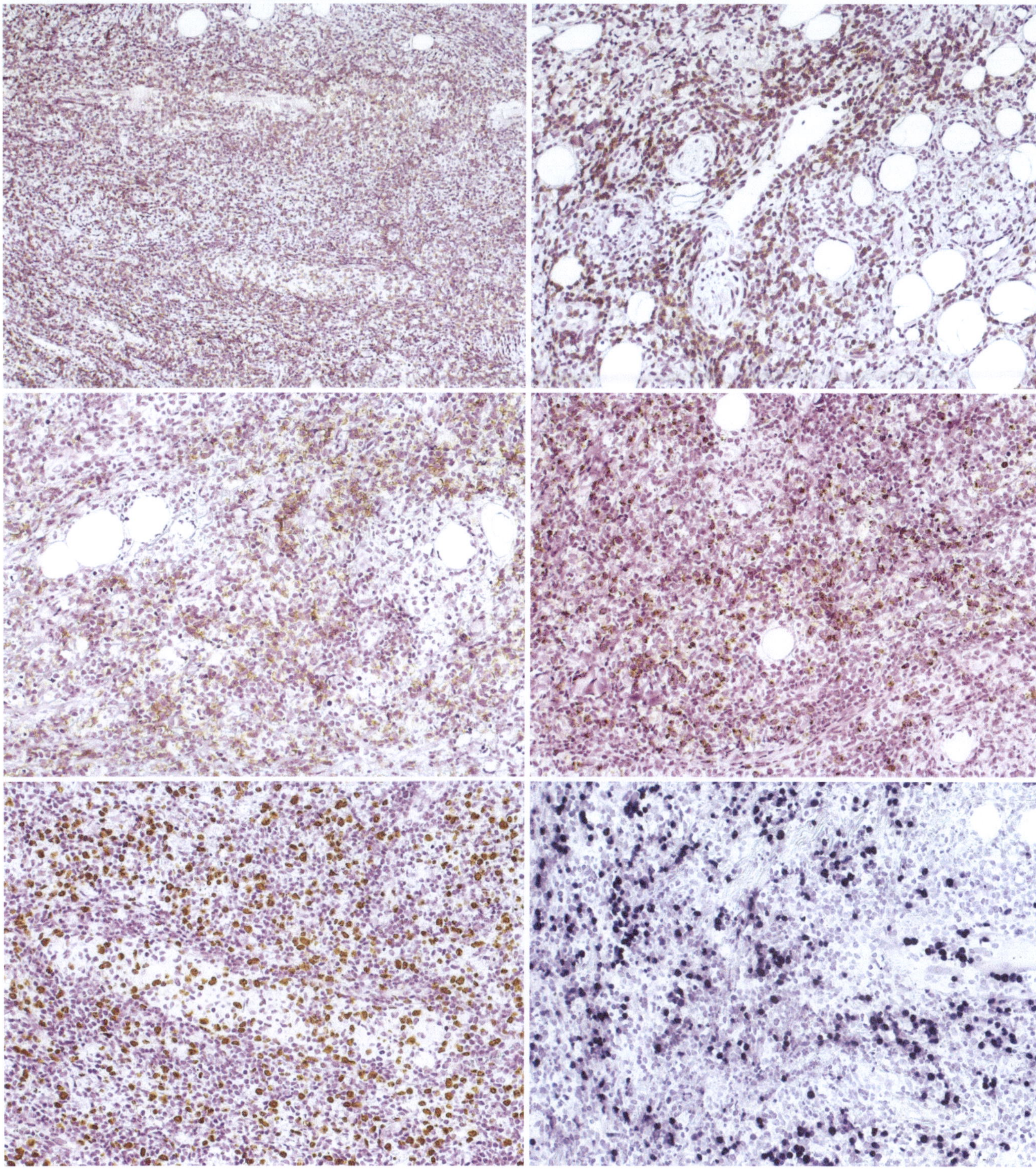

Fig. 43.13 Immunohistochemical features of extranodal NK/T-cell lymphoma of the same patient illustrated in Fig. 43.12. (**a**) Diffuse expression of CD3 (DAB; 100×). (**b**) Note the angiocentric distribution of CD3-positive tumor cells (DAB; 200×). (**c**) Expression of CD56 (DAB; 200×). (**d**) Granzyme B expression (DAB; 200×). (**e**) High proliferative rate demonstrated by Ki67 expression (DAB; 200×). (**f**) Presence of EBV confirmed by in situ hybridization (EBER; 200×)

Sources

1. Pontes HA, Pontes FS, Silva BS, Fonseca FP, Andrade BA, Rizo VH, et al. Extranodal nasal NK/T-cell lymphoma: a rare oral presentation and FASN, CD44 and GLUT-1 expression. Braz Dent J. 2013;24(3):284–8. https://doi.org/10.1590/0103-6440201302202.
2. Haverkos BM, Pan Z, Gru AA, Freud AG, Rabinovitch R, Wu-Welliver M, et al. Extranodal NK/T cell lymphoma, nasal type (ENKTL-NT): an update on epidemiology, clinical presentation, and natural history in North American and European cases. Curr Hematol Malig Rep. 2016;11(6):514–27. https://doi.org/10.1007/s11899-016-0355-9.
3. Sánchez-Romero C, Paes de Almeida O, Díaz Molina JP, Carlos R. Pediatric nasal NK/T-cell lymphoma microscopically mimicking carcinoma. Int J Dermatol. 2020;59(3):373–6. https://doi.org/10.1111/ijd.14722.
4. Sánchez-Romero C, Bologna-Molina R, Paes de Almeida O, Santos-Silva AR, Prado-Ribeiro AC, Brandão TB, et al. Extranodal NK/T cell lymphoma, nasal type: an updated overview. Crit Rev Oncol Hematol. 2021;159:103237. https://doi.org/10.1016/j.critrevonc.2021.103237.
5. de Arruda JAA, Abrantes TC, Cunha JLS, Roza ALOC, Agostini M, Abrahão AC, et al. Mature T/NK-cell lymphomas of the oral and maxillofacial region: a multi-institutional collaborative study. J Oral Pathol Med. 2021;50(6):548–57. https://doi.org/10.1111/jop.13205.
6. Sun KM, Wong YH, Cheung KC, Yuen CM, Chan YT, Lai WJ, et al. Update on molecular diagnosis in extranodal NK/T-cell lymphoma and its role in the era of personalized medicine. Diagnostics (Basel). 2022;12(2):409. https://doi.org/10.3390/diagnostics12020409.
7. Dong G, Liu X, Wang L. Genomic profling identifes distinct genetic subtypes in extra-nodal natural killer/T-cell lymphoma. Leukemia. 2022;36(8):2064–75. https://doi.org/10.1038/s41375-022-01623-z.
8. Quintanilla-Martinez L, Swerdlow SH, Tousseyn T, Barrionuevo C, Nakamura S, Jaffe ES. New concepts in EBV-associated B, T, and NK cell lymphoproliferative disorders. Virchows Arch. 2023;482(1):227–44. https://doi.org/10.1007/s00428-022-03414-4.
9. Zhang X, Liang K, Chen H, Liu L, Liu R, Wang C, et al. Genomic analysis reveals molecular characterization of CD30(+) and CD30(−) extranodal natural killer/T-cell lymphomas (ENKTLs). Hum Pathol. 2024;152:105650. https://doi.org/10.1016/j.humpath.2024.105650.
10. Chang YC, Tsai HJ, Huang TY, Su NW, Su YW, Chang YF, et al. Analysis of mutation profiles in extranodal NK/T--cell lymphoma: clinical and prognostic correlations. Ann Hematol. 2024 Aug;103(8):2917–30. https://doi.org/10.1007/s00277-024-05698-9.
11. Ito Y, Marouf A, Kogure Y, Koya J, Liévin R, Bruneau J, et al. Comprehensive genetic profiling reveals frequent alterations of driver genes on the X chromosome in extranodal NK/T-cell lymphoma. Cancer Res. 2024;84(13):2181–201. https://doi.org/10.1158/0008-5472.CAN-24-0132.
12. Yeh SA, Chiu LC, Lin HC, Li HJ, Lin SF, Su YC. Trends in the incidence of the Epstein-Barr virus-associated malignancies extranodal NK/T-cell lymphoma and nasopharyngeal carcinoma in Taiwan. PLoS One. 2024;19(12):e0315380. https://doi.org/10.1371/journal.pone.0315380.
13. Kaewboot W, Norasetthada L, Tantiworawit A, Chai-Adisaksopha C, Hantrakool S, Rattanathammethee T, et al. Clinical manifestations, prognostic factors, and outcomes of extranodal natural killer T-cell lymphoma: a single-center experience in Thailand. Hematol Rep. 2024;16(4):769–80. https://doi.org/10.3390/hematolrep16040073.
14. Lee J, Yoon SE, Kim SJ, Kim WS, Cho J. Mutational characteristics of extranodal NK/T-cell lymphoma analyzed in relation to clinical prognostic indices. Ann Hematol. 2024;103(12):5749–57. https://doi.org/10.1007/s00277-024-06035-w.
15. Do KH, Do TA, Nguyen TV, Le DT, Phan LV, Nguyen CV. Clinical and paraclinical features, outcome, and prognosis of extranodal natural killer/T-cell lymphoma, nasal type: a retrospective study of 31 Vietnamese patients. Int J Hematol Oncol Stem Cell Res. 2024;18(3):262–73. https://doi.org/10.18502/ijhoscr.v18i3.16107.

Peripheral T-Cell Lymphoma, Not Otherwise Specified

44

José Narciso Rosa Assunção Júnior, Javier Rendon Henao, and Felipe Paiva Fonseca

44.1 General Overview and Clinical Presentation

Peripheral T-Cell lymphoma (PTCL) accounts for 12–26% of all non-Hodgkin lymphomas, representing many different subtypes; therefore, this is a highly heterogeneous group of lymphomas derived from mature, post-thymic or "peripheral" T- and natural killer cells. The analysis of clinical, morphologic, immunophenotypic, and genetic features is necessary for achieving a precise final diagnosis according to the current guidelines of the World Health Organization. However, approximately 30% of these neoplasms cannot be further classified and are, therefore, diagnosed as *not otherwise specified (NOS)*, which represents a diagnosis made by exclusion, similar to diffuse large B-cell lymphoma not otherwise specified.

PTCL NOS derives from mature CD4+ or CD8+ αβ TCR T lymphocytes, but the etiology of this high-grade neoplasm remains unknown and is very difficult to establish given the biological heterogeneity of PTCL NOS. However, positivity for EBV can be observed in scattered B cells in some cases, suggesting that this virus may play some pathogenetic role in a small subset of cases. Much work has been done to better understand the molecular basis and the pathogenesis of this tumor as an attempt to identify new subgroups that would have the potential to reclassify or substratify cases previously diagnosed as PTCL NOS. In addition to the recognition of new entities that were removed from this umbrella term, like T Follicular Helper lymphoma (TFH lymphoma) and primary nodal EBV-positive NK/T-cell lymphoma, cases of PTCL NOS have been further classified according to different molecular groups as either PTCL-TBX21 or PTCL-GATA3. This recommendation is based on the characteristics of their gene expression profiles and clinical behavior. It is believed that PTCL-TBX21 cases that more closely resemble the genetic landscape of Th1 cells have a better prognosis, demonstrate less genomic complexity, have a higher frequency of epigenetic events in genes like *TET1*, *TET3*, and *DNMT3A*, and express TBX21 and CXCR3 proteins by immunohistochemistry. On the other hand, PTCL-GATA3 cases more closely resemble the genetic features of Th2 cells, have a poorer prognosis, a higher genomic complexity, and more often exhibit mutations in *TP53*, *PTEN*, *RB1*, *CDKN2A/B*, *PRDM1*, *STAT3* and *MYC*, and express GATA3 and CCR4 proteins by immunohistochemistry. However, the clinical application of this stratification remains to be further validated.

Most of the patients affected by PTCL NOS are adults, with a predominance of male patients. The lymph nodes are the most affected locations and patients demonstrate asymptomatic swellings in most cases, but virtually any site can be affected. The skin and the gastrointestinal tract are the two most affected extranodal locations. In advanced-stage disease, the presence of B symptoms like fever, weight loss and night sweating is common, but the involvement of the central nervous system and bone marrow is unusual. Moreover, affected patients may also develop paraneoplastic manifestations, represented by pruritus and hemophagocytic syndrome.

In the oral cavity, this heterogeneous and aggressive neoplasm represents the most common T-cell lymphoma in many epidemiological studies, except for those studies developed in Central/South America and Asia, where extranodal NK/T-cell

J. N. R. Assunção Júnior (✉)
Serviço de Estomatologia do Hospital Infantil Gonzaga, Santos, Brazil

Serviço de Estomatologia da Santa Casa da Misericórdia de Santos, Santos, Brazil

Faculdade de Odontologia da Universidade São Judas Tadeu – Campus Unimonte, Santos, Brazil
e-mail: narciso@alumni.usp.br

J. R. Henao
Department of Hematopathology and Flow Cytometry, Ayudas Diagnósticas Sura Center, Cartagena, Colombia

F. P. Fonseca
Department of Oral Surgery and Pathology, School of Dentistry, Universidade Federal de Minas Gerais, Belo Horizonte, Brazil

© The Author(s), under exclusive license to Springer Nature Switzerland AG 2025

F. P. Fonseca et al. (eds.), *Lymphoproliferative and Granulomatous Disorders of the Oral Cavity*,
https://doi.org/10.1007/978-3-031-98844-8_44

lymphoma frequently predominates. Oral presentation of PTCL NOS is usually in accordance with its aggressive behavior, manifesting as destructive, painful, ulcerative swellings, with variable necrotic regions. The palate and the gingiva are the most affected locations. The palatine tonsils may also be affected. Oral PTCL NOS may have variable osseous involvement due to neoplastic infiltration of the surrounding maxillary and/or mandibular bones, radiographically presenting as ill-defined radiolucent images. In the maxilla it may not be possible to determine if the neoplasm originates from the oral cavity or from the maxillary sinus.

The prognosis of patients affected by PTCL NOS is usually very poor, with 5-year overall survival rates ranging from 20% to 30%. Therapy varies, but higher intensity approaches are the most used, while stem cell transplantation has been shown to be contributory for patients' survival. Disease stage and International Prognostic Index (IPI) seem to be the most reproducible prognostic factors, but several other molecular and clinical parameters may variably impact patients' survival and response to chemotherapy (Fig. 44.1).

44.2 Microscopic Findings

- The tumor cells exhibit a diffuse growth pattern.
- Tumor cells infiltrate and destroy adjacent normal structures.
- Neoplastic cells are usually polymorphic, ranging from small to medium to large atypical cells.
- Cellular pleomorphism is usually high, with hyperchromatism or vesicular nuclei, and evident nucleoli.
- Scattered Reed-Sternberg-like cells may be found.
- Numerous typical and atypical mitotic figures are found.
- Necrotic regions can also be observed in many cases.
- Angiocentricity and epidermotropism may be present in some patients.
- An inflammatory background is often present, including small lymphocytes, eosinophils, plasma cells, large B cells and macrophages.
- Clusters of macrophages can be seen in the lymphoepithelioid variant of PTCL NOS, also known as Lennert lymphoma.
- PTCL-TBX21 tends to be more polymorphic than PTCL-GATA3 and contains a background of reactive inflammatory cells.
- Cases of PTCL-GATA3 tend to lack a prominent inflammatory background and show either sheets of medium-sized tumor cells with abundant clear cytoplasm or clusters or sheets of large tumor cells (Figs. 44.2, 44.3, 44.4, 44.5, and 44.6).

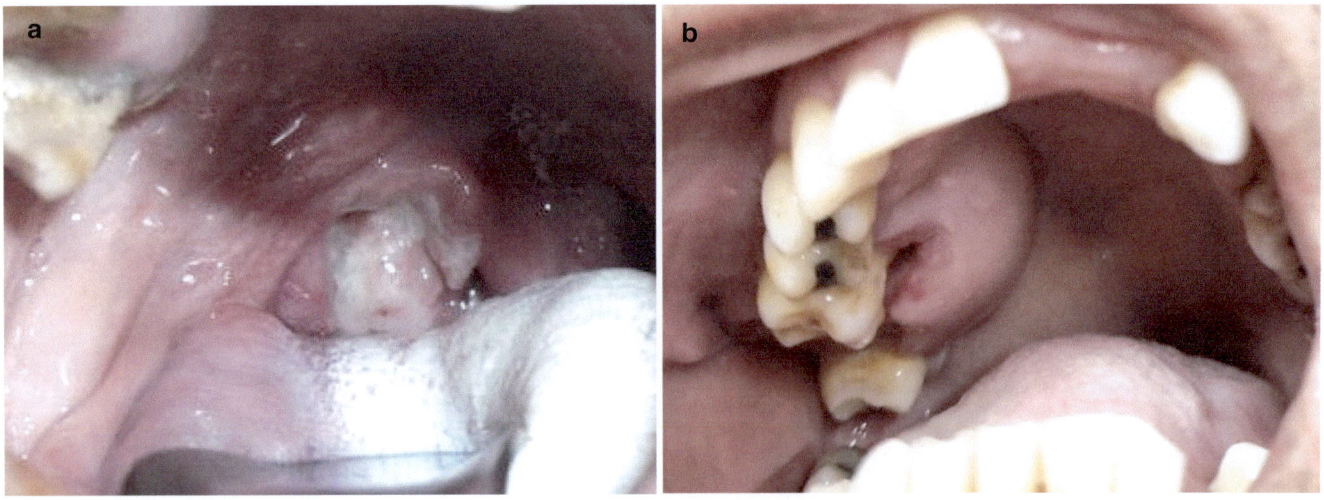

Fig. 44.1 Clinical presentation of peripheral T-cell lymphoma not otherwise specified affecting the oral cavity. (**a**) Painful swelling with necrotic regions affecting the right tonsil and extending towards the soft palate. (**b**) Destructive neoplasm affecting the maxillary sinus, causing extensive bone destruction and leading to hard palate and upper alveolar process involvement. The investigation of EBV was negative and contributed to excluding the diagnosis of an extranodal NK/T-cell lymphoma

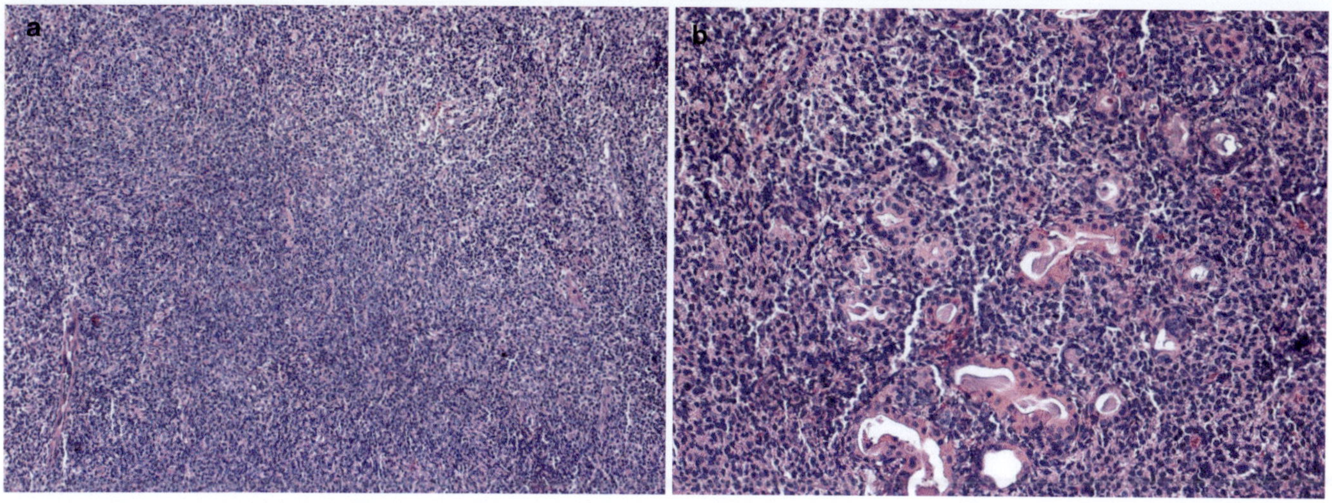

Fig. 44.2 Microscopic features of peripheral T-cell lymphoma not otherwise specified affecting the oral cavity. (**a**) Diffuse proliferation of neoplastic cells in the lamina propria (H&E; 50×). (**b**) The neoplastic cells infiltrated the normal surrounding tissues, like the glandular structures (H&E; 100×)

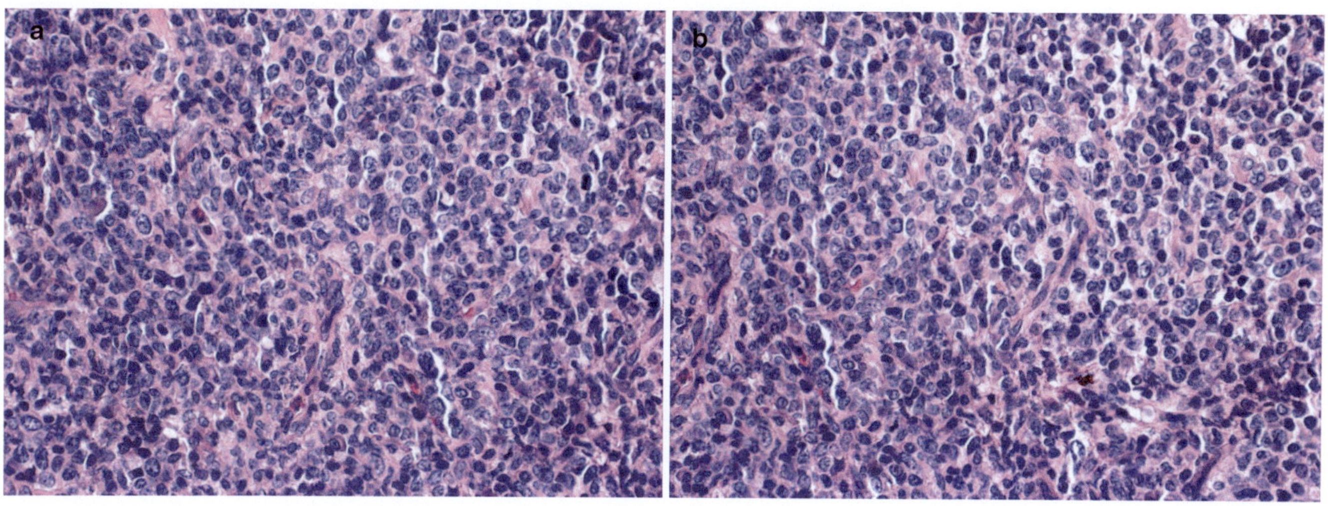

Fig. 44.3 Microscopic features of peripheral T-cell lymphoma not otherwise specified affecting the oral cavity. (**a**) This neoplasm is composed of a cellular population that exhibits a highly polymorphic aspect. The neoplastic cells range from small to medium to large. Mitotic figures are commonly found (H&E; 200×). (**b**) Tumor cells can be hyperchromatic or may present dispersed chromatin with prominent nucleoli (H&E; 200×)

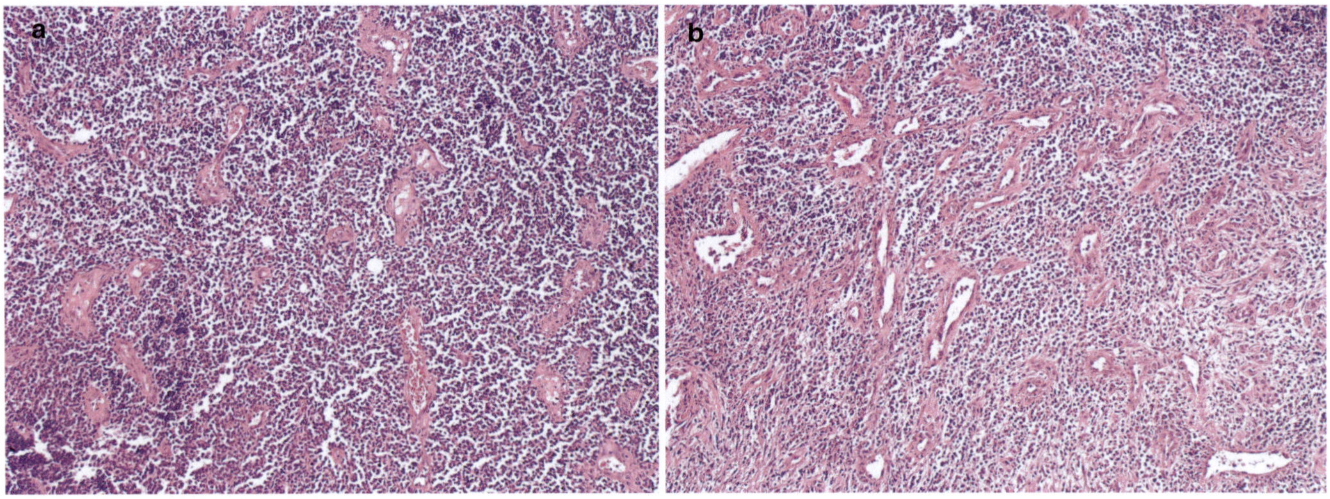

Fig. 44.4 Microscopic features of peripheral T-cell lymphoma not otherwise specified affecting the hard palate. (**a**) Diffuse proliferation of neoplastic cells loosely arranged in a scarcely fibrotic stroma (H&E; 50×). (**b**) Tumor cells surround blood vessels of different size and shape (H&E; 50×)

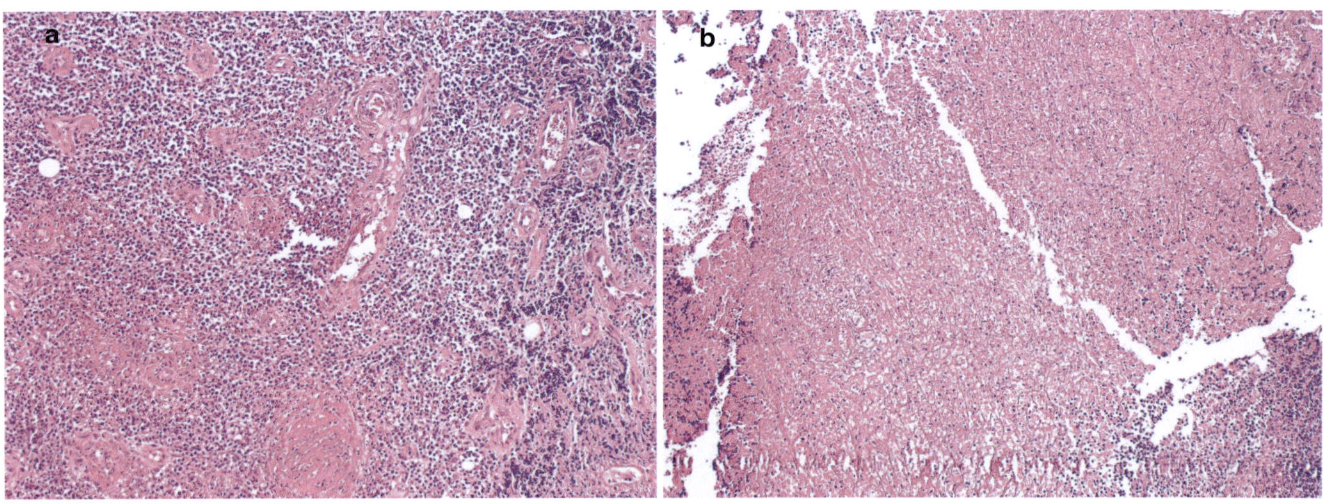

Fig. 44.5 Microscopic features of peripheral T-cell lymphoma not otherwise specified affecting the hard palate. (**a**) In some regions it is possible to observe the presence of an angiocentric distribution with destruction of the blood vessel leading to an eosinophilic fibrinous necrosis (H&E; 50×). (**b**) Areas of tissue necrosis are a common finding in peripheral T-cell lymphoma NOS, given its high-grade nature (H&E; 50×)

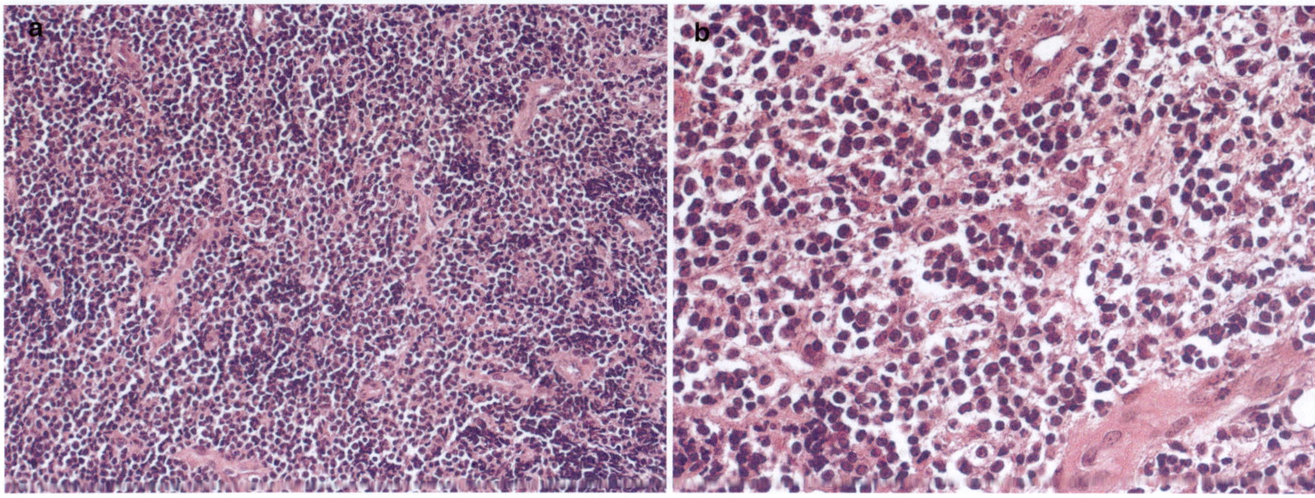

Fig. 44.6 Microscopic features of peripheral T-cell lymphoma not otherwise specified affecting the hard palate. (**a**) Neoplastic cells exhibit a high-grade of pleomorphism, with cells ranging from small to large size and predominantly exhibiting a hyperchromatic nucleus (H&E; 100×). (**b**) The variable cell cytology can be observed in this image. Tumor cells range from small to large, with pleomorphism and hyperchromatism (H&E; 200×)

44.3 Immunohistochemistry and/or Genetics

Immunohistochemical reactions are necessary not only to demonstrate the T-cell lineage origin of the neoplasm by the expression of CD3 and/or CD45RO, but also to exclude other more specific diagnostic possibilities. Expression of CD56 and cytotoxic granules like TIA-1, Granzyme B and Perforin may be found, and positive cases should be differentiated from extranodal NK/T-cell lymphoma, which, however, is consistently positive for EBV, whereas this virus is only present in scattered B lymphocytes of some PTCL NOS cases. The occurrence of a possible T follicular helper phenotype must be ruled out by investigating CD10, BCL6, CD279/PD1, CXCL13, ICOS markers and at least two of these markers should be positive to indicate this cellular origin. Approximately 50% of the cases show CD30 expression, but usually without the strong membranous and Golgi accentuation patterns found in anaplastic large cell lymphoma. The majority of the PTCL NOS cases are CD4-positive/CD8-negative, although cases exhibiting a double-negative, double-positive and CD8-positive/CD4-negative cases can also be diagnosed. ALK protein is negative, and aberrant expression of B cell markers like CD20, PAX5 and CD79a may be seen in exceptional cases. Proliferative index is usually very high, although variable, and loss of BCL2 expression may occur.

Molecular landscape of PTCL NOS is very complex and heterogeneous with karyotypic abnormalities like gains of 7q and 8q and alterations observed in different genes like *TP63*, *CDKN2A*, *PTEN*, *TP53*, *PLCG1*, *CD28*, and *VAV1*, meanwhile Gene expression profiling was used to categorized *PTCL NOS as* PTCL-TBX21 or PTCL-GATA3 groups, which is more routinely approached on surgical pathology laboratories using immunohistochemistry (Table 44.1; Figs. 44.7, 44.8, and 44.9).

Table 44.1 Summary of the main immunohistochemical reactions used for PTCL NOS diagnosis

Antibody/probe	Main result	Pattern	Objective
CD20	Negative	Membrane	To exclude a B-cell lymphoma
CD3	Positive	Membrane	To demonstrate the T-cell origin
CD45RO	Positive	Membrane	To demonstrate the T-cell origin
CD4/CD8	Double positive/negative	Membrane	To characterize the tumor
CD56	Variable	Membrane	To characterize the tumor
CD43	Positive	Membrane	To characterize the tumor
Granzyme B/TIA-1/Perforin	Variable	Cytoplasm	To characterize the tumor and to exclude NK/T lymphoma
CD10/BCL6/CD279/CXCL13/ICOS	Negative	Variable	To investigate a possible TFH lymphoma
CD21	Negative	Membrane	To investigate a possible AITL
CD30	Variable	Membrane[a]	To investigate a possible ALCL
ALK	Negative	Variable	To investigate a possible ALK+ ALCL
TBX21 and CXCR3	Variable	Cytoplasm	To stratify tumors according to cell of origin (Th1)
GATA3 and CCR4	Variable	Cytoplasm	To stratify tumors according to cell of origin (Th2)
CD25	Negative	Membrane	To investigate a possible ATLL
FOXP3	Negative	Nucleus	To investigate a possible ATLL
Ki67	High (~80%)	Nucleus	To demonstrate the proliferative index of the neoplasm
EBER[b]	Positive in a few cases	Nucleus	To demonstrate the presence of EBV in a few B cells
HTLV-1	Negative[c]	–	To investigate a possible ATLL

The main results for EBV and HTLV-1 detection are also described

TFH T follicular helper, *AITL* angioimmunoblastic T-cell lymphoma, *ALCL* Anaplastic large cell lymphoma, *ATLL* Adult T cell leukemia/lymphoma

[a]The dot-like staining pattern found in ALCL is usually absent in PTCL NOS

[b]*In situ* hybridization

[c]The molecular search for HTLV-1 is more reliable than serological tests

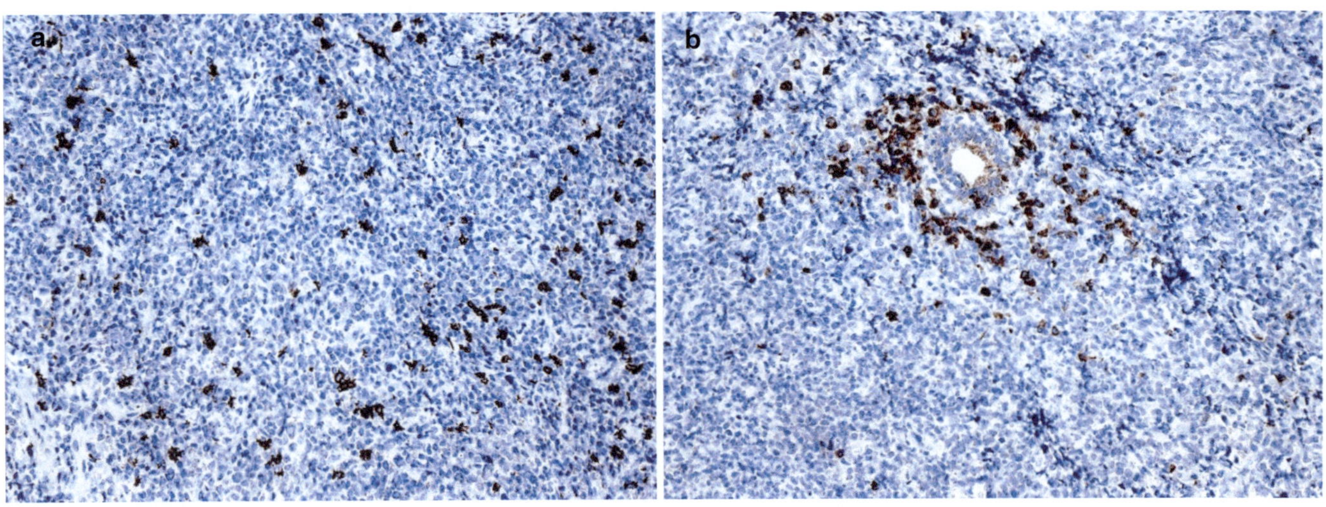

Fig. 44.7 Immunohistochemical findings of peripheral T-cell lymphoma not otherwise specified affecting the oral cavity. (**a**) The neoplastic cells are negative for the mature B-cell markers CD20 (DAB; 100×). and (**b**) CD79a. However, a subset of cases may exhibit an aberrant expression for some B-cell antigens (DAB; 100×)

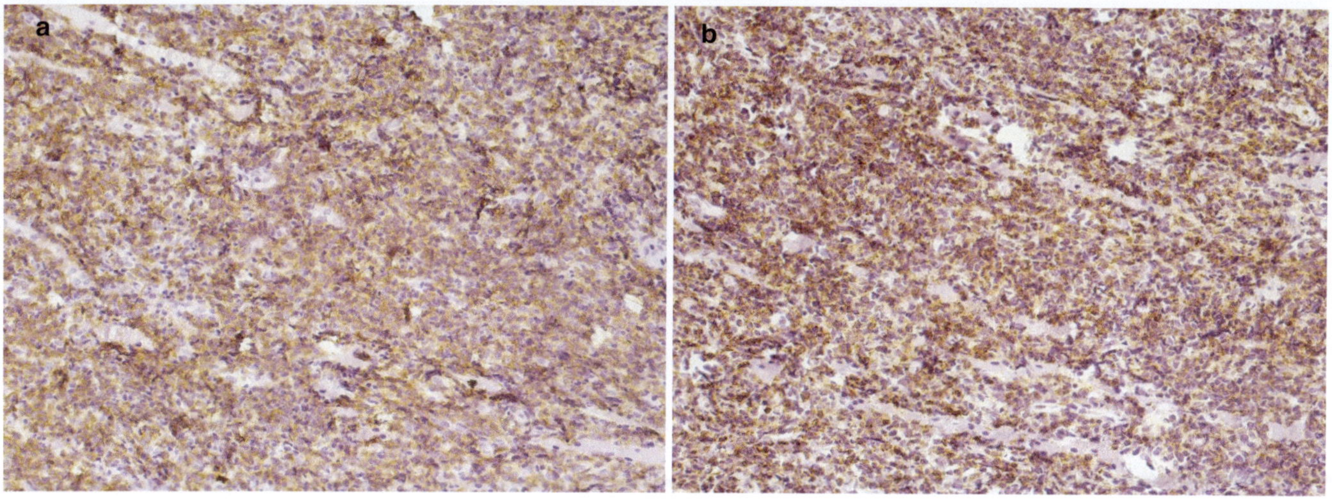

Fig. 44.8 Immunohistochemical findings of peripheral T-cell lymphoma not otherwise specified affecting the oral cavity (DAB; 100×). (**a**) Diffuse expression of CD3 in tumor cells. (**b**) The expression of CD45RO further confirms the T-cell nature of this neoplasm (DAB; 100×)

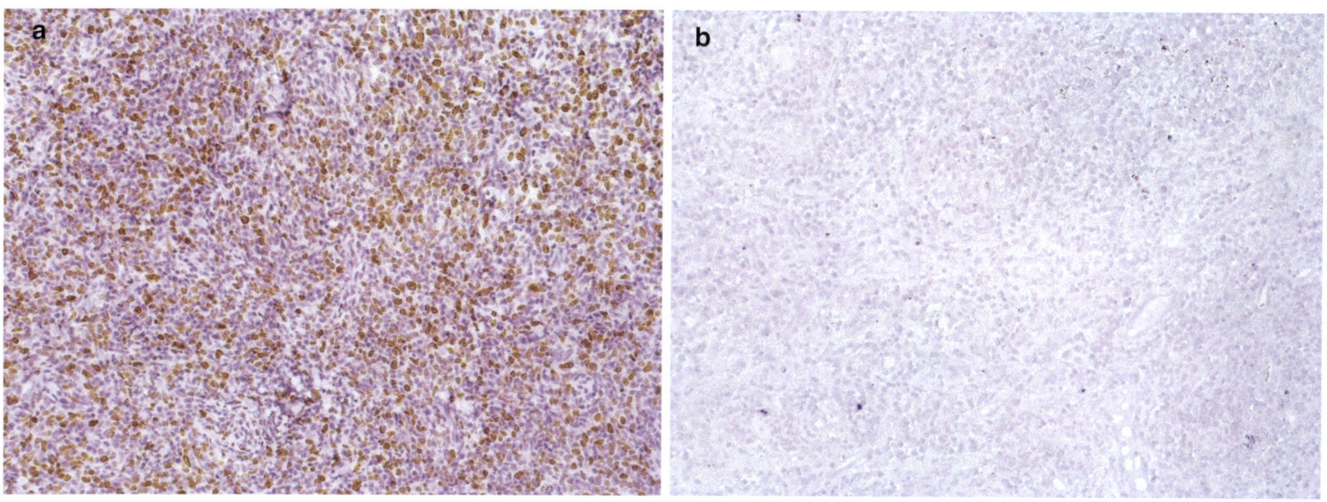

Fig. 44.9 Immunohistochemical findings and in situ hybridization for EBV detection of peripheral T-cell lymphoma not otherwise specified affecting the oral cavity. (**a**) This heterogeneous group of neoplasms usually presents a very high proliferative index measured by Ki67 (DAB; 100×). (**b**) EBV can be present in the B lymphocytes of a subset of peripheral T-cell lymphoma not otherwise specified, although the majority of the cases are negative, as illustrated in this example (DAB; 100×)

Sources

1. Iqbal J, Wright G, Wang C. Gene expression signatures delineate biological and prognostic subgroups in peripheral T-cell lymphoma. Blood. 2014;123:2915–23. https://doi.org/10.1182/blood-2013-11-536359.
2. Jeon YK. Clinicopathological analysis of a case series of peripheral T-cell lymphomas, not otherwise specified, of lymphoepithelioid variant (Lennert's lymphoma). A Central European single-center study-reply. Hum Pathol. 2016;53:194–5. https://doi.org/10.1016/j.humpath.2015.12.034.
3. Gafencu GA, Selicean SE, Petrushev B, Cucuianu A, Dima D, Frinc I, et al. Clinicopathological analysis of a case series of peripheral T-cell lymphomas, not otherwise specified, of lymphoepithelioid variant (Lennert's lymphoma). A Central European single-center study. Hum Pathol. 2016;53:192–4. https://doi.org/10.1016/j.humpath.2015.12.033.
4. Amador C, Greiner TC, Heavican TB. Reproducing the molecular subclassification of peripheral T-cell lymphoma-NOS by immunohistochemistry. Blood. 2019;134:2159–70. https://doi.org/10.1182/blood.2019000779.
5. Basha BM, Bryant SC, Rech KL, Feldman AL, Vrana JA, Shi M, et al. Application of a 5 marker panel to the routine diagnosis of peripheral t-cell lymphoma with T-follicular helper phenotype. Am J Surg Pathol. 2019;43(9):1282–90. https://doi.org/10.1097/PAS.0000000000001315.
6. Montes-Mojarro IA, Kim WY, Fend F, Quintanilla-Martinez L. Epstein-Barr virus positive T and NK-cell lymphoproliferations: morphological features and differential diagnosis. Semin Diagn Pathol. 2020;37(1):32–46. https://doi.org/10.1053/j.semdp.2019.12.004.
7. de Arruda JAA, Schuch LF, Conte Neto N, de Souza LL, Rodrigues-Fernandes CI, Abreu LG, et al. Oral and oropharyngeal lymphomas: a multi-institutional collaborative study. J Oral Pathol Med. 2021;50(6):603–12. https://doi.org/10.1111/jop.13211.

8. de Arruda JAA, Abrantes TC, Cunha JLS, Roza ALOC, Agostini M, Abrahão AC, et al. Mature T/NK-cell lymphomas of the oral and maxillofacial region: a multi-institutional collaborative study. J Oral Pathol Med. 2021;50(6):548–57. https://doi.org/10.1111/jop.13205.
9. Satou A, Takahara T, Tsuzuki T. Pathological and molecular features of nodal peripheral T-cell lymphomas. Diagnostics (Basel). 2022;12(8):2001. https://doi.org/10.3390/diagnostics12082001.
10. Eriksen PRG, Clasen-Linde E, Brown PN, Haunstrup L, Christoffersen M, Asdahl P, et al. NK- and T-cell lymphoma of the nasal cavity and paranasal sinuses in Denmark 1980–2017: a nationwide cohort study. Leuk Lymphoma. 2022;63(11):2579–88. https://doi.org/10.1080/10428194.2022.2087069.
11. Feldman AL, Laurent C, Narbaitz M, Nakamura S, Chan WC, de Leval L, et al. Classification and diagnostic evaluation of nodal T- and NK-cell lymphomas. Virchows Arch. 2023;482(1):265–79. https://doi.org/10.1007/s00428-022-03412-6.
12. Oliveira EM, de Cáceres CVBL, Santos-Silva AR, Vargas PA, Lopes MA, Pontes HAR, et al. Clinical diagnostic approach for oral lymphomas: a multi-institutional, observational study based on 107 cases. Oral Surg Oral Med Oral Pathol Oral Radiol. 2023;136(4):427–35. https://doi.org/10.1016/j.oooo.2023.03.011.
13. Oliveira EM, Cáceres CVBL, Fernandes-Rodrigues CI, Penafort PVM, Legarrea JMA, Gomes NR, et al. Oral manifestations of peripheral T cell lymphoma, not otherwise specified: case series and review of the current literature. Oral Surg Oral Med Oral Pathol Oral Radiol. 2024;139:e37–45. https://doi.org/10.1016/j.oooo.2024.08.011.
14. Ding S, Chen J, Su J, Liu J, Yin W, Qi F. Clinicopathological diagnosis of Lennert lymphoma: a case report and review of the literature. Diagn Pathol. 2024;19(1):111. https://doi.org/10.1186/s13000-024-01533-x.
15. Pichler AS, Amador C, Fujimoto A, Takeuchi K, de Jong D, Iqbal J, et al. Advances in peripheral T cell lymphomas: pathogenesis, genetic landscapes and emerging therapeutic targets. Histopathology. 2025;86(1):119–33. https://doi.org/10.1111/his.15376.

Anaplastic Large Cell Lymphoma

45

Ciro Dantas Soares,
Cinthia Veronica Bardalez Lopez de Caceres,
Guilherme Rossi Assis de Mendonça,
and Felipe Paiva Fonseca

45.1 General Overview and Clinical Presentation

Anaplastic large cell lymphoma (ALCL) is a high-grade lymphoma consisting of large T cells with abundant cytoplasm and pleomorphic, often horseshoe-shaped or reniform nuclei that show uniform strong expression of CD30 protein. It comprises two systemic subtypes that more frequently affect the lymph nodes, more often in the cervical and inguinal regions, and are differentiated based on the presence of mutations in the *ALK* (anaplastic lymphoma kinase) gene (*ALK*-positive ALCL and *ALK*-negative ALCL). Primary cutaneous ALCL and breast implant-associated ALCL, even in the presence of nodal or extranodal dissemination, should be considered different entities.

ALK-positive ALCL by definition carries chromosomal translocation involving the *ALK* gene that is fused with different partner genes, more often with *NPM1*, which results from t(2;5)(p23;q35) and leads to a strong nuclear and cytoplasmic constitutive expression of *NPM1::ALK* fusion oncoprotein. Depending on different fusion partners of the *ALK* gene, distinct immunohistochemical expression patterns of the oncogenic protein may be seen. This lymphoma subtype is also defined by the expression of CD30 in the membrane and as a perinuclear Golgi accentuation pattern. It accounts for approximately 3% of all non-Hodgkin lymphomas and it is more commonly diagnosed in the first three decades of life, accounting for 10–15% of pediatric and adolescent non-Hodgkin lymphomas. There is a slight male predominance. Extranodal cases account for up to 60% of all cases, more commonly affecting the bone, soft tissue, lungs and liver. The involvement of the central nervous system is uncommon and bone marrow is affected in approximately 15% of the cases.

ALK-positive ALCL demonstrates a more favorable clinical course and prognosis than its *ALK*-negative counterpart, which is also characterized by the strong and diffuse CD30 membrane positivity, but lacking *ALK* translocation and its oncoprotein expression. Instead, *ALK*-negative ALCL has been shown to carry several other mutations involving *JAK1*, *STAT3*, *TP53*, *TP63* and other genes. Moreover, tumors carrying mutations in the *DUSP22* gene may represent a specific subtype of *ALK*-negative ALCL with particular microscopic features and molecular mechanisms. However, there is still a lack of definitive evidence to justify the inclusion of a new official ALCL subtype. Adult patients aged 40–60 years are the most affected individuals by *ALK*-negative ALCL with a slight male predominance. Lymph nodes are also the most affected site, although approximately 50% of the cases may develop in extranodal sites like soft tissues, liver, spleen and the gastrointestinal tract. In both *ALK*-positive and *ALK*-negative ALCL, tumors are most often diagnosed in advanced stages and B symptoms are usually present.

ALCL manifesting in the oral and maxillofacial region is very unusual, with approximately 30 cases reported in the literature, and most of the available reports represent extension of a primary nodal disease or a widely disseminated process, although rare examples of primary oral ALCL have also been described. The tumors usually present as rapidly growing, painful, ulcerated swellings that may cause variable degrees of trismus. Some cases may manifest as lobulated tumors. Patients usually have a mean age of 53.7 years, ranging from 12 to 77 years, depending on the presence of *ALK* translocation as described above, with predilection for females. The gingiva/alveolar ridge is the most commonly affected site, followed by the palate. The occurrence of

C. D. Soares (✉)
Laboratório de Patologia Getúlio Sales, Natal, Brazil

C. V. B. L. de Caceres · F. P. Fonseca
Department of Oral Surgery and Pathology, School of Dentistry, Universidade Federal de Minas Gerais, Belo Horizonte, Brazil

G. R. A. de Mendonça
Department of Pathology, School of Medical Sciences, University of Campinas, Campinas, Brazil

© The Author(s), under exclusive license to Springer Nature Switzerland AG 2025
F. P. Fonseca et al. (eds.), *Lymphoproliferative and Granulomatous Disorders of the Oral Cavity*,
https://doi.org/10.1007/978-3-031-98844-8_45

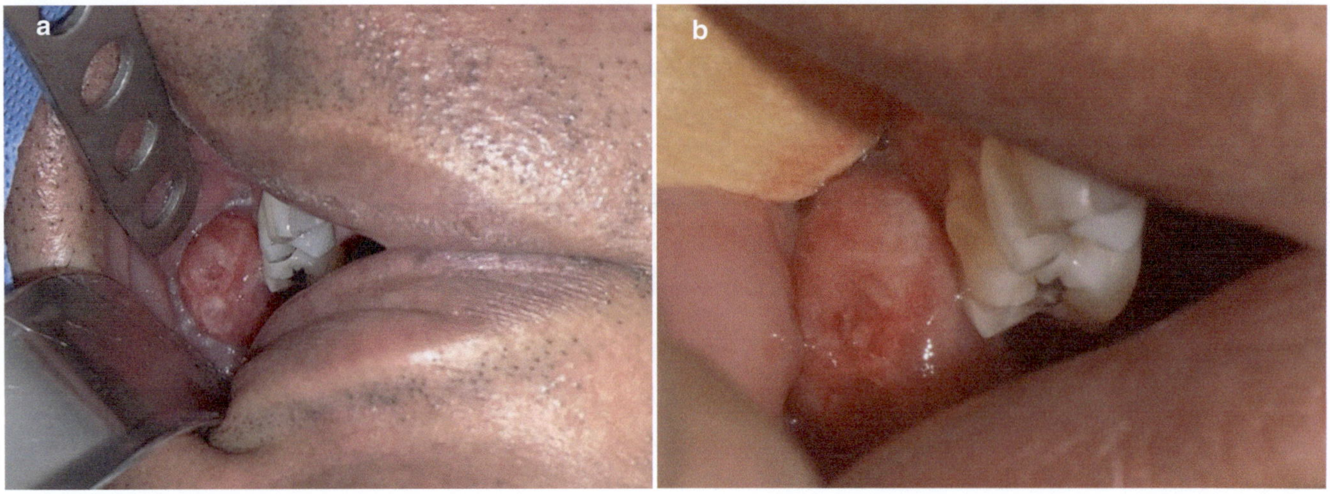

Fig. 45.1 Clinical presentation of an ALK-negative anaplastic large cell lymphoma affecting the oral cavity. (**a**) The neoplasm originated from the lymph node and disseminated to the oral cavity. (**b**) The disease manifested as a painful swelling, affecting the cheek mucosa and caused a significant trismus

gnathic bone destruction can also be found in radiographic examinations as poorly defined radiolucent images.

Using a large series of extranodal ALCL, Nguyen et al. (2018) investigated the prognostic impact of primary site of the tumor, demonstrating that patients affected by primary ALCL of the central nervous system and chest/abdomen/pelvis had a significantly shorter overall survival than individuals affected by primary tumors of the head and neck, bone, and cutaneous/subcutaneous tissue. Overall survival of patients affected by *ALK*-positive ALCL may achieve 80% after 5 years of follow-up and their prognosis is better than that observed for *ALK*-negative ALCL patients, who have a mean survival ranging from 30% to 40%. Chemotherapy schemes, including the combined use of Brentuximab vedotin, an anti-CD30 drug, have significantly improved the prognosis of affected patients (Fig. 45.1).

45.2 Microscopic Findings

- The tumors exhibit a diffuse growth pattern or clusters of neoplastic cells.
- Tumor cells infiltrate and destroy adjacent normal structures.
- Presence of tissue necrosis is frequent.
- The presence of large cells with eccentric horseshoe-shaped or kidney-shaped nuclei, with an eosinophilic region near the nucleus (hallmark cells) is typically found in ALCL cases.
- Multiple evident nucleoli and abundant amphophilic cytoplasm.
- Depending on the plane of section, pseudonuclear inclusions or invaginations can be observed (doughnut cells).
- The starry-sky pattern is uncommonly observed.
- Mitotic figures are frequent.
- A small cell variant is known.
- Different histologic patterns can be found: common pattern (60%), lymphohistiocytic pattern (10%), small-cell pattern (5–10%), Hodgkin-like pattern (3%) and composite pattern (15%).
- *ALK*-negative DUSP22+ ALCL was shown to have a specific morphological pattern characterized by sheets of more medium-sized cells with a monotonous appearance. Doughnut cells are often prominent in this subtype (Table 45.1; Figs. 45.2, 45.3, and 45.4).

Table 45.1 Histologic subtypes of ALCL

Common	Lymphohistiocytic	Small-cell	Hodgkin-like	Composite	Others
Large cells Eosinophilic cytoplasm Multiple nuclei Reed-Stenberg-like cells Dispersed chromatin Multiple small or large nucleoli Intrasinusoidal growth	Presence of histiocytes Neoplastic cells are smaller Located around blood vessels	Small to medium-sized neoplastic cells Centrally located nucleus (fried egg-like cells) Signet-ring-like cells	Nodular growth and often associated with fibrosis, mimicking nodular sclerosis Hodgkin lymphoma (NSHL) Lack of immunophenotypic criteria for NSHL	Presence of more than one pattern	Multinucleated giant neoplastic cells Sarcomatous features Hypocellular appearance Myxoid aspect

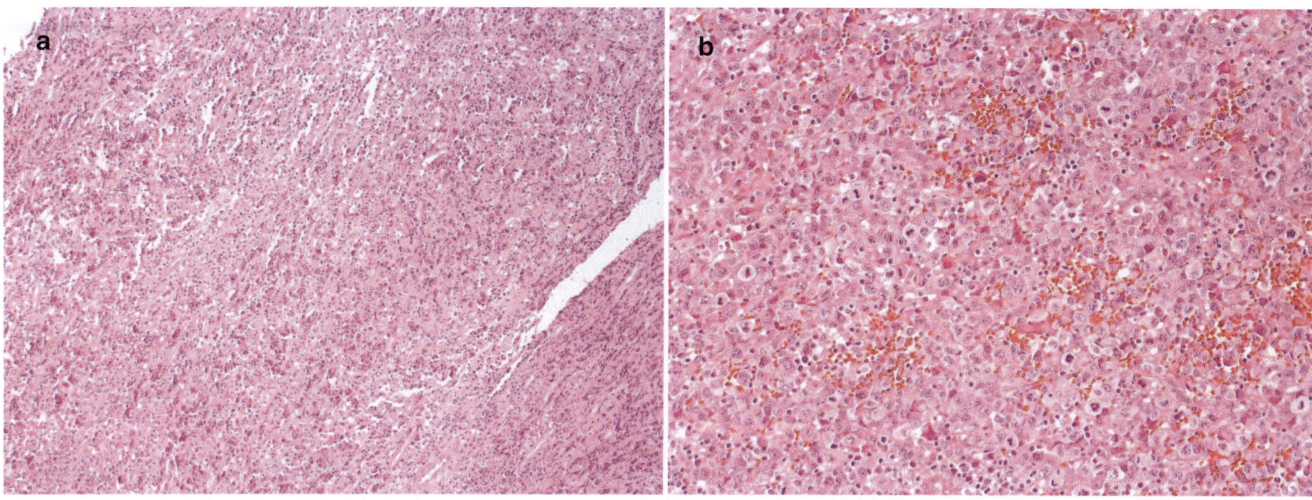

Fig. 45.2 Microscopic findings of ALCL affecting the oral cavity. (**a**) The neoplasm exhibited a diffuse growth pattern and contained a population of reactive smaller cells (H&E; 50×). (**b**) Observe the sheet-like proliferation of neoplastic cells with many mitotic figs. (H&E; 100×)

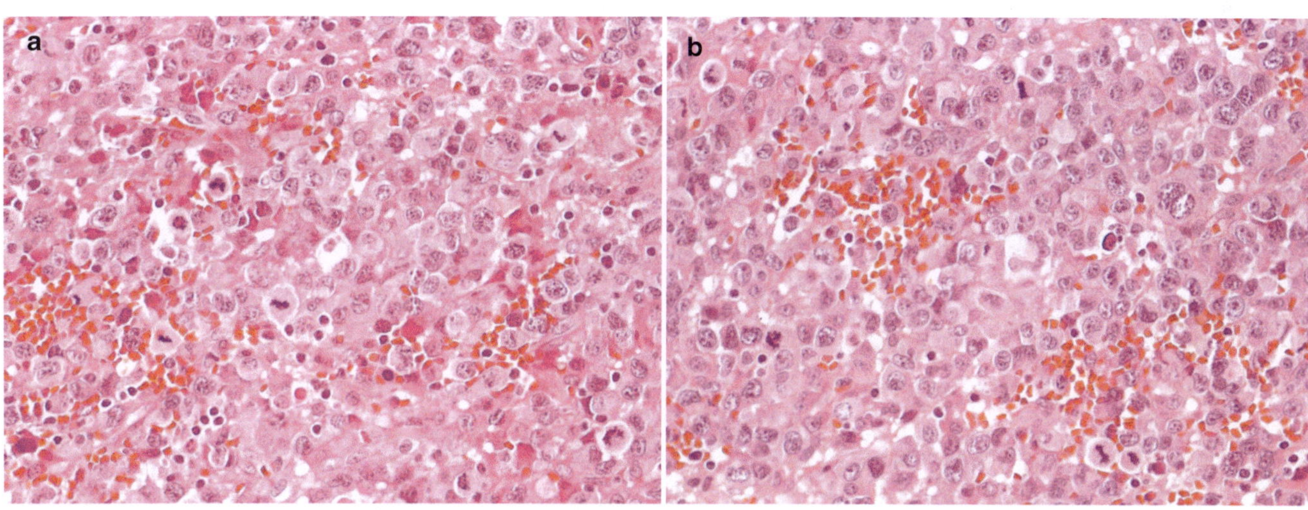

Fig. 45.3 Microscopic findings of ALCL affecting the oral cavity. (**a**) The neoplasm was composed of large cells exhibiting a high degree of pleomorphism and abundant eosinophilic cytoplasm. An epithelioid and a plasmablastic appearance could be observed. Some of the so-called hallmark cells can be found (H&E; 200×). (**b**) Atypical mitotic figures were common; sparse doughnut cells are present and pleomorphic cells are easily observed (H&E; 200×)

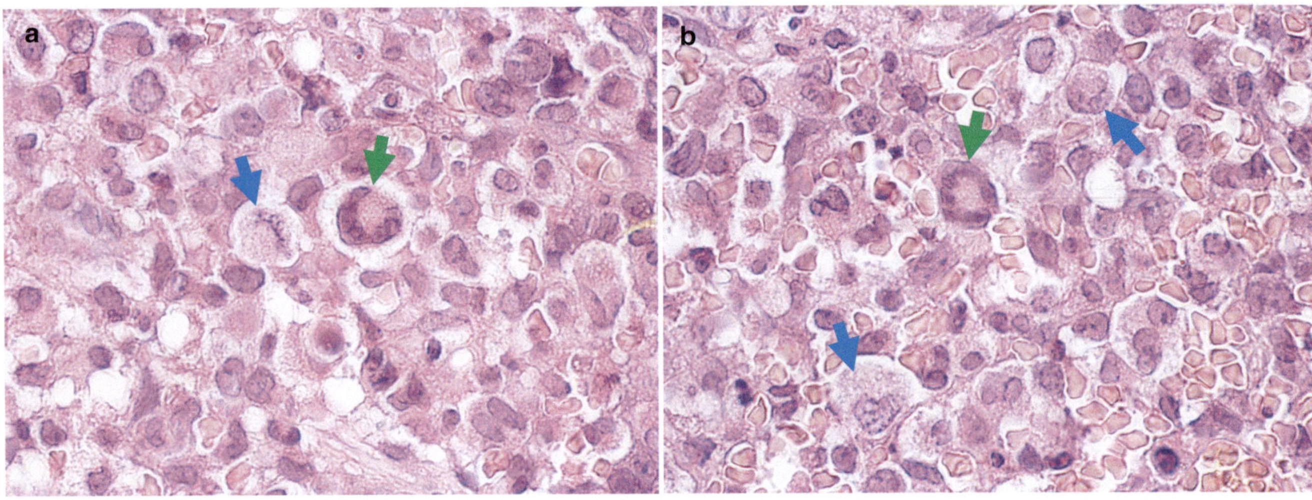

Fig. 45.4 Microscopic findings of ALCL affecting the oral cavity. (**a**) High magnification image illustrating the large pleomorphic cells. Note the presence of a horseshoe-shaped cell (green arrow) and mitotic figure (blue arrow) (H&E; 1000×). (**b**) Doughnut cells can also be appreciated in this image (green arrow). Observe the presence of many pleomorphic cells (blue arrow) (H&E; 1000×)

45.3 Immunohistochemistry and/or Genetics

Immunohistochemical reactions using the pan-T-cell marker CD3 are usually not useful in demonstrating the lineage of differentiation of the neoplastic cells, since ALCL loses the expression of this protein in approximately 75% of the cases. Other T-cell markers can also be lost, like CD5 and CD7. A notable number of cases express CD2 and CD4, albeit their expression may also be downregulated. Therefore, other markers like CD45RO and cytotoxic granulations (Granzyme B, TIA-1 and perforin) can be very useful to demonstrate the cellular lineage of differentiation. The CD8 is only rarely positive. Although CD43 can also be used, it is a less specific marker and not reliable for determining lineage differentiation. In rare instances, the null cell phenotype is encountered, and assessment of clonal rearrangements of T-cell receptor (TCR) may be needed. The typical strong and diffuse CD30 expression in the membrane and as a dot-like staining in the Golgi region is mandatory for the diagnosis, but the expression of CD30 may be lost after treatment with Brentuximab vedotin in some patients. ALK protein expression is present in *ALK*-positive ALCL, but its expression pattern varies depending on the gene partner involved in *ALK* translocation, although a strong and diffuse nuclear and cytoplasmic expression is the most commonly observed pattern (Table 45.2).

EBER is consistently negative and Ki67 is usually very high. The microscopic features together with the absence of LCA (CD45), CD20 and CD3, in addition to the simultaneous expression of EMA, may lead to a misdiagnosis of carcinoma. Molecular landscape of ALCL is complex, but it has been more thoroughly understood during the last decades, with *ALK*-positive ALCL demonstrating chromosomal abnormalities in the *ALK* gene that has approximately 20 different gene partners, and *ALK*-negative cases harboring multiple alterations including rearrangements of *DUSP22, TP63, JAK2, FRK, MYC, ROS1* and *TYK2* genes; mutations of *JAK1, STAT3* and *MSCE* genes; and aberrant expression of *ERBB4* (Table 45.3; Figs. 45.5, 45.6, 45.7, 45.8, and 45.9).

Table 45.2 Most frequent molecular features of ALK-positive anaplastic large cell lymphoma [14, 16]

Genetic event	Oncogenic protein	Immunohistochemistry staining pattern	Frequency
t(2;5)(p23;q35)	*NPM::ALK*	Diffuse nucleus, cytoplasm	84%
t(1;2)(q25; p23)	*TPM3::ALK*	Strong cytoplasmic and membranous	13%
inv(2)(p23q35)	*ATIC::ALK*	Diffuse cytoplasmic	1%
t(2;19)(p23;p13)	*TPM4::ALK*	Diffuse cytoplasm	<1%
t(2;3)(p23;q21)	*TFG::ALK*	Diffuse cytoplasmic	<1%
t(2;17)(p23;q25)	*RNF213::ALK*	Diffuse cytoplasmic	<1%
t(2;17)(p23;q23)	*CLTC::ALK*	Granular cytoplasmic	<1%
t(X;2)(q11; p23)	*MSN::ALK*	Membranous	<1%
t(2;22)(p23;q11)	*MYH9::ALK*	Diffuse cytoplasmic	<1%
t(2;19)(p23;q33)	*TRAF1::ALK*	Diffuse cytoplasmic	<1%
t(2;11)(p23;q11)	*EEF1G::ALK*	Diffuse cytoplasmic	<1%
t(2;9)(p23;q33)	*PABPC1::ALK*	Diffuse cytoplasmic	<1%

Table 45.3 Summary of the main immunohistochemical reactions used for ALCL diagnosis

Antibody/ probe	Most frequent results	Pattern	Objective
CD20	Negative	Membrane	To exclude a possible B-cell origin of the neoplasm
CD2	Occasionally positive; may be negative	Membrane	The loss of this marker is sometimes seen in ALCL, but its positivity favors a T-cell phenotype
CD3	Usually negative	Membrane	The loss of this marker is commonly seen in ALCL
CD5	Usually negative	Membrane	The loss of this marker is commonly seen in ALCL
CD7	Usually negative	Membrane	The loss of this marker is commonly seen in ALCL
CD4	Occasionally positive; may be negative	Membrane	The loss of this marker is sometimes seen in ALCL, but its positivity favors a T-cell phenotype
CD8	Usually negative	Membrane	This marker is usually negative in ALCL, but rare positive cases exist
CD45RO	Positive	Membrane	To demonstrate the leukocyte lineage of the neoplasm
CD56	Negative	Membrane	To exclude an extranodal NK/T-cell lymphoma
EMA	Usually positive	Membrane/ cytoplasm	Positive in a variable number of the cases
Granzyme B	Positive	Cytoplasm	To demonstrate the expression of cytotoxic antigens by the neoplasm
TIA-1	Positive	Cytoplasm	To demonstrate the expression of cytotoxic antigens by the neoplasm
Perforin	Positive	Cytoplasm	To demonstrate the expression of cytotoxic antigens by the neoplasm
CD30	Positive	Membrane/Golgi	Consistently positive in ALCL
ALK	Positive or negative	Variable	To determine the diagnosis of ALK+ or ALK− ALCL
CD25	Positive	Membrane	To characterize the immunophenotype of ALCL
Ki67	~60–70%	Nucleus	To demonstrate the proliferative index of the neoplasm
EBER[a]	Negative	–	To demonstrate the absence of EBV
HTLV-1	Negative	–	To differentiate this neoplasm from ATLL
ALK[b]	Positive or negative	–	To characterize the genetic landscape of the neoplasm
TP63[b]	Positive in ALK-ALCL	–	To characterize the genetic landscape of the neoplasm
DUSP22[b]	Positive in ALK-ALCL	–	To characterize the genetic landscape of the neoplasm
JAK/STAT[b]	Positive in ALK-ALCL	–	To characterize the genetic landscape of the neoplasm

The main results for EBV detection and some important molecular findings are also described

ATLL Adult T-cell leukemia/lymphoma, *ALK−* ALK negative

[a]Investigated by in situ hybridization

[b]Investigated by fluorescent in situ hybridization

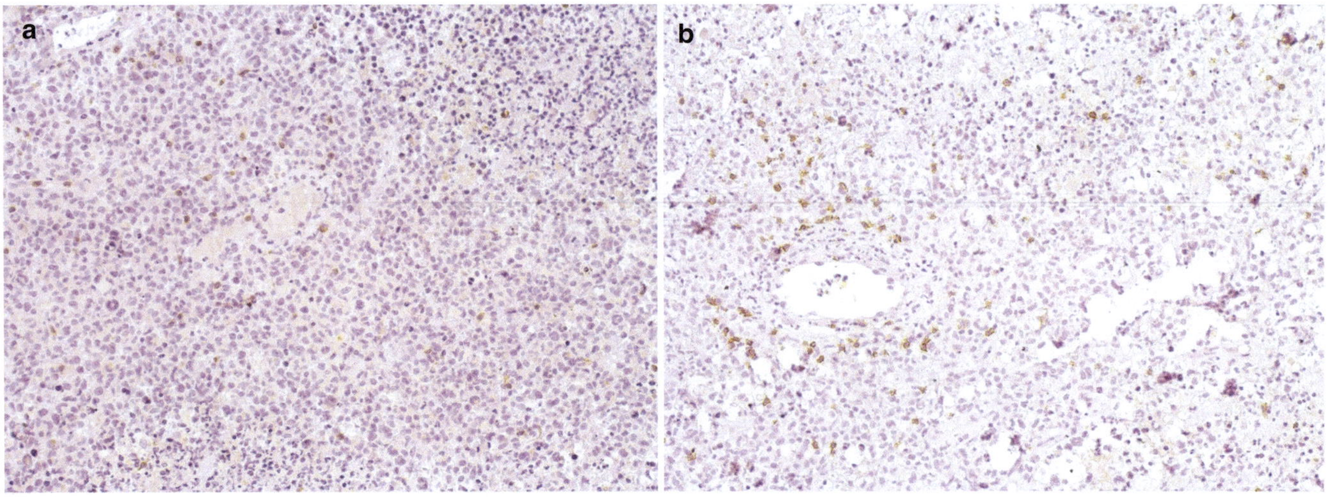

Fig. 45.5 Immunohistochemical findings of ALCL. (**a**) Tumor cells usually lose the expression of pan-T cell markers like CD3, which stains reactive cells (DAB; 100×). (**b**) The expression of CD4 may also be lost (DAB; 100×)

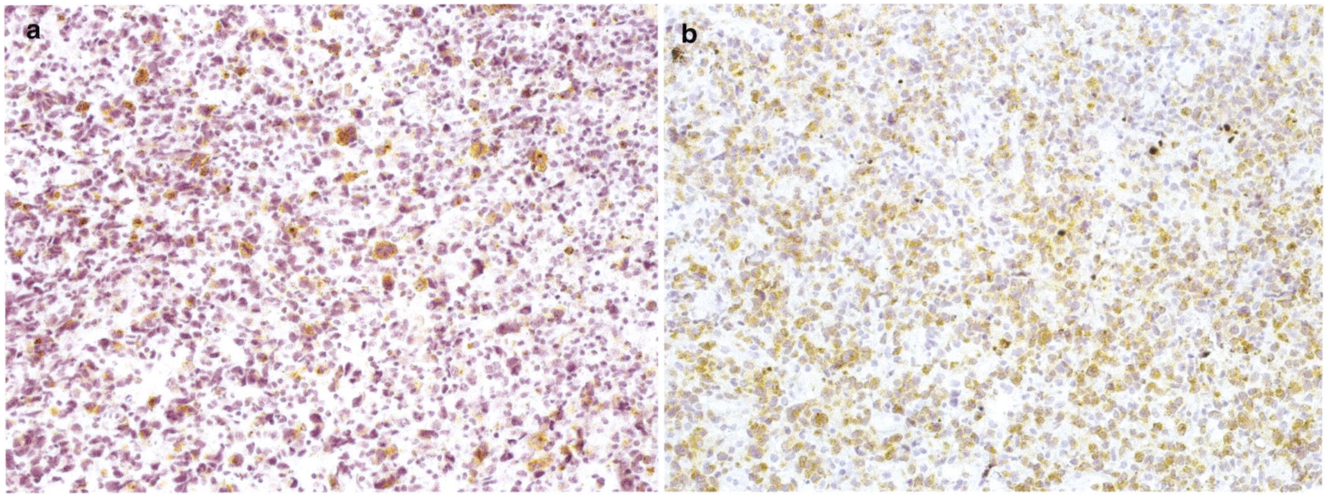

Fig. 45.6 Immunohistochemical findings of ALCL. (**a**) The cytotoxic immunophenotype of ALCL can be demonstrated by the expression of cytotoxic granules. In this image the granular expression of granzyme B can be seen in the cytoplasm of tumor cells (DAB; 100×). (**b**) Perforin is another important cytotoxic granule that can be investigated (DAB; 100×)

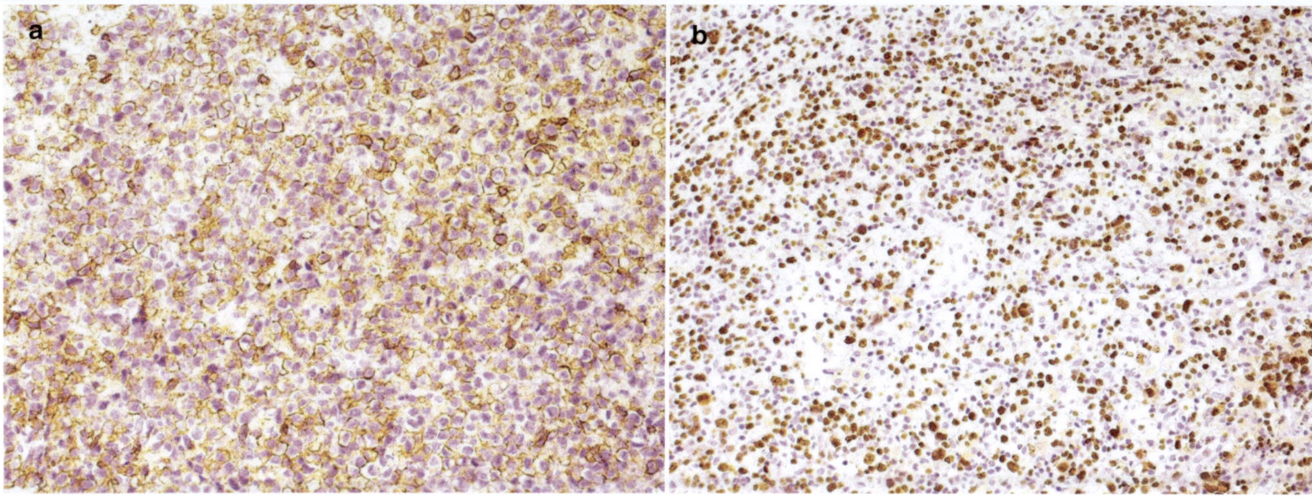

Fig. 45.7 Immunohistochemical findings of ALCL. (**a**) The expression of CD43 is common in ALCL, but despite representing a T cell marker, its low specificity does not allow it to be used to determine the lineage of differentiation of the neoplasm (DAB; 100×). (**b**) The Ki67 proliferative index of ALCL is usually very high (DAB; 400×)

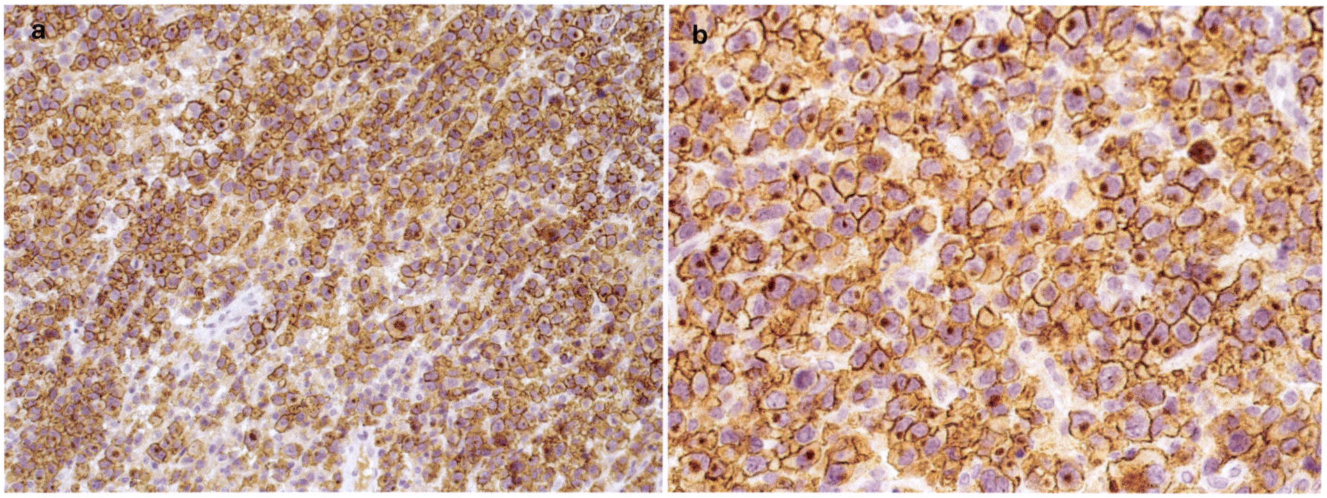

Fig. 45.8 Immunohistochemical findings of ALCL. (**a**) The strong and diffuse membrane expression of CD30 with accentuation in the Golgi region is considered a hallmark of ALCL and it is also important for treatment approaches (DAB; 100×). (**b**) Note the Golgi-like staining pattern of CD30 (DAB; 400×)

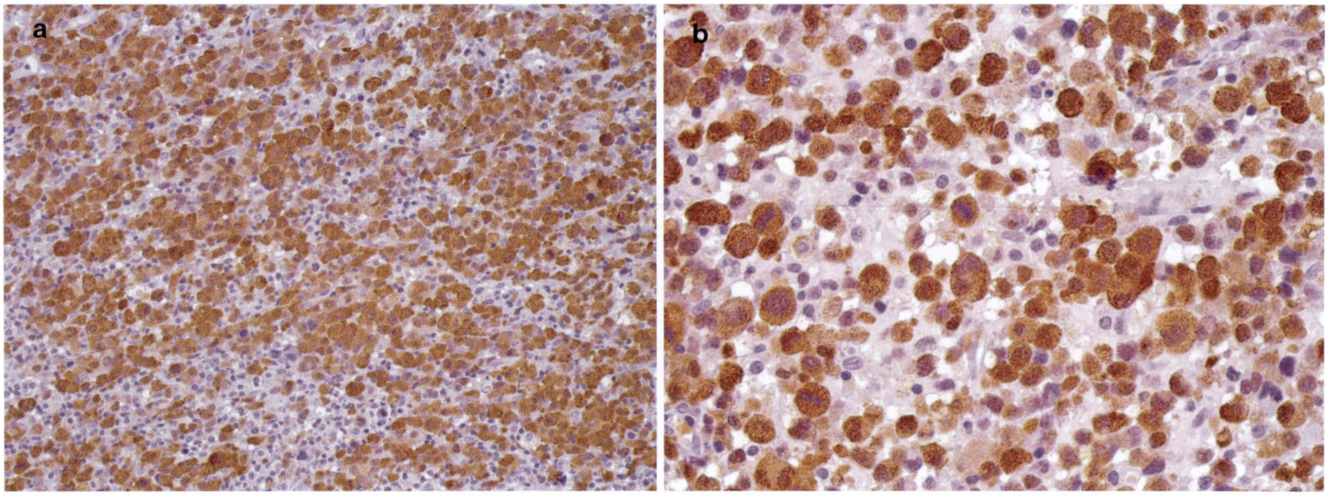

Fig. 45.9 Immunohistochemical findings of ALCL. (**a**) The expression of ALK protein is strongly and diffusely observed in this example of ALK-positive ALCL affecting the oral cavity (DAB; 100×). (**b**) Note the nuclear and cytoplasmic expression pattern indicative of the t(2;5)(p23;q35) translocation involving *NPM::ALK* genes (DAB; 400×)

Sources

1. Matsumoto N, Ohki H, Mukae S, Amano Y, Harada D, Nishimura S, et al. Anaplastic large cell lymphoma in gingiva: case report and literature review. Oral Surg Oral Med Oral Pathol Oral Radiol Endod. 2008;106(4):e29–34. https://doi.org/10.1016/j.tripleo.2008.05.037.
2. Sciallis AP, Law ME, Inwards DJ, McClure RF, Macon WR, Kurtin PJ, et al. Mucosal CD30-positive T-cell lymphoproliferations of the head and neck show a clinicopathologic spectrum similar to cutaneous CD30-positive T-cell lymphoproliferative disorders. Mod Pathol. 2012;25(7):983–92. https://doi.org/10.1038/modpathol.2012.38.
3. Grandhi A, Boros AL, Berardo N, Reich RF, Freedman PD. Two cases of CD30+, anaplastic lymphoma kinase (ALK)-negative anaplastic large cell lymphoma with oral manifestations. Oral Surg Oral Med Oral Pathol Oral Radiol. 2013 Feb;115(2):e41–7. https://doi.org/10.1016/j.oooo.2012.04.010.
4. Wang W, Cai Y, Sheng W, Lu H, Li X. The spectrum of primary mucosal CD30-positive T-cell lymphoproliferative disorders of the head and neck. Oral Surg Oral Med Oral Pathol Oral Radiol. 2014;117(1):96–104. https://doi.org/10.1016/j.oooo.2013.10.002.
5. Nguyen KA, Su C, Bai HX, Zhang Z, Xiao R, Karakousis G, et al. Disease site as a determinant of survival outcome in patients with systemic anaplastic lymphoma kinase positive anaplastic large cell lymphoma with extranodal involvement: an analysis of 1306 cases from the US National Cancer Database. Br J Haematol. 2018;181(2):196–204. https://doi.org/10.1111/bjh.15145.
6. de Andrade BAB, Fontes MD, Roza ALOC, Vargas PA, Agostini M, Canedo NHS, et al. Anaplastic large cell lymphoma with oral manifestation: a series of four cases and literature review. Head Neck Pathol. 2020;14(4):991–1000. https://doi.org/10.1007/s12105-020-01176-6.
7. de Arruda JAA, Abrantes TC, Cunha JLS, Roza ALOC, Agostini M, Abrahão AC, et al. Mature T/NK-cell lymphomas of the oral and maxillofacial region: a multi-institutional collaborative study. J Oral Pathol Med. 2021;50(6):548–57. https://doi.org/10.1111/jop.13205.
8. Pina-Oviedo S, Ortiz-Hidalgo C, Carballo-Zarate AA, Zarate-Osorno A. ALK-negative anaplastic large cell lymphoma: current concepts and molecular pathogenesis of a heterogeneous group of large T-cell lymphomas. Cancers (Basel). 2021;13(18):4667. https://doi.org/10.3390/cancers13184667.
9. Parkhi M, Bal A, Das A, Kashyap D, Bhardwaj S, Prakash G, et al. ALK-negative anaplastic large cell lymphoma (ALCL): prognostic implications of molecular subtyping and JAK-STAT pathway. Appl Immunohistochem Mol Morphol. 2021;29(9):648–56. https://doi.org/10.1097/PAI.0000000000000936.
10. Khanlari M, Li S, Miranda RN, Iyer S, Konoplev S, Lin P, Yin CC, et al. Small cell/lymphohistiocytic morphology is associated with peripheral blood involvement, CD8 positivity and retained T-cell antigens, but not outcome in adults with ALK+ anaplastic large cell lymphoma. Mod Pathol. 2022;35(3):412–8. https://doi.org/10.1038/s41379-021-00944-1.
11. Feldman AL, Laurent C, Narbaitz M, Nakamura S, Chan WC, Leval L, et al. Classification and diagnostic evaluation of nodal T- and NK-cell lymphomas. Virchows Arch. 2023;482:265–79.
12. Lewis NE, Sardana R, Dogan A. Mature T-cell and NK-cell lymphomas: updates on molecular genetic features. Int J Hematol. 2023;117(4):475–91. https://doi.org/10.1007/s12185-023-03537-7.
13. Qiu L, Tang G, Li S, Vega F, Lin P, Wang SA, et al. DUSP22 rearrangement is associated with a distinctive immunophenotype but not outcome in patients with systemic ALK-negative anaplastic large cell lymphoma. Haematologica. 2023;108(6):1604–15. https://doi.org/10.3324/haematol.2022.281222.
14. Wu R, Lim MS. Updates in pathobiological aspects of anaplastic large cell lymphoma. Front Oncol. 2023;13:1241532. https://doi.org/10.3389/fonc.2023.1241532.
15. Xie W, Medeiros LJ, Fan G, Li S, Xu J. Systemic ALK-negative anaplastic large cell lymphoma: insights into morphologic, immunophenotypic, genetic and molecular characteristics. Hum Pathol. 2024;156:105671. https://doi.org/10.1016/j.humpath.2024.105671.
16. Elenitoba-Johnson K, Ott G, Takeuchi K, Klapper W, Lamant-Rochaix L, d-Amore ESG, et al. ALK-positive anaplastic large cell lymphoma. In: WHO Classification of Tumours Editorial Board. Haematolymphoid tumours, WHO classification of tumours series, vol. 11. 5th ed. Lyon: International Agency for Research on Cancer; 2024. https://publications.iarc.who.int/637.
17. Shaw TI, Pounds S, Cao X, Ma J, Palacios G, Mason J, et al. Comprehensive genomic analysis reveals molecular heterogeneity in pediatric ALK-positive anaplastic large cell lymphoma. Leukemia. 2025;39(1):199–210. https://doi.org/10.1038/s41375-024-02468-4.

Mycosis Fungoides and Sezary Syndrome

46

José Candido Xavier-Junior, Ciro Dantas Soares, and Felipe Paiva Fonseca

46.1 General Overview and Clinical Presentation

Mycosis fungoides is an epidermotropic T-cell lymphoma that primarily affects the skin, representing the most common primary cutaneous T-cell lymphoma subtype, accounting for approximately 38–50% of all cases. Mycosis fungoides clinical findings are widely variable, and its classical presentation frequently demonstrates a non-aggressive, slowly growing cutaneous lesion in the form of a pruritic and erythematous flat patch that develops most often in non-sun-exposed areas, whose diagnosis can be extremely difficult due to strong similarities with other reactive cutaneous conditions. Sometimes only after long periods of follow-up, the disease evolves to more advanced clinical stages characterized by plaques or tumors. Large cell transformation of mycosis fungoides is defined by the presence of at least 25% of atypical large cells or by the presence of nodules of large atypical cells, showing at least four times the size of a small lymphocyte and conspicuous nucleoli. It frequently occurs in the tumor stage and occasionally in the plaque stage. Extracutaneous manifestations are rare and the lymph nodes, liver, spleen and lungs are the most commonly affected sites. There is a slight male predominance and patients are usually in their 50s. Considering the mycosis fungoides subtypes, according to the new classification of the World Health Organization, it can be diagnosed as classical, folliculotropic, granulomatous slack skin disease and Pagetoid reticulosis.

In contrast to this frequent indolent behavior of mycosis fungoides, Sezary syndrome represents a leukemic disease associated with immunosuppression. In comparison, Sezary syndrome shows a more aggressive behavior and poorer prognosis for affected patients, with an approximate 5-year survival rate of 30% with currently available treatment modalities. Originally described in 1938 as a lymphocytosis typically consisting of neoplastic cells exhibiting grooved and cerebriform nuclei, Sezary syndrome is known to be closely related to mycosis fungoides; however, they are considered separate entities. This leukemic disease usually arises de novo and is characterized by erythroderma (involving >80% of the body surface), generalized lymphadenopathy and the presence of clonally related T cells in the skin, peripheral blood and/or lymph nodes defined by clonal TCR gene rearrangements. Patients may also demonstrate other manifestations like pruritus, alopecia, ectropion, palmar or plantar hyperkeratosis, lichenification, and onychodystrophy. Male patients are the most affected, usually among the elderly population. While mycosis fungoides neoplastic cells may derive from resident cutaneous memory T cells, those from Sezary syndrome seem to originate from central memory T cells. In peripheral blood the absolute number of Sezary cell should be ≥1000/ mL or flow cytometry can identify CD4+ T-cell population with CD4/CD8 >10 or an expanded CD4+ T-cell population with an abnormal phenotype (CD4+/CD7− T cells ≥40% or CD4+/CD26− T cells ≥30%). The genetic landscape of mycosis fungoides and Sezary syndrome is considered complex, and a large number of numerical or structural abnormalities have been described for both entities, with some degree of similarity among themselves.

The occurrence of oral manifestations in both disorders is very uncommon, but well-documented cases are available in the literature. In the large majority of the cases reported cutaneous lesions precede the diagnosis of oral lesions by

J. C. Xavier-Junior (✉)
School of Medicine, Centro Universitário Católico Unisalesiano Auxilium, Araçatuba, Brazil

Pathology Institute of Araçatuba, Araçatuba, Brazil

C. D. Soares
Laboratório de Patologia Getúlio Sales, Natal, Brazil

F. P. Fonseca
Department of Oral Surgery and Pathology, School of Dentistry, Universidade Federal de Minas Gerais, Belo Horizonte, Brazil

© The Author(s), under exclusive license to Springer Nature Switzerland AG 2025
F. P. Fonseca et al. (eds.), *Lymphoproliferative and Granulomatous Disorders of the Oral Cavity*,
https://doi.org/10.1007/978-3-031-98844-8_46

approximately 8 years of duration. Although very rare, exclusive oral manifestations have already been described, and these cases require a high degree of suspicion from clinicians and pathologists. In an autopsy-based study with patients diagnosed with mycosis fungoides, it was observed that oral tongue involvement was present in about 18.6% of the individuals, suggesting that oral cavity can be more frequently affected in advanced cases, and although oral involvement has been associated with a poorer survival, they have now a better prognosis due to improvements in the therapeutic options. Mycosis fungoides affecting the oral cavity is more common in males, with a mean age of 59.7 years, but with a wide range (from 9 to 80 years old). Multiple oral lesions are more frequently diagnosed than solitary manifestations, and the tongue, palate and gingiva are the most affected locations. The clinical presentation varies significantly from ulcers to erythematous plaques to nodules or tumors, which leads to a broad list of differential diagnoses.

Clinical stage is considered the most important prognostic factor for patients affected by mycosis fungoides and Sezary syndrome. Moreover, the clinical presence of plaques (vs patches only), histopathologic evidence of large cell transformation, elevated serum lactate dehydrogenase levels, and severe pruritus at the time of diagnosis have also been associated with reduced survival. Treatment will also mainly depend on disease stage and may vary from topical therapies with steroids, topical nitrogen mustard, phototherapy and topical bexarotene, to systemic therapies with oral bexarotene, interferon-alpha, alemtuzumab, to different chemotherapy schemes associated or not with the use of radiotherapy.

46.2 Microscopic Findings

- The main morphological features of classical mycosis fungoides and less frequently in Sezary syndrome are:
- Prominent, diffuse infiltrate of atypical lymphocytes showing cerebriform and hyperchromatic nuclei, sometimes surrounded by clear halos.
- In the patch and plaque stages, tumor cells are often located at the epidermal/dermal interface.
- Epidermotropism and subepidermal fibrosis are very common findings (Figs. 46.1 and 46.2).
- In the tumor stage a deeper infiltrate with reduced epidermotropism is present and ulceration can occur.

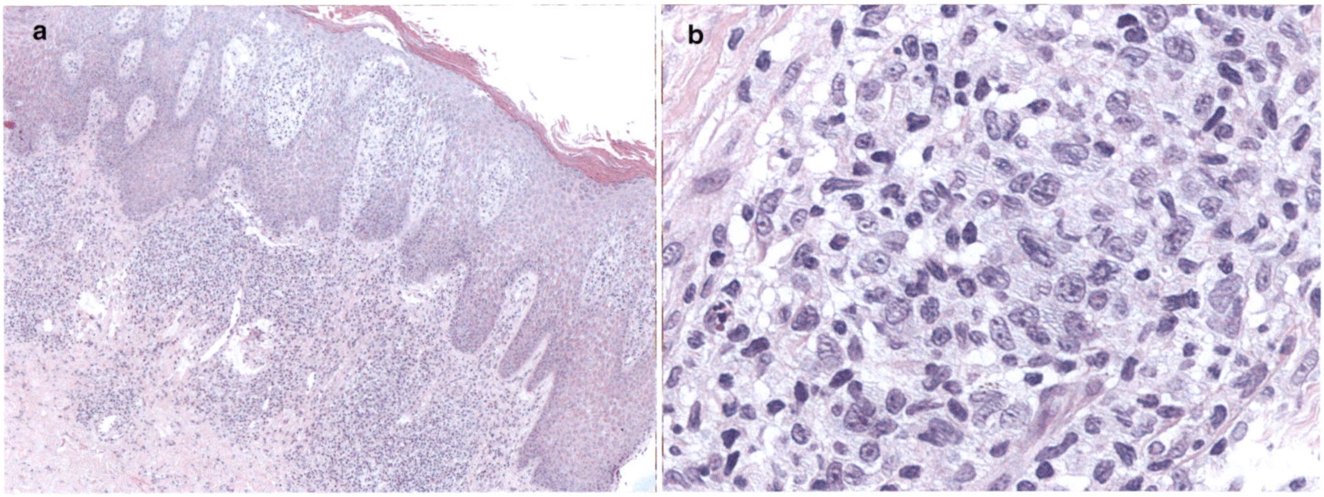

Fig. 46.1 Microscopic features of mycosis fungoides affecting the labial and perioral region. (**a**) Neoplastic cells are located near the overlying epithelium, which is referred to as epidermotropism and represents a typical finding of mycosis fungoides (H&E; 50×). (**b**) Neoplastic cells are predominantly medium-sized and typically exhibit a cerebriform aspect (H&E; 200×)

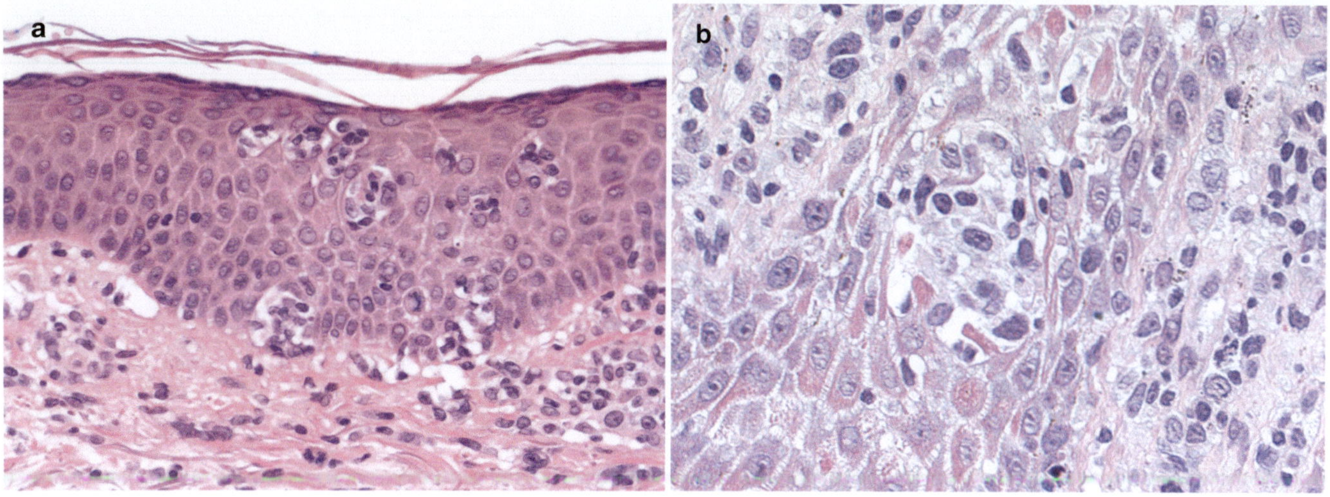

Fig. 46.2 Microscopic features of mycosis fungoides affecting the labial and perioral region. (**a**) Neoplastic cells infiltrate the overlying squamous epithelium and give rise to the so-called Pautrier microabscesses (H&E; 100×). (**b**) Observe in this image an aggregate of atypical neoplastic cells inside the epithelium (Paltrier microabscess) (H&E; 200×)

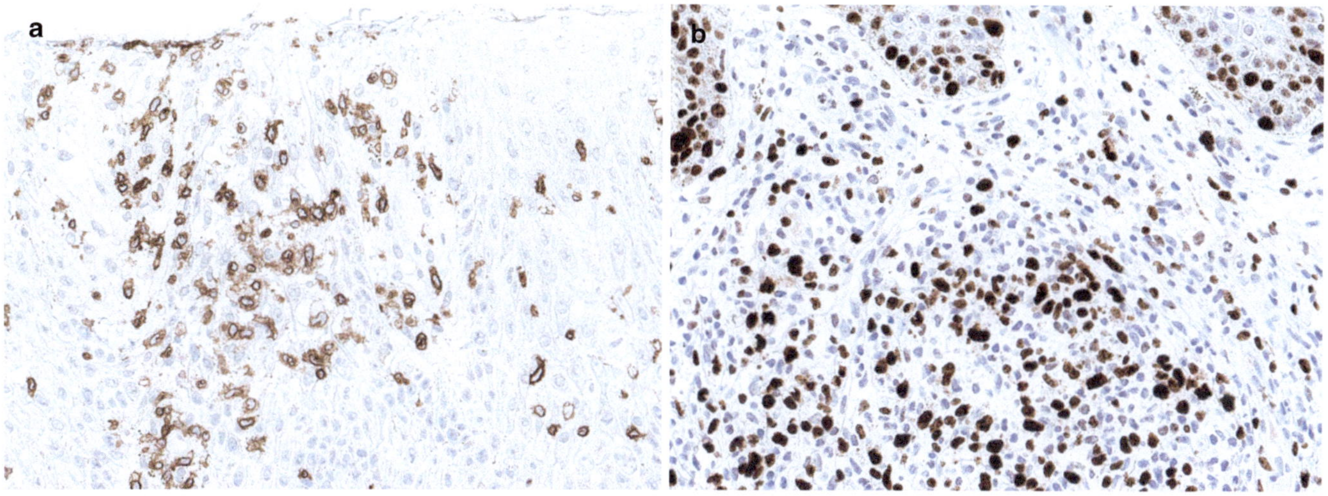

Fig. 46.3 Immunohistochemical findings of mycosis fungoides affecting the labial and perioral region. (**a**) Neoplastic cells exhibited a strong CD3 expression (DAB; 100×). (**b**) Mycosis fungoides exhibits a variable Ki67proliferative index (DAB; 100×)

- Formation of intraepithelial aggregates of tumor cells (Pautrier microabscesses) ispathognomonic, but these are not found in every case.
- Early skin and oral lesions rarely demonstrate these typical findings.
- Interface change, when it is present, is focal and minimal.
- The disorder is comprised of small to medium-sized T lymphocytes.
- Cleaved nuclei leading to the so-called "cerebriform" cells are a typical finding.
- Infiltration of the overlying epithelium is common.
- Several microscopic variants are recognized for mycosis fungoides (Figs. 46.3 and 46.4), but they are more often applied to cutaneous manifestations of the disease, not being clinicopathological variants in fact (Table 46.1; Figs. 46.5 and 46.6).

Note: Skin biopsy of patients with Sezary syndrome frequently presents nonspecific findings with superficial atypical lymphocytes and variable epidermotropism. It is important to highlight Sezary syndrome is not a dermatopathological diagnosis.

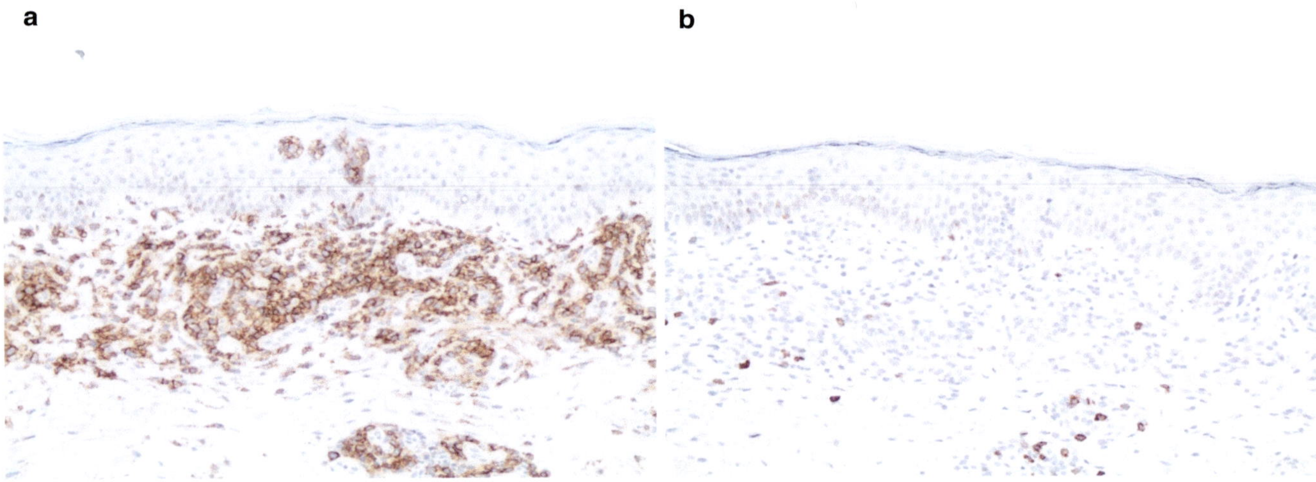

Fig. 46.4 Immunohistochemical findings of mycosis fungoides affecting the labial and perioral region. (**a**) Neoplastic cells are also more often positive for CD4 (DAB; 100×). (**b**) The loss of CD7 expression by tumor cells is very consistent with the diagnosis of mycosis fungoides (DAB; 100×)

Table 46.1 Clinicopathological variants of mycosis fungoides

Folliculotropic	Pagetoid reticulosis	Granulomatous slack skin disease
Head and neck	Distal extremities	Skin folds
Presence of mucinous degeneration of the hair follicle	Intraepidermal proliferation of atypical cells	Granulomatous infiltrate in the skin
Atypical cells infiltrate the hair follicles	This term is applied only for localized lesions on acral skin	Loss of elastic fibers
		Proliferation of clonal CD4+ cells

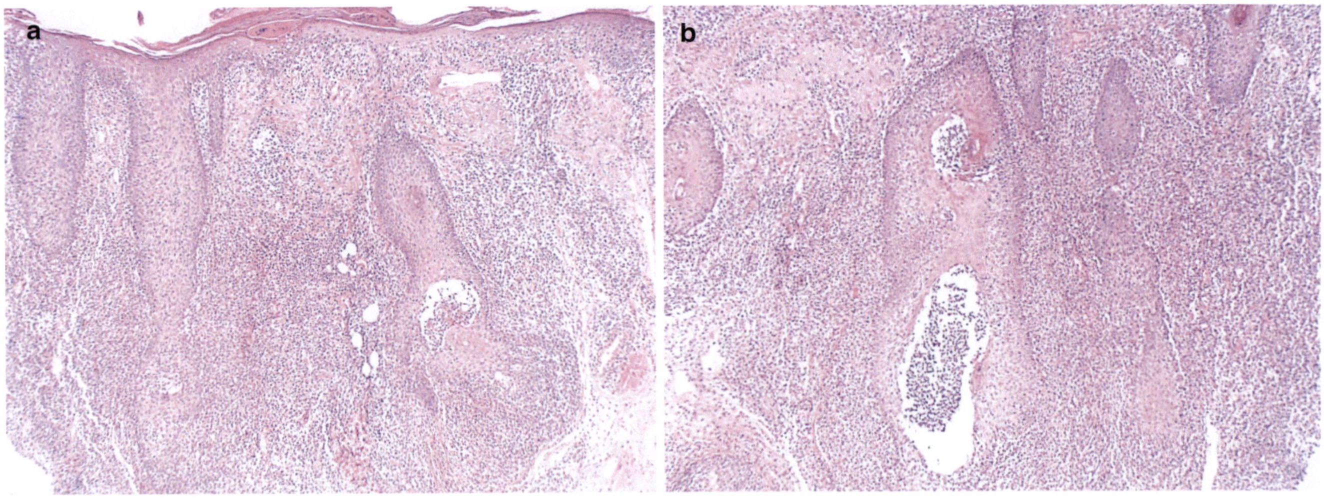

Fig. 46.5 Microscopic features of mycosis fungoides affecting the skin. (**a**) Diffuse infiltration of neoplastic cells in the dermis with the presence of a typical epidermotropism (H&E; 40×). (**b**) Note the infiltrative pattern of neoplastic cells in the epithelium (H&E; 100×)

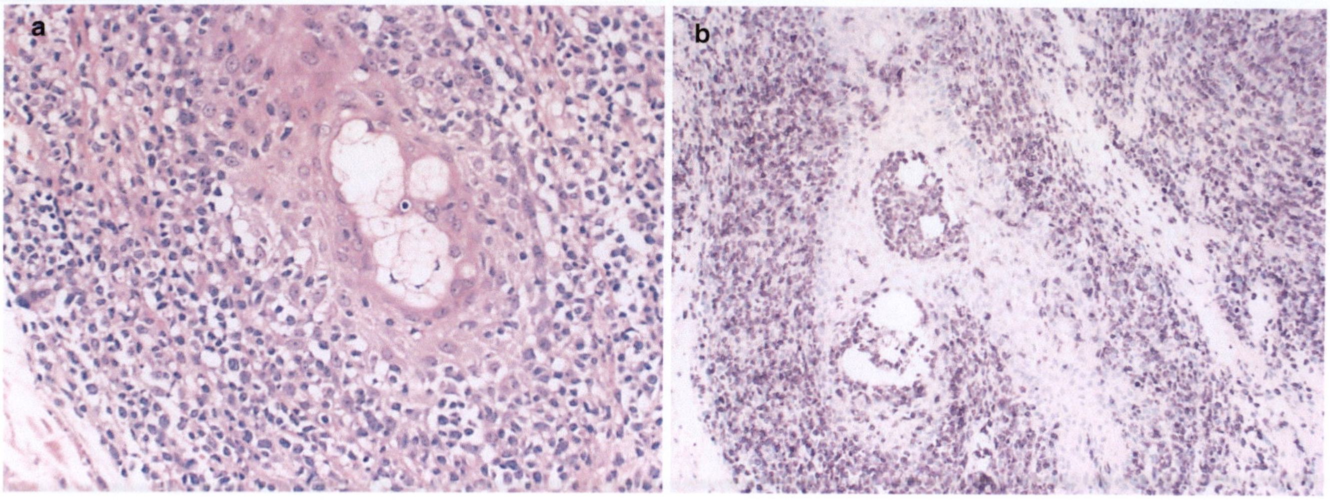

Fig. 46.6 Microscopic and immunohistochemical features of mycosis fungoides affecting the skin. (**a**) Neoplastic cells are predominantly small with indented nuclei. Note the infiltrative pattern of tumor cells towards the epithelium (H&E; 200×). (**b**) Tumor cells expressing CD3 protein (DAB; 100×)

46.3 Immunohistochemistry and/or Genetics

Immunohistochemical reactions typically show that tumor cells are CD4+/CD8−, although some CD8+ cases are known, and very often exhibit the aberrant loss of typical T-cell markers like CD2, CD3, CD5 and CD7. Cytotoxic granule expression is negative in most of the early-stage cases, but it can be positive in more advanced ones. Variable expression is also observed for CD56 and CD30 proteins. Large transformed cells can be CD30 positive, but this expression has no clinical meaning in early-stage disease. Nuclear expression of STAT3 can be found in many cases of mycosis fungoides and Sezary syndrome. In some cases, to differentiate Pautrier microabscess from Langerhans cell proliferation (a common finding in inflammatory conditions), CD1a can be helpful. The EBV is not found in this tumor. The genetic basis of both entities is still being better evaluated, but it has been proven to be very complex with alterations in multiple molecular pathways (Table 46.2; Figs. 46.3, 46.4, 46.7, and 46.8).

Table 46.2 Summary of the main immunohistochemical reactions used for mycosis fungoides/Sezary syndrome diagnosis

Antibody/probe	Most frequent results	Pattern	Objective
CD20	Negative	Membrane	To exclude a B-cell nature of the tumor
CD2	Often aberrantly lost	Membrane	Its frequent aberrant loss is useful to characterize the neoplasm
CD3	Positive (it can be lost)	Membrane	To demonstrate the T-cell nature of the tumor, but it can also be lost
CD45RO	Positive (it can be lost)	Membrane	To demonstrate the T-cell nature of the tumor, but it can also be lost
CD4	Positive in a larger subset of T cells	Membrane	To demonstrate the T-cell nature of the tumor
CD8	Positive in a smaller subset of T cells	Membrane	To demonstrate the T-cell nature of the tumor
CD5	Often aberrantly lost	Membrane	Its frequent aberrant loss is useful to characterize the neoplasm
CD7	Often aberrantly lost	Membrane	Its frequent aberrant loss is useful to characterize the neoplasm
CD56	Variably positive	Membrane	To characterize the immunophenotype of the tumor
STAT3	Positive	Nucleus	To characterize the immunophenotype of the tumor
CD30	Variably positive	Membrane	To characterize the immunophenotype of the tumor
Ki67	~60–70%	Nucleus	To demonstrate the proliferative index of the tumor
EBER[a]	Negative	Nucleus	To exclude the presence of EBV, which is useful for the differential diagnosis

The EBV status is also described
[a]Investigated by in situ hybridization

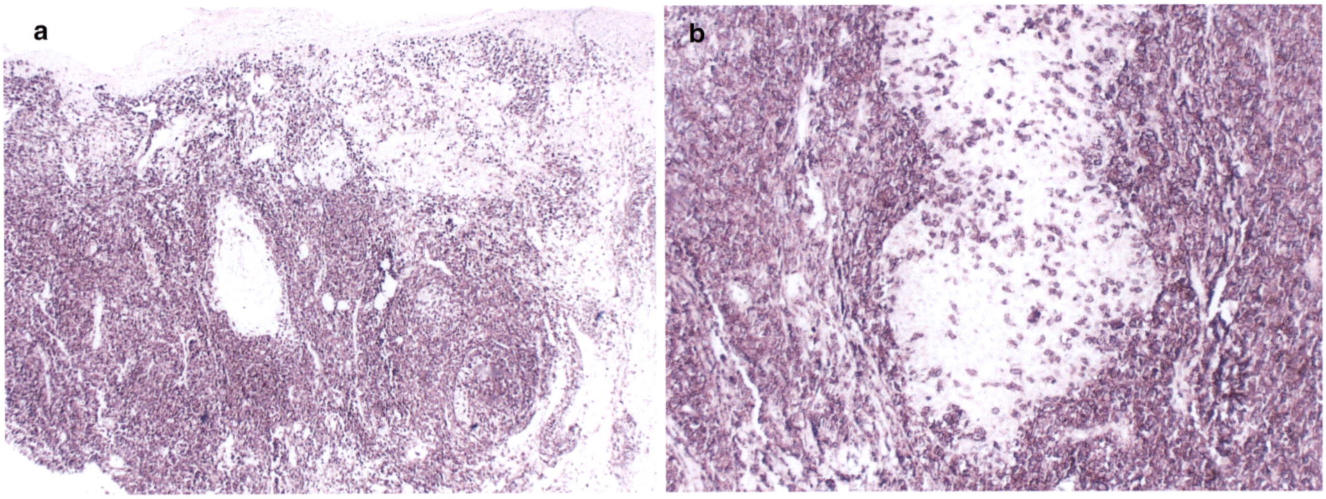

Fig. 46.7 Immunohistochemical findings of mycosis fungoides affecting the skin. (**a**) Neoplastic cells are strongly positive for CD4 (DAB; 100×). (**b**) Observe the tumor cells infiltrating the epithelium and expressing CD4 protein (DAB; 200×)

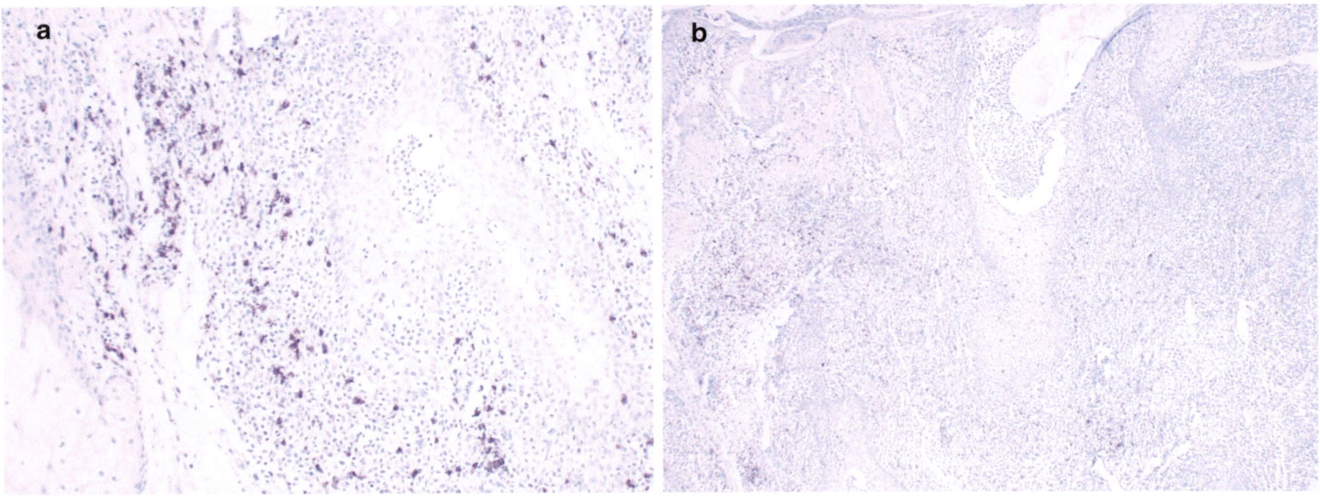

Fig. 46.8 Immunohistochemical findings of mycosis fungoides affecting the skin. (**a**) Expression of CD8 protein is a smaller subset of neoplastic cells (DAB; 200×). (**b**) Lack of CD7 protein expression (DAB; 100×)

Sources

1. Fraser-Andrews EA, Mitchell T, Ferreira S, Seed PT, Russell-Jones R, Calonje E, et al. Molecular staging of lymph nodes from 60 patients with mycosis fungoides and Sézary syndrome: correlation with histopathology and outcome suggests prognostic relevance in mycosis fungoides. Br J Dermatol. 2006;155(4):756–62. https://doi.org/10.1111/j.1365-2133.2006.07428.x.
2. Steffen C. The man behind the eponym dermatology in historical perspective: Albert Sézary and the Sézary syndrome. Am J Dermatopathol. 2006;28:357–67. https://doi.org/10.1097/00000372-200608000-00014.
3. Goldsmith SM, Seo BL, Kumara de Silva R, Parachuru P, Rich AM, Seymour GJ. Oral mycosis fungoides: report with immune profile. Oral Surg Oral Med Oral Pathol Oral Radiol. 2014;118:e48–52. https://doi.org/10.1016/j.oooo.2013.10.005.
4. Postorino M, Pupo L, Provenzano I, Del Principe MI, Buccisano F, Franceschini L, et al. A case of oral mycosis fungoides successfully treated by combination of alemtuzumab and chemotherapy. Ann Hematol. 2016;95:153–4. https://doi.org/10.1007/s00277-015-2503-z.
5. van Santen S, Roach RE, van Doorn R, Horváth B, Bruijn MS, Sanders CJ, et al. Clinical staging and prognostic factors in folliculotropic mycosis fungoides. JAMA Dermatol. 2016;152(9):992–1000. https://doi.org/10.1001/jamadermatol.2016.1597.
6. Sultan AS, Mostoufi B, Papadimitriou JC, Koka R, Basile J, Younis RH. Large cell transformation of oral mycosis fungoides. Head Neck Pathol. 2018;12:247–51. https://doi.org/10.1007/s12105-017-0840-z.
7. Rosebush MS, Allen CM, Accurso BT, Baiocchi RA, Cordell KG. Oral mycosis fungoides: a report of three cases and review of the literature. Head Neck Pathol. 2019;13:492–9. https://doi.org/10.1007/s12105-018-0923-5.
8. de la Fuente EG, Rodriguez-Peralto JL, Ortiz PL, Barrientos N, Vanaclocha F, Iglesias L. Oral involvement in mycosis fungoides: report of two cases and a literature review. Acta Derm Venereol. 2000;80(4):299–301. https://doi.org/10.1080/000155500750012234.
9. Bayramgürler D, Kazan D, Eruyar T, Demirkesen C, Demirbaş A. The oral cavity and gastric involvement in mycosis fungoides while on systemic bexarotene therapy: a rare case report. Dermatol Ther. 2022;35(4):e15349. https://doi.org/10.1111/dth.15349.
10. Farabi B, Seminario-Vidal L, Jamgochian M, Akay BN, Atak MF, Rao BK, et al. Updated review on prognostic factors in mycosis fungoides and new skin lymphoma trials. J Cosmet Dermatol. 2022;21(7):2742–8. https://doi.org/10.1111/jocd.14528.
11. Jung JM, Yoo H, Lim DJ, Won CH, Chang SE, Lee MW, et al. Clinicoprognostic implications of head and neck involvement by mycosis fungoides: a retrospective cohort study. J Am Acad Dermatol. 2022;86(6):1258–65. https://doi.org/10.1016/j.jaad.2021.03.056.
12. Miyashiro D, Sanches JA. Mycosis fungoides and Sézary syndrome: clinical presentation, diagnosis, staging, and therapeutic management. Front Oncol. 2023;14(13):1141108. https://doi.org/10.3389/fonc.2023.1141108.
13. Lee H. Mycosis fungoides and Sézary syndrome. Blood Res. 2023;58(S1):66–82. https://doi.org/10.5045/br.2023.2023023.
14. WHO Classification of Tumours Editorial Board. Haematolymphoid tumours [Internet], WHO classification of tumours series, vol. 11. 5th ed. Lyon: International Agency for Research on Cancer; 2024. Available from: https://tumourclassification.iarc.who.int/chapters/6.
15. Shrestha S, Newsom K, Chaffin JM, Seifert RP. Pathogenic variants of mycosis fungoides identified using next-generation sequencing. J Hematop. 2024;17(4):209–14. https://doi.org/10.1007/s12308-024-00607-5.
16. Moon IJ, Won CH, Chang SE, Park CS, Yoon DH, Song SY, et al. Prevalence, clinical features, and survival outcome trends of 627 patients with primary cutaneous lymphoma over 29 years: a retrospective review from single tertiary center in Korea. Sci Rep. 2024;14(1):20118. https://doi.org/10.1038/s41598-024-71210-y.
17. Cascardo CA, Mansour MR, Oska S, Sundram U. Histopathologic comparisons of discoid lupus erythematosus and folliculotropic mycosis fungoides in a series of 43 cases. J Cutan Pathol. 2025;52(2):126–31. https://doi.org/10.1111/cup.14752.

Index

© The Editor(s) (if applicable) and The Author(s), under exclusive license to Springer Nature Switzerland AG 2025

F. P. Fonseca et al. (eds.), *Lymphoproliferative and Granulomatous Disorders of the Oral Cavity*,
https://doi.org/10.1007/978-3-031-98844-8

MIX
Papier aus verantwortungsvollen Quellen
Paper from responsible sources
FSC® C105338

If you have any concerns about our products,
you can contact us on
ProductSafety@springernature.com

In case Publisher is established outside the EU,
the EU authorized representative is:
Springer Nature Customer Service Center GmbH
Europaplatz 3, 69115 Heidelberg, Germany

Printed by Libri Plureos GmbH
in Hamburg, Germany